TREATMENT OF THE OBESE PATIENT

CONTEMPORARY ENDOCRINOLOGY

P. Michael Conn, SERIES EDITOR

Genomics in Endocrinology: DNA Microarray Analysis in Endocrine Health and Disease, edited by STUART HANDWERGER AND BRUCE ARONOW, 2007

Controversies in Treating Diabetes: Clinical and Research Aspects, edited by DEREK LEROITH AND AARON I. VINIK, 2007

Autoimmune Diseases in Endocrinology, edited by ANTHONY P. WEETMAN, 2007

When Puberty is Precocious: Scientific and Clinical Aspects, edited by ORA H. PESCOVITZ AND EMILY C. WALVOORD, 2007

Insulin Resistance and Polycystic Ovarian Syndrome: Pathogenesis, Evaluation and Treatment, edited by JOHN E. NESTLER, EVANTHIA DIAMANTI-KANDARAKIS, RENATO PASQUALI, AND D. PANDIS, 2007

Hypertension and Hormone Mechanisms, edited by ROBERT M. CAREY, 2007

The Leydig Cell in Health and Disease, edited by ANITA H. PAYNE AND MATTHEW PHILLIP HARDY, 2007

Treatment of the Obese Patient, edited by ROBERT F. KUSHNER AND DANIEL H. BESSESEN, 2007

Androgen Excess Disorders in Women: Polycystic Ovary Syndrome and Other Disorders, Second Edition, edited by RICARDO AZZIS, JOHN E. NESTLER, AND DIDIER DEWAILLY, 2006

Evidence-Based Endocrinology, edited by VICTOR M. MONTORI, 2006

Stem Cells in Endocrinology, edited by LINDA B. LESTER, 2005

Office Andrology, edited by PHILLIP E. PATTON AND DAVID E. BATTAGLIA, 2005

Male Hypogonadism: Basic, Clinical, and Therapeutic Principles, edited by STEPHEN J. WINTERS, 2004

Androgens in Health and Disease, edited by CARRIE J. BAGATELL AND WILLIAM J. BREMNER, 2003

Endocrine Replacement Therapy in Clinical Practice, edited by A. WAYNE MEIKLE, 2003

Early Diagnosis of Endocrine Diseases, edited by ROBERT S. BAR, 2003

Type I Diabetes: Etiology and Treatment, edited by MARK A. SPERLING, 2003

Handbook of Diagnostic Endocrinology, edited by JANET E. HALL AND LYNNETTE K. NIEMAN, 2003

Pediatric Endocrinology: A Practical Clinical Guide, edited by SALLY RADOVICK AND MARGARET H. MACGILLIVRAY, 2003

Diseases of the Thyroid, 2nd ed., edited by LEWIS E. BRAVERMAN, 2003

Developmental Endocrinology: From Research to Clinical Practice, edited by ERICA A. EUGSTER AND ORA HIRSCH PESCOVITZ, 2002

Osteoporosis: Pathophysiology and Clinical Management, edited by ERIC S. ORWOLL AND MICHAEL BLIZIOTES, 2002

Challenging Cases in Endocrinology, edited by MARK E. MOLITCH, 2002

Selective Estrogen Receptor Modulators: Research and Clinical Applications, edited by ANDREA MANNI AND MICHAEL F. VERDERAME, 2002

Transgenics in Endocrinology, edited by MARTIN MATZUK, CHESTER W. BROWN, AND T. RAJENDRA KUMAR, 2001

Assisted Fertilization and Nuclear Transfer in Mammals, edited by DON P. WOLF AND MARY ZELINSKI-WOOTEN, 2001

Adrenal Disorders, edited by ANDREW N. MARGIORIS AND GEORGE P. CHROUSOS, 2001

Endocrine Oncology, edited by STEPHEN P. ETHIER, 2000

Endocrinology of the Lung: Development and Surfactant Synthesis, edited by CAROLE R. MENDELSON, 2000

Sports Endocrinology, edited by MICHELLE P. WARREN AND NAAMA W. CONSTANTINI, 2000

Gene Engineering in Endocrinology, edited by MARGARET A. SHUPNIK, 2000

Endocrinology of Aging, edited by JOHN E. MORLEY AND LUCRETIA VAN DEN BERG, 2000

Human Growth Hormone: Research and Clinical Practice, edited by ROY G. SMITH AND MICHAEL O. THORNER, 2000

Hormones and the Heart in Health and Disease, edited by LEONARD SHARE, 1999

Menopause: Endocrinology and Management, edited by DAVID B. SEIFER AND ELIZABETH A. KENNARD, 1999

The IGF System: Molecular Biology, Physiology, and Clinical Applications, edited by RON G. ROSENFELD AND CHARLES T. ROBERTS, JR., 1999

Neurosteroids: A New Regulatory Function in the Nervous System, edited by ETIENNE-EMILE BAULIEU, MICHAEL SCHUMACHER, AND PAUL ROBEL, 1999

TREATMENT OF THE OBESE PATIENT

Edited by

ROBERT F. KUSHNER, MD

Department of Medicine, Northwestern University, Feinberg School of Medicine, Chicago, IL

DANIEL H. BESSESEN, MD

Division of Endocrinology, University of Colorado at Denver and Health Sciences Center, Denver, CO

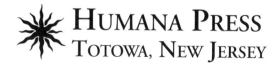 HUMANA PRESS
TOTOWA, NEW JERSEY

MT

© 2007 Humana Press Inc.
999 Riverview Drive, Suite 208
Totowa, New Jersey 07512
humanapress.com

This publication is printed on acid-free paper. ∞

ANSI Z39.48-1984 (American National Standards Institute) Permanence of Paper for Printed Library Materials.

Production Editor: Amy Thau

Cover design by Donna Niethe

For additional copies, pricing for bulk purchases, and/or information about other Humana titles, contact Humana at the above address or at any of the following numbers: Tel: 973-256-1699; Fax: 973-256-8341; E-mail: orders@humanapr.com or visit our website at http://humanapress.com

Printed in the United States of America. 10 9 8 7 6 5 4 3 2 1
eISBN 10: 1-59745-400-1
eISBN 13: 978-1-59745-400-1

Treatment of the obese patient / edited by Robert F. Kushner, Daniel
   H. Bessesen.
      p. ; cm. -- (Contemporary endocrinology)
   Includes bibliographical references and index.
   ISBN 10: 1-58829-735-7 (alk. paper)
   ISBN 13: 978-1-58829-735-8 (alk. paper)
   1. Obesity.   I. Kushner, Robert F., 1953-   . II. Bessesen, Daniel
H., 1956-   . III. Series: Contemporary endocrinology (Totowa, N.J.
: Unnumbered)
   [DNLM: 1. Obesity--therapy.   WD 210 T7842 2007]
   RC628.T696 2007
   616.3'9806--dc22
                                          2006026833

PREFACE

The rising prevalence of obesity among children and adults is one of the most significant threats to our nation's health as we enter the 21st century. Among a host of disorders associated with obesity that affect multiple organ systems, the escalating prevalence of type 2 diabetes and conditions associated with the metabolic syndrome and cardiovascular disease are the most worrisome. For these reasons, it is increasingly important for clinical endocrinologists and other health care providers to be informed about breakthroughs in obesity research and to become engaged in the clinical care of the obese patient. Although our medical journals and the popular press are including more and more articles about obesity-related topics, there is a need to sort, synthesize, and interpret this information into a single readable text. Thus, the primary purpose of this volume of Contemporary Endocrinology, entitled *Treatment of the Obese Patient*, is to inform clinicians of recent scientific advances in obesity research and to provide an up-to-date review of current treatment issues and strategies. To provide the most useful and authoritative text, we have selected chapter authors who are not only experts in their fields of study but who are also able to translate important and emerging concepts to the practicing clinician.

The volume is divided into two parts. Part 1 covers new discoveries in the physiological control of body weight, as well as the pathophysiology of obesity. The most exciting breakthroughs in obesity research over the past decade have come from a growing appreciation of the critical pathways that control food intake, energy expenditure, and peripheral nutrient metabolism including the emerging evidence of the role of adipose tissue as an endocrine organ. Each of these evolving areas is covered in its entirety in this volume. Chapters 1 through 3 address the neuroregulation of appetite, the role of gut peptides in providing peripheral signals of nutrient balance to the brain, and the new biology of the endocannabanoid system. In Chapters 4 and 5, the pathophysiology of adipokines and role of free fatty acids, insulin, and ectopic fat in the metabolic dysregulation of obesity are reviewed. Chapter 6 examines the provocative role of fetal origins and birth weight in the causation of obesity. Finally, Chapters 7 and 8 provide a comprehensive review of new developments in body composition in health and disease, and the role of alterations of energy expenditure in the development of obesity.

In Part 2, we turn to a range of issues that are central to the clinical management of obese patients. This section begins with an informative review of the socioeconomic aspects of obesity. Chapters 10 through 12 address the comprehensive assessment and evaluation of the obese adult patient, the pathophysiology and approach to the patient with polycystic ovarian syndrome, and management of the obese patient with diabetes. Chapters 13 through 15 provide an excellent review and discussion of three dietary approaches that have been advocated in the treatment of obesity—energy density, glycemic index, and low-carbohydrate diets. The role of physical activity is covered in Chapter 16. Communication, counseling, and motivational interviewing, keys to changing patient behavior, are considered in Chapter 17. Chapters 18 through 20 turn our attention to new developments in the pharmacotherapy of obesity, surgical approaches and outcomes, and management of micronutrient deficiencies in the postbariatric surgical patient. Lessons learned from individuals who have succeeded in losing weight and maintaining a reduced obese state long term: members of the National Weight Control Registry are discussed in Chapter 21. Lastly, a succinct summary of evaluation and management of the pediatric obese patient is reviewed in Chapter 22.

Treatment of the Obese Patient is a timely and informative text for all health care providers facing the challenges of helping their patients manage their weight. Our intention is to provide a resource that will both stimulate and engage clinicians to take part more successfully in the obesity-care process. We hope we have accomplished this goal.

Robert F. Kushner, MD
Daniel H. Bessesen, MD

Contents

Preface v

Contributors ix

PART I. PHYSIOLOGY AND PATHOPHYSIOLOGY

  1 Neuroregulation of Appetite 3
     Ofer Reizes, Stephen C. Benoit, and Deborah J. Clegg

  2 Gut Peptides 27
     Vian Amber and Stephen R. Bloom

  3 Endocannabinoids and Energy Homeostasis 49
     Stephen C. Woods and Daniela Cota

  4 Obesity and Adipokines 69
     Nicole H. Rogers, Martin S. Obin, and Andrew S. Greenberg

  5 Free Fatty Acids, Insulin Resistance, and Ectopic Fat 87
     David E. Kelley

  6 Critical Importance of the Perinatal Period in the Development
     of Obesity 99
     Barry E. Levin

  7 Measurement of Body Composition in Obesity 121
     Jennifer L. Kuk and Robert Ross

  8 Energy Expenditure in Obesity 151
     Leanne M. Redman and Eric Ravussin

PART II. CLINICAL MANAGEMENT

  9 Socioeconomics of Obesity 175
     Roland Sturm and Yuhua Bao

  10 Assessment of the Obese Patient 195
     Daniel H. Bessesen

  11 Polycystic Ovary Syndrome 219
     Romana Dmitrovic and Richard S. Legro

  12 Weight Management in Diabetes Prevention:
     *Translating the Diabetes Prevention Program
     Into Clinical Practice* 243
     F. Xavier Pi-Sunyer

  13 Reductions in Dietary Energy Density as a
     Weight Management Strategy 265
     *Jenny H. Ledikwe, Heidi M. Blanck, Laura Kettel Khan,
     Mary K. Serdula, Jennifer D. Seymour, Beth C. Tohill,
     and Barbara J. Rolls*

14   Glycemic Index, Obesity, and Diabetes 281
     Cara B. Ebbeling and David S. Ludwig

15   Low-Carbohydrate Diets 299
     Angela P. Makris and Gary D. Foster

16   Physical Activity and Obesity 311
     *John M. Jakicic, Amy D. Otto, Kristen Polzien,
        and Kelli K. Davis*

17   Motivational Interviewing in Medical Settings: *Application
        to Obesity Conceptual Issues and Evidence Review* 321
     Ken R. Resnicow and Abdul Shaikh

18   Weight-Loss Drugs: *Current and on the Horizon* 341
     George A. Bray and Frank L. Greenway

19   Surgical Approaches and Outcomes:
        Treatment of the Obese Patient 369
     George L. Blackburn and Vivian M. Sanchez

20   Managing Micronutrient Deficiencies in the Bariatric
        Surgical Patient 379
     Robert F. Kushner

21   Lessons Learned From the National Weight Control Registry 395
     *James O. Hill, Holly R. Wyatt, Suzanne Phelan,
        and Rena R. Wing*

22   Pediatric Obesity 405
     Lawrence D. Hammer

     Index 425

CONTRIBUTORS

VIAN AMBER, MBChB, MSc, PhD, MRCPath • *Department of Metabolic Medicine, Imperial College London, Hammersmith Campus, London, UK*

YUHUA BAO, PhD • *RAND Corporation, Santa Monica, CA*

STEPHEN C. BENOIT, PhD • *Department of Psychiatry, Obesity Research Center, University of Cincinnati, Cincinnati, OH*

DANIEL H. BESSESEN, MD • *Division of Endocrinology, University of Colorado at Denver and Health Sciences Center, Denver, CO*

GEORGE L. BLACKBURN, MD, PhD • *Division of Nutrition, Center for the Study of Nutrition Medicine, Harvard Medical School, Boston, MA*

HEIDI M. BLANCK, PhD • *Division of Nutrition and Physical Activity, Centers for Disease Control and Prevention, National Center for Chronic Disease Prevention and Health Promotion, Atlanta, GA*

STEPHEN R. BLOOM, MBChB, MA, FRCP, FRCPath, DSc, MD • *Department of Metabolic Medicine, Imperial College London, Hammersmith Campus, London, UK*

GEORGE A. BRAY, MD • *Pennington Biochemical Research Center, Louisiana State University System, Baton Rouge, LA*

DEBORAH J. CLEGG, PhD • *Department of Psychiatry, Obesity Research Center, University of Cincinnati, Cincinnati OH*

DANIELA COTA, MD • *Department of Psychiatry, University of Cincinnati Medical Center, Cincinnati, OH*

KELLI K. DAVIS, MS • *Department of Health and Physical Activity, Physical Activity and Weight Management Research Center, University of Pittsburgh, Pittsburgh, PA*

ROMANA DMITROVIC, MD • *Reproductive Endocrinology Research Center, Pennsylvania State University College of Medicine, Hershey, PA*

CARA B. EBBELING, PhD • *Division of Endocrinology, Department of Medicine, Children's Hospital Boston, Boston, MA*

GARY D. FOSTER, PhD • *Center for Obesity Research and Education, Temple University School of Medicine, Philadelphia, PA*

ANDREW S. GREENBERG, MD • *Jean Mayer USDA Human Nutrition Research Center on Aging, Tufts University, Boston, MA*

FRANK L. GREENWAY, MD • *Pennington Biochemical Research Center, Louisiana State University, Baton Rouge, LA*

LAWRENCE D. HAMMER, MD • *Center for Healthy Weight, Lucile Packard Children's Hospital and Department of Pediatrics, Stanford University School of Medicine, Palo Alto, CA*

JAMES O. HILL, PhD • *Center for Human Nutrition, University of Colorado at Denver and Health Sciences Center, Denver, CO*

JOHN M. JAKICIC, PhD • *Department of Health and Physical Activity, Physical Activity and Weight Management Research Center, University of Pittsburgh, Pittsburgh, PA*

DAVID E. KELLEY, MD • *Division of Endocrinology and Metabolism, University of Pittsburgh School of Medicine, Pittsburgh, PA*

LAURA KETTEL KHAN, PhD • *Division of Nutrition and Physical Activity, Centers for Disease Control and Prevention, National Center for Chronic Disease Prevention and Health Promotion, Atlanta, GA*

JENNIFER L. KUK, MSc • *School of Kinesiology and Health Studies, Queen's University, Kingston, ON, Canada*

ROBERT F. KUSHNER, MD • *Department of Medicine, Northwestern University Feinberg School of Medicine, Chicago, IL*

JENNY H. LEDIKWE, PhD • *Department of Nutritional Sciences, The Pennsylvania State University, University Park, PA*

RICHARD S. LEGRO, MD • *Department of Obstetrics and Gynecology, Pennsylvania State University College of Medicine, Hershey, PA*

BARRY E. LEVIN, MD • *Department of Neurosciences, New Jersey Medical School/ University of Medicine and Dentistry of New Jersey, and Neurology Service, VA Medical Center, East Orange, NJ*

DAVID S. LUDWIG, MD, PhD • *Division of Endocrinology, Department of Medicine, Children's Hospital Boston, Boston, MA*

ANGELA P. MAKRIS, PhD, RD • *Center for Obesity Research and Education, Temple University School of Medicine, Philadelphia, PA*

MARTIN S. OBIN, PhD • *Jean Mayer USDA Human Nutrition Research Center on Aging, Tufts University, Boston, MA*

AMY D. OTTO, PhD, LDN • *Department of Health and Physical Activity, Physical Activity and Weight Management Research Center, University of Pittsburgh, Pittsburgh, PA*

SUZANNE PHELAN, PhD • *Department of Psychiatry and Human Behavior, Weight Control and Diabetes Research Center, Brown Medical School, Providence, RI*

F. XAVIER PI-SUNYER, MD, MPH • *Obesity Research Center, Columbia University College of Physicians and Surgeons, New York, NY*

KRISTEN POLZIEN, PhD • *Department of Kinesiology, University of Massachusetts, Amherst, MA*

ERIC RAVUSSIN, PhD • *Health and Performance Enhancement Division, Pennington Biomedical Research Center, Baton Rouge, LA*

LEANNE M. REDMAN, PhD • *Health and Performance Enhancement Division, Pennington Biomedical Research Center, Baton Rouge, LA*

OFER REIZES, PhD • *Department of Cell Biology, Lerner Research Institute, Cleveland Clinic Foundation, Cleveland, OH*

KEN R. RESNICOW, PhD, MHS • *Department of Health Behavior and Health Education, School of Public Health, University of Michigan, Ann Arbor, MI*

NICOLE H. ROGERS, MS • *Jean Mayer USDA Human Nutrition Research Center on Aging, Tufts University, Boston, MA*

BARBARA J. ROLLS, PhD • *Department of Nutritional Sciences, The Pennsylvania State University, University Park, PA*

ROBERT ROSS, PhD • *School of Kinesiology and Health Studies, Queen's University, Kingston, ON, Canada*

VIVIAN M. SANCHEZ, MD • *Department of Surgery, Beth Israel Deaconess Medical Center, Harvard Medical School, Boston, MA*

MARY K. SERDULA, MD • *Division of Nutrition and Physical Activity, Centers for Disease Control and Prevention, National Center for Chronic Disease Prevention and Health Promotion, Atlanta, GA*

JENNIFER D. SEYMOUR, PhD • *Division of Nutrition and Physical Activity, Centers for Disease Control and Prevention, National Center for Chronic Disease Prevention and Health Promotion, Atlanta, GA*

ABDUL R. SHAIKH, PhD, MHS • *Behavioral Research Program, Division of Cancer Control and Population Sciences, National Cancer Institute, Bethesda, MD*

ROLAND STURM, PhD • *RAND Corporation, Santa Monica, CA*

BETH C. TOHILL, PhD • *Division of Nutrition and Physical Activity, Centers for Disease Control and Prevention, National Center for Chronic Disease Prevention and Health Promotion, Atlanta, GA*

RENA R. WING, PhD • *Department of Psychiatry and Human Behavior, Weight Control and Diabetes Research Center, Brown Medical School, Providence, RI*

STEPHEN C. WOODS, PhD • *Department of Psychiatry, University of Cincinnati Medical Center, Cincinnati, OH*

HOLLY R. WYATT, MD • *Center for Human Nutrition, University of Colorado at Denver and Health Sciences Center, Denver, CO*

I PHYSIOLOGY AND PATHOPHYSIOLOGY

1

Neuroregulation of Appetite

Ofer Reizes, PhD, Stephen C. Benoit, PhD, and Deborah J. Clegg, PhD

CONTENTS

INTRODUCTION
THE DUAL-CENTERS HYPOTHESIS
CONTROL OF ENERGY INTAKE
INTEGRATION OF ADIPOSITY SIGNALS
CENTRAL SIGNALS RELATED TO ENERGY HOMEOSTASIS
CATABOLIC EFFECTOR SYSTEMS
CONCLUSIONS
REFERENCES

Summary

This chapter reviews current literature on hormonal and neural signals critical for the regulation of individual meals and body fat. Body weight is regulated via an ongoing process called energy homeostasis, or the long-term matching of food intake to energy expenditure. Reductions from an individual's "normal" weight owing to a lack of sufficient food lowers levels of adiposity signals (leptin and insulin) reaching the brain from the blood, activates anabolic hormones that stimulate food intake, and decreases the efficacy of meal-generated signals (such as cholecystokinin) that normally reduce meal size. A converse sequence of events happens when individuals gain weight, adiposity signals are increased, catabolic hormones are stimulated, and the consequence is a reduction in food intake and a normalization of body weight. The brain also functions as a "fuel sensor" and thereby senses nutrients and generates signals and activation of neuronal systems and circuits that regulate energy homeostasis. This chapter focuses on how these signals are received and integrated by the central nervous system.

Key Words: Hypothalamus; arcuate nucleus; body weight regulation; neuropeptides; central nervous system (CNS); obesity.

INTRODUCTION

Body weight (or, more accurately, body adiposity) is a tightly regulated variable. To maintain body fat stores over long periods of time, caloric intake must precisely match expenditure. Such a process relies on the complex interactions of many different physiological systems. As an example, one negative feedback system is composed of hormonal signals derived from adipose tissue that inform the central nervous system (CNS)

From: *Contemporary Endocrinology: Treatment of the Obese Patient*
Edited by: R. F. Kushner and D. H. Bessesen © Humana Press Inc., Totowa, NJ

about the status of peripheral energy stores. These signals from adipose tissue or peripheral fat stores form one side of the hypothesized feedback loop. The receiving side of this regulatory system includes one or more central effectors that translate adiposity information into appropriate subsequent ingestive behavior. When the system detects low levels of adipose hormones, food intake is increased, whereas energy expenditure is decreased. On the other hand, in the presence of high adiposity signals, food intake is reduced and energy expenditure increased. In this way, the negative feedback system can maintain energy balance or body adiposity over long periods of time by signals in the CNS.

THE DUAL-CENTERS HYPOTHESIS

Historically, the conceptual framework that dominated thinking about the role played by the hypothalamus in the control of food intake was the dual-centers hypothesis proposed by Stellar in 1954 (1). In the same year that the discovery of leptin refocused attention on the role of the hypothalamus in energy balance, *Psychological Review* honored this article as one of the 10 most influential articles it had published in a century of publications. Stellar eloquently argued that the hypothalamus is the central neural structure involved in "motivation" generally and in the control of food intake more specifically. This control is divided into two conceptual categories controlled by two separate hypothalamic structures. The first category was "satiety" and was thought to be controlled by the ventromedial hypothalamus (VMH). The most important data that contributed to this hypothesis were that bilateral lesions of the VMH resulted in rats that ate more than controls and became obese. These lesioned rats were thought to have a defect in satiety; therefore, the VMH was described as being a "satiety" center. Additionally, experimentally the lesion could be replicated by electrical stimulation of the VMH, which also caused the animals to stop eating—in other words, these experiments demonstrated a role for the VMH in enhancing satiety. In contrast to the VMH, the lateral hypothalamic area (LHA) was thought to be the "hunger" nucleus, as lesions of the LHA resulted in rats that under-ate and lost body weight. Additionally, electrical stimulation of the LHA caused eating in sated animals. Therefore, the VMH was thought to be the satiety center and the LHA was considered the hunger center. This characterization of the brain was called the dual-centers hypothesis and was the dominant conceptualization of how the CNS controlled food intake for almost 30 yr.

CNS Regulation of Food Intake

CNS regulation of food intake was originally thought to be controlled by the VMH and the LHA; however, several challenges were made to this early hypothesis. The first was a realization that there are limitations to our understanding of the neurocircuitry using the lesions as an experimental approach to understanding CNS function. Conclusions made about larger lesion studies were difficult to interpret because lesions usually destroyed all fibers in the nuclei, not just those fibers of specific interest. An additional problem was that there are consequences of the lesion not directly tested. For example, although lesions of the VMH result in hyperphagic and obese rats, they also result in rapid and dramatic increases in insulin secretion from pancreatic β-cells (2). Indeed, exogenous peripheral insulin administration results in increased food intake, and repeated administration can result in rapid weight gain (3). Therefore, in addition to regulating

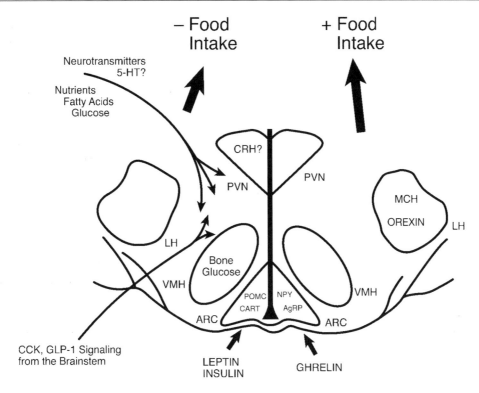

Fig. 1. Cartoon drawing of a coronal section of the brain. It represents the key nuclei in the hypothalamus that influence food intake and body weight regulation. There are peripheral signals, leptin, insulin, and ghrelin, which interact with the hypothalamus; these are depicted with arrows pointing to the arcuate nucleus. Additionally, there are signals that originate in the brainstem, CCK and GLP-1; these are depicted with an arrow and are denoted as arising from the brain stem. Last, there are nutrients and neurostransmitters that interact with many of the hypothalamic nuclei, and there are arrows that represent their interactions. The hypothalamic nuclei are represented as shapes, and these shapes are labeled as: arcuate (ARC), ventromedial nucleus (VMH), paraventricular nucleus (PVN), and lateral hypothalamus (LH). The concept conveyed here is that there are orexigenic (anabolic) neuropeptides that stimulate food intake, and there are anorexigenic (catabolic) neuropeptides, nutrients, and neurostransmitters that decrase food intake.

"satiety," the VMH also appears to have an important role in the regulation of insulin secretion *(2)*. Further research supported the VMH's role in regulating additional functions other then satiety. In particular, later data indicated that it was not cell bodies in the VMH but rather fibers running from the paraventricular nucleus (PVN) to the brainstem that were critical for the effect of VMH lesions on insulin secretion *(4,5)*. So although the changes in insulin secretion were potentially responsible for the effects of VMH lesions on food intake and body weight, this control of insulin secretion may not be directly mediated by the VMH.

Another challenge to the dual-centers hypothesis came from work out of Grill's lab, which focused on transection of the neuraxis at different levels by utilizing the chronic decerebrate rat. The chronic decerebrate rat has a complete transection of the neuraxis at the mesodiencephalic junction that isolates the caudal brainstem, severing all neural input from more rostral structures such as the hypothalamus. Hence, neither the VMH nor LHA (nor any other hypothalamic nuclei, for that matter) could exert direct influence on the motor neurons in the brainstem critical for executing ingestive behavior (6). Despite a complete loss of neural input from the hypothalamus, the chronic decerebrate animal has the ability to engage in consummatory behavior and to adjust that behavior in response to both external and internal stimuli. Chronic decerebrate rats respond appropriately to taste stimuli (6–9). More importantly, chronic decerebrate rats demonstrate satiety, and the size of the meals is influenced in the same manner as in a normal rat (6,8). The caudal brainstem is therefore sufficient to integrate internal regulatory signals that limit meal size into ongoing ingestive behavior independent of the hunger and satiety centers of the hypothalamus. These data suggest that there are several regions in the CNS that mediate the control of food intake and that no single brain area constitutes either a "hunger" or a "satiety" center.

CNS Regulation by Adiposity Signals and Effector Pathways

These challenges to the dual-centers hypothesis led to new models for understanding the role of the hypothalamus in the control of food intake. Other research has focused on emphasizing factors and signaling pathways that control long-term energy balance. Adult mammals typically match their caloric intake to their caloric expenditure in a remarkably accurate fashion. In the 1950s Kennedy postulated that animals could regulate their energy balance by monitoring the major form of energy storage in the body, adipose mass (10). When caloric intake exceeds caloric expenditure, fat stores are expanded; when caloric expenditure exceeds caloric intake, fat stores are reduced. In other words, if the size of the adipose mass could be monitored, energy intake and energy expenditure could be adjusted to keep adipose mass constant and thereby keep the energy equation balanced over long periods of time.

There are at least two peripherally derived hormones that provide key afferent information to the CNS for body weight regulation. Leptin, a peptide hormone secreted from adipocytes in proportion to fat mass, has received tremendous attention during the last decade. Considerable evidence has been derived that implicates leptin as one of the body's adiposity signals (11–14). Leptin levels in the blood correlate directly with body fat, and peripheral or central administration of leptin reduces food intake and increases energy expenditure.

Importantly, leptin levels are better correlated with subcutaneous fat than with visceral fat in humans, such that the reliability of leptin as an adiposity signal varies with the distribution of body fat. There is a sexual dimorphism with respect to the way in which body fat is distributed. Males tend to have more body fat located in the visceral adipose depot, whereas females tend to have more fat in the subcutaneous depot. Because females tend to have more subcutaneous fat than males, on the average, leptin is therefore a better correlate of total adiposity in females than in males (15). Further, when energy balance is suddenly changed (for example, if an individual is fasted for a day), plasma leptin levels decrease far more than body adiposity in the short term (16–18). Hence, although much has been written about leptin as an adiposity signal, it is not ideal in and of itself, suggesting that other signals may exist. One candidate is the pancreatic hormone, insulin.

Insulin is well known for its role in regulating glucose homeostasis; however, an often under-represented role for insulin is as an adiposity signal. Plasma insulin levels also directly correlate with adiposity, and although leptin is a better correlate of subcutaneous adiposity, insulin correlates better with visceral adiposity *(19–22)*. Moreover, when energy balance changes, there are changes in plasma insulin that closely follow changes in homeostasis *(23)*. Therefore, both leptin and insulin can be considered adiposity signals, each indicating something different to the brain; insulin is a correlate of visceral adiposity and leptin is a correlate of subcutaneous adiposity and, together or separately, they are markers of changes of metabolic status.

CONTROL OF ENERGY INTAKE

Food intake in mammals, including humans, occurs in distinct bouts or meals, and the number and size of meals over the course of a day comprises the meal pattern. Food intake is thought to be regulated by signals from the gut, brainstem, and hypothalamus. Most humans are quite habitual in that they eat approximately the same number of meals, and at the same time of day *(24,25)*. Factors or signals that control when meals occur are different from those that control when they end—i.e., different factors control meal onset and meal size *(25,26)*. Historically, meal onset was thought to be a reflexive response to a reduction in the amount or availability of some parameter related to energy. Changes in glucose levels were posited to stimulate meals; this was coined the "glucostatic" theory. This theory put forth the idea that a reduction of glucose utilization by sensor cells in the hypothalamus of the brain caused the sensation of "hunger" and a tendency to start a meal *(27,28)*. An additional hypothesis was generated about what stimulates "hunger"; this was associated with changes in fuel, either from changes in body heat, upon fat utilization by the liver, or upon the generation of adenosine triphosphate (ATP) and other energy-rich molecules by cells in the liver and/or brain *(29–32)*.

Food intake may be stimulated for reasons other than simple changes in energy substrates. An alternative hypothesis for meal generation is that most meals are initiated at times that are convenient or habitual, and thus based on social or learned factors as opposed to fluxes of energy within the body *(33)*. In this schema, the regulatory control over food intake is exerted on how much food is consumed once a meal is started rather than on when the meal occurs *(34,35)*. Therefore, individuals have flexibility over their individualized meal patterns, and this is influenced by their environment and lifestyle. Hence, there are factors and signals that are regulatory controls that determine meal size, and this is generally equated with the phenomenon of satiety or fullness *(26)*.

Satiety

Meals are considered to be regulated—there are initiation and cessation cues that signal the beginning and completion of the meal, respectively. If the cessation cue is controlled by signals that arise from the brain and gut, then the individual must have a means of measuring reliably how much food has been eaten—i.e., the number of calories consumed, or perhaps the precise mix of carbohydrates, lipids, and proteins, and/or other food-related parameters. Consumption must be monitored as the meal progresses so the person knows when to say "I'm full" and put down the fork *(26)*. Some parameters or signals might provide the important feedback during an ongoing meal. These signals may be in the form of vision, smell, or taste to gauge the amount of energy consumed. However, several types of experiments have found that any such input is minimal at best.

To determine whether the gut conveys a signal to end the meal, animals have been experimentally implanted with a gastric fistula *(36)*. When the fistula is closed, swallowed food enters the stomach, is processed normally, and moves into the duodenum.

When the fistula is open, swallowed food enters the stomach and then exits the body via the fistula, in a process called sham eating. In both instances the visual, olfactory, and taste inputs are the same, but the amount eaten varies considerably. When the fistula is closed (representing what happens in a normal meal), animals eat normal-sized meals; when the fistula is open (representing the experimental condition, or sham eating), animals continue eating for long intervals and consume very large meals (36–38). Hence, whatever signals an individual uses to gauge how many calories have been consumed must arise no more proximally than the distal stomach and/or small intestine.

As ingested food interacts with the stomach and intestine, it elicits the secretion of an array of gut peptides and other signals that function to coordinate and optimize the digestive process. In 1973 Gibbs and Smith and their colleagues reported that the gut peptide, cholecystokinin (CCK), acts as a satiety signal, suggesting that this peptide may regulate the size of meals. When purified or synthetic CCK is administered to rats or humans prior to a meal, it dose-dependently reduced the size of that meal (39–43). Further support of a role of endogenous CCK in eliciting satiety is indicated by the observation that the administration of specific CCK-1 receptor antagonists prior to a meal causes increased meal size in animals and humans (44–47) and reduces the subjective feeling of satiety in humans (44).

Endogenous factors that reduce the size of meals are considered satiety signals. There are several different gut peptides that normally contribute to reductions in meal size and number (48,49). Besides CCK, gastrin-releasing peptide (GRP) (50), neuromedin B (51), enterostatin (52,53), somatostatin (54), glucagon-like peptide (GLP)-1 (55,56), apolipoprotein A-IV (57), and peptide YY (PYY)3-36 (58) are all peptides secreted from the gastrointestinal system that have been reported to reduce meal size when administered systemically. Amylin (59,60) and glucagon (61,62) secreted from the pancreatic islets during meals also have this property.

These peptides signal the central nervous system via multiple mechanisms but all contribute to the phenomenon of satiety. The mechanism thought to be used by most is to activate receptors on vagal afferent fibers passing to the hindbrain (e.g., CCK [63–65], glucagon [66,67]), or to stimulate the hindbrain directly at sites with a relaxed blood–brain barrier (e.g., amylin [68,69]). Signals from different peptides, as well as signals related to stomach distension, are thought to be integrated either within the vagal fibers themselves or in the hindbrain, as they generate an overall signal that ultimately causes the individual to stop eating (70–73).

In summary, when food is eaten, it interacts with receptors lining the stomach and intestine, causing the release of peptides and other factors that coordinate the process of digestion with the particular food being consumed. Some of the peptides provide a signal to the nervous system, and as the integrated signal accumulates, it ultimately creates the sensation of fullness and contributes to cessation of eating.

An important and generally unanswered question concerns whether satiety signals have therapeutic value to treat obesity. Thus, if satiety signals reduce individual meals (e.g., by administering CCK prior to each meal), individuals may adjust by increasing their frequency of eating, thereby maintaining total daily intake essentially constant (74,75). CCK and the other gut-derived satiety signals have very short half-lives, on the order of one or a few minutes. Of note, rats with a genetic ablation of functional CCK-1 receptors gradually become obese over their lifetimes (76). Hence, long-acting analogs of the satiety signals may have efficacy in causing weight loss. This is an area of considerable research activity at present.

INTEGRATION OF ADIPOSITY SIGNALS

The information about total body fat derived from insulin and leptin must be integrated with satiety signals as well as with other signals related to learning, social situations, stress, and other factors, for the control system to be maximally efficient. Although the nature of these interactions is not well understood, several generalizations or conclusions can be made. For one, the negative feedback circuits related to body fat and meal ingestion can easily be overridden by situational events. As an example, even though satiety signals might indicate that no more food should be eaten during an ongoing meal, the sight, smell, and perceived palatability of an offered dessert can stimulate further intake. Likewise, even though an individual is severely underweight and food is available, the influence of stressors can preclude significant ingestion. Because of these kinds of interactions, trying to relate food intake within an individual meal to recent energy expenditure or to fat stores is futile, at least in the short term. Rather, the influence of homeostatic signals becomes apparent only when intake is considered over longer intervals. That is, if homeostatic signals predominated, a relatively large intake in one meal should be compensated by reduced intake in the subsequent meal. However, detailed analyses have revealed that such compensation, if it occurs at all, is apparent in humans only when intervals of one or more days are considered (77,78). This phenomenon was initially demonstrated in a rigorous experiment using rabbits, where weekly intake correlated better with recent energy expenditure than did intake after 1 or 3 d (79).

Homeostatic controls over food intake act by changing the sensitivity to satiety signals. The adiposity signals insulin and leptin alter sensitivity to CCK. Hence, when an individual has gained excess weight, more insulin and leptin stimulate the brain, and this in turn renders CCK more efficacious at reducing meal size (80–84). This association continues until the individual or animal becomes obese and resistant to the adiposity signals leptin and insulin.

The feeding circuitry is integrated. As discussed above, satiety signals that influence meal size interact with vagal afferent fibers and continue into the hindbrain (85,86), where meal size is ultimately determined (87). At the same time, the hypothalamic arcuate nucleus receives adiposity signals (leptin and insulin) as well as information related to ongoing meals from the hindbrain. Through integration of these multiple signals, metabolism and ingestion are monitored (11–14,88).

Importantly, leptin and insulin fill distinct niches in the endocrine system. Although leptin has been implicated in several systemic processes, such as angiogenesis, the primary role of leptin appears to be as a negative-feedback adiposity signal that acts in the brain to suppress food intake and net catabolic effector (22,89,90). Consistent with this, animals lacking leptin or functional leptin receptors are grossly obese. Insulin (as previously mentioned), in contrast, has a primary action in the periphery to regulate blood glucose and stimulate glucose uptake by most tissues. Analogous to leptin, however, deficits in insulin signaling are also associated with hyperphagia in humans, and animals that lack normal insulin signaling in the brain are also obese (22,89–92).

The potential for redundancy between leptin and insulin has been highlighted by several recent studies in which leptin and insulin have been found to share both intracellular and neuronal signaling pathways. The melanocortin system has long been thought to mediate the central actions of leptin (see "Melanocortins" section), though recent studies indicate insulin stimulated the expression of the melanocortin agonist precursor peptide pro-opiomelanocortin (POMC) in fasted rats and insulin-induced hypophagia is blocked by a non-specific melanocortin receptor antagonist *(93–98)*. Furthermore, phosphatidylinositol-3-OH kinase (PI(3)K), an intracellular mediator of insulin signaling *(99)*, appears to play a crucial role in the leptin-induced anorexia signal transduction pathway as well *(99)*. Leptin functionally enhances or "sensitizes" some actions of insulin. The underlying molecular mechanisms for the insulin-sensitizing effects of leptin are unclear, and studies are conflicting regarding the effect of leptin on insulin-stimulated signal transduction. Whereas the long form of the leptin receptor has the capacity to activate the JAK/STAT3 *(100,101)* and mitogen-activated protein kinase (MAPK) pathways, leptin is also able to stimulate tyrosine phosphorylation of insulin receptor substrate (IRS-1) *(101)*, and to increase transcription of fos, jun *(102)*.

CENTRAL SIGNALS RELATED TO ENERGY HOMEOSTASIS

Neural circuits in the brain that control energy homeostasis can be subdivided into those that receive sensory information (afferent circuits), those that integrate the information, and those that control motor, autonomic, and endocrine responses (efferent circuits). Peptides such as insulin, leptin, and CCK—i.e., adiposity and satiety signals—are afferent signals that influence food intake. Additional, more direct, metabolic signals arise within the brain itself and also influence food intake, and these are discussed below.

Substrates such as glucose and/or fatty acids are utilized in most cells in the body and can be captured or released as energy. As oxygen combines with these substrates in the mitochondria of the cell, water and carbon dioxide are produced, and the substrate's energy is transferred into molecules such as ATP that can be used as needed to power cellular processes. Most cells in the body have complex means of maintaining adequate ATP generation because they are able to oxidize either glucose or fatty acids. Hence, if one or the other substrate becomes low, enzymatic changes occur to increase the ability of the cell rapidly to take up and oxidize the alternate fuel. Compromising the formation of ATP disables cells, and when it occurs in the brain, generates a signal that leads to increased eating *(32,103–105)*.

It has been posited that specific cells/neurons in the brain function as fuel sensors and thereby generate signals that interact with other neuronal systems to regulate energy homeostasis *(32,105)*. The brain is sensitive to changes in glucose utilization because neurons primarily use glucose for energy. Recently, it has been demonstrated that in addition to sensing changes in glucose levels, the brain also responds to and uses fatty acids as sensor to influence food intake.

When energy substrates are abundant, most cells throughout the body have the ability to synthesize fatty acids from acetyl CoA (TCA cycle intermediate) and malonyl CoA via the cellular enzyme, fatty acid synthase (FAS). When FAS activity is inhibited locally in the brain by the drug C75, animals eat less food and over the course of a few days, selectively lose body fat *(106–108)*. One interpretation of these findings is that there are some hypothalamic cells that have the ability to sense changes in fatty acids, and these are the critical populations of cells that are responsible for energy homeostasis *(109)*. The anorexic activity of C75 appears to require brain carbohydrate metabolism *(110)*, further supporting a critical role of key hypothalamic cells in the regulation of energy homeostasis. Consistent with this, increases of either carbohydrate or long-chain fatty acid availability locally in the arcuate nucleus leads to reduced food intake and signals are sent to the liver to reduce the secretion of energy-rich fuels into the blood

Table 1
Neuropeptides/Hormones/Nutrients/Neurotransmitters

	Anabolic	Catabolic
Melanin-concentrating hormone (MCH)	√	
Hypocretin–orexin	√	
Neuropeptide Y (NPY)	√	
Agouti-related protein (AgRP)	√	
Ghrelin	√	
Cocaine–amphetamine-related transcript (CART)		√
Corticotropin-releasing hormone (CRH) and urocortin		√
Proglucagon (GLP-1, GLP-2)		√
Serotonin		√
Ciliary neurotrophic factor (CNTF)		√
Pro-opiomelanocortin (POMC)		√

(111). These findings further support the concept that some brain neurons can utilize either glucose or lipids for energy and hence function as overall energy sensors (e.g., *see* refs. *31,32,112*).

These nutrient-sensing cells in the brain have begun to be more fully characterized. As previously mentioned, there are glucose-sensing neurons/cells, and these appear to contain receptors and enzymes that are consistent with another type of cell that senses changes in glucose, the pancreatic β-cells. Like β-cells, certain populations of neurons and glia detect changes in glucose levels and generate signals that influence metabolism and behavior *(113,114)*. In further support of an integrated system, there is evidence that the same or proximally close neurons contain receptors for leptin and insulin. What can be imagined from the current findings is that the brain is a critical "nutrient-sensing"organ; there is a population of neurons that collectively sample different classes of energy-rich molecules (i.e., glucose and fatty acids) as well as hormones whose levels reflect adiposity throughout the body (i.e., insulin and leptin). These same neurons appear also to be sensitive to the myriad neuropeptides known to be important regulators of energy homeostasis *(32)*, which will be described more fully below.

Anabolic Effector Systems

NEUROPEPTIDE Y

Neuropeptide Y (NPY) is one of the most potent stimulators of food intake *(115–117)*, and is proposed to be an anabolic effector that induces positive energy balance. NPY is a highly expressed peptide in the mammalian CNS *(118,119)*, and is well conserved across species. Hypothalamic NPY neurons are found primarily in the arcuate (ARC) and dorsomedial nuclei, and in neurons such as the PVN *(120–125)*. Endogenous release of NPY is regulated by energy balance. Specifically, in the ARC, food deprivation, food restriction, or exercise-induced negative energy balance each results in upregulation of NPY mRNA in the ARC and increased NPY protein. Repeated administration of NPY results in sustained hyperphagia and rapid body weight gain *(126,127)*. The response of the NPY system to negative energy balance is mediated, at least in part, by the falls in both insulin and leptin that accompany negative energy balance. Central insulin or central/peripheral leptin infusion attentuates the effect of negative energy balance and reduced NPY mRNA levels in the ARC *(128–131)*.

The ARC NPY system has received the most experimental attention; however, there is also evidence that implicates the dorsal medial hypothalamus (DMH) NPY system in the regulation of food intake. The role of NPY in the DMH in regulation of body weight is most evident in several genetic murine obesity models, such as in tubby and agouti *lethal yellow* mice, where these animals are hyperphagic, yet have no elevations in ARC NPY mRNA, but do have elevations in DMH NPY mRNA *(132–134)*. Rats that do not make a specific receptor for the classic gut-satiety factor, CCK, have elevated body fat mass *(135)*, with elevated NPY mRNA in the DMH but not the ARC. There is growing evidence that points to the hypothesis that there are multiple inputs that determine NPY activity in both the ARC and DMH.

There has been considerable controversy about the importance of the NPY system because mice with a targeted deletion of the NPY gene do not show a dramatic phenotype in terms of their regulation of energy balance *(136)*. Interestingly, when NPY-deficient mice are crossed with obese *ob/ob* mice, the resultant mice with both NPY and leptin deficiency weigh less than *ob/ob* mice that have an intact NPY system, indicating that the NPY system contributes significantly to the obesity of *ob/ob* mice *(137)*. This is consistent with data showing elevated NPY levels in the hypothalamus of *ob/ob* mice. However, a number of other murine models of obesity have no apparent difference when crossed with NPY-deficient mice *(138)*. Thus one conclusion that could be reached from experiments on NPY-deficient mice suggests that NPY's importance may not be as great as the physiological evidence has indicated. Alternatively, NPY-deficient mice may compensate for developing in the absence of NPY signaling *(139,140)*.

A recent report has further demonstrated the critical role of NPY neurons in the arcuate nucleus. Bruning and colleagues induced targeted expression of a toxin receptor to neurons expressing agouti-related protein (AgRP) *(141)*. NPY and AgRP (discussed in Melanocortin section) are coexpressed in a subset of arcuate nuclei. These are the critical NPY/AgRP neurons that are believed to mediate many of the effects of leptin and insulin on food intake. Using this technique, the investigators were able to induce cell death specifically in these neurons in a temporal manner *(141)*. In contrast to the embryonic deletion of the neurons, mice with adult targeted deletion of the NPY/AgRP neurons stopped eating and lost significant amounts of body adiposity. Indeed, the embryonic ablation of these neurons is consistent with ablation of the individual NPY and AgRP neuropeptides. This elegant study confirms the important role of these cells in the normal regulation of energy balance. Although they are compelling, the data point to the importance of the neurons, not the unique neuropeptides NPY and AgRP *(141)*.

There are several NPY receptors that are critical for the physiological effects observed following NPY administration. Both the Y1 and Y5 receptors have significant expression in areas of the hypothalamus that are sensitive to the orexigenic effects of NPY. However, both pharmacological *(142–147)* and transgenic approaches to assessing the relative contributions of Y1 and Y5 receptors have resulted in conflicting data. There remains some speculation for the existence of an unidentified NPY receptor that contributes significantly to the feeding response *(148)*. Over the years, the NPY receptors have attracted a significant interest by the biotechnology and pharmaceutical industries *(149)*. Despite this industry investment, NPY antagonists have failed to show significant efficacy in preclinical obesity models *(150)*. Therefore, it is unlikely that we will see NPY pharmacological agents in the clinic in the near future.

MELANIN-CONCENTRATING HORMONE

As previously described, the LHA was known as an area critical for the regulation of food intake and fluid intake and was first reviewed in Stellar's original papers in the 1940s and 1950s. There are at least two peptides released from the LHA that appear to mediate these effects: melanin-concentrating hormone (MCH) and orexin (*see* "Hypocretin/Orexin"). MCH regulates food intake and its expression is increased in obese *ob/ob* mice *(151)*. When MCH is delivered into the ventricular system it potently increases food intake *(152,153)* and water intake *(154)*. Unlike NPY, repeated administration of MCH does not result in increased body weight *(155)*. Importantly, mice with targeted deletion of MCH have reduced food intake and decreased body weight and adiposity *(156)*, unlike the NPY-null mice. Recent evidence indicates that MCH is potently regulated by estrogen and may be an important component of mediating the effects of estrogen on food intake and energy balance *(157)*. Because there are MCH projections and receptors that are broadly distributed throughout the neuraxis, and combined with the fact that the MCH knockout animal is lean, it is likely that MCH has a significant role in the regulation of food intake. Several MCH antagonists have been described in the literature and all appear to reduce body weight, food intake, and fat mass *(158,159)*. Indeed, several pharmaceutical companies have begun evaluation of MCH-selective antagonists in humans *(160)*.

HYPOCRETIN/OREXIN

"Hypocretins" *(161)* and "orexins" *(162)* are two names given to the same peptide. Hypocretin is the more commonly used term in sleep/wake cycle research, whereas orexin is more commonly used in food intake research. The orexins consist of two peptides (ORX-A and ORX-B) and two receptors, and although the cell bodies are located in close proximity to MCH-expressing neurons in the LHA, the two systems do not colocalize to any significant extent *(163)*. Considerable evidence indicates that central administration of ORX-A increases food intake *(164,165)*. Like MCH, orexins have a broad distribution pattern and a variety of evidence links the ORX system directly to the control of arousal *(166,167)*.

In further support of the CNS being an integrated system, the LHA is positioned to receive information about nutrients and information concerning the levels of adiposity signals that are transmitted to the LHA via projections from the ARC. There are significant hypothalamic connections among the ARC, the PVN, and the LHA. Projections from the ARC synapse on both MCH and ORX neurons in the LHA *(168)*. NPY and melanocortin neurons from the ARC interact in a specific way with MCH and the ORX systems in the LHA *(164,165,169,170)*, suggesting that it is tied to energy homeostasis. Additionally, ORX mRNA in the LHA is inhibited by leptin *(162)* and increased by decreased glucose utilization *(171)*.

GHRELIN

Ghrelin is the endogenous ligand for the growth hormone secretagog receptor *(172,173)*. Endocrine cells of the stomach secrete ghrelin, and consistent with its role as an anabolic effector, centrally and peripherally administered ghrelin results in increased food intake in both rats *(174,175)* and humans *(176)*. Ghrelin infusion results in dramatic obesity, and circulating ghrelin levels are increased during fasting and rapidly decline after nutrients are provided to the stomach *(172,173;* for review, *see* ref. *177)*. Ghrelin binds to the growth hormone secretagog receptor, which is found in the arcuate nucleus of the hypothalamus. NPY-producing cells in the ARC are critical mediators of the effect of ghrelin *(178–181)*. Finally, clinical evidence points to elevated levels of ghrelin in weight-reduced patients *(182)* with the notable exception of patients who have been successfully treated for obesity by gastric bypass, in whom circulating ghrelin levels are close to undetectable *(183)*.

As previously discussed, there are numerous peptides secreted from the stomach and intestines that influence food intake. Gastrointestinal signals are thought to be released to restrain the consumption of excess calories and to minimize the increase of postprandial blood glucose *(34)*. Gastrointestinal signals reduce meal size and provide signals as to the complexity of macronutrients consumed. The fact that only one gastrointestinal peptide stimulates food intake speaks to the importance of limiting meal size. The ghrelin signaling pathway has received much publicity in the media and attention by pharmaceutical companies *(184)*. The data suggest that ghrelin antagonists may be potent inhibitors of food intake and good weight loss agents *(185)*. Indeed, several studies indicate that antagonists may be potent food intake inhibitors in lean rodents, though evidence in high-fat-fed diet-induced obese rodents is lacking *(186)*.

CATABOLIC EFFECTOR SYSTEMS

Catabolic systems are those that are activated during positive energy balance. These systems oppose those previously described, which are activated during negative energy balance. When animals or humans consume calories in excess of their requirements, body weight is gained. Additionally, if animals are forced to consume calories in excess of their needs, voluntary food intake drops to near zero and the animals gain body weight *(187,188)*. These data provide further evidence that body weight is tightly regulated. Hence animals not only have potent regulatory responses to being in negative energy balance, but they also possess regulatory responses to being in positive energy balance. Catabolic systems are defined here as those that are activated during positive energy balance and that act to reduce energy intake and/or to increase energy expenditure and thereby restore energy stores to its defended levels.

Cocaine–Amphetamine-Related Transcript

Cocaine–amphetamine-related transcript (CART) *(189)* was first identified as a gene whose expression is regulated by cocaine and amphetamine. CART is expressed in many of the POMC-expressing neurons in the ARC. CART expression is reduced during negative energy balance and is stimulated by leptin *(190)*. Exogenous administration of CART peptide fragments into the ventricular system potently reduces food intake *(190–192)* and ventricular administration of antibodies to CART produce significant increases in intake, implicating a role for endogenous CART in the inhibition of food intake *(190)*. However, at these same doses, CART also produces a number of other behavioral actions that make its exact role in the control of food intake unclear *(193)*. CART is a very prevalent peptide and its distinct role in the regulation of food intake and body weight is further confused by data indicating that when delivered specifically into the arcuate nucleus, CART actually produces an increase in food intake *(194)*.

Corticotropin-Releasing Hormone and Urocortin

Corticotropin-releasing hormone (CRH) is synthesized in the PVN and LHA and is negatively regulated by levels of glucocorticoids. CRH is a key controller of the hypothalamic–pituitary axis (HPA), which regulates glucocorticoid secretion from the adrenal gland. Administration of CRH into the ventricular system potently reduces food intake, increases energy expenditure, and reduces body weight *(195,196)*. As previously mentioned, when animals are overfed, they voluntarily reduced their food intake, and CRH mRNA in the PVN is also potently increased by involuntary overfeeding *(188)*. The role of CRH in the regulation of food intake and body is complex owing to the presence of a binding protein within the CNS and evidence that inhibition of this binding protein results in decreased food intake *(197)*.

Urocortin is a second peptide in the CRH family. Urocortin administration reduces food intake but unlike what occurs following CRH, reductions in food intake are not associated with other aversive effects *(198)*. Urocortin is produced in the caudal brainstem and has prominent projections to the PVN *(199)*. Given the central importance of the CRH system to activity of the HPA axis, the important role of peripheral glucocorticoids in controlling metabolic processes, and the inverse relationship between peripheral leptin and glucocorticoid levels, unraveling the complicated relationship of the CRH/urocortin systems in control of energy balance remains a critical but elusive goal. (For a more thorough review of the CRH system and energy balance *see* refs. *200,201*)

Proglucagon-Derived Peptides

Preproglucagon is a peptide made both in the periphery and in the CNS. Preproglucagon encodes two peptides with described central activity: glucagon-like-peptide 1 (GLP-1) and glucagon-like-peptide 2 (GLP-2). Both peptides are made in the L-cells of the distal intestine and have well-described functions in the periphery, with GLP-1 critical for enhancing nutrient-induced insulin secretion *(202)* and GLP-2 playing an important role in maintenance of the gut mucosa *(203)*. Preproglucagon is also made in a distinct population of neurons in the nucleus of the solitary tract, with prominent projections to the PVN and DMH *(204,205)* as well as to the spinal cord. Preproglucagon neurons appear to be targets of leptin, as peripheral leptin administration induces fos expression, a marker of neuronal activation, in them *(206,207)*. Both GLP-1 and GLP-2 have distinct receptors, with the GLP-1 receptor found predominantly in the PVN and the GLP-2 receptor in the DMH. When administered into the ventricular system, GLP-1 produces a profound reduction in food intake and antagonists to the GLP-1 receptor increase food intake *(208,209)*. However, exogenous GLP-1 administration is also associated with a number of the symptoms of visceral illness *(210,211)*, and GLP-1 receptor antagonists can block the visceral illness effects of the toxin LiCl *(212,213)*. GLP-2 administration is associated with a less potent anorectic response but one that appears not to be accompanied by the symptoms of visceral illness associated with GLP-1 *(214)*. The interaction of these two cosecreted peptides is yet to be determined.

Serotonin

Serotonin has been implicated in body weight and food intake regulation, based on animal and human studies *(215)*. Serotonin affects feeding behavior by promoting satiation and also appears to play a role in carbohydrate intake *(216)*. The activity of serotonin is observed in several hypothalamic nuclei in the medial hypothalamus, notably the

PVN, VMHl, suprachiasmatic, and LHA of the hypothalamus nuclei *(217)*. There are at least 14 serotonin receptor subtypes, but the receptor subtypes implicated in feeding include $5HT_{1A}$, $5HT_{1B}$, $5HT_{2C}$, $5HT_{1D}$, $5HT_{2A}$, and $5HT_3$ *(218)*. Importantly, enhancement or stimulation of serotonergic activity leads to decreased food intake, whereas attenuation or inhibition of serotonergic activity leads to increased food intake. Indeed, clinical evidence for the importance of the serotonergic system derives from the highly efficacious drugs dexfenfluramine and fenfluramine *(215)*. Both were dual-acting 5HT-reuptake and 5HT-releasing agents that were potent satiety drugs used as obesity therapeutics. They were withdrawn from the clinic because of untoward effects on the heart valve, perhaps related to their activity at peripheral $5HT_{2B}$ receptor stimulation. Newer serotonergic agonists are being developed to selectively stimulate the $5HT_{2C}$ receptor subtype *(219)*. In fact, $5HT_{2C}$ null mice are obese and hyperphagic *(220)*. Finally, recent data show that serotonergic signaling, specifically $5HT_{2C}$ receptors, requires melanocortinergic signaling to inhibit feeding *(221)*.

Ciliary Neurotrophic Factor and Axokine

Ciliary neurotrophic factor (CNTF) is a neuronal survival factor shown to induce weight loss in rodents and humans *(222,223)*. CNTF leads to a reduction in food intake and body weight apparently via activating pathways that mimic leptin, though unlike leptin, CNTF is active in leptin-resistant diet-induced obese mice *(224)*. Interestingly, CNTF-treated rodents and humans lose weight and maintain the reduced body weight for a long period after cessation of treatment. The implication of these observations suggests that CNTF resets the body weight "set point," or changes the weight the body defends. But the reason was not understood, although recent data from the Flier laboratory shed light on a potential mechanism for the maintenance of the weight loss *(225)*. Flier and colleagues showed that CNTF induces neuronal cell proliferation in hypothalamic feeding centers. The new cells show functional leptin responsiveness. The data provide an explanation for the prolonged weight loss maintenance but do not explain how CNTF induces satiety and leads to weight loss. Initial data in rodents appeared to indicate that CNTF somehow suppresses the appetite-enhancing neuropeptide NPY *(226)*.

Melanocortins

The action of leptin, and possibly insulin, on feeding behavior is transduced by the melanocortin signaling pathway in the hypothalamus *(227)*. The arcuate nuclei in the hypothalamus contain two distinct populations of neurons that highly express the leptin receptor. These neurons are the POMC and agouti-related protein (AgRP)/NPY neurons, which project onto neurons in the paraventricular and lateral hypothalamic area known to express the melanocortin receptors. The POMC-containing neurons secrete the melanocortin agonist α-MSH, whereas the AgRP/NPY-containing neurons secrete the melanocortin antagonist AgRP. Leptin appears to reciprocally regulate these nuclei. Low leptin levels lead to increased expression of AgRP and reduced expression of POMC and α-MSH. In contrast, high leptin levels lead to increased expression of POMC and reduced expression of AgRP.

The importance of the melanocortin signaling pathway in feeding behavior and body weight was originally uncovered by mouse fanciers characterizing coat color phenotypes in the mouse *(228)*. One of these mutations, named agouti *lethal yellow*, had a yellow coat color and was obese. Over the past decade, the details of this unusual mutation were elucidated, as well as its relevance to human obesity. The signaling system involves the melanocortin receptor and two functionally opposing ligands, an agonist derived from the POMC peptide and an antagonist, AgRP *(229,230)*. Inactivating mutations in the receptor as well as the activating ligand, α–MSH, lead to hyperphagia and obesity in both rodents and humans *(231–233)*. Likewise, overexpression of the antagonist, AgRP, also leads to obesity in rodents *(234)*.

There are five mammalian melanocortin receptor subtypes involved in diverse physiological processes such as feeding behavior, energy balance, pigmentation, and stress response *(235,236)*. The melanocortin-3 and -4 receptors (MC3R, MC4R) are expressed in the brain and implicated in body weight and feeding behavior regulation. The MC1R is expressed in the skin and implicated in skin and hair pigmentation. The MC2R is expressed in the adrenal gland and implicated in the stress response, part of the hypothalamic–pituitary adrenal (HPA) axis. Finally, the MC5R is ubiquitously expressed in the periphery and implicated in sebaceous gland physiology.

The melanocortin receptors, particularly the MC4R, have attracted significant pharmaceutical attention *(237)*. Indeed, pharmacological validation for the role of the melanocortin receptors in feeding behavior derives based on the peptide nonspecific melanocortin agonist melanotan II (MTII) *(238,239)*. Rodent and human studies with MTII indicate that melanocortin agonism leads to reduced food intake. The melanocortin receptors are involved in a variety of physiological process, thus identifying a selective agonist has been quite complicated. Despite significant biotechnology and pharmaceutical interest, pharmacological modulators of MC4R are not likely to appear in the clinic in the near future.

Syndecan-3

Syndecan-3, a neuronal heparan sulfate proteoglycan (HSPG), was recently identified as a modulator of feeding behavior by acting as a coreceptor for the melanocortin receptors in the hypothalamus *(240)*. Syndecan-3 expression is regulated by nutritional status; ablation of the gene leads to reduced food intake and resistance to high-fat diet-induced obesity *(241)*. The finding was quite unexpected, but provides a novel mechanism for regulating body weight. Syndecan-3 is a member of a family of four type I transmembrane HSPGs that act as coreceptors for diverse cell surface receptors *(242)*. As coreceptors, the syndecans modulate a variety of cellular and physiological processes. Syndecan function is regulated by transcriptional, post-transcriptional, and post-translational processes. Syndecans are also regulated by cleavage of their extracelluar domain in a process commonly referred to as shedding *(243)*. Release of the extracellular domain can inactivate the signaling modulated by the syndecans.

Regulation of feeding behavior by syndecan-3 is likely modulated by cleavage of its extracellular domain by shedding *(244)*. Transgenic expression of syndecan-1, a homolog of syndecan-3, in the hypothalamus leads to hyperphagia and obesity in mice *(240)*. Notably, the hypothalamic expressed syndecan-1 cannot be shed, suggesting loss of feeding regulation. In fact, injection of shedding inhibitors into the hypothalamus of normal rodents leads to hyperphagia. Syndecan-3 is poised to play a role in the hypothalamic regulation of feeding behavior modulated by synaptic plasticity. Recent data from the Horvath and Simmerly laboratories indicate that rewiring of the arcuate nuclei in the hypothalamus occurs in response to leptin *(245,246)*. The data indicate that excitatory and inhibitory synapses on the POMC and AgRP/NPY neurons can rapidly change in response to adiposity signals such as leptin. Syndecan-3 has been implicated in synaptic plasticity changes involved in hippocampus-dependent memory *(247)*. Therefore, it is likely that syndecan-3 can also play a related role in the synaptic plasticity changes occurring in the hypothalamus.

CONCLUSIONS

The research and topics presented in this review are by no means the entirety of work into the CNS regulation of food intake and appetite. In fact, there are rich areas of investigation that we have been able to mention only briefly. The important conclusion from all of this work is, however, that the regulation system—and specifically the CNS control of this regulation—is diverse and yet exquisitely integrated. From signals arising in the gastrointestinal tract, to hormones that convey adiposity information, to the multiple nuclei in the brain that receive and coordinate the behavioral response, each part of the system represents not an independent entity, but rather an important piece of a complex whole.

REFERENCES

1. Stellar E. The physiology of motivation. Psychol Rev 1954;61:5–22.
2. Powley TL. The ventromedial hypothalamic syndrome, satiety, and a cephalic phase hypothesis. Psychol Rev 1977;84:89–126.
3. Sclafani A. The role of hyperinsulinema and the vagus nerve in hypothalamic hyperphagia reexamined. Diabetologia 1981;20(Suppl):402–410.
4. Bray GA, Sclafani A, Novin D. Obesity-inducing hypothalamic knife cuts: effects on lipolysis and blood insulin levels. Am J Physiol 1982;243(3):R445–R449.
5. Aravich PF, Sclafani A. Paraventricular hypothalamic lesions and medial hypothalamic knife cuts produce similar hyperphagia syndromes. Behav Neurosci 1983;97(6):970–983.
6. Grill HJ, Norgren R. Chronically decerebrate rats demonstrate satiation but not bait shyness. Science 1978;201(4352):267–269.
7. Grill HJ, Norgren R. The taste reactivity test. II. Mimetic responses to gustatory stimuli in chronic thalamic and chronic decerebrate rats. Brain Res 1978;143(2):281–297.
8. Grill HJ, Smith GP. Cholecystokinin decreases sucrose intake in chronic decerebrate rats. Am J Physiol 1988;254: R853–R856.
9. Flynn FW, Grill HJ. Intraoral intake and taste reactivity responses elicited by sucrose and sodium chloride in chronic decerebrate rats. Behav Neurosci 1988;102(6):934–941.
10. Kennedy GC. The role of depot fat in the hypothalamic control of food intake in the rat. Proc R Soc Lond (Biol) 1953;140:579–592.
11. Ahima RS, et al. Leptin regulation of neuroendocrine systems. Front Neuroendocrinol 2000;21:263–307.
12. Cone RD, et al. The arcuate nucleus as a conduit for diverse signals relevant to energy homeostasis. Int J Obes Relat Metab Disord 2001;25 Suppl 5:S63–S67.
13. Elmquist JK, Elias CF,. Saper CB From lesions to leptin: hypothalamic control of food intake and body weight. Neuron 1999;22:221–232.
14. Schwartz MW, et al. Central nervous system control of food intake. Nature 2000;404:661–671.
15. Havel PJ, et al. Gender differences in plasma leptin concentrations. Nat Med 1996;2(9):949–950.
16. Ahren B, et al. Regulation of plasma leptin in mice: influence of age, high-fat diet and fasting. Am J Physiol 1997;273:R113–R120.
17. Havel PJ, Mechanisms regulating leptin production: Implications for control of energy balance. Am J Clin Nutr 1999;70:305–306.
18. Buchanan C, et al. Central nervous system effects of leptin. Trends Endocrinol Metab 1998;9(4):146–150.
19. Bjorntorp P. Metabolic implications of body fat distribution. Diabetes Care 1991;14(12):1132–1143.
20. Bjorntorp P. Abdominal fat distribution and the metabolic syndrome. J Cardiovasc Pharmacol 1992;20 Suppl 8:S26–S28.

21. Bjorntorp P. Body fat distribution, insulin reistance, and metabolic diseases. Nutrition 1997;13:795–803.
22. Woods SC, et al. Signals that regulate food intake and energy homeostasis. Science 1998;280:1378–1383.
23. Schwartz, MW, et al. Insulin in the brain: a hormonal regulator of energy balance. Endocrine Rev 1992;13:387–414.
24. de Castro JM, Stroebele N. Food intake in the real world: implications for nutrition and aging. Clin Geriatr Med 2002;18:685–697.
25. de Castro JM. The control of eating behavior in free living humans. In: Stricker EM, Woods SC, eds. Handbook of Neurobiology. Neurobiology of Food and Fluid Intake, vol. 14, no. 2 Kluwer Academic/Plenum Publishers, New York: 2004; pp. 467–502.
26. de Graaf C, et al. Biomarkers of satiation and satiety. Am J Clin Nutr 2004;79:946–961.
27. Mayer J. Regulation of energy intake and the body weight: The glucostatic and lipostatic hypothesis. Ann NY Acad Sci 1955;63:14–42.
28. Mayer J, Thomas DW Regulation of food intake and obesity. Science 1967;156:328–337.
29. Friedman MI. Fuel partitioning and food intake. Am J Clin Nutr 1998;67(Suppl 3):513S–518S.
30. Friedman MI. An energy sensor for control of energy intake. Proc Nutr Soc 1997;56(1A):41–50.
31. Langhans W. Metabolic and glucostatic control of feeding. Proc Nutr Soc 1996;55:497–515.
32. Peters A, et al. The selfish brain: competition for energy resources. Neurosci Biobehav Rev 2004;28:143–180.
33. Strubbe JH, Woods SC. The timing of meals. Psychol Rev 2004;111:128–141.
34. Woods SC, Strubbe JH. The psychobiology of meals. Psychonom Bull Rev 1994;1:141–155.
35. Woods SC, et al. Food intake and the regulation of body weight. Ann Rev Psychol 2000;51:255–277.
36. Davis JD, Campbell CS. Peripheral control of meal size in the rat. Effect of sham feeding on meal size and drinking rate. J Comp Physiol Psychol 1973;83(3):379–87.
37. Davis JD, Smith GP. Learning to sham feed: behavioral adjustments to loss of physiological postingestional stimuli. Am J Physiol 1990;259(6 Pt 2):R1228–R1235.
38. Gibbs J, Young RC, Smith GP. Cholecystokinin elicits satiety in rats with open gastric fistulas. Nature 1973;245:323–325.
39. Gibbs J, Young RC, Smith GP. Cholecystokinin decreases food intake in rats. J Comp Physiol Psychol 1973;84:488–495.
40. Kissileff HR, et al. Cholecystokinin decreases food intake in man. Am J Clin Nutr 1981;34:154–160.
41. Muurahainenn N, et al. Effects of cholecystokinin-octapeptide (CCK-8) on food intake and gastric emptying in man. Physiol Behav 1988;44:644–649.
42. Moran TH, Schwartz GJ. Neurobiology of cholecystokinin. Crit Rev Neurobiol 1994;9:1–28.
43. Smith GP, Gibbs J. The development and proof of the cholecystokinin hypothesis of satiety. In: Dourish CT, et al., eds. Multiple Cholecystokinin Receptors in the CNS, Oxford University Press, Oxford: 1992; pp. 166–182.
44. Beglinger C, et al. Loxiglumide, a CCK-A receptor antagonist, stimulates calorie intake and hunger feelings in humans. Am J Physiol 2001;280:R1149–R1154.
45. Hewson G, et al. The cholecystokinin receptor antagonist L364,718 increases food intake in the rat by attenuation of endogenous cholecystokinin. Br J Pharmacol 1988;93:79–84.
46. Moran TH, et al. Blockade of type A, but not type B, CCK receptors postpones satiety in rhesus monkeys. Am J Physiol 1993;265:R620–R624.
47. Reidelberger RD, O'Rourke MF. Potent cholecystokinin antagonist L-364,718 stimulates food intake in rats. Am J Physiol 1989;257:R1512–R1518.
48. Kaplan JM, Moran TH. Gastrointestinal signaling in the control of food intake. In: Stricker EM, Woods SC, eds. Handbook of Behavioral Neurobiology. Neurobiology of Food and Fluid Intake, vol. 4, no. 2, Kluwer Academic/Plenum Publishers, New York: 2004; pp. 273–303.
49. Smith GP, ed. Satiation: From Gut to Brain. Oxford University Press, New York: 1998.
50. Stein LJ, Woods SC. Gastrin releasing peptide reduces meal size in rats. Peptides 1982;3(5):833–835.
51. Ladenheim EE, Wirth KE, Moran TH. Receptor subtype mediation of feeding suppression by bombesin-like peptides. Pharmacol Biochem Behav 1996;54(4):705–711.
52. Okada S, et al. Enterostatin (Val-Pro-Asp-Pro-Arg), the activation peptide of procolipase, selectively reduces fat intake. Physiol Behav 1991;49:1185–1189.
53. Shargill NS, et al. Enterostatin suppresses food intake following injection into the third ventricle of rats. Brain Res 1991;544:137–140.

54. Lotter EC, et al. Somatostatin decreases food intake of rats and baboons. J Comp Physiol Psychol 1981;95(2):278–287.
55. Larsen PJ, et al, Systemic administration of the long-acting GLP-1 derivative NN2211 induces lasting and reversible weight loss in both normal and obese rats. Diabetes 2001;50:2530–2539.
56. Naslund E, et al. Energy intake and appetite are suppressed by glucagon-like peptide-1 (GLP-1) in obese men. Int J Obes Relat Metab Disord 1999;23(3):304–311.
57. Fujimoto K, et al. Effect of intravenous administration of apolipoprotein A-IV on patterns of feeding, drinking and ambulatory activity in rats. Brain Res 1993;608:233–237.
58. Batterham RL, et al. Gut hormone PYY(3-36) physiologically inhibits food intake. Nature 2002;418(6898):650–654.
59. Chance WT, et al. Anorexia following the intrahypothalamic administration of amylin. Brain Res 1991;539(2):352–354.
60. Lutz T., Del Prete E, Scharrer E. Reduction of food intake in rats by intraperitoneal injection of low doses of amylin. Physiol Behav 1994;55(5):891–895.
61. Geary N. Glucagon and the control of meal size. In: Smith GP, ed. Satiation. From Gut to Brain. Oxford University Press, New York: 1998; pp. 164–197.
62. Salter JM, Metabolic effects of glucagon in the Wistar rat. Am J Clin Nutr 1960;8:535–539.
63. Davison JS, Clarke GD. Mechanical properties and sensitivity to CCK of vagal gastric slowly adapting mechanoreceptors. Am J Physiol 1988;255(1 Pt 1):G55–G61.
64. Lorenz DN, Goldman SA. Vagal mediation of the cholecystokinin satiety effect in rats. Physiol Behav 1982;29(4):599–604.
65. Moran TH, et al. Vagal afferent and efferent contributions to the inhibition of food intake by cholecystokinin. Am J Physiol 1997;272(4 Pt 2):R1245–R1251.
66. Geary N, Le Sauter J, Noh U. Glucagon acts in the liver to control spontaneous meal size in rats. Am J Physiol 1993;264:R116–R122.
67. Langhans W. Role of the liver in the metabolic control of eating: what we know — and what we do not know. Neurosci Biobehav Rev 1996;20:145–153.
68. Lutz TA, Del Prete E, Scharrer E. Subdiaphragmatic vagotomy does not influence the anorectic effect of amylin. Peptides 1995;16(3):457–462.
69. Lutz TA, et al. Lesion of the area postrema/nucleus of the solitary tract (AP/NTS) attenuates the anorectic effects of amylin and calcitonin gene-related peptide (CGRP) in rats. Peptides 1998;19(2): 309–317.
70. Edwards GL, Ladenheim EE, Ritter RC. Dorsomedial hindbrain participation in cholecystokinin-induced satiety. Am J Physiol 1986;251:R971–R977.
71. Moran TH, Ladenheim EE, Schwartz GJ. Within-meal gut feedback signaling. Int J Obes Rel Metab Disord 2001;25 Suppl 5:S39–S41.
72. Moran TH, Kinzig KP. Gastrointestinal satiety signals II. Cholecystokinin. Am J Physiol Gastrointest Liver Physiol 2004;286(2):G183–G188.
73. Rinaman L, et al. Cholecystokinin activates catecholaminergic neurons in the caudal medulla that innervate the paraventricular nucleus of the hypothalamus in rats. J Comp Neurol 1995;360:246–256.
74. West DB, Fey D, Woods SC. Cholecystokinin persistently suppresses meal size but not food intake in free-feeding rats. Am J Physiol 1984;246:R776–R787.
75. West DB, et al. Lithium chloride, cholecystokinin and meal patterns: evidence the cholecystokinin suppresses meal size in rats without causing malaise. Appetite 1987;8:221–227.
76. Moran TH, et al. Disordered food intake and obesity in rats lacking cholecystokinin A receptors. Am J Physiol 1998;274(3 Pt 2):R618–R625.
77. Birch LL, et al. The variability of young children's energy intake. N Engl J Med 1991;324:232–235.
78. de Castro JM. Prior day's intake has macronutrient-specific delayed negative feedback effects on the spontaneous food intake of free-living humans. J Nutr 1998 ;128:61–67.
79. Gasnier A, Mayer A. Recherche sur la régulation de la nutrition. II. Mécanismes régulateurs de la nutrition chez le lapin domestique. Annals Physiologie Physicoichemie et Biologie 1939;15:157–185.
80. Barrachina MD, et al. Synergistic interaction between leptin and cholecystokinin to reduce short-term food intake in lean mice. Proc Natl Acad Sci USA 1997;94:10,455–10,460.
81. Figlewicz DP, et al. Intraventricular insulin enhances the meal-suppressive efficacy of intraventricular cholecystokinin octapeptide in the baboon. Behav Neurosci 1995;109:567–569.
82. Matson CA, et al. Synergy between leptin and cholecystokinin (CCK) to control daily caloric intake. Peptides 1997;18:1275–1278.

83. Matson CA, et al. Cholecystokinin and leptin act synergistically to reduce body weight. Am J Physiol 2000;278:R882–R890.
84. Riedy CA, et al. Central insulin enhances sensitivity to cholecystokinin. Physiol Behav 1995;58:755–760.
85. Schwartz GJ, Moran TH. Sub-diaphragmatic vagal afferent integration of meal-related gastrointestinal signals. Neurosci Biobehav Rev 1996;20:47–56.
86. Schwartz GJ, et al. Relationships between gastric motility and gastric vagal afferent responses to CCK and GRP in rats differ. Am J Physiol 1997;272(6 Pt 2):R1726–R1733.
87. Grill HJ, Kaplan JM. The neuroanatomical axis for control of energy balance. Front Neuroendocrinol 2002;23(1):2–40.
88. Flier JS. Obesity wars: molecular progress confronts an expanding epidemic. Cell 2004;116:337–350.
89. Porte DJ, et al. Obesity, diabetes and the central nervous system. Diabetologia 1998;41:863–881.
90. Woods SC, et al. Insulin and the blood-brain barrier. Curr Pharmaceut Des 2003;9:795–800.
91. Tartaglia LA, et al. Identification and expression cloning of a leptin receptor, OB-R. Cell 1995;83:1263–1271.
92. Bruning JC, et al. Role of brain insulin receptor in control of body weight and reproduction. Science 2000;289(5487):2122–2125.
93. Seeley R, et al. Melanocortin receptors in leptin effects. Nature 1997;390(Nov 27):349.
94. Ollmann M, et al. Antagonism of central melanocortin receptors in vitro and in vivo by agouti-related protein. Science 1997;278(Oct 3):135–138.
95. Rossi M, et al. A C-terminal fragment of agouti-related protein increases feeding and antagonizes the effect of alpha-melanocyte stimulating hormone in vivo. Endocrinology 1998;139(Oct):4428–4431.
96. Hagan MM, et al. Long-term orexigenic effects of AgRP-(83-132) involve mechanisms other than melanocortin receptor blockade. Am J Physiol 2000;279:R47–R52.
97. Fan W, et al. Role of melanocortinergic neurons in feeding and the agouti obesity syndrome. Nature 1997;385(Jan 9):165–168.
98. Hagan M, et al. Role of the CNS melanocortin system in the response to overfeeding. J Neurosci 1999;19(Mar 15):2362–2367.
99. Niswender KD, Schwartz MW. Insulin and leptin revisited: adiposity signals with overlapping physiological and intracellular signaling capabilities. Front Neuroendocrinol 2003;24:1–10.
100. Tartaglia LA. The leptin receptor. J Biol Chem 1997;272:6093–6096.
101. Vaisse C, et al. Leptin activation of Stat3 in the hypothalamus of wild-type and ob/ob mice but not db/db mice. Nat Genet 1996;14(1):95–97.
102. Cohen B, Novick D, Rubinstein M. Modulation of insulin activities by leptin. Science 1996;274(5290):1185–1188.
103. Ainscow EK, et al. Dynamic imaging of free cytosolic ATP concentration during fuel sensing by rat hypothalamic neurones: evidence for ATP-independent control of ATP-sensitive K(+) channels. J Physiol 2002;544:429–445.
104. Even P, Nicolaidis S. Spontaneous and 2DG-induced metabolic changes and feeding: The ischymetric hypothesis. Brain Res Bull 1985 ;15:429–435.
105. Nicolaidis S, Even P. Mesure du métabolisme de fond en relation avec la prise alimentaire: Hypothese iscymétrique. Comptes Rendus Academie de Sciences, Paris 1984;298:295–300.
106. Clegg DJ, et al. Comparison of central and peripheral administration of C75 on food intake, body weight, and conditioned taste aversion. Diabetes 2002;51(11):3196–3201.
107. Kumar MV, et al. Differential effects of a centrally acting fatty acid synthase inhibitor in lean and obese mice. Proc Natl Acad Sci USA 2002;99:1921–1925.
108. Loftus TM, et al. Reduced food intake and body weight in mice treated with fatty acid synthase inhibitors. Science 2000;288:2299–2300.
109. Obici S, et al. Inhibition of hypothalamic carnitine palmitoyltransferase-1 decreases food intake and glucose production. Nat Med 2003;9:756–761.
110. Wortman MD, et al. C75 inhibits food intake by increasing CNS glucose metabolism. Nat Med 2003;9:483–485.
111. Obici S, et al. Central administration of oleic acid inhibits glucose production and food intake. Diabetes 2002 ;51(2):271–275.
112. Nicolaidis S. Mecanisme nerveux de l'equilibre energetique. Journees Annuelles de Diabetologie de l'Hotel-Dieu 1978;1: 152–156.
113. Levin BE, Dunn-Meynell AA, Routh VH. Brain glucose sensing and body energy homeostasis: role in obesity and diabetes. Am J Physiol 1999;276:R1223–R1231.

114. Levin BE. Glucosensing neurons as integrators of metabolic signals. EWCBR 2002;22:67.
115. Clark JT, et al. Neuropeptide Y and human pancreatic polypeptide stimulate feeding behavior in rats. Endocrinology 1984;115(1):427–429.
116. Stanley BG, Leibowitz SF. Neuropeptide Y injected into the paraventricular hypothalamus: a powerful stimulant of feeding behavior. Proc Natl Acad Sci USA 1984;82:3940–3943.
117. Seeley RJ, Payne, CJ, Woods SC. Neuropeptide Y fails to increase intraoral intake in rats. Am J Physiol 1995;268:R423–R427.
118. Allen YS, et al. Neuropeptide Y distribution in the rat brain. Science 1983;221:877–879.
119. Minth CD, Andrews PC, Dixon JE. Characterization, sequence and expression of the cloned human neuropeptide Y gene. J Biol Chem 1986;261(26):11,975–11,979.
120. Mizuno TM, et al. Fasting regulates hypothalamic neuropeptide Y, agouti-related peptide, and proopiomelanocortin in diabetic mice independent of changes in leptin or insulin. Endocrinology 1999;140(10):4551–4557.
121. Sahu A, et al. Neuropeptide Y release from the parventricular nucleus increases in association with hyperphagia in streptozotocin-induced diabetic rats. Endocrinology 1992;131(6):2979–2985.
122. Marks JL, et al. Effect of fasting on regional levels of neuropeptide Y mRNA and insulin receptors in the rat hypothalamus: An autoradiographic study. Mol Cell Neurosci 1992;3:199–205.
123. Sahu A, et al. Neuropeptide Y concentration in microdissected hypothalamic regions and in vitro release from the medial basal hypothalamus-preoptic area of streptozotocin-diabetic rats with and without insulin substitution therapy. Endocrinology 1990;126:192–198.
124. Kalra SP, et al. Neuropeptide Y secretion increases in the paraventricular nucleus in association with increased appetite for food. Proc Natl Acad Sci USA 1991;88:10,931–10,935.
125. Sahu A, Kalra PS, Kalra SP. Food deprivation and ingestion induce reciprocal changes in neuropeptide Y concentrations in the paraventricular nucleus. Peptides 1988;9:83–86.
126. Stanley BG, et al. Neuropeptide Y chronically injected into the hypothalamus: A powerful neurochemical inducer of hyperphagia and obesity. Peptides 1986;7:1189–1192.
127. McMinn JE, et al. NPY-induced overfeeding suppresses hypothalamic NPY mRNA expression: potential roles of plasma insulin and leptin. Regulat Peptides 1998;75–76:425–431.
128. Sipols AJ, Baskin DG, Schwartz MW. Effect of intracerebroventricular insulin infusion on diabetic hyperphagia and hypothalamic neuropeptide gene expression. Diabetes 1995;44:147–151.
129. Sipols AJ, Baskin DG, Schwartz MW. The importance of central nervous system insulin deficiency to diabetic hyperphagia. Diabetes 1993;42(Suppl 1):152.
130. Stephens TW, et al. The role of neuropeptide Y in the antiobesity action of the obese gene product. Nature 1995;377:530–534.
131. Schwartz MW, et al. Specificity of leptin action on elevated blood glucose levels and hypothalamic neuropeptide Y gene expression in ob/ob mice. Diabetes 1996; 45:531–535.
132. Bernardis LL, Bellinger LL. The dorsomedial hypothalamic nucleus revisited: 1998 update. Proc Soc Exp Biol Med 1998;218(4):284–306.
133. Kesterson RA, et al. Induction of neuropeptide Y gene expression in the dorsal medial hypothalamic nucleus in two models of the agouti obesity syndrome. Mol Endocrinol 1997;11(5):630–637.
134. Guan XM, et al. Induction of neuropeptide Y expression in dorsomedial hypothalamus of diet-induced obese mice. Neuroreport 1998;9(15):3415–3419.
135. Bi S, Ladenheim EE, Moran TH. Elevated neuropeptide Y expression in the dorsomedial hypothalamic nucleus may contribute to the hyperphagia and obesity in OLETF rats with CCKA receptor deficit. Annual Meeting of the Society for Neuroscience, New Orleans, LA: 2000.
136. Erickson JC, Clegg KE, Palmiter RD. Sensitivity to leptin and susceptibility to seizures of mice lacking neuropeptide Y. Nature 1996;381:415–418.
137. Erickson JC, Hollopeter G, Palmiter RD. Attenuation of the obesity syndrome of ob/ob mice by the loss of neuropeptide Y. Science 1996;274(5293):1704–1707.
138. Hollopeter G, Erickson JC, Palmiter RD. Role of neuropeptide Y in diet-, chemical- and genetic-induced obesity of mice. Int J Obes Relat Metab Disord 1998;22(6):506–512.
139. Palmiter RD, et al. Life without neuropeptide Y. Recent Prog Horm Res 1998;53:163–199.
140. Woods SC, et al. NPY and food intake: Discrepancies in the model. Regul Peptides 1998;75–76:403–408.
141. Gropp E, et al. Agouti-related peptide-expressing neurons are mandatory for feeding. Nat Neurosci 2005;8(10):1289–1291.
142. Criscione L, et al. Food intake in free-feeding and energy-deprived lean rats is mediated by the neuropeptide Y5 receptor. J Clin Invest 1998;102(12):2136–2145.

143. Marsh DJ, et al. Role of the Y5 neuropeptide Y receptor in feeding and obesity (see comments). Nat Med 1998;4(6):718–721.
144. Kanatani A, et al, Role of the Y1 receptor in the regulation of neuropeptide Y-mediated feeding: comparison of wild-type, Y1 receptor-deficient, and Y5 receptor-deficient mice. Endocrinology 2000;141(3):1011–1016.
145. Tang-Christensen M, et al. Central administration of Y5 receptor antisense decreases spontaneous food intake and attenuates feeding in response to exogenous neuropeptide Y. J Endocrinol 1998;159(2):307–312.
146. Larsen PJ, et al. Activation of central neuropeptide Y Y1 receptors potently stimulates food intake in male rhesus monkeys [In Process Citation]. J Clin Endocrinol Metab 1999;84(10):3781–3791.
147. Hellig M, et al. In vivo downregulation of neuropeptide Y (NPY) Y1-receptors by i.c.v. antisense oligodeoxynucleotide administration is associated with signs of anxiety in rats. Soc Neurosci Abstr 1992;18:1539.
148. O'Shea D, et al. Neuropeptide Y induced feeding in the rat is mediated by a novel receptor. Endocrinology 1997;138(1):196–202.
149. Zimanyi IA, Fathi Z, Poindexter GS. Central control of feeding behavior by neuropeptide Y. Curr Pharm Des 1998;4(4):349–366.
150. Levens NR, Della-Zuana O. Neuropeptide Y Y5 receptor antagonists as anti-obesity drugs. Curr Opin Investig Drugs 2003;4(10):1198–1204.
151. Qu D, et al. A role for melanin-concentrating hormone in the central regulation of feeding behaviour. Nature 1996;380(6571):243–247.
152. Ludwig D, et al. Melanin-concentrating hormone: a functional melanocortin antagonist in the hypothalamus. Am J Physiol 1998;274(Apr):E627–E633.
153. Sanchez M, Baker B, Celis M. Melanin-concentrating hormone (MCH) antagonizes the effects of alpha-MSH and neuropeptide E-I on grooming and locomotor activities in the rat. Peptides 1997;18:393–396.
154. Clegg DJ, et al. Intraventricular melanin-concentrating hormone stimulates water intake independent of food intake. Am J Physiol Regul Integr Comp Physiol, 2003;284(2):R494–R499.
155. Rossi M, et al. Melanin-concentrating hormone acutely stimulates feeding, but chronic administration has no effect on body weight. Endocrinology 1997;138(1):351–355.
156. Shimada M, et al. Mice lacking melanin-concentrating hormone are hypophagic and lean. Nature 1998;396(Dec 17):670–674.
157. Mystkowski P, et al. Hypothalamic melanin-concentrating hormone and estrogen-induced weight loss [In Process Citation]. J Neurosci 2000;20(22):8637–8642.
158. Mashiko S, et al. Antiobesity effect of a melanin-concentrating hormone 1 receptor antagonist in diet-induced obese mice. Endocrinology 2005;146(7):3080–3086.
159. Takekawa S, et al. T-226296: a novel, orally active and selective melanin-concentrating hormone receptor antagonist. Eur J Pharmacol 2002;438(3):129–135.
160. Kowalski TJ, McBriar MD. Therapeutic potential of melanin-concentrating hormone-1 receptor antagonists for the treatment of obesity. Expert Opin Investig Drugs 2004;13(9):1113–1122.
161. de Lecea L, et al. The hypocretins: hypothalamus-specific peptides with neuroexcitatory activity. Proc Natl Acad Sci USA 1998;95:322–327.
162. Sakurai T, et al. Orexins and orexin receptors: a family of hypothalamic neuropeptides and G protein-coupled receptors that regulate feeding behavior. Cell 1998;92(4):573–585.
163. Broberger C, et al. Hypocretin/orexin- and melanin-concentrating hormone-expressing cells form distinct populations in the rodent lateral hypothalamus: relationship to the neuropeptide Y and agouti gene-related protein systems. J Comp Neurol 1998;402:460–474.
164. Yamanaka A, et al. Orexin-induced food intake involves neuropeptide Y pathway. Brain Res 2000;859(2):404–409.
165. Rauch M, et al. Orexin A activates leptin-responsive neurons in the arcuate nucleus [In Process Citation]. Pflugers Arch 2000;440(5):699–703.
166. Peyron C, et al. Neurons containing hypocretin (orexin) project to multiple neuronal systems. J Neurosci 1998;18:9996–10,015.
167. Kilduff TS, Peyron C. The hypocretin/orexin ligand-receptor system: implications for sleep and sleep disorders. Trends Neurosci 2000;23(8):359–365.
168. Elias CF, et al. Chemically defined projections linking the mediobasal hypothalamus and the lateral hypothalamic area. J Comp Neurol 1998;402(4):442–459.

169. Tritos NA, et al. Functional interactions between melanin-concentrating hormone, neuropeptide Y, and anorectic neuropeptides in the rat hypothalamus. Diabetes 1998;47:1687–1692.

170. Jain MR, et al. Evidence that NPY Y1 receptors are involved in stimulation of feeding by orexins (hypocretins) in sated rats. Regul Peptides 2000;87(1–3):19–24.

171. Sergeyev V, et al. Effect of 2-mercaptoacetate and 2-deoxy-D-glucose administration on the expression of NPY, AGRP, POMC, MCH and hypocretin/orexin in the rat hypothalamus. Neuroreport 2000;11(1):117–121.

172. Kojima M, et al. Ghrelin is a growth-hormone-releasing acylated peptide from stomach. Nature 1999;402(6762):656–660.

173. Kojima M, Hosoda H, Kangawa K. Purification and distribution of ghrelin: the natural endogenous ligand for the growth hormone secretagogue receptor. Horm Res 2001;56(Suppl 1):93–97.

174. Tschöp M, Smiley DL, Heiman ML. Ghrelin induces adiposity in rodents. Nature 2000;407(6806): 908–913.

175. Kamegai J, et al. Central effect of ghrelin, an endogenous growth hormone secretagogue, on hypothalamic peptide gene expression. Endocrinology 2000;141(12):4797–4800.

176. Wren AM, et al. Ghrelin enhances appetite and increases food intake in humans. J Clin Endocrinol Metab 2001;86(12):5992.

177. Horvath TL, et al. Minireview: ghrelin and the regulation of energy balance—a hypothalamic perspective. Endocrinology 2001;142(10):4163–4169.

178. Asakawa A, et al. Ghrelin is an appetite-stimulatory signal from stomach with structural resemblance to motilin. Gastroenterology 2001;120(2):337–345.

179. Kamegai J, et al. Chronic central infusion of ghrelin increases hypothalamic neuropeptide Y and Agouti-related protein mRNA levels and body weight in rats. Diabetes 2001;50(11):2438–2443.

180. Nakazato M, et al. A role for ghrelin in the central regulation of feeding. Nature 2001;409(6817):194–198.

181. Wang L, Saint-Pierre DH, Tache Y. Peripheral ghrelin selectively increases Fos expression in neuropeptide Y-synthesizing neurons in mouse hypothalamic arcuate nucleus. Neurosci Lett 2002;325(1):47–51.

182. Tschöp M, et al. Circulating ghrelin levels are decreased in human obesity. Diabetes 2001;50(4):707–709.

183. Cummings DE, et al. Plasma ghrelin levels after diet-induced weight loss or gastric bypass surgery. N Engl J Med 2002;346(21):1623–1630.

184. Horvath TL, Diano S, Tschop M. Ghrelin in hypothalamic regulation of energy balance. Curr Top Med Chem 2003;3(8):921–927.

185. Asakawa A, et al. Antagonism of ghrelin receptor reduces food intake and body weight gain in mice. Gut 2003;52(7):947–952.

186. Beck B, Richy S, Stricker-Krongrad A. Feeding response to ghrelin agonist and antagonist in lean and obese Zucker rats. Life Sci 2004;76(4):473–478.

187. Bernstein IL, Lotter EC, Kulkosky PJ. Effect of force-feeding upon basal insulin levels in rats. Proc Soc Exp Biol Med 1975;150:546–548.

188. Seeley RJ, et al. Behavioral, endocrine and hypothalamic responses to involuntary overfeeding. Am J Physiol 1996;271:R819–R823.

189. Elias CF, et al. Leptin activates hypothalamic CART neurons projecting to the spinal cord. Neuron 1998;21:1375–1385.

190. Kristensen P, et al. Hypothalamic CART is a new anorectic peptide regulated by leptin. Nature 1998;393:72–76.

191. Lambert PD, et al. CART peptides in the central control of feeding and interactions with neuropeptide Y. Synapse 1998;29:293–298.

192. Vrang N, et al. Recombinant CART peptide induces c-Fos expression in central areas involved in control of feeding behaviour. Brain Res 1999;818:499–509.

193. Kask A, et al. Anorexigenic cocaine- and amphetamine-regulated transcript peptide intensifies fear reactions in rats. Brain Res 2000;857(1–2):283–285.

194. Abbott CR, et al. Evidence of an orexigenic role for cocaine- and amphetamine-regulated transcript after administration into discrete hypothalamic nuclei. Endocrinology 2001;142(8):3457–3463.

195. Krahn DD, Gosnell BA. Behavioral effects of corticotropin-releasing factor: localization and characterization of central effects. Brain Res 1988;443:63–69.

196. Arase K, et al. Effects of corticotropin releasing factor on food intake and brown adipose tissue thermogenesis in rats. Am J Physiol 1988;255:E255–E259.

197. Heinrichs S, et al. Corticotropin-releasing factor-binding protein ligand inhibitor blunts excessive weight gain in genetically obese Zucker rats and rats during nicotine withdrawal. Proc Natl Acad Sci USA 1996;93(Dec 24):15,475–15480.

198. Spina M, et al. Appetite-suppressing effects of urocortin, a CRF-related neuropeptide. Science 1996;273(Sep 13):1561–1564.

199. Vaughan J, et al. Urocortin, a mammalian neuropeptide related to fish urotensin I and to corticotropin-releasing factor (see comments). Nature 1995;378(Nov 16):287–292.

200. Richard D, Huang Q, Timofeeva E. The corticotropin-releasing hormone system in the regulation of energy balance in obesity. Int J Obes Relat Metab Disord 2000;24(Suppl 2):S36–S39.

201. Heinrichs SC, Richard D. The role of corticotropin-releasing factor and urocortin in the modulation of ingestive behavior. Neuropeptides 1999;33(5):350–359.

202. D'Alessio DA, et al. Elimination of the action of glucagon-like peptide 1 causes an impairment of glucose tolerance after nutrient ingestion by healthy baboons. J Clin Invest 1996;97(1):133–138.

203. Drucker DJ, et al. Biologic properties and therapeutic potential of glucagon-like peptide-2. JPEN J Parenter Enteral Nutr 1999;23(5 Suppl):S98–S100.

204. Drucker DJ, Glucagon-like peptides. Diabetes 1998;47(2):159–169.

205. van Dijk G, Thiele TE. Glucagon-like peptide-1 (7-36) amide: a central regulator of satiety and interoceptive stress. Neuropeptides 1999;33(5):406–414.

206. Goldstone AP, et al. Effect of leptin on hypothalamic GLP-1 peptide and brain-stem pre-proglucagon mRNA. Biochem Biophys Res Commun 2000;269(2):331–335.

207. Elmquist JK, et al. Leptin activates neurons in ventrobasal hypothalamus and brainstem. Endocrinology 1997;138:839–842.

208. Turton MD, et al. A role for glucagon-like peptide-1 in the central regulation of feeding (see comments). Nature 1996;379(6560):69–72.

209. Tang-Christensen M, et al. Central administration of GLP-1-(7-36) amide inhibits food and water intake in rats. Am J Physiol 1996;271(4 Pt 2):R848–R856.

210. Van Dijk G, et al. Central infusions of leptin and GLP-1-(7-36) amide differentially stimulate c-FLI in the rat brain. Am J Physiol 1996;271(4 Pt 2):R1096–R1100.

211. Thiele TE, et al. Central infusion of GLP-1, but not leptin, produces conditioned taste aversions in rats. Am J Physiol 1997;272(2 Pt 2):R726–R730.

212. Thiele TE, et al. Central infusion of glucagon-like peptide-1-(7-36) amide (GLP-1) receptor antagonist attenuates lithium chloride-induced c-Fos induction in rat brainstem. Brain Res 1998;801(1–2):164–170.

213. Seeley RJ, et al. The role of CNS GLP-1-(7-36) amide receptors in mediating the visceral illness effects of lithium chloride. J Neurosci 2000;20:1616–1621.

214. Tang-Christensen M, et al. The proglucagon-derived peptide, glucagon-like peptide-2, is a neurotransmitter involved in the regulation of food intake. Nat Med 2000;6(7):802–807.

215. Halford JC, et al. Serotonin (5-HT) drugs: effects on appetite expression and use for the treatment of obesity. Curr Drug Targets 2005;6(2):201–213.

216. Lawton CL, Blundell JE. The effect of d-fenfluramine on intake of carbohydrate supplements is influenced by the hydration of the test diets. Behav Pharmacol 1992;3(5):517–523.

217. Leibowitz SF, Alexander JT. Hypothalamic serotonin in control of eating behavior, meal size, and body weight. Biol Psychiatry 1998;44(9):851–864.

218. Pierce PA, et al. 5-Hydroxytryptamine receptor subtype messenger RNAs in human dorsal root ganglia: a polymerase chain reaction study. Neuroscience 1997;81(3):813–819.

219. Miller KJ, Serotonin 5-ht2c receptor agonists: potential for the treatment of obesity. Mol Interv 2005;5(5):282–291.

220. Nonogaki K, et al. Leptin-independent hyperphagia and type 2 diabetes in mice with a mutated serotonin 5-HT2C receptor gene. Nat Med 1998;4(10):1152–1156.

221. Heisler LK, et al. Activation of central melanocortin pathways by fenfluramine. Science 2002;297(5581):609–611.

222. Ettinger MP, et al. Recombinant variant of ciliary neurotrophic factor for weight loss in obese adults: a randomized, dose-ranging study. JAMA 2003;289(14):1826–1832.

223. Anderson KD, et al. Activation of the hypothalamic arcuate nucleus predicts the anorectic actions of ciliary neurotrophic factor and leptin in intact and gold thioglucose-lesioned mice. J Neuroendocrinol 2003;15(7):649–660.

224. Kelly JF, et al. Ciliary neurotrophic factor and leptin induce distinct patterns of immediate early gene expression in the brain. Diabetes 2004;53(4):911–920.

225. Kokoeva MV, Yin H, Flier JS. Neurogenesis in the hypothalamus of adult mice: potential role in energy balance. Science 2005;310(5748):679–683.

226. Pu S, et al. Neuropeptide Y counteracts the anorectic and weight reducing effects of ciliary neuro-tropic factor. J Neuroendocrinol 2000;12(9):827–832.

227. Cone RD, Anatomy and regulation of the central melanocortin system. Nat Neurosci 2005;8(5):571–578.

228. Yen T, et al. Obesity, diabetes, and neoplasia in yellow A(vy)/- mice: ectopic expression of the agouti gene. FASEB J 1994;8(May):479–488.

229. Zimanyi IA, Pelleymounter MA. The role of melanocortin peptides and receptors in regulation of energy balance. Curr Pharm Des 2003;9(8):627–641.

230. Stutz AM, Morrison CD, Argyropoulos G. The agouti-related protein and its role in energy homeo-stasis. Peptides 2005;26(10):1771–1781.

231. Yaswen L, et al. Obesity in the mouse model of pro-opiomelanocortin deficiency responds to periph-eral melanocortin. Nat Med 1999;5(9):1066–1070.

232. Krude H, et al. Severe early-onset obesity, adrenal insufficiency and red hair pigmentation caused by POMC mutations in humans. Nat Genet 1998;19(2):155–157.

233. Huszar D, et al. Targeted disruption of the melanocortin-4 receptor results in obesity in mice. Cell 1997;88(1):131–141.

234. Ollmann MM, et al. Antagonism of central melanocortin receptors in vitro and in vivo by agouti-related protein. Science 1997;278(5335):135–138.

235. Cone RD, et al. The melanocortin receptors: agonists, antagonists, and the hormonal control of pigmentation. Rec Prog Hormone Res 1996;51:287–320.

236. Seeley RJ, Drazen DL, Clegg DJ. The critical role of the melanocortin system in the control of energy balance. Annu Rev Nutr 2004;24:133–149.

237. Boyce RS, Duhl DM. Melanocortin-4 receptor agonists for the treatment of obesity. Curr Opin Investig Drugs 2004;5(10):1063–1071.

238. Bluher S, et al. Ciliary neurotrophic factorAx15 alters energy homeostasis, decreases body weight, and improves metabolic control in diet-induced obese and UCP1-DTA mice. Diabetes 2004; 53(11):2787–2796.

239. Dorr RT, et al. Evaluation of melanotan-II, a superpotent cyclic melanotropic peptide in a pilot phase-I clinical study. Life Sci 1996;58(20):1777–1784.

240. Reizes O, et al. Transgenic expression of syndecan-1 uncovers a physiological control of feeding behavior by syndecan-3. Cell 2001;106(1):105–116.

241. Strader AD, et al.,Mice lacking the syndecan-3 gene are resistant to dietary-induced obesity. J Clin Invest 2004;114:1354–1360.

242. Park PW, Reizes O, Bernfield M. Cell surface heparan sulfate proteoglycans: selective regulators of ligand-receptor encounters. J Biol Chem 2000;275(39):29,923–29,926.

243. Bernfield M, et al. Functions of cell surface heparan sulfate proteoglycans. Annu Rev Biochem 1999;68:729–777.

244. Reizes O, et al. Syndecan-3 modulates food intake by interacting with the melanocortin/AgRP path-way. Ann NY Acad Sci 2003;994:66–73.

245. Pinto S, et al. Rapid rewiring of arcuate nucleus feeding circuits by leptin. Science 2004;304(5667): 110–115.

246. Bouret SG, Draper SJ, Simerly RB. Trophic action of leptin on hypothalamic neurons that regulate feeding. Science 2004;304(5667):108–110.

247. Kaksonen M, et al. Syndecan-3-deficient mice exhibit enhanced LTP and impaired hippocampus-dependent memory. Mol Cell Neurosci 2002;21(1):158–172.

2

Gut Peptides

*Vian Amber, MBChB, MSc, PhD, MRCPath,
and Stephen R. Bloom, MBChB, MA, FRCP,
FRCPath, DSc, MD*

Contents

INTRODUCTION
HYPOTHALAMIC CIRCUITRY
ANOREXIGENIC GUT PEPTIDES
OREXIGENIC GUT PEPTIDES
GUT HORMONE SYNERGISM AND/OR ANTAGONISM
CONCLUSION
REFERENCES

Summary

Obesity occurs as a result of excessive energy intake and /or reduced energy expenditure. The hypothalamus is the principal region in the central nervous system that regulates appetite and energy homeostasis by incorporating neural and hormonal signals from the periphery. A large number of such hormones (gut peptides) are synthesized and secreted by cells in the gastrointestinal tract in addition to its function as a digestive system. Increasing evidence supports the role of gut peptides as short-term satiety signals regulating appetite and food intake. The anorexigenic gut peptides include PYY, PP, oxyntomodulin (OXM), GLP-1, and CCK. They are secreted mainly from the intestine, inhibit appetite, and promote satiety, whereas ghrelin, the only orexigenic peptide produced by the stomach, increases food intake. In this chapter we discuss the pathophysiology of gut peptides in health and disease.

Key Words: Gut peptides; polypeptide YY (PYY); oxyntomodulin; glucagon-like protein (GLP)-1; ghrelin; obesity; neuropeptide Y (NPY); pro-opiomelanocortin (POMC).

INTRODUCTION

The main function of the gut is digestion and absorption of food through mechanical and enzymatic processes. However, the gastrointestinal (GI) system produces and secretes gut peptides by nerve and gland cells in the mucosa. These exert diverse physiologic functions including gut motility, acid secretion, appetite control, and regulation of food intake. The latter is accomplished in consortium with neuronal signals and psychological and habitual behavior, which may result in a considerable variation in

From: *Contemporary Endocrinology: Treatment of the Obese Patient*
Edited by: R. F. Kushner and D. H. Bessesen © Humana Press Inc., Totowa, NJ

energy intake and energy expenditure on a day-to-day basis. However, for body weight to remain constant in the long term, there should be a tight control between energy intake and energy expenditure. An imbalance in energy homeostasis would thus result in either excessive fat storage and obesity or weight loss and cachexia.

The hypothalamus is the principal region in the central nervous system that regulates energy intake and energy expenditure. It contains several nuclei that elicit multiple activities, including appetite control, when stimulated or inhibited. Integrated complex neural and hormonal signals are communicated to the appetite centers in the hypothalamus from a peripheral satiety system that includes the gut and adipose tissue. The neuroregulation of appetite is discussed in detail in Chapter 1. In this chapter we concentrate on the role of gut peptides as short term regulators of appetite. The long-term signals from adipose tissue that encode energy stores are discussed in Chapters 4 and 5.

Gut peptides act in a paracrine fashion, via the circulation, and/or act directly on the CNS. They also act as a gut nutriment sensor by signaling the appetite centers in the brain via the vagal or sympathetic afferents. In addition, many of the gut peptides and their receptors are also produced locally as neurotransmitters in the CNS regulating food intake.

Several gut hormones produced by the intestine and pancreas have been shown to inhibit food intake (anorexigenic) (Table 1). These include peptide YY3-36 (PYY3-36), pancreatic polypeptide (PP), cholecystokinin (CCK), oxyntomodulin (OXM), and glucagon-like peptide (GLP)-1, whereas ghrelin, produced in the stomach, is the only gut peptide known to stimulate feeding (orexigenic). In the past decade, numerous studies have made great advances in our understanding of the important sensing and signaling roles of gut peptides in the regulation of food intake and energy homeostasis.

This chapter discusses the pathophysiological roles of orexigenic and anorexigenic gut peptides in the regulation of food intake.

HYPOTHALAMIC CIRCUITRY

Central Pathways

In addition to neuroregulation, discussed in the previous chapter, the hypothalamus integrates chemical and humoral signals from the gut, and hormonal signals from the periphery (adipose tissue), for the regulation of appetite and energy homeostasis. It contains several nuclei—the lateral nuclei, ventromedial nucleus (VMN), dorsomedial nucleus (DMN), paraventricular nucleus (PVN), perifornical, and arcuate nuclei—and anatomically, it is in close proximity to the brain stem, amygdala, and higher brain centers that are involved in appetite control. Despite its small size—only 1% of the brain mass—it plays a major role in bridging peripheral signals with central pathways that control the vegetative and (neuro)endocrine functions of the body.

The arcuate nucleus (ARC), positioned at the base of the hypothalamus with an "incomplete" blood–brain barrier, is subjected to direct exposure to factors in the general circulation such as gut peptides. It contains two subsets of neurons: a stimulatory neuron (orexigenic) containing neuropeptide Y (NPY) and agouti-related peptide (AgRP), and an inhibitory neuron (anorexigenic) containing pro-opiomelanocortin (POMC) (Fig. 1). The latter is a precursor of α-melanocyte-stimulating hormone (α-MSH), and cocaine- and amphetamine-regulated transcript (CART). The α-MSH produces its anorexigenic effects mainly via melanocortin receptors (MCRs). Of the five identified MCRs, MC3R

Table 1
Anorexigenic and Orexigenic Gut Hormones

Peptide	Sites of synthesis	Stimulus	Actions	Mediation of action	Molecular forms
Anorexigenic					
OXM	L-cells of distal ileum and colon Pancreas CNS	Meal Calorie content Fat	Inhibits food intake Inhibits gastric acid secretion Inhibits gastric motility Reduces pancreatic enzyme secretion	GLP-1 receptor Glucagon receptor Suppression of ghrelin	—
GLP-1	L-cells of distal small ileum, colon Pancreas CNS	Meal	Incretin effect on insulin secretion Suppresses glucagon release Promotes pancreatic β-cell growth Inhibits food intake Delays gastric emptying Inhibits gastric secretion Inhibits lipase secretion	GLP-1 receptor	GLP-17-36 GLP 17-37
PYY3-36	L-cells of distal ileum, colon, rectum CNS	Meal Fat and protein Calorie content CCK, gastric acid, bile acid, bombesin, IGF-1	Inhibits food intake Reduces gastric motility Inhibits gallbladder secretion Inhibits pancreatic secretion	Y2 receptor Inhibits NPY	PYY 1-36 PYY 3-36
PP	PP-cells in islets of Langerhans CNS		Inhibits pancreatic enzyme secretion Inhibits food intake Gallbladder relaxation	Y4 receptors	—
CCK	I-cells of duodenum, jejunum CNS Enteric nerve ending	Food ingestion, protein, fat	Stimulates pancreatic exocrine secretion Stimulates gallbladder contraction Delays gastric emptying Inhibits gastric acid secretion Reduces food intake Increases satiety Stimulates bowel motility	CCK A CCK B	Multiple Intestinal CCK-33, CCK-8
Orexigenic					
Ghrelin	Stomach, small bowel, colon Hypothalamus	Fasting	Promotes GH release Increases food intake Promotes gastric motility Promotes PP release	GHS receptor	—

CCK, cholecystokinin; CNS, central nervous system; GHS, growth hormone secretagogue; GLP-1 glucagon-like peptides-1; PP, pancreatic polypeptide; PYY, peptide YY.

29

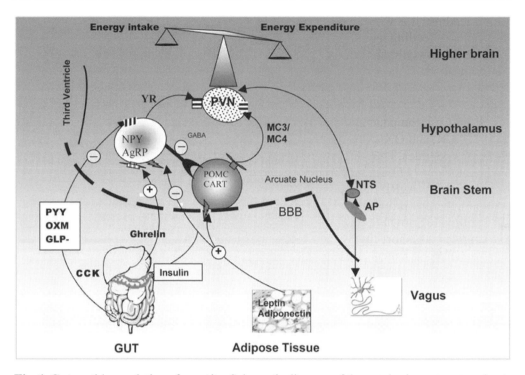

Fig. 1. Gut peptide regulation of appetite. Schematic diagram of the gut–brain, gut–gut, and gut–adipose tissue interactions. MC3/MC4 R, melanocortin 3 and 4 receptors; YR, Y receptors; NPY/AgRP, neuropeptide Y and agouti-related peptide neurons in the arcuate nucleus in the hypothalamus; POMC/CART, pro-opiomelanocortin and cocaine–amphetamine-regulated peptide; PVN, paraventricular nucleus; NTS, nucleus tractus solitarius; AP, area postrema; BBB, blood–brain barrier.

and MC4R, present in high density in the PVN, have been shown to be important in the regulation of food intake *(1)*. α-MSH is a natural endogenous agonist, whereas AgRP is an endogenous antagonist of the MC3/MC4 receptors *(2)*. Disruption of the MCR pathway has been shown to be associated with extreme obesity *(4)*. In fact, transgenic animals lacking the POMC gene, having MC4R mutations, or overexpressing AgRP have been shown to be hyperphagic and obese *(3,4)*. In humans, MC4 receptor mutations have been shown to be the most common known cause of single gene (monogenic) obesity *(5,6)*. On the other hand, NPY, with a shorter half-life compared with AgRP, is proposed to exert its effect via Y receptors. Six subtypes of these have been described (Y1–Y6) (Table 2) *(7–10)*. NPY has a higher affinity to Y1 and Y5 receptors. These are available in high abundance in the nucleus tractus solitarius (NTS), from which NPY neurons project to the PVN.

Neuron projections from the arcuate nucleus extend to the PVN and DMN (Fig. 1). Activated neuronal pathways in the PVN signal the NTS, which also integrates signals from the sympathetic and vagal afferent fibers. The PVN also coordinates input from melanin-concentrating hormone (MCH)-producing neurons in the lateral hypothalamus and other brain areas, such as the area postrema, brainstem, and amygdala, that have impact on food intake. The latter has some areas that increase feeding and other areas that inhibit feeding. It is worth noting that areas in the brainstem and amygdala control the mechanics of feeding including salivation, taste, chewing, and swallowing. Destruction of these areas would thus cause the animal to lose its recognition for the type and/or quality of food.

Peripheral Signals

Insulin from the pancreas, leptin from adipose tissue, and gut peptides (PYY3-36, GLP-1, CCK, and OXM) from the gastrointestinal tract (GIT) are known anorexigenic hormones/peptides. They directly inhibit NPY/AgRP and stimulate POMC/CART in the arcuate nucleus (11). Reciprocal to this is the orexigenic gut peptide ghrelin. Ghrelin stimulates NPY/AgRP and inhibits POMC/CART (discussed in "Ghrelin Mechanism of Action"), thereby promoting meal initiation and increasing food intake. Whereas leptin and insulin are known to be long-term regulators of adiposity and energy expenditure, gut peptides are short-lived signals controlling food intake. They are sensed by the hypothalamus on a meal-to-meal and/or day-to-day basis along with other neural, mechanical, and nutrient gut sensing signals. Here we discuss the anorexigenic and orexigenic gut peptides.

ANOREXIGENIC GUT PEPTIDES

PP Fold Family of Peptides

The PP fold family of peptides include peptide YY (PYY) and PP from the gut and NPY from the central nervous system. These peptides are structurally similar. They are all small (36 amino acid) peptides containing several tyrosine residues. They are characterized by a specific tertiary structure known as the PP fold, and they become biologically active following COOH-terminal amidation. The PP fold tertiary structure consists of a characteristic u-shape double helix: one α and one polyproline, connected by a β-turn unit. The PP fold peptides appear to exert their effects through the Y receptors (Y1–Y6), which are classified according to their affinity to PYY, PP, and NPY fragments and analogs (7) (Table 2). Although they are all seven-domain transmembrane receptors that inhibit adenylate cyclase by coupling to G-proteins, the Y1 receptor also increases intracellular calcium and the Y2 receptor regulates calcium and potassium channels. Y1 through Y5 are present centrally in the brain, and peripherally in the intestine, pancreas, heart, muscle, and blood vessels. However, the Y6 receptors are found mainly in the periphery (intestine, muscle, heart, and spleen) and are nonfunctional in man. They have diverse functions including stimulation/suppression of appetite, reduction of intestinal secretion, vasoconstriction, and analgesia. Table 1 summarizes the distribution and functions of these receptors.

PYY

PYY, a gut-derived peptide, was first isolated from porcine intestine (12). Although it is virtually absent in the stomach, it is widely expressed in the intestine. It is produced by the L-cells throughout the intestine, but predominantly in the ileum and colon, with the highest levels being produced in the rectum (13,14). PYY is colocalized with GLP-I and has a 42% and 70% amino acid homology with PP and NPY, respectively. There is evidence that PYY is also produced by the pancreas (though not in humans), adrenal medulla, and the CNS (hypothalamus, medulla, pons, and spinal cord) (14).

Table 2
Affinity, Distribution, and Actions of the Known Y Receptor Superfamily

Receptor	High-affinity peptide	Low-affinity peptide	Distribution actions	Proposed
Y1	NPY, PYY	PP	Cortex DRG Amygdala Hypothalamus Blood vessels	Analgesia Anxiolysis ↑ Appetite Vasoconstriction
Y2 (Presynaptic)	NPY, PYY, PYY (3-36)	PP	Hypothalamus DRG Hippocampus Intestine	Anorexia Analgesia ↑ Memory ↓ Secretion
Y4	PP, NPY (2-36), NPY (3-36), PYY, NPY/PYY	NPY/PYY fragments PYY (3-36)	Hypothalamus Amygdala Thalamus Intestine, pancreas, heart, muscle	↑Appetite
Y5	NPY, PYY, NPY (2-36), NPY (3-36), PYY (3-36), NPY/PYY	NPY/PYY fragments	Hypothalamus Thalamus NTS	↑ Appetite ↑ ACTH
Y6 (mouse)	PP, NPY/PYY	C-terminal NPY fragments	Intestine Spleen	
Y6	A truncated non-functional receptor in man produced by deletion in sixth TM domain			Heart, muscle, intestine, spleen

DRG- dorsal root ganglion; NTS, nucleus tractus solitarius

PYY is released into the circulation 15 min following food ingestion. Once in circulation, the native form PYY1-36 undergoes N-terminal, Tyr-pro, truncation by the action of dipeptidyl peptidase IV (DPPIV) to produce the 34-amino-acid form, PYY3-36 (15). This is the active circulating form of PYY, which has been shown to cross the incomplete blood–brain barrier around the base of the hypothalamus by nonsaturable mechanisms. Postprandial plasma levels of PYY3-36 plateau after 1 to 2 h, but remain elevated for up to 6 h.

PYY3-36 is released into the circulation in proportion to the number of calories ingested (16) but not to gastric distension. Meal composition has also been shown to affect PYY release. Higher plasma levels of PYY are achieved after isocaloric meals of fat compared with those of proteins and carbohydrates (17,18). A number of other factors have been shown to stimulate PYY release, including CCK, gastric acid, bile acid infusion to ileum and colon, insulin-like growth factor (IGF)-1, bombesin, and calcitonin gene-related peptide. Neural signals—for example, vagal stimuli—have also been implicated (19,20). Evidence to support the latter is the increase in PYY levels in response to the presence of food in the duodenum, before its arrival to the L-cells in the ileum. In contrast, release of the peptide is inhibited during fasting (9,21), and by GLP-1 (22).

PYY Actions. PYY has numerous actions on the gut. It delays gastric emptying and gastric and pancreatic secretions, and increases the absorption of fluid and electrolytes in the ileum after a meal. PYY also inhibits food intake. This has been discovered recently. The peripheral administration of PYY, first reported to reduce appetite in 1993, has gained further support from subsequent animal and human studies. Indeed, in the past decade, a number of studies have demonstrated the anorexigenic effects of PYY3-36. In mice, administration of PYY3-36, peripherally *(8,23–25)*, and centrally, by direct injection to the arcuate nucleus *(8)*, was shown to acutely reduce food intake. This reduction in food intake was shown to continue on chronic peripheral administration of the peptide, resulting in reduced weight gain *(8)*.

In contrast, PYY administration to the third, lateral, or fourth cerebral ventricles potently stimulates food intake in rodents. These findings may indicate, on the one hand, that PYY might exert its effects through multiple complex pathways resulting in variable effects, depending on its location being central or peripheral. On the other hand, it might indicate that perhaps the PYY molecule undergoes configurational changes during its passage through the blood–brain barrier, resulting in alteration in its effect.

Mechanism of Action. PYY has been shown to exert its effects primarily through binding to the Y receptors. Though it has some affinity to Y1 and Y5 receptors, it particularly binds with higher affinity to the Y2 receptors *(9,26)*. The anorexigenic effect of PYY3-36 is absent in Y2 receptor knockout mice *(8,27)* and was shown to be completely blocked by a Y2 receptor antagonist *(26,28)*. Peripheral administration of PYY 3-36 has been shown to cause c-fos activation, a marker of neuronal activation, and expression in the arcuate nucleus *(8)*. Involvement of the melanocortin system has been proposed to explain this effect of PYY via the Y2 receptors. Y2 is a presynaptic inhibitory receptor of the orexigenic NPY neurons and mRNA expression/release in the arcuate nucleus. NPY neurons inhibit POMC neurons via GABA mediation. Therefore, inhibition of the NPY neurons results in a reciprocal activation of POMC neurons. Inhibition of NPY and activation of POMC induces appetite suppression *(29)*. However, this cannot fully explain PYY3-36's mechanism of action. The anorectic effects of peripheral PYY3-36 were retained in POMC knockout mice doubting the necessity of melanocortin peptides for the action of PYY3-36. In support of this, MC4R knockout and agouti mice are shown to be sensitive to the anorectic effects of peripherally administered PYY3-36 *(24)*. These findings support the notion that PYY may exert its effect through multiple pathways. Therefore, it is tempting to propose that although the Y1 and Y5 receptors have lower affinities for PYY, they might override the actions of Y2 receptors when they are exposed directly to increasing amounts of PYY. This might be the reason for the contrasting actions of PYY when injected to different parts of the brain. The reduction in the orexigenic effects of centrally administered PYY in both Y1 and Y5 receptor knockout mice *(30)* further supports this. In addition, the area postrema appears to be yet another mechanism through which PYY3-36 exerts its effect. For example, in rats, ablation of the area postrema results in an increase in the acute anorectic effects of PYY3-36 *(31)*.

PYY3-36 has also been shown to inhibit food intake in man. A single infusion of PYY3-36 caused a 30% and 31% reduction in food intake in a free-choice meal 2 h postinfusion *(8,21)* in both obese and lean individuals. Subjective hunger feeling was also reduced with the reduction in calorie intake without changes in gastric emptying *(21)*. The appetite reducing effect of PYY3-36 persisted for 24 h in both lean and obese subjects, despite PYY3-36 levels retuning to basal levels, which implies that PYY3-36 may be an important physiological postprandial satiety signal. This supports the findings in the animal studies and suggests that, unlike leptin, PYY resistance *(17,32)* seems unlikely. Therefore, much interest has been put into PYY3-36's role in the pathogenesis of obesity and its possible future therapeutic role as an antiobesity treatment *(17)*. The effects of PYY3-36 have been the subject of immense scrutiny and controversy *(33–35)*, however, with some laboratories claiming inability to reproduce the experiments in the animal studies. Interestingly and more recently, the acute inhibitory effect of PYY3-36 on food intake was confirmed by other studies in rodents *(23,31)* and primates *(36)*. Halatchev et al. confirmed that intraperitoneal (IP) administration of PYY3-36 inhibits food intake in a dose-dependent manner in rodents in both dark-phase food intake and following a fast *(24)*. In addition, the cumulative effect of chronic injection of PYY on food intake and weight reductions was also reproduced *(37)*. Several factors are likely to contribute to this controversy and the outcome of these delicate behavioral studies. These include different methodologies and protocols, different strains of animals, variable immunoassay methods of PYY measurements, poor handling techniques, and stress conditions under which the experiments are conducted. In fact, the stress caused by handling and IP injections has been shown to cause a 32% reduction in food intake in nonacclimatized mice compared with acclimatized mice *(38)*. Acute stress is also known to increase NPY neuron expression, which is likely to override the anorectic effects of PYY3-36.

Insulin sensitivity has also been shown to be improved by PYY3-36. In animal models of diabetes, long-term peripheral administration of PYY 3-36 has been shown to improve glycemic control *(37)* as a consequence to reduced food intake, body weight, and visceral fat.

Although all the above support a possible therapeutic role of PYY in obesity, in practice this is still not established based on the current knowledge on the identified molecular configuration of the peptide thus far.

PYY Levels in Normal Physiology and Disease. PYY3-36 is inversely related to body mass index (BMI). Obese patients have relatively lower basal levels of PYY3-36 compared with lean subjects. Even though attenuated, the postprandial response of PYY3-36 in these patients is still present *(9,21)*. However, fasting levels are not elevated in morbidly obese patients, suggesting that the latter is a specific metabolic state *(33)*. PYY levels are subject to diurnal variation. It has been shown to be higher during night sleep (in nonshift workers), which may explain why we do not feel hungry during sleep. Interestingly, levels have been shown to be higher in lean subjects as compared with obese ones during sleeping hours. This may partly contribute to the latter's diverse eating habits.

On the other hand, higher PYY concentrations were shown in the cerebrospinal fluid (CSF) of patients with eating disorders such as bulimia nervosa and binge-eating disorders *(39)*. However, the occurrence of low levels of PYY in patients with anorexia nervosa might fall into a different complex psychological entity.

PYY3-36 appears to increase in a number of gastrointestinal conditions and following abdominal surgery *(40–42)*. These conditions are usually associated with wasting status and reduced body weight, which further supports PYY's role as an anorexigenic peptide and a satiety agent. Higher levels of PYY have also been demonstrated in diseases such as malabsorption syndromes including tropical sprue, chronic pancreatitis, and celiac disease *(43)*, following small-intestinal surgery, and with acute gut infection and inflammatory bowel disease *(44)*. In these conditions elevated levels of PYY 3-36 have been suggested to contribute to the recovery of the disease process. PYY is known to reduce gastric motility, secretion and gallbladder contractility, and bile acid secretion. This delays gastric emptying and subsequently the passage of nutrients to the diseased intestine thereby promoting a natural rest to the gut. This will also allow the gut's adaptation to the new condition *(33,40)*. Levels are also elevated in other cachectic conditions, such as cardiac cachexia *(45)* and in cachexia associated with chronic kidney disease (CKD) *(46)*. Clearance of PYY through the impaired renal function might be partly the culprit in the latter.

PANCREATIC POLYPEPTIDE

PP, discovered well before PYY *(47)*, is another anorexigenic peptide, produced by the PP cells of the islets of Langerhans *(48,49)* and, to a lesser extent, by the exocrine pancreas, colon, and rectum. PP immunoreactivity has also been shown in adrenal medulla (in rats) and porcine hypothalamic extracts, and PP mRNA has been detected by RT-PCR in rat brain.

PP level is subject to diurnal variation, being lowest early in the morning and highest in the evening. As with PYY, it is released in response to meal ingestion in proportion to caloric content of the meal. The release of the peptide is biphasic; although it increases with consecutive meals *(50)*, the total amount released remains constant based on the caloric load. Once in the circulation PP levels remain elevated up to 6 h.

PP release is stimulated by gastric distension; for example, water ingestion has been shown to significantly increase PP release. Vagal tone also appears to regulate PP release both postprandially and throughout the day. Propantheline has been shown to block both the diurnal (in fasting) and the postprandial levels of PP by 60%. The latter is shown to be abolished by vagotomy.

Circulating levels of PP are increased by ghrelin, motilin, secretin *(51–53)* and adrenergic stimulation, and are reduced by somatostatin and its analogs *(54)*. PP level has an inverse relationship with BMI, with higher levels in anorectic than in obese subjects *(55,56)*. This supports its role as an anorexigenic peptide; however, not all studies have been able to confirm this. Transgenic mice, with overexpression of PP, have reduced food intake and low lean body mass *(48)*. However, obese animal models show lower sensitivity to the effects of PP compared with the high sensitivity observed in lean animals. Peripheral administration of PP reduces food intake in animals *(57)* as well as in humans *(58,59)*. In 10 healthy volunteers calorie intake was reduced by 21% within 2 h and 33% within 24 h post-PP infusion at a rate of 10 pmol/kg/min *(58)*. In patients with Prader-Willi syndrome, iv infusion of PP was shown to reduce food intake *(59)*.

It is thought that PP exerts its anorectic effects on the ARC nucleus. Unlike PYY, there is no evidence to support PP's ability to cross the blood barrier. This may be partly attributable to the difference between the N-terminal moieties of the two peptides. C-fos expression and PP accumulation has been shown in area postrema following iv administration of PP. Y4 receptors, to which PP has a high affinity and are highly expressed in the area postrema, are suggested to be mediating this effect. Y5 receptors are also postulated to mediate the anorectic effects of PP, as no response is observed in Y5 receptor knockout mice. However, results from other studies are conflicting, as Y5 antisense oligonucleotides do not appear to block the PP anorectic effects. Other postulated mechanisms for the anorectic effects of PP are via the NPY and the orexin pathway, suppression of ghrelin, and vagal neurons. Both NPY and mRNA expression are reduced following peripheral PP administration, and PP has reduced effect following vagotomy. PP administration also reduced ghrelin expression in the stomach.

As with PYY, PP becomes orexigenic when directly administered into the third ventricle, although the mechanism of this is not known.

Cholecystokinin

CCK, originally isolated from the intestine, has been extensively investigated and reviewed with regard to its role as a regulator of food intake *(60,61)*. Multiple forms of CCK, varying in length from 8 to 83 amino acids, have been isolated from the intestine, blood, and brain *(60)*. Though they differ in size, they originate from a single gene resulting in the formation of different molecular forms by post-translational processing *(60,62)*. CCK is produced primarily by the I-cells in the duodenum and jejunum and, to a lesser extent, in the ilial mucosa *(60)*. CCK-58, -33, -22, and -8 are the main forms that are released from I-cells into the plasma. However, CCK is also produced in the brain, in which it is one of the most abundant peptides, and by the enteric nerve endings, where they act as neurotransmitters. The biologically active form of CCK shares a sequence (carboxy terminus) homology with gastrin *(60)*. Two receptors have been identified for CCK: CCK_A (CCK 1) receptor in the GI tract and CCK_B (CCK 2) receptor in the brain, through which the peptide exerts its biological actions *(63,64)* (*see* "Mechanism of Action" below).

CCK is a known satiety peptide; it slows gastric emptying and inhibits gastric acid secretion, but stimulates intestinal motility and gallbladder contraction, and increases pancreatic exocrine secretion. All these help the digestion process. CCK is known to inhibit food intake in humans and rodents *(65,66)*. The food inhibitory actions of CCK are enhanced by gastric distension, which implies that chemoreceptors are involved. However, the duration of its action is short, with a half-life of only 1 to 2 min. Therefore, no anorectic effect is observed if CCK is administered more than 15 min before meal intake *(62)*. In addition, chronic administration of CCK, although it reduces food intake, increases meal frequency. Consequently, long-term administration does not appear to have any effects on body weight *(60)*. This suggests that CCK is a short-term inhibitor of food intake.

MECHANISM OF ACTION

CCK exerts its effect via the CCK A and B receptors. Both are seven-domain transmembrane receptors from the G protein-coupled receptor superfamily. The CCK A receptor, primarily alimentary, mediates gallbladder contraction, relaxation of the sphincter of Oddi, pancreatic growth, and enzyme secretion. It delays gastric emptying, and inhibits gastric acid secretion by binding to sulfated CCK peptides. CCK A receptors have also been found in the pituitary, myenteric plexus, and areas of the midbrain. CCK B is the predominant receptor in the brain, but is also found in the stomach and pancreas. It is less restrictive, with a structure identical to the gastrin receptor, and binds nonsulfated CCK peptides *(67)*.

In addition, circulating CCK sends satiety signals to the ARC via the vagal stimuli through the NTS and area postrema, and/or directly by crossing the blood–brain barrier. Peripheral administration of CCK, at doses sufficient to inhibit food intake, has been shown to induce synthesis of c-fos in brainstem, NTS and the dorsal vagal nucleus *(68)*.

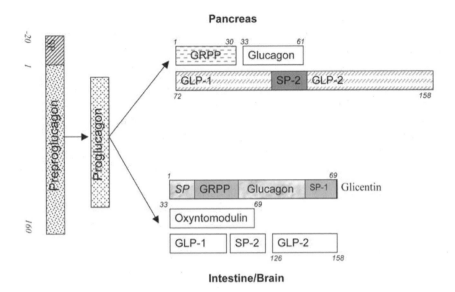

Fig. 2. Preproglucagon products. GRPP, glicentin-related pancreatic polypeptide; GLP-1, glucagon-like peptide -1 (7-36); GLP-2, glucagon-like peptide-2; SP-1, spacer peptide-1; SP-2, spacer peptide-2; SP, signal peptide.

Vagotomy blocks the effect of CCK on food intake indicating neuronal requirement for the mediation of CCK action to the CNS. Rats lacking functional CCK A receptors are diabetic, hyperphagic, and obese *(69,70)*, whereas receptor-deficient mice have been shown to have normal body weight.

Proglucagon Gene Products

Post-translational processing of preproglucagon results in the production of several peptides in the gut, pancreas, and brain (Fig. 2). These include oxyntomodulin (OXM) and GLP-1 and GLP-2 peptides, which are involved in the regulation of food intake. Prohormone convertase enzymes 1 and 2 cleave preproglucagon and produce different products, depending on the tissue. In the pancreas, glicentin-related pancreatic polypeptide (GRPP), glucagon, and GLP-1 and GLP-2 are produced. The latter two are cosecreted as a large inactive peptide. However, in the intestine and the brain, where the post-translational processing is similar, glicentin, glucagon, GLP-1, and GLP2 are produced. Glucagon remains in the large inactive peptide, whereas glicentin is cleaved to GRPP, with an inactive N-terminal, and oxyntomodulin (Fig. 2) *(17)*.

Oxyntomodulin

Oxyntomodulin is a 37-amino-acid peptide produced in the L-cells of the small intestine along with GLP-1 and GLP-2 *(71)* (Fig. 2).

OXM shows a diurnal variation, with the lowest levels being early in the morning and higher levels peaking in the evening *(72)*. Similar to the rest of the anorexigenic peptides, it is released in proportion to food ingestion and calorie intake *(71)*. Raised plasma levels of OXM have been shown to inhibit gastric acid secretion and motility in both humans and rodents. It also stimulates intestinal glucose uptake and decreases pancreatic enzyme secretion in rats.

Recent evidence supports an anorexigenic role for OXM in both animals and humans. In animals, central administration of OXM has been shown to acutely inhibit food intake *(73,74)*, and chronic intracerebroventricular (ICV) and IP administration reduces both food intake and weight gain *(74,75)*. The latter is thought to be the effect of reduced food intake as well as increased energy expenditure *(75)*. In humans, Cohen and coworkers *(76)* demonstrated a significant reduction in hunger scores and calorie intake (in a free-choice buffet meal by 19.3%) following parentral administration of OXM. More recently, Wynne et al. *(77)* have confirmed that the appetite inhibitory effect of OXM is long-lasting, resulting in significant weight reduction. In this study, subcutaneous injections of OXM three times per day for 30 d, in a double-blind placebo-controlled trial in 26 overweight human volunteers, was shown to significantly reduce weight (5.5 lb in the active group compared with 1 lb in those on placebo)*(77)*. Exercise and diet were fixed in both groups. Weight reduction in those subjects was shown to be associated with decreased leptin and increased adiponectin levels *(77)*.

It has been shown that OXM exerts its actions via the GLP-1 and glucagon receptors *(78)*. Therefore, exendin 9-39, which can act either as a GLP-2 receptor antagonist and/ or a GLP-1 agonist, can block the actions of both GLP-1 and OXM *(17)*. GLP-1R is present in the NTS and the arcuate nucleus in addition to its widespread presence peripherally. It is present in the gastrointestinal tract, lung, pancreas, and heart. Interestingly, exendin 9-39 administration into the arcuate nucleus abolishes the peripheral effects of OXM but not that of GLP-1 *(74)*. This suggests an arcuate site of action for OXM, whereas GLP-1 acts via the brain stem. Further evidence suggests different neuronal activation between OXM and GLP-1. OXM has a lower affinity (2-fold) to GLP-1 receptors compared with GLP-1 *(79)*. This may suggest that other mechanisms might be involved in mediating the anorexigenic effects of OXM. Activation of the neuronal c-fos expression in the arcuate nucleus, but not in the brainstem region, was observed following IP administration of OXM and exendin 9-39 *(75,78)*. This pattern of activation is different from that seen following GLP-1 administration *(74)*.

An additional mechanism whereby OXM may exert its effect on appetite is via suppression of ghrelin. In rodents and humans, peripheral administration of OXM results in reduction of circulating ghrelin by 20% *(74)* and 44% *(76)*, respectively.

The human studies on OXM effect on appetite control may indicate a novel potential role that OXM may have as an antiobesity therapeutic agent. However, more studies research is required to develop the drug into a more user-friendly format *(77)*.

GLUCAGON-LIKE PEPTIDE-1

Along with OXM, GLP-1 is also produced by post-translational processing of preproglucagon in the L-cells in the distal ileum *(80)*. Postprandially, GLP-1 is rapidly secreted in response to food intake *(81,82)*. Two equally potent forms (GLP-17-37 and GLP-17-36) have been identified, which undergo rapid inactivation and cleavage by dipeptidyl peptidase IV (DPP IV). As a consequence GLP-1's half-life becomes very short (1–2 min) in the circulation.

Similar to OXM, GLP-1 secretion is regulated by both nutritional and neural/hormonal signals, and its action is mediated via GLP-1R. Actions of GLP-1 on the CNS are complex and are mediated via the dorsal vagal complex acting through the area postrema *(83)*. In rats, similar to OXM, GLP-1 results in c-fos, a marker of neuronal activation, expression in the brainstem *(74)*.

GLP-1 Actions. In addition to its central actions, including the transduction of aversive signals, regulation of learning and memory, and neuroprotection, GLP-1 acts as a regulatory peptide in appetite control. GLP-1 inhibits food intake *(84,85)*, reduces gastric secretion and motility, and increases gastric satiety. Central administration of GLP-1 in rodents has been shown to inhibit food intake, which, if continued, results in weight loss *(84)*. Seemingly peripheral administration causes reduced food intake *(85–87)*.

Human studies have shown that peripheral administration of GLP-1 inhibits food intake in normal *(88)*, diabetic *(89)*, and nondiabetic obese men *(90)* in a dose-dependent manner. Subcutaneous injection of GLP-1 in obese subjects over 5 d was shown to cause a 15% reduction in calorie intake *(90)* and 0.5 kg weight loss. Although low levels have been shown in obese subjects that normalize after weight loss *(86)*, the anorectic effects of GLP-1 have been shown to be preserved in obesity *(90)*. GLP-1 also decreases gastric emptying, resulting in increased satiety, which may further explain its effect on food intake *(91)*.

GLP-1 is an incretin mimetic that has been found to upregulate insulin gene expression *(92)*. It promotes meal-induced insulin secretion, resulting in reduced blood glucose level. Lower blood glucose level is also achieved via a GLP-1 inhibitory effect on glucagon secretion and reduced gastric emptying. The latter slows the rate of nutrient transit to the small intestine, leading to decreased glycemic excursion after meal ingestion *(91,93)*. Both intravenous and subcutaneous infusions have been shown to normalize blood glucose levels in poorly controlled diabetics. HbA1c was shown to be reduced by 1.3% over a 6-wk period of subcutaneous infusion of GLP-1 in addition to a 2-kg weight loss *(94)*. GLP-1 also stimulates B-cell proliferation and promotes islet cell neogenesis *(95)*. This is thought to be mediated through GLP-1R.

The collective actions of GLP-1 resulting in inhibition of food intake, reduction in weight, a glucose-dependent reduction in blood glucose level, and improvement in diabetes control made it an ideal candidate in the treatment of diabetes. Its therapeutic application is of immense importance in diabetic patients who are increasingly overweight and suffer from drug-related hypoglycaemia.

OREXIGENIC GUT PEPTIDES

Ghrelin

Ghrelin, the endogenous ligand for the growth hormone secretagog receptor (GHS-R), was discovered in 1999 *(96,97)*. It is produced from preproghrelin peptide in the oxyntic gland in the fundus of the stomach, but not in the pylorus *(97)*. Ghrelin is also produced, though to a lower extent, in the small and large intestine *(96)*. Various ghrelin variants are produced from alternative splicing, but the mature molecule is a 28-amino-acid peptide with an octanoyl acyl group on its third amino acid residue. This is acquired after post-translational modification and is essential for its action on appetite *(98)*. There is evidence for ghrelin expression in other tissues, including the hypothalamus, pancreas, lungs, ovaries, and testes. In the hypothalamus ghrelin expression is shown in the ARC adjacent to the orexigenic neurons; NPY and AgRP, PVN, DMN, and VMN; however, its physiological role needs to be established *(99,100)*. Circulating levels change throughout the day in relations to meals, increasing during fasting, peaking just before food intake, and decreasing postprandially *(101–104)*. Ghrelin reaches trough levels 60 to 120 min after food intake. As with other peptides, levels are subject to diurnal variations, being high at night and declining in the early hours of the morning along with leptin levels. The postprandial decline of ghrelin is proportional to calorie intake and nutrient sensing but not stomach volume load. In keeping with this, glucose, but not water/saline, infusion into the stomach caused suppression of ghrelin *(105)*. However, no changes in ghrelin level were observed without normal gastric emptying, which suggests a requirement for a postgastric factor. The effect of glucose on ghrelin is independent of insulin actions. Further studies in humans showed that carbohydrate, and to a lesser extent fat, reduces, whereas protein appears to stimulate, ghrelin levels in normal *(106)* and type 1 diabetic patients *(107)*. However, the micronutrient content and calorie load can not wholly explain the postprandial suppression of ghrelin; other factors might be involved. Whereas leptin, GHRH, testosterone, thyroid hormone, and parasympathetic activity upregulate ghrelin, insulin, somatostatin, growth hormone, and PYY3-36 result in its downregulation.

GHRELIN ACTION

Ghrelin has a number of known effects, including release of growth hormone (GH), ACTH, and prolactin, increasing gastric motility, acid secretion in the cephalic phase response of food intake *(108)*, and promoting cell proliferation. Since its discovery, accumulating evidence supports its orexigenic effects and its role in the regulation of body weight. In both animal and human studies ghrelin has been shown to contribute in signaling the preprandial hunger and meal initiation *(97,109)*. In animals, acute administration of ghrelin increases food intake *(110,111)*, whereas chronic administration results in hyperphagia and obesity *(112)*. It is worth noting that the effects of ghrelin on food intake and adiposity are independent of its effect on GH. Central administration of ghrelin, by direct injection into the ICV or ARC, stimulates food intake and can be inhibited by pretreatment with ghrelin antagonists/antibodies. This suggests that ghrelin is an endogenous regulator of food intake. Ghrelin shows similar effects in humans; following intravenous ghrelin administration, appetite and food intake increase by 28% in normal volunteers, though this effect is short-lived *(113)*. However, satiety is not changed postprandially following ghrelin administration *(113)*.

MECHANISM OF ACTION

Evidence supports ghrelin exerting its effects mainly via the orexigenic peptides NPY/AgRP in the hypothalamus. ICV injection of ghrelin increases NPY/AgRP gene expression and blocks the anorexic actions of leptin. NPY/AgRP antibodies or NPY Y1 receptor antagonists abolish ghrelin-induced feeding, but ghrelin antibodies do not inhibit NPY-induced feeding. Electrophysiological studies have shown that ghrelin activates NPY neurons and inhibits POMC, with the former being postsynaptic and the latter a presynaptic effect. Peripheral administration of ghrelin also results, though reduced, in c-fos expression primarily at the ARC site. This suggests that ghrelin might reach the ARC through the incomplete blood–brain barrier at the base of the hypothalamus. In keeping with this, animals with damaged ARC show GH response, though reduced, but no feeding effects after ghrelin administration.

Ghrelin neurons are expressed elsewhere in the brain. An increase in c-fos activation following central ghrelin administration has been shown in the ARC, PVN, DMN, the lateral hypothalamus, and the area postrema and NTS in the brainstem *(114,115)*. The central ghrelin neurons also terminate on orexin-containing neurons within the lateral hypothalamus (LH) *(116)*, which have been shown to be stimulated following ICV ghrelin injection.

Despite the above evidence supporting its orexigenic effect, ghrelin appears not to be the only factor in meal initiation and food intake. Recently, ghrelin infusions in six men and one woman with previous complete truncal vagotomy had no effect on food intake *(117)*. This suggests that an intact vagal nerve is required for ghrelin's stimulatory effect.

GHRELIN IN PHYSIOLOGY AND DISEASE

In addition to calorie intake and meal composition, ghrelin levels appear to be influenced by the nutritional status of the individual. The basal level is shown to be reduced in chronic obesity with an attenuated postprandial response *(118–120)*. The latter may explain persistent eating habits in obese patients. Paradoxically, the level is increased during fasting, cachexia *(121)*, in states of malnutrition, and in patients with anorexia nervosa *(122)*. Interestingly, and contrary to these findings, ghrelin levels are reduced after a Roux-en-Y gastric bypass, but not other forms of antiobesity surgery, despite massive weight loss *(33)*. One explanation might be that the surgery involves the removal of the ghrelin-secreting part of the stomach *(33,123)*, although the real mechanism is still unknown. However, in addition to the mechanical restriction owing to reduced stomach size and hence reduced meal portions, it has been hypothesized that the decreased ghrelin level in these patients might be the reason for maintaining their weight loss.

GUT HORMONE SYNERGISM AND/OR ANTAGONISM

From the previous sections it is evident that multiple factors are involved in the regulation of food intake and energy homeostasis in which gut hormones appear to play a central role. Here we propose three different interactive processes (Fig. 1): gut–brain interaction; gut–gut interaction; and gut–adipose interaction.

Gut–Brain Interaction

Gut peptides increase/reduce food intake by binding to specific neurons in the appetite centers in the brain. This can be via specific known or even yet unknown receptors, direct effect from the circulation, and/or through neuronal activation outside the blood–brain barrier. Peripheral and central administration of both the orexigenic and anorexigenic gut peptides results in c-fos activation in the arcuate nucleus. Suppression/activation of NPY neurons and NPY mRNA expression and reciprocal effect in POMC neurons following gut peptide administration is associated with altered feeding control. Several receptors that are involved in mediating the actions of gut peptides in the hypothalamus and brainstem have now been identified (Table 2). In support of this, receptor knockout animals have defective food intake and body weight. Similarly, defects in MC4 receptors have been described in human forms of obesity. However, the central effect of these gut peptides is abolished in vagotomized animals, indicating the importance of neural pathways in connecting the signals to the hypothalamus and other appetite centers in the brain.

Gut–Gut Interaction

Three mechanisms appear to regulate this: first, the effect of nutrients, and meal size, and composition on the release of gut peptides; second, the synergistic and antagonistic actions of gut peptides; and third, the effect of gut peptides on gut secretion, motility, and gastric emptying.

In addition to external cues, following food ingestion, various factors affect the release and circulating levels of gut peptides and thereby their effect on the appetite centers in the brain. Nutriment sense within the gut *(17)* influences PYY, PP, and OXM release, whereas stomach distension influences the release of PP and CCK, which indicates the effects of chemoreceptors. A higher calorie intake results in a more sustained release of PYY and consequently a reduction in calorie intake in the subsequent 12 to 24 h. Reciprocal to this, ghrelin is suppressed postprandially proportional to meal caloric content, assisting and further promoting satiety and meal termination.

Gut hormones appear to act both in synergism and antagonism. Interestingly, increasing evidence suggest that whichever way they work they appear to complement each other to promote satiety. Some gut peptides share structural homology (PYY3-36 and PP), cosecreted from the same cell line (PYY3-36, OXM and GLP-1), and have been shown to be products of the same gene (OXM and GLP-1). These are all known anorexigenic peptides. Exendin, a GLP-1 receptor agonist, and PYY act synergistically, but through different mechanisms to reduce food intake *(124)*. CCK is well known to produce early satiety *(60,62)*, but the meal-to-meal duration is longer than what can be explained by CCK levels. Therefore, it is in order to suggest a sequential release and suppression of gut hormones to sustain the diurnal pattern of food intake. For example, ghrelin peaks before food ingestion and is suppressed postprandially, during which CCK, one of the earliest peptides released, promotes early satiety, whereas persistence of PYY3-36 and OXM levels prevent the animal (human) from continuous eating and reduce subsequent calorie intake in the following 12 to 24 h *(21,76)*. In contrast, GLP-1 has been shown to suppress PYY3-36 *(22)*; however, the short half-life of GLP-1 in circulation might be yet another explanation for the persistent release of PYY. Similarly, OXM has been suggested to exert its anorexigenic effect, at least partly, through the suppression of ghrelin. To some extent, this may explain the suppression of ghrelin postprandially in addition to its suppression by nutriment sense in the gut.

Another action of gut peptides PYY, OXM, and PP is the reduction of gastric motility. This will delay gastric emptying, and consequently the persistence of food/nutrients in the gut. The latter may produce a satiating effect through three mechanisms: (1) activation of chemoreceptors; (2) activation of the vagal afferents; and (3) persistence release of PYY and OXM.

Gut–Adipose Interaction

Gut hormones have been shown to interact with long-term signals from adipose tissue. GLP-1 is known to improving insulin sensitivity and, thereby, glycemic control. In rodents, peripheral administration of PYY3-36 for 4 wk resulted in improved glycemic control; reduce body weight and visceral fat *(33)*. Recently, Wynne et al. *(77)* showed a significant reduction in leptin and an increment in adiponectin, markers of adiposity, associated with reduced body weight in 14 patients who had subcutaneous OXM injections for 4 wk.

CONCLUSION

Obesity causes premature death of about 2 million people a year worldwide, and its prevalence is rising. The decision to eat or not and/or alterations in energy expenditure are central to the dilemma of increased body adiposity. The appetite centers in the brain receive neural, humoral, and hormonal signals from the periphery for the regulation of food intake and energy homeostasis.

Gut peptides are secreted from the gastrointestinal tract either before or after each meal. They can act synergistically or antagonistically to each other, but in a sequential manner and in consortium with neural and long-term signals from adipose tissue. Recent advances in establishing their identification, characterization, and their increasingly recognized effect on appetite and gastrointestinal motility has contributed tremendously to our understanding of the central regulation of appetite and energy homeostasis. We are now entering a new era for discovering their novel potential roles as single agents or, perhaps more likely, in combination in the treatment of obesity.

REFERENCES

1. Barsh GS, Farooqi IS, O'Rahilly S. Genetics of body-weight regulation. Nature 2000;404(6778):644–651.
2. Butler AA, Cone RD. Knockout studies defining different roles for melanocortin receptors in energy homeostasis. Ann NY Acad Sci 2003;994:240–245.
3. Butler AA, Kesterson RA, Khong K, et al. A unique metabolic syndrome causes obesity in the melanocortin-3 receptor-deficient mouse. Endocrinology 2000;141(9):3518–3521.
4. Butler AA, Cone RD. The melanocortin receptors: lessons from knockout models. Neuropeptides 2002;36(2–3):77–84.
5. Farooqi IS, Yeo GS, Keogh JM, et al. Dominant and recessive inheritance of morbid obesity associated with melanocortin 4 receptor deficiency. J Clin Invest 2000;106(2):271–279.
6. Farooqi IS, O'Rahilly S. Monogenic obesity in humans. Annu Rev Med 2005;56:443–458.
7. Larhammar D. Structural diversity of receptors for neuropeptide Y, peptide YY and pancreatic polypeptide. Regul Pept 1996;65(3):165–174.
8. Batterham RL, Cowley MA, Small CJ, et al. Gut hormone PYY(3-36) physiologically inhibits food intake. Nature 2002;418(6898):650–654.
9. Batterham RL, Bloom SR. The gut hormone peptide YY regulates appetite. Ann NY Acad Sci 2003; 994:162–168.
10. Broberger C, Landry M, Wong H, Walsh JN, Hokfelt T. Subtypes Y1 and Y2 of the neuropeptide Y receptor are respectively expressed in pro-opiomelanocortin- and neuropeptide-Y-containing neurons of the rat hypothalamic arcuate nucleus. Neuroendocrinology 1997;66(6):393–408.
11. Sahu A. Interactions of neuropeptide Y, hypocretin-I (orexin A) and melanin-concentrating hormone on feeding in rats. Brain Res 2002;944(1–2):232–238.
12. Tatemoto K. Isolation and characterization of peptide YY (PYY), a candidate gut hormone that inhibits pancreatic exocrine secretion. Proc Natl Acad Sci USA 1982;79(8):2514–2518.
13. Adrian TE, Ferri GL, Bacarese-Hamilton AJ, et al. Human distribution and release of a putative new gut hormone, peptide YY. Gastroenterology 1985;89(5):1070–1077.
14. Ekblad E, Sundler F. Distribution of pancreatic polypeptide and peptide YY. Peptides 2002;23(2):251–261.
15. Eberlein GA, Eysselein VE, Schaeffer M, et al. A new molecular form of PYY: structural characterization of human PYY(3-36) and PYY(1-36). Peptides 1989;10(4):797–803.
16. Pedersen-Bjergaard U, Host U, Kelbaek H, et al. Influence of meal composition on postprandial peripheral plasma concentrations of vasoactive peptides in man. Scand J Clin Lab Invest 1996;56(6): 497–503.
17. Small CJ, Bloom SR. Gut hormones as peripheral anti obesity targets. Curr Drug Targets CNS Neurol Disord 2004;3(5):379–388.
18. Lin HC, Chey WY. Cholecystokinin and peptide YY are released by fat in either proximal or distal small intestine in dogs. Regul Pept 2003;114(2–3):131–135.
19. Abbott CR, Monteiro M, Small CJ, et al. The inhibitory effects of peripheral administration of peptide YY(3-36) and glucagon-like peptide-1 on food intake are attenuated by ablation of the vagal-brainstem-hypothalamic pathway. Brain Res 2005;1044(1):127–131.
20. Koda S, Date Y, Murakami N, et al. The role of the vagal nerve in peripheral PYY3-36-induced feeding reduction in rats. Endocrinology 2005;146:2369–2375.
21. Batterham RL, Cohen MA, Ellis SM, et al. Inhibition of food intake in obese subjects by peptide YY3-36. N Engl J Med 2003;349(10):941–948.
22. Naslund E, Bogefors J, Skogar S, et al. GLP-1 slows solid gastric emptying and inhibits insulin, glucagon, and PYY release in humans. Am J Physiol 1999;277(3 Pt 2):R910–R916.

23. Challis BG, Pinnock SB, Coll AP, et al. Acute effects of PYY3-36 on food intake and hypothalamic neuropeptide expression in the mouse. Biochem Biophys Res Commun 2003;311(4):915–919.
24. Halatchev IG, Ellacott KL, Fan W, et al. Peptide YY3-36 inhibits food intake in mice through a melanocortin-4 receptor-independent mechanism. Endocrinology 2004;145(6):2585–2590.
25. Chelikani PK, Haver AC, Reidelberger RD. Intravenous infusion of peptide YY(3-36) potently inhibits food intake in rats. Endocrinology 2005;146(2):879–888.
26. Abbott CR, Small CJ, Kennedy AR, et al. Blockade of the neuropeptide Y Y2 receptor with the specific antagonist BIIE0246 attenuates the effect of endogenous and exogenous peptide YY(3-36) on food intake. Brain Res 2005;1043(1–2):139–144.
27. Batterham RL, Bloom SR. The gut hormone peptide YY regulates appetite. Ann NY Acad Sci 2003; 994:162–168.
28. Scott V, Kimura N, Stark JA, et al. Intravenous peptide YY3-36 and Y2 receptor antagonism in the rat: effects on feeding behavior. J Neuroendocrinol 2005;17(7):452–457.
29. Le Roux CW, Bloom SR. Peptide YY, appetite and food intake. Proc Nutr Soc 2005;64(2):213–216.
30. Kanatani A, Mashiko S, Murai N et al. Role of the Y1 receptor in the regulation of neuropeptide Y-mediated feeding: comparison of wild-type, Y1 receptor-deficient, and Y5 receptor-deficient mice. Endocrinology 2000;141(3):1011–1016.
31. Cox JE, Randich A. Enhancement of feeding suppression by PYY(3-36) in rats with area postrema ablations. Peptides 2004;25(6):985–989.
32. Batterham RL, Bloom SR. The gut hormone peptide YY regulates appetite. Ann NY Acad Sci 2003; 994:162–168.
33. Hanusch-Enserer U, Roden M. News in gut-brain communication: a role of peptide YY (PYY) in human obesity and following bariatric surgery? Eur J Clin Invest 2005;35(7):425–430.
34. McGowan BM, Bloom SR. Peptide YY and appetite control. Curr Opin Pharmacol 2004;4(6):583–588.
35. Tschop M, Castaneda TR, Joost HG, et al. Physiology: does gut hormone PYY3-36 decrease food intake in rodents? Nature 2004; 430(6996):1.
36. Moran TH, Smedh U, Kinzig KP, et al. Peptide YY(3-36) inhibits gastric emptying and produces acute reductions in food intake in rhesus monkeys. Am J Physiol Regul Integr Comp Physiol 2005;288(2): R384–R388.
37. Pittner RA, Moore CX, Bhavsar SP, et al. Effects of PYY[3-36] in rodent models of diabetes and obesity. Int J Obes Relat Metab Disord 2004;28(8):963–971.
38. Dhillo WS, Bloom SR. Gastrointestinal hormones and regulation of food intake. Horm Metab Res 2004;36(11–12):846–851.
39. Monteleone P, Martiadis V, Rigamonti AE, et al. Investigation of peptide YY and ghrelin responses to a test meal in bulimia nervosa. Biol Psychiatry 2005;57(8):926–931.
40. Inamura M. Effects of surgical manipulation of the intestine on peptide YY and its physiology. Peptides 2002;23(2):403–407.
41. Naslund E, Gryback P, Hellstrom PM, et al. Gastrointestinal hormones and gastric emptying 20 years after jejunoileal bypass for massive obesity. Int J Obes Relat Metab Disord 1997;21(5):387–392.
42. Adrian TE, Savage AP, Fuessl HS, et al. Release of peptide YY (PYY) after resection of small bowel, colon, or pancreas in man. Surgery 1987;101(6):715–719.
43. Wahab PJ, Hopman WP, Jansen JB. Basal and fat-stimulated plasma peptide YY levels in celiac disease. Dig Dis Sci 2001;46(11):2504–2509.
44. Adrian TE, Savage AP, Bacarese-Hamilton AJ, et al. Peptide YY abnormalities in gastrointestinal diseases. Gastroenterology 1986;90(2):379–384.
45. Le Roux CW, Ghatei MA, Gibbs JS, Bloom SR. The putative satiety hormone PYY is raised in cardiac cachexia associated with primary pulmonary hypertension. Heart 2005;91(2):241–242.
46. Mitch WE. Cachexia in chronic kidney disease: a link to defective central nervous system control of appetite. J Clin Invest 2005;115(6):1476–1478.
47. Larsson LI, Sundler F, Hakanson R. Immunohistochemical localization of human pancreatic polypeptide (HPP) to a population of islet cells. Cell Tissue Res 1975;156(2):167–171.
48. Ueno N, Inui A, Iwamoto M, et al. Decreased food intake and body weight in pancreatic polypeptide-overexpressing mice. Gastroenterology 1999;117(6):1427–1432.
49. McLaughlin CL, Baile CA. Obese mice and the satiety effects of cholecystokinin, bombesin and pancreatic polypeptide. Physiol Behav 1981;26(3):433–437.

50. Track NS, McLeod RS, Mee AV. Human pancreatic polypeptide: studies of fasting and postprandial plasma concentrations. Can J Physiol Pharmacol 1980;58(12):1484–1489.

51. Mochiki E, Inui A, Satoh M, et al. Motilin is a biosignal controlling cyclic release of pancreatic polypeptide via the vagus in fasted dogs. Am J Physiol 1997;272(2 Pt 1):G224–G232.

52. Peracchi M, Tagliabue R, Quatrini M, Reschini E. Plasma pancreatic polypeptide response to secretin. Eur J Endocrinol 1999;141(1):47–49.

53. Arosio M, Ronchi CL, Gebbia C, et al. Stimulatory effects of ghrelin on circulating somatostatin and pancreatic polypeptide levels. J Clin Endocrinol Metab 2003;88(2):701–704.

54. Parkinson C, Drake WM, Roberts ME, et al. A comparison of the effects of pegvisomant and octreotide on glucose, insulin, gastrin, cholecystokinin, and pancreatic polypeptide responses to oral glucose and a standard mixed meal. J Clin Endocrinol Metab 2002;87(4):1797–1804.

55. Uhe AM, Szmukler GI, Collier GR, et al. Potential regulators of feeding behavior in anorexia nervosa. Am J Clin Nutr 1992;55(1):28–32.

56. Fujimoto S, Inui A, Kiyota N, et al. Increased cholecystokinin and pancreatic polypeptide responses to a fat-rich meal in patients with restrictive but not bulimic anorexia nervosa. Biol Psychiatry 1997;41(10):1068–1070.

57. Asakawa A, Inui A, Yuzuriha H, et al. Characterization of the effects of pancreatic polypeptide in the regulation of energy balance. Gastroenterology 2003;124(5):1325–1336.

58. Batterham RL, Le Roux CW, Cohen MA, et al. Pancreatic polypeptide reduces appetite and food intake in humans. J Clin Endocrinol Metab 2003;88(8):3989–3992.

59. Berntson GG, Zipf WB, O'Dorisio TM, et al. Pancreatic polypeptide infusions reduce food intake in Prader-Willi syndrome. Peptides 1993;14(3):497–503.

60. Liddle RA. Cholecystokinin: its role in health and disease. Curr Opin Endocrinol Diabetes 2003;10(1):50–54.

61. Moran TH. Gut peptides in the control of food intake: 30 years of ideas. Physiol Behav 2004;82(1): 175–180.

62. Rehfeld JF. Clinical endocrinology and metabolism. Cholecystokinin. Best Pract Res Clin Endocrinol Metab 2004;18(4):569–586.

63. Wank SA, Pisegna JR, de Weerth A. Brain and gastrointestinal cholecystokinin receptor family: structure and functional expression. Proc Natl Acad Sci USA 1992;89(18):8691–8695.

64. Wank SA. Cholecystokinin receptors. Am J Physiol 1995;269(5 Pt 1):G628–G646.

65. Beglinger C, Degen L. Fat in the intestine as a regulator of appetite—role of CCK. Physiol Behav 2004;83(4):617–621.

66. Kissileff HR, Carretta JC, Geliebter A, et al. Cholecystokinin and stomach distension combine to reduce food intake in humans. Am J Physiol Regul Integr Comp Physiol 2003;285(5):R992–R998.

67. Moran TH, Kinzig KP. Gastrointestinal satiety signals II. Cholecystokinin. Am J Physiol Gastrointest Liver Physiol 2004;286(2):G183–G188.

68. Zittel TT, Glatzle J, Kreis ME, et al. C-fos protein expression in the nucleus of the solitary tract correlates with cholecystokinin dose injected and food intake in rats. Brain Res 1999;846(1):1–11.

69. Schwartz GJ, Whitney A, Skoglund C, et al. Decreased responsiveness to dietary fat in Otsuka Long-Evans Tokushima fatty rats lacking CCK-A receptors. Am J Physiol 1999;277(4 Pt 2):R1144–R1151.

70. Moran TH, Katz LF, Plata-Salaman CR, Schwartz GJ. Disordered food intake and obesity in rats lacking cholecystokinin A receptors. Am J Physiol 1998;274(3 Pt 2):R618–R625.

71. Ghatei MA, Uttenthal LO, Christofides ND, et al. Molecular forms of human enteroglucagon in tissue and plasma: plasma responses to nutrient stimuli in health and in disorders of the upper gastrointestinal tract. J Clin Endocrinol Metab 1983;57(3):488–495.

72. Le Quellec A, Kervran A, Blache P, et al. Oxyntomodulin-like immunoreactivity: diurnal profile of a new potential enterogastrone. J Clin Endocrinol Metab 1992;74(6):1405–1409.

73. Dakin CL, Gunn I, Small CJ, et al. Oxyntomodulin inhibits food intake in the rat. Endocrinology 2001;142(10):4244–4250.

74. Dakin CL, Small CJ, Batterham RL, et al. Peripheral oxyntomodulin reduces food intake and body weight gain in rats. Endocrinology 2004;145(6):2687–2695.

75. Dakin CL, Small CJ, Park AJ, et al. Repeated ICV administration of oxyntomodulin causes a greater reduction in body weight gain than in pair-fed rats. Am J Physiol Endocrinol Metab 2002;283(6): E1173–E1177.

76. Cohen MA, Ellis SM, Le Roux CW, et al. Oxyntomodulin suppresses appetite and reduces food intake in humans. J Clin Endocrinol Metab 2003;88(10):4696–4701.

77. Wynne K, Park AJ, Small CJ, et al. Subcutaneous oxyntomodulin reduces body weight in overweight and obese subjects: a double-blind, randomized, controlled trial. Diabetes 2005;54(8):2390–2395.

78. Baggio LL, Huang Q, Brown TJ, et al. Oxyntomodulin and glucagon-like peptide-1 differentially regulate murine food intake and energy expenditure. Gastroenterology 2004;127(2):546–558.

79. Fehmann HC, Jiang J, Schweinfurth J, et al. Stable expression of the rat GLP-I receptor in CHO cells: activation and binding characteristics utilizing GLP-I(7-36)-amide, oxyntomodulin, exendin-4, and exendin(9-39). Peptides 1994;15(3):453–456.

80. Holst JJ. Glucagonlike peptide 1: a newly discovered gastrointestinal hormone. Gastroenterology 1994;107(6):1848–1855.

81. Drucker DJ, Lovshin J, Baggio L, et al. New developments in the biology of the glucagon-like peptides GLP-1 and GLP-2. Ann NY Acad Sci 2000;921:226–232.

82. Drucker DJ. Minireview: the glucagon-like peptides. Endocrinology 2001;142(2):521–527.

83. Tang-Christensen M, Vrang N, Larsen PJ. Glucagon-like peptide containing pathways in the regulation of feeding behavior. Int J Obes Relat Metab Disord 2001;25 Suppl 5:S42–S47.

84. Meeran K, O'Shea D, Edwards CM, et al. Repeated intracerebroventricular administration of glucagon-like peptide-1-(7-36) amide or exendin-(9-39) alters body weight in the rat. Endocrinology 1999;140(1):244–250.

85. Verdich C, Flint A, Gutzwiller JP, et al. A meta-analysis of the effect of glucagon-like peptide-1 (7-36) amide on ad libitum energy intake in humans. J Clin Endocrinol Metab 2001;86(9):4382–4389.

86. Verdich C, Toubro S, Buemann B, et al. The role of postprandial releases of insulin and incretin hormones in meal-induced satiety—effect of obesity and weight reduction. Int J Obes Relat Metab Disord 2001;25(8):1206–1214.

87. Flint A, Raben A, Ersboll AK, et al. The effect of physiological levels of glucagon-like peptide-1 on appetite, gastric emptying, energy and substrate metabolism in obesity. Int J Obes Relat Metab Disord 2001;25(6):781–792.

88. Gutzwiller JP, Goke B, Drewe J, et al. Glucagon-like peptide-1: a potent regulator of food intake in humans. Gut 1999;44(1):81–86.

89. Gutzwiller JP, Drewe J, Goke B, et al. Glucagon-like peptide-1 promotes satiety and reduces food intake in patients with diabetes mellitus type 2. Am J Physiol 1999;276(5 Pt 2):R1541–R1544.

90. Naslund E, Barkeling B, King N, et al. Energy intake and appetite are suppressed by glucagon-like peptide-1 (GLP-1) in obese men. Int J Obes Relat Metab Disord 1999;23(3):304–311.

91. Willms B, Werner J, Holst JJ, et al. Gastric emptying, glucose responses, and insulin secretion after a liquid test meal: effects of exogenous glucagon-like peptide-1 (GLP-1)-(7-36) amide in type 2 (noninsulin-dependent) diabetic patients. J Clin Endocrinol Metab 1996;81(1):327–332.

92. MacDonald PE, El Kholy W, Riedel MJ, et al. The multiple actions of GLP-1 on the process of glucose-stimulated insulin secretion. Diabetes 2002;51 Suppl 3:S434–S442.

93. Wishart JM, Horowitz M, Morris HA, et al. Relation between gastric emptying of glucose and plasma concentrations of glucagon-like peptide-1. Peptides 1998;19(6):1049–1053.

94. Zander M, Madsbad S, Madsen JL, et al. Effect of 6-week course of glucagon-like peptide 1 on glycaemic control, insulin sensitivity, and beta-cell function in type 2 diabetes: a parallel-group study. Lancet 2002;359(9309):824–830.

95. Egan JM, Bulotta A, Hui H, et al. GLP-1 receptor agonists are growth and differentiation factors for pancreatic islet beta cells. Diabetes Metab Res Rev 2003;19(2):115–123.

96. Kojima M, Hosoda H, Date Y, et al. Ghrelin is a growth-hormone-releasing acylated peptide from stomach. Nature 1999;402(6762):656–660.

97. Ariyasu H, Takaya K, Tagami T, et al. Stomach is a major source of circulating ghrelin, and feeding state determines plasma ghrelin-like immunoreactivity levels in humans. J Clin Endocrinol Metab 2001;86(10):4753–4758.

98. Kojima S, Nakahara T, Nagai N, et al. Altered ghrelin and peptide YY responses to meals in bulimia nervosa. Clin Endocrinol (Oxf) 2005;62(1):74–78.

99. Cowley MA, Smith RG, Diano S, et al. The distribution and mechanism of action of ghrelin in the CNS demonstrates a novel hypothalamic circuit regulating energy homeostasis. Neuron 2003;37(4):649–661.

100. Cummings DE, Foster-Schubert KE, Overduin J. Ghrelin and energy balance: focus on current controversies. Curr Drug Targets 2005;6(2):153–169.

101. Asakawa A, Inui A, Kaga T, et al. Ghrelin is an appetite-stimulatory signal from stomach with structural resemblance to motilin. Gastroenterology 2001;120(2):337–345.
102. Cummings DE, Purnell JQ, Frayo RS, et al. A prerandial rise in plasma ghrelin levels suggests a role in meal initiation in humans. Diabetes 2001;50(8):1714–1719.
103. Kojima M, Kangawa K. Ghrelin: structure and function. Physiol Rev 2005;85(2):495–522.
104. Williams DL, Cummings DE. Regulation of ghrelin in physiologic and pathophysiologic states. J Nutr 2005;135(5):1320–1325.
105. Shiiya T, Nakazato M, Mizuta M, et al. Plasma ghrelin levels in lean and obese humans and the effect of glucose on ghrelin secretion. J Clin Endocrinol Metab 2002;87(1):240–244.
106. Le Roux CW, Patterson M, Vincent RP, et al. Postprandial plasma ghrelin is suppressed proportional to meal calorie content in normal-weight but not obese subjects. J Clin Endocrinol Metab 2005;90(2):1068–1071.
107. Murdolo G, Lucidi P, Di Loreto C et al. Insulin is required for prandial ghrelin suppression in humans. Diabetes 2003;52(12):2923–2927.
108. Masuda Y, Tanaka T, Inomata N, et al. Ghrelin stimulates gastric acid secretion and motility in rats. Biochem Biophys Res Commun 2000;276(3):905–908.
109. Date Y, Kojima M, Hosoda H, et al. Ghrelin, a novel growth hormone-releasing acylated peptide, is synthesized in a distinct endocrine cell type in the gastrointestinal tracts of rats and humans. Endocrinology 2000;141(11):4255–4261.
110. Tang-Christensen M, Vrang N, Ortmann S, et al. Central administration of ghrelin and agouti-related protein (83-132) increases food intake and decreases spontaneous locomotor activity in rats. Endocrinology 2004;145(10):4645–4652.
111. Wren AM, Small CJ, Fribbens CV, et al. The hypothalamic mechanisms of the hypophysiotropic action of ghrelin. Neuroendocrinology 2002;76(5):316–324.
112. Wren AM, Small CJ, Abbott CR, et al. Ghrelin causes hyperphagia and obesity in rats. Diabetes 2001;50(11):2540–2547.
113. Wren AM, Seal LJ, Cohen MA, et al. Ghrelin enhances appetite and increases food intake in humans. J Clin Endocrinol Metab 2001;86(12):5992.
114. Shintani M, Ogawa Y, Ebihara K, et al. Ghrelin, an endogenous growth hormone secretagogue, is a novel orexigenic peptide that antagonizes leptin action through the activation of hypothalamic neuropeptide Y/Y1 receptor pathway. Diabetes 2001;50(2):227–232.
115. Hewson AK, Dickson SL. Systemic administration of ghrelin induces Fos and Egr-1 proteins in the hypothalamic arcuate nucleus of fasted and fed rats. J Neuroendocrinol 2000;12(11):1047–1049.
116. Toshinai K, Date Y, Murakami N, et al. Ghrelin-induced food intake is mediated via the orexin pathway. Endocrinology 2003;144(4):1506–1512.
117. Le Roux CW, Neary NM, Halsey TJ, et al. Ghrelin does not stimulate food intake in patients with surgical procedures involving vagotomy. J Clin Endocrinol Metab 2005;90(8):4521–4524.
118. Le Roux CW, Patterson M, Vincent RP, et al. Postprandial plasma ghrelin is suppressed proportional to meal calorie content in normal-weight but not obese subjects. J Clin Endocrinol Metab 2005;90(2):1068–1071.
119. Shiiya T, Nakazato M, Mizuta M, et al. Plasma ghrelin levels in lean and obese humans and the effect of glucose on ghrelin secretion. J Clin Endocrinol Metab 2002;87(1):240–244.
120. Tschop M, Weyer C, Tataranni PA, et al. Circulating ghrelin levels are decreased in human obesity. Diabetes 2001;50(4):707–709.
121. Nagaya N, Uematsu M, Kojima M, et al. Elevated circulating level of ghrelin in cachexia associated with chronic heart failure: relationships between ghrelin and anabolic/catabolic factors. Circulation 2001;104(17):2034–2038.
122. Otto B, Cuntz U, Fruehauf E, et al. Weight gain decreases elevated plasma ghrelin concentrations of patients with anorexia nervosa. Eur J Endocrinol 2001;145(5):669–673.
123. Cummings DE, Weigle DS, Frayo RS, et al. Plasma ghrelin levels after diet-induced weight loss or gastric bypass surgery. N Engl J Med 2002;346(21):1623–1630.
124. Talsania T, Anini Y, Siu S, et al. Peripheral exendin-4 and peptide YY3-36 synergistically reduce food intake through different mechanisms in mice. Endocrinology 2005;146(9):3748–3756.

3

Endocannabinoids and Energy Homeostasis

Stephen C. Woods, PhD, and Daniela Cota, MD

CONTENTS

INTRODUCTION
THE ENDOCANNABINOID SYSTEM
ENDOCANNABINOID BIOLOGY
ENDOCANNABINOIDS AND REGULATION OF ENERGY BALANCE
ENDOCANNABINOID SYSTEM AND PERIPHERAL METABOLISM
CLINICAL USE OF CB1 AGONISTS
CONCLUSION
REFERENCES

Summary

The body's endogenous endocannabinoid system includes two endogenous agonists for cannabinoid-(CB)-1 receptors, anadamide and 2-arachidonoyl-glycerol (2-AG). Both of these endocannabinoids (ECs) are fatty acid signals derived from cell membranes. They exert a coordinated action at multiple tissues to promote increased food intake, lipogenesis, and storage of fat. Endocannabinoids interact with multiple hypothalamic circuits and transmitter systems to stimulate food intake in general, and they also act in reward areas of the brain to selectively enhance intake of palatable foods. Activation of CB1 receptors increases enzyme activity that causes *de novo* fatty acids to be formed in the liver and circulating lipids to be taken up by fat cells. All these actions are reversed in animals lacking CB1 receptors, and there is growing evidence that activity of the endocannabinoid system is tonically increased in animal and human obesity. Acute or chronic administration of selective synthetic CB1 antagonists to overweight or obese individuals causes weight loss, reduced waist circumference, and an improved lipid and glycemic profile. Developing ligands for endocannabinoid receptors is an important novel therapeutic strategy for the treatment of metabolic dysregulation.

Key Words: Satiety; lipogenesis; obesity; anandamide; 2-arachidonoyl-glycerol; CB1 receptors; food intake; leptin.

INTRODUCTION

Energy Homeostasis

Energy homeostasis is a term that encompasses the collective processes whose goal is to provide adequate supplies of energy to the body's organs. This includes stocking fuel storage depots such as fat and liver cells with ample supplies, as well as recruiting

From: *Contemporary Endocrinology: Treatment of the Obese Patient*
Edited by: R. F. Kushner and D. H. Bessesen © Humana Press Inc., Totowa, NJ

the stored energy back from these depots and distributing them to tissues as needed. It also includes procuring new sources of energy, whether by the consumption of food or by the de novo synthesis of utilizable high-energy molecules by liver and other tissues. All these processes are controlled by a complex and highly integrated network of cells in strategic locations in the body that continuously monitor the energy use and anticipated energy needs of each tissue; at the same time, the network continuously monitors energy available in storage depots, what will be entering the blood from ingested food still within the gastrointestinal system, and energy that may be available to eat in the external environment. Myriad neural and hormonal signals participate in this regulation, with the goal of ensuring that active tissues have what they need when they need it.

The previous decades saw tremendous growth in our understanding of many of the signals involved in energy homeostasis. Dozens of neurotransmitters, neuropeptides, and other signals were newly described and found to fit the general model depicted in Fig. 1. Information relevant to the regulation of energy intake and metabolism is detected by sensory cells in strategic organs, and they in turn generate signals that are relayed to other cells, especially to the brain, so that any necessary action can be taken. Most signals transferring information between cells in the body are derived from modified amino acids (e.g., glutamate and γ-aminobutyric acid [GABA]) or biogenic amines (e.g., serotonin, acetylcholine, and the catecholamines), or are composed of chains of amino acids formed into biologically active peptides. Lipids in the form of steroids have long been known to be important signaling molecules, and other signaling lipids in the form of modified fatty acids have recently been added to the list. Finally, energy-rich molecules themselves, including glucose and some fatty acids, are also recognized to function as key signals in this system. For a review, *see* ref. *(1)*.

Energy Homeostasis and the Endocannabinoid System

In this chapter we review the endocannabinoid system. It represents a novelly described and quite different kind of intercellular signaling system within the body, and we focus on how it influences energy homeostasis as well as how it might be exploited to treat obesity and its complications. Although synthetic and plant-derived cannabinoids such as Δ^9-tetrahydrocannabinol (Δ^9-THC) have long been recognized to influence food intake, it is only relatively recently that endogenous cannabinoids (endocannabinoids [ECs]) generated within the body have been identified, and it is very recently that the scope of their influence on energy homeostasis has started to become revealed, along with potential therapeutic implications.

THE ENDOCANNABINOID SYSTEM

The endocannabinoid system includes cannabinoid receptors called CB1 and CB2 that are located on cell membranes, along with the endogenous ligands that bind to them and the enzymes that synthesize, degrade, and/or reuptake the ligands. Key ligands include the endogenous agonists anandamide and 2-arachidonoyl-glycerol (2-AG). Exogenous compounds can also access and bind to the same receptors, and numerous plant-derived and synthetic CB1 and CB2 agonists and antagonists are available for research and under consideration for therapeutic purposes. Marijuana (*Cannabis sativa*) has long been recognized to stimulate hunger and food intake in addition to its other effects, and Δ^9-THC, its active principle, is an agonist at CB1 receptors in the brain.

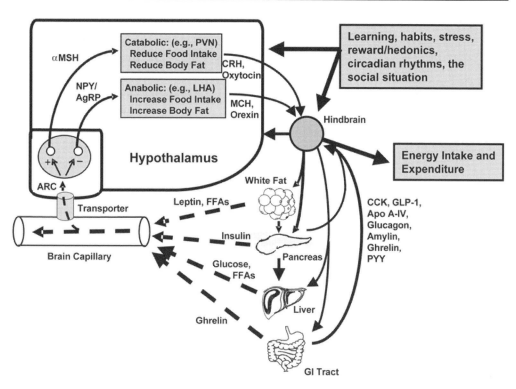

Fig. 1. Model of signals controlling energy homeostasis. During meals, signals such as cholecystokinin (CCK), glucagon-like peptide (GLP)-1, apolipoprotein A-IV (apo A-IV), peptide-YY (PYY), and others that arise from the digestive viscera (stomach, intestine, pancreas, and liver) trigger nerve impulses in sensory nerves traveling to the hindbrain, where they influence meal size. Other signals related to meals such as amylin and ghrelin, and signals related to body fat content such as leptin and insulin, collectively called adiposity signals, circulate in the blood to the brain. Adiposity signals are transported through the blood–brain barrier in the region of the hypothalamic arcuate nucleus (ARC) and interact with catabolic neurons that synthesize proopiomelanocortin (POMC) and secrete α-MSH, or with anabolic neurons that secrete NPY and AgRP. These neurons in turn project to other hypothalamic areas including the paraventricular nuclei (PVN) and the lateral hypothalamic area (LHA). The net output of the PVN is catabolic and includes transmitters such as corticotropin-releasing hormone (CRH) and oxytocin. Signals from the PVN enhance the potency of satiety signals in the hindbrain. The net output of the LHA, on the other hand, is anabolic, and includes melanin-concentrating hormone (MCH) and the orexins. These signals suppress the activity of the satiety signals.

Cannabinoid Receptors

CB1 was the first cannabinoid receptor to be characterized; it is found in the central nervous system, adipose tissue, the liver and many other tissues *(2,3)*. CB2 receptors were subsequently identified and are localized mainly in the immune system; and they share a 48% homology with CB1 *(4–6)*. Both are 7-transmembrane-spanning $G-_{i/o}$ receptors (negatively coupled to adenylyl cyclase and positively coupled to mitogen-activated protein kinase) *(3,5)*. CB1 receptors are also positively coupled to inwardly rectifying potassium channels and negatively coupled to several subtypes of calcium channels *(7,8)*.

Distribution of Cannabinoid Receptors

CB1 receptors are among the most abundant G protein-coupled receptors in the brain, having similar densities as receptors for GABA and glutamate-gated ion channels *(5,9)*. The distribution of CB1 receptors in the central nervous system is heterogeneous, with higher densities in the basal ganglia, hippocampus, and cerebellum *(10)*. Although CB1 expression in the hypothalamus, a key integrative area in the regulation of energy homeostasis, is relatively low, activation of hypothalamic CB1 has profound effects *(9)*. Within the brain, CB1 receptors are expressed by glial astrocytes as well as by neurons *(11)*. Activation of CB1 on astrocytes increases available energy to local neuronal circuits, and the administration of cannabinoid agonists increases overall energy metabolism in the brain *(12)*.

CB1 receptors are also expressed by peripheral nerves and are located on nerve terminals innervating the gastrointestinal tract (as well as within the enteric nervous system *[13–15]*), as well as other organs involved in energy regulation, including white adipose tissue, liver, and skeletal muscle *(16–20)*. There are several recent reviews of the characteristics and functions of CB receptors *(3,5,6,21)*.

Although CB2 receptors are located mainly in tissues of the immune system *(22)*, they have recently also been identified in neurons in several regions of the brain *(23)*. It may therefore be the case that CB1 and CB2 within the brain have differing functions, and that selective CB1 or CB2 ligands could be used to differentiate manipulation of the neural circuits controlling energy homeostasis from those controlling mood, memory, or other behaviors influenced by ECs. Consistent with this, selective CB1 and CB2 ligands were found to differentially influence emesis in ferrets *(23)*.

Endogenous Cannabinoid Ligands

All ECs identified so far are amides, esters, or ethers of arachidonic acid, a long-chain polyunsaturated fatty acid that is a constituent of cell membranes *(3)*. ECs bind both CB1 and CB2 receptors with differential selectivity. Anandamide (the ethanolamide of arachidonic acid) was the first described EC *(24)*, and 2-AG was identified later *(25)*. Other putative ECs that have been identified include noladin ether (ether-linked analog of 2-AG), virhodamine (ester of arachidonic acid and ethanolamine), and N-arachidonoyl dopamine *(3)*. Neither the mechanisms of synthesis and deactivation, nor the specific functions, have been characterized for these other compounds *(21)*.

ENDOCANNABINOID BIOLOGY

Synthesis and Degradation

Both anandamide and 2-AG are synthesized from cell membrane phospholipids, and their biosynthetic pathways have been recently reviewed *(3,5,26,27)*. Unlike the case for many neural signals that are synthesized and stored in vesicles until needed, ECs are made *de novo* as neurons become hyperactive *(28)*, and they are immediately released into the extracellular space of synapses (*see* Fig. 2). As they bind to CB1, a sequence of intracellular events is elicited, and the ECs are then rapidly eliminated via reuptake and degradation by neurons and glial cells *(27,29–31)*. This model of EC synthesis, action, and degradation has been described as an "on demand" process that is utilized by neurons mainly during periods of high-frequency membrane stimulation *(28)* or sudden bursts of

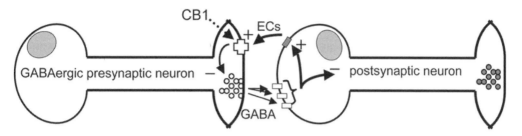

Fig. 2. Model of GABAergic neuron that expresses CB1 receptors. Action potentials in the presynaptic GABAergic neuron cause depolarization of the nerve terminal where synaptic vesicles containing GABA are stored. Some of the GABA is then released into the synaptic cleft, and it diffuses to the postsynaptic neuron and interacts with GABA receptors. This initiates two events. One is inhibition of the postsynaptic neuron, and the other is stimulation of synthesis of endocannabinoids (ECs) from the postsynaptic membrane. The ECs diffuse retrogradely across the synaptic cleft and interact with CB1 receptors on the presynaptic membrane. This has the effect of reducing the amount of GABA released during subsequent depolarizations of the presynaptic membrane. The consequence of this is that there is less inhibition of the postsynaptic membrane as a result of the action of the ECs.

action potentials *(32)*; however, there may be important exceptions to this generality in some areas of the brain.

Distribution

The concentrations of ECs within the brain vary considerably by area *(10,33)*. 2-AG is around two orders of magnitude more abundant than anandamide in most brain areas, with the highest levels of both occurring in the brainstem, hippocampus, and striatum *(34)*; the two can be synthesized in the same tissues independent of one another *(5)*. Both anandamide and 2-AG are also produced in several peripheral tissues, including skin, gut, liver, adipose tissue, and testis *(26,34)*. Anandamide circulates in the blood, where it is bound to albumin *(35)*. Anandamide and 2-AG each bind to both CB1 and CB2 receptors, although with differing affinities. 2-AG is a full agonist at CB1, whereas anandamide is a partial CB1 agonist *(36)*. Anandamide also binds to the transient receptor potential vanilloid receptor 1 (TRPV1 or capsaicin receptor) *(37)*.

Function as Retrograde Neurotransmitter

Many CNS CB1 receptors are localized presynaptically on GABAergic interneurons *(33,38)*. Endocannabinoids released from postsynaptic membranes therefore must diffuse or be transported retrogradely, back across the synaptic cleft, in order to interact with CB1 and thereby decrease the release of presynaptic neurotransmitter, as diagrammed in Fig. 2. The generally accepted model is that when electrical activity in the form of repeated action potentials and consequent depolarization in the presynaptic neuron (a GABAergic neuron in the example in Fig. 2) becomes especially high and sustained, the continuous bombardment of the postsynaptic membrane (by GABA) results in the accumulation of intracellular Ca^{2+} in the postsynaptic neuron. One important consequence of the elevated calcium is that enzymes that synthesize ECs become activated in the postsynaptic neuron's cell membrane, generating anandamide and/or 2-AG. These EC molecules then rapidly diffuse retrogradely back across the synapse, where they bind to CB1 receptors on the presynaptic membrane. Activation of CB1 results in reduced transmitter (GABA) release from the presynaptic neuron in response to further action potentials. Hence, when activity passing across the synapse from the pre- to the postsynaptic neuron becomes sufficiently high, the EC system can be recruited to provide a kind of brake, decreasing the amount of neurotransmitter (GABA in the example) reaching the postsynaptic cell.

Continuing with the same example, because GABA typically has a net inhibitory effect on postsynaptic neurons, as activity in the GABAergic neuron increases, and as the amount of GABA released into the synapse consequently increases, the degree of inhibition of the postsynaptic cell caused by GABA also increases. As this intensifies, intracellular calcium in the postsynaptic cell activates the EC system with the net effect of causing less GABA to be released, consequently reducing the degree of inhibition of the postsynaptic cell. To provide a perhaps more relevant (albeit hypothetical) example, increased activity in a particular presynaptic neuron might be sensitive to signals from the gastrointestinal system during a meal, signals that are integrated with other kinds of information to elicit satiation and ultimately stop ingestion at some point during the meal. This is accomplished through the release of GABA onto (postsynaptic) neurons in circuits that function to prolong the meal. However, on occasions when the food being eaten tastes particularly palatable, or when the social situation is particularly pleasing, other inputs to the same postsynaptic neuron might increase its level of intracellular Ca^{2+}. Hence, when meal-inhibitory inputs in the form of GABA start arriving, the postsynaptic neuron is more likely to initiate the synthesis and release of ECs, ultimately reducing GABA release from the presynaptic neuron. This in turn would result in disinhibition of the postsynaptic neuron with the consequence that the duration of the meal would be prolonged. Conversely, providing a CB1 antagonist would effectively block the disinhibition, resulting in reduced food intake in the same situations. The important point is that activity at CB1 receptors determines the amount of neurotransmitter released from certain presynaptic neurons. Because many CB1 receptors are located on GABAergic neurons, cannabinoid agonists generally have a disinhibiting effect, whereas CB1 antagonists have a net inhibitory effect on those same circuits.

Although CB1 receptors are located on many GABAergic neurons, where they are involved with what has been termed a depolarization-induced suppression of inhibition, they are also found on neurons that have excitatory influences on postsynaptic cells — i.e., some glutamatergic neurons also express CB1, which is therefore involved with depolarization-induced suppression of excitation *(39)*.

Constitutive Release of ECs

Research on EC biology is progressing at a rapid rate. One consequence is that exceptions to the general model proposed above have become apparent. For example, although increased intracellular calcium is necessary for EC synthesis and release in most neuronal circuits *(40)*, others appear to be calcium-independent *(41,42)*. More pertinent to this review, although ECs are generally thought to be synthesized and released only when presynaptic neurons become highly activated, there is evidence for constitutive release, in the absence of external stimulation, in both the hippocampus *(43)* and the arcuate nucleus (ARC) in the hypothalamus *(44)*. In the latter case, neurons in the ARC that synthesize pro-opiomelanocortin (POMC) and that initiate a net catabolic response, including reducing food intake when activated, have been reported to secrete ECs constitutively, in the absence of external stimulation. These locally released ECs in turn suppress presynaptic GABAergic inputs to the same POMC cells. In this situation, the POMC cells are chronically disinhibiting themselves *(44)*. What is particularly intriguing is that when exogenous cannabinoid agonists are administered, they elicit a somewhat different profile of actions than the constitutively released cannabinoids—whereas the endogenously released ECs suppress only the inhibitory GABAergic inputs to the POMC cells, exogenously administered cannabinoids additionally suppress excitatory glutamatergic inputs to the same POMC neurons *(44)*. The adiposity hormone, leptin, has important actions on these same POMC neurons in the ARC. Leptin directly stimulates the POMC neurons *(45)*, and the ability of leptin to reduce food intake depends on the melanocortin transmitters released by the POMC neurons *(46)*. Leptin also reduces EC activity in the ARC, and obese animals deficient in leptin have elevated hypothalamic, but not cerebellar, ECs levels *(47)*, implying that ECs may normally exert a net anabolic tone in the hypothalamus, and especially within the ARC, that favors food intake and fat storage.

ENDOCANNABINOIDS AND REGULATION OF ENERGY BALANCE

Early animal studies demonstrated that systemic or oral administration of Δ^9-THC potently increases food intake. Administration of CB1 antagonists, conversely, blocks the orexigenic action of exogenous cannabinoid agonists and also decreases food intake and body weight in laboratory animals (reviewed in ref. *16*). Based on these promising observations, considerable research is currently under way to elucidate the mechanisms of action of endocannabinoids and to determine the feasibility of using cannabinoid antagonists to treat obesity and its complications *(48,49)*.

Anabolic Actions of Cannabinoids

The endocannabinoid system influences energy balance at many sites in the brain and throughout the body, with the net and highly coordinated effect being anabolic—i.e., increased EC activity enhances food intake and favors the storage of fat. Within the brain, ECs are located in both hypothalamic (where they influence caloric homeostasis by stimulating food intake) and extrahypothalamic (where they influence reward mechanisms, in part by increasing the hedonic value of food) circuits. Both networks contribute to excessive eating when EC activity is high. Within peripheral organs including adipose tissue, liver, and skeletal muscle, locally produced ECs are also anabolic, contributing to lipogenesis and fat storage and reduced energy expenditure. In the gastrointestinal system, ECs are thought to increase fuel absorption and decrease satiety. Hence, the endocannabinoid system is a multileveled, highly coordinated cell-signaling system that biases behavioral and metabolic processes to favor becoming obese. Importantly, the same system is thought to have an important role in facilitating food intake and energy storage during the early stages of life, including facilitating suckling in newborns *(50)*. Consistent with all this, genetic polymorphisms of components of the endocannabinoid system have been associated with overweight and obesity in humans *(51)*.

ENDOCANNABINOID SYSTEM AND THE HYPOTHALAMUS

Arcuate Nucleus. As reviewed in other chapters in this book, the hypothalamus is an important integrative center for the control of energy homeostasis (*see* Fig. 1). Neurons in the hypothalamic ARC are sensitive to the circulating adiposity signals, leptin and insulin *(45,52,53)*, and the ARC in turn projects to many other sites in the hypothalamus and elsewhere in the brain. Two categories of ARC neurons are particularly relevant to this review. ARC POMC neurons synthesize the catabolic neurotransmitter, α-melano-cyte-stimulating hormone (α-MSH), which acts at melanocortin receptors to elicit reduced food intake and body weight. Increased leptin and/or insulin, a signal of increased body fat, stimulates POMC neurons, initiating the catabolic response. As discussed above, POMC cells in the ARC release ECs *(44)*, and leptin inhibits endocannabinoid activity there, facilitating its overall catabolic action *(47)*. The levels of hypothalamic ECs are increased in genetically obese rodents with defective leptin signaling, and treatment of these genetically obese mice with a CB1 antagonist attenuates their hyperphagia and retards their weight gain, implying that overactivation of the endocannabinoid system may be a contributing factor in some animal models of genetic obesity *(47)*.

Other ARC neurons synthesize the anabolic neurotransmitters neuropeptide Y (NPY) and agouti-related protein (AgRP). NPY acts on Y receptors throughout the hypothalamus to stimulate food intake, whereas AgRP antagonizes α-MSH, thus attenuating the catabolic action of POMC cells (*see* reviews in refs. *52,54,55*). It has recently been reported that cannabinoid agonists increase the secretion of NPY in the hypothalamus *(56)*, consistent with ECs increasing food intake. The important point is that hypothalamic circuits controlling energy homeostasis are highly complex, utilizing both anabolic and catabolic transmitters. Understanding the role of the EC system in influencing these circuits is still in its infancy.

Several general statements can be made, however. Hypothalamic 2-AG levels increase during fasting, decline as animals are re-fed, and return to normal values when animals eat to satiation *(57,58)*, consistent with a role in modulating appetite *(59)*. CB1 mRNA has been colocalized with many hypothalamic neuropeptides involved in energy regulation, including corticotropin-releasing hormone (CRH), cocaine–amphetamine-regulated transcript (CART), prepro-orexin, and melanin-concentrating hormone (MCH) *(16)*, and as discussed above, CB1s are also expressed by GABAergic neurons entering the ARC *(44)*.

Intrahypothalamic Cannabinoids Increase Food Intake. Intrahypothalamic administration of Δ^9-THC increases food intake in laboratory rats *(60,61)* and facilitates eating elicited by electrical stimulation of the brain *(62)*. Anandamide also increases food intake when injected into the hypothalamus *(63,64)*, and pretreatment with the selective CB1 antagonist SR141716 (rimonabant) administered intrahypothalamically attenuates anandamide-induced hyperphagia *(63)*. Anandamide also stimulates food intake when administered systemically *(65)*.

CB1 Knockout Animals. Animals lacking CB1 (CB1$^{-/-}$ mice) have reduced food intake, decreased body weight, and a lean phenotype *(16,66,67)*. The brains of these mice have increased levels of neuropeptides that suppress food intake *(16)*, and they do not become obese on a high-fat diet *(66)*. CB1$^{-/-}$ mice have increased sensitivity to the catabolic action of leptin *(66)* and they do not increase their food intake as much as control mice when administered orexigenic compounds such as NPY *(47 68)*. These findings suggest that activation of CB1 is necessary for NPY's orexigenic action. SR 141716 also attenuates the hyperphagia elicited by ghrelin *(69)* and by orexin A *(70)*, and CB1s are coexpressed with orexin 1 receptors *(71)*. Hence, the actions of several orexigenic peptides within the hypothalamus, including NPY, orexin 1, and ghrelin, are facilitated by ECs.

As discussed above, ECs are also important in the hypothalamic POMC/melanocortin system. Administration of SR141716 attenuates the orexigenic effect of melanocortin antagonists (72), but the administration of melanocortin agonists does not block the action of cannabinoid agonists, suggesting that endocannabinoids act "downstream" of melanocortins (72). The important point is that ECs interact with many levels of the neurocircuitry in the hypothalamus and other locations in the brain that control food intake (67).

ENDOCANNABINOID SYSTEM AND BRAIN REWARD SYSTEMS

Limbic System. Brain areas that control hedonic or reward aspects of food, sometimes referred to as "liking" (pleasure/palatability) and "wanting" (appetite/incentive motivation) perceptions associated with the availability and variety of food, include many corticolimbic structures (73–75). This complex system is composed of a series of synaptically interconnected circuits linking the prefrontal cortex, the amygdala, the ventral tegmental area, the nucleus accumbens, and the ventral pallidum. This integrated network connects forebrain, hindbrain, and midbrain areas with hypothalamic areas and is thus able to modulate food intake (74,75).

Palatability. It is widely hypothesized that the rewarding properties of popular foods represent an important obstacle for effective weight control in Western societies. Because of this, systems that control the mechanisms of hedonics and reward value of food are obvious targets for novel pharmacological agents. In the 1970s anecdotal observations of humans smoking marijuana indicated that they have increased appetite and often have induced cravings for palatable foods (reviewed in ref. 76). Studies in rats found increased preference for palatable foods such as sucrose following administration of Δ^9-THC (77). Rats treated with Δ^9-THC in fact overconsume food, eating as much in single meals as rats that have been fasted for a day (78). These observations are consistent with the hypothesis that ECs help mediate palatability or other positive aspects of food (79). This hypothesis has gained support through studies with CB1 antagonists. Systemic SR141716 specifically reduces intake of alcohol, sucrose, and other sweet foods in animals (80–82), and in some reports cannabinoid antagonists reduce the intake of bland foods as well (83 84).

Both anandamide and 2-AG levels are increased in limbic areas of rats that have been fasted, whereas only 2-AG is increased in the hypothalamus (58), indicating both that brain ECs are responsive to fasting and that there are differences in the response between the caloric homeostasis and reward areas of the brain. When rats are ingesting a palatable food, hypothalamic 2-AG levels decrease (85). Rats maintained on a palatable diet for 10 wk, besides becoming obese, express less CB1 mRNA in several limbic areas (85). Further evidence for a direct role of the endocannabinoid system in reward circuits is that when 2-AG was administered directly into the shell of the nucleus accumbens, a limbic area with particularly high levels of CB1 and that is strongly associated with reward processes, a rapid and profound hyperphagia was elicited (58).

Dopamine and Serotonin. The neurotransmitter dopamine (DA) is recognized to be an important mediator of the rewarding effects of food and drugs of abuse (73). CB1 has recently been observed to be coexpressed with dopamine D1 and D2 receptors within the limbic system (86), and marijuana selectively increases DA release in the nucleus accumbens *(87)*. Consistent with this, increased DA and EC levels have been correlated with the craving for palatable foods *(88)*. Serotonin, another neurotransmitter involved with both reward and food intake *(89)*, also interacts with the endocannabinoid system *(90)*. Serotonin 5-HT1B receptors are coexpressed with CB1 in several limbic areas *(86)*, and the combined administration of SR141716 and dexfenfluramine (a drug that increases serotonin activity) have additive effects in reducing food intake *(91)*. Consistent with this, drugs that modulate serotonin activity are frequently prescribed to treat depression, obesity, and/or eating-related disorders *(92)*.

Opioids. ECs also interact with endogenous opioid circuits *(88,93)*. There is considerable anatomical overlap of CB1, opioid receptors, and their respective endogenous ligands in brain areas involved with food intake and reward mechanisms *(10,94,95)*. Levels of endogenous opioids are increased in the hypothalamus following administration of Δ^9-THC to rats *(96,97)*. Conversely, rats chronically treated with the exogenous opioid, morphine, have decreased 2-AG and CB1 in several limbic areas *(98)*. Interactions between the endocannabinoid and opioid systems have been hypothesized to be a critical component for the rewarding aspects of the intake of food and also to provide a molecular basis for drug or food dependence *(99)*. As an example, the administration of selective CB1 agonists increases consumption of palatable beverages in rats; this effect is blocked by the opioid receptor antagonist naloxone *(81)*. When subthreshold doses of naloxone and SR 141716 are combined, they potently suppress food intake and significantly attenuate the hyperphagia caused by the administration of Δ^9-THC *(100)*. There are also synergistic interactions between cannabinoid and opioid antagonists *(101,102)*.

In sum, the endocannabinoid system is positioned in the brain to have a profound influence over the ingestion of food. Within the hypothalamus, ECs interact with circuitry controlling caloric homeostasis and the regulation of body weight, exerting a net anabolic effect. Within the limbic area of the brain, ECs interact with circuitry controlling hedonic or reward aspects of food, again acting to increase ingestion, especially of palatable foods. An important point is that pharmacological manipulation of EC activity, in either direction, has profound effects on food intake.

ENDOCANNABINOID SYSTEM AND PERIPHERAL METABOLISM

CB1 is present in several tissues related to energy homeostasis as well as in peripheral nerve terminals *(14,103)*, consistent with the hypothesis that peripheral metabolic mechanisms might be directly modulated by the endocannabinoid system independent of and in addition to modulation by central pathways.

Sustained Weight Loss With Chronic Cannabinoid Stimulation

When mice are fed a palatable high-fat diet, they overeat and become obese. In one series of experiments, mice maintained on the palatable diet and chronically administered the CB1 antagonist (SR 141716) ate less food *(104–106)*. What is particularly important is that the anorectic action of the antagonists lessened and then disappeared altogether over a week or two in spite of continued dosing, indicating apparent tolerance to the behavioral action *(105)*. Nonetheless, there was a sustained—and, in fact, increased—reduction of body weight and body fat mass over the next several weeks despite the fact that food intake was normal, strongly implying that other actions of the CB1 antagonists were continuing to exert metabolic effects *(104,105)*. At the end of the experiments, mice receiving the CB1 antagonists chronically had reduced body weight, body fat, plasma leptin, and plasma insulin, and an improved lipid profile *(104,105)*, perhaps through the ability of the drug to increase adiponectin expression and secretion from adipose tissue *(17,107)*. Adiponectin, unlike other adipokines, improves insulin sensitivity and induces fatty acid oxidation in muscle and liver *(108)*.

Perhaps related to these findings, experiments using $CB1^{-/-}$ mice revealed that the lean phenotype is caused predominantly by a decrease in caloric intake when the mice are young, whereas peripheral metabolic factors are the major cause of maintaining the lean phenotype in the adults *(16)*. As discussed previously, $CB1^{-/-}$ mice are resistant to diet-induced obesity. They maintain their lean phenotype and they do not develop hyperglycemia or insulin resistance *(66)*. The key point from these experiments is that chronic treatment with a selective CB1 antagonist causes reduction of body fat as well as improvement in many symptoms commonly associated with metabolic syndrome, and although there is an early transient reduction of food intake when animals are started on the antagonist, it cannot account for the sustained improvement in metabolic parameters. The strong inference is that selective CB1 antagonists act directly through other than behavioral means to accomplish this. Consistent with this, chronic treatment with the CB1 antagonist altered gene expression profiles in both white and brown adipose tissue to favor fat oxidation and increased thermogenesis *(106)*.

Adipose Tissue

White adipocytes express CB1 receptors *(16,17,20)*, and in vitro experiments demonstrate that the CB1 agonist WIN-55,212 stimulates adipocyte differentiation and increases the activity of lipoprotein lipase; both actions are blocked by pretreatment with SR 141716 (16). These findings imply that EC activity in white fat has the potential to facilitate growth of new fat cells as well as an enhanced ability to remove fat from circulating lipoproteins and deposit it into fat cells. Furthermore, as adipocytes mature, they express a greater amount of CB1, and CB1 expression is higher in adipocytes of obese as opposed to lean animals *(17)*. Studies in humans also indicate that mature adipocytes have increased CB1 expression as compared to preadipocytes. However, in contrast with the observations reported in obese animals, obese humans have decreased CB1 expression in their adipose tissue relative to lean humans *(20)*.

Energy Expenditure

There is also evidence that ECs reduce energy expenditure. The administration of the CB1 antagonist SR141716 reportedly increases glucose uptake and basal oxygen consumption of skeletal muscle from genetically obese mice *(19)*, and chronic administration of SR141716 elicits increased expression of genes for thermogenesis in brown adipose tissue *(106)*.

Gastrointestinal Tract

The gastrointestinal tract is an important source of signals generated during meals that help to create satiation and limit meal size *(109–111)*. Most meal-generated satiation and satiety signals reach the hindbrain via vagal afferent nerves, and the signal is then relayed to the hypothalamus and other areas in the brain that control food intake. The vagal sensory signals also activate reflexes that travel in vagal efferent nerves back to the gastrointestinal tract. CB1 has been localized in all parts of these circuits, including

Table 1
Key Characteristics and Actions of the Endocannabinoid System

- Endocannabinoids are fatty acid signals derived from arachidonic acid in cell membranes.
- Endocannabinoid agonists act at CB1 receptors in the brain and other organs to cause a net anabolic effect.
- In the brain, endocannabinoids stimulate caloric intake, especially intake of palatable foods, by functioning as retrograde inhibitors of synaptic activity.
- In liver, adipose tissue, skeletal muscle, and the gastrointestinal system, endocannabinoids facilitate the formation and storage of lipids, decrease satiety, and decrease energy expenditure.
- Obesity is characterized by increased levels of endocannabinoids and their receptors; acute or chronic administration of selective CB1 antagonists causes weight loss, loss of body fat, and improved glucose and lipid profiles in overweight and obese patients.

being expressed in vagal afferent nerves *(112)*, neurons in the dorsal vagal complex *(113)*, and vagal efferent nerves *(114)*. The observation that cholecystokinin (CCK) inhibits the expression of CG1 on vagal afferents *(112)* is consistent with CCK's role as a satiety signal that reduces food intake *(109–111)*. In the small intestine, anandamide levels are greatly increased after animals have been fasted, and this effect is reversed when the animals are re-fed *(14)*, again consistent with a role of ECs in influencing food intake via modulation of gastrointestinal signals. ECs in fact modulate many aspects of gastrointestinal function, including gastric emptying and intestinal peristalsis *(15)*.

Liver

There is also evidence that ECs are active in the liver. ECs are produced in the liver *(18)*, where they help regulate hepatic blood flow *(115)*. Activation of CB1 in hepatic tissue increases *de novo* fatty acid synthesis through the induction of lipogenic enzymes *(18)*, and high-fat diet obese mice have increased activity of this hepatic lipogenic pathway as well as elevated expression of CB1 and increased anandamide levels *(18)*.

To summarize, the picture of EC activity that has been developing over the past several years is one of a diverse intercellular communication system that creates a net anabolic tone or bias. This is manifest in the brain as an increased tendency to consume more food, and especially hedonically pleasing food. In several organs including adipose tissue, the liver, skeletal muscle, and the gut, ECs favor the intake of food and the formation and storage of fat while simultaneously decreasing energy expenditure. The observation that the administration of CB1 antagonists to normal and especially obese animals reverses many of these actions implies that CB1 antagonists may be useful for treating obesity and related metabolic complications. These points are summarized in Table 1.

An important and as yet unanswered question is whether the improvement seen in metabolic parameters in adipose tissue, liver, and elsewhere when CB1 antagonists are administered is caused by the drug's blocking the action of constitutively released ECs, or whether the CB1 receptors are "autoactive," providing a constant anabolic tone. Evidence for the latter is that CB1 have been reported to be precoupled to G-protein signaling systems *(116)*, and there is evidence that the CB1 antagonist that was used in the chronic experiments, SR 141716, is an inverse agonist as well as an antagonist at CB1 receptors *(117)*.

CLINICAL USE OF CB1 ANTAGONISTS

SR 141716

The selective CB1 antagonist SR 141716 (rimonabant or Acomplia; Sanofi-Synthelabo), when administered to marijuana smokers, caused weight loss in over-weight and obese subjects without causing adverse side effects *(118)*. Based on this and the promising studies on animals (reviewed previously), SR 141716 has been used in randomized, double-blind clinical trials to determine its efficacy in treating obesity and related metabolic complications. Several Phase III clinical trials named RIO (Rimonabant In Obesity) were initiated starting in 2001 and included more than 6600 overweight or obese patients with or without comorbidities who were given SR141716 (5 or 20 mg) or placebo for up to 2 yr *(119 – 121)*. All subjects were on a calorie-restricted diet and underwent a run-in period of diet alone prior to being randomized to drug or placebo conditions.

RIO Trials

RIO-North America investigated the absolute change in weight during the first year of treatment and the prevention of weight gain after rerandomization in the second year *(119)*, whereas RIO-Europe evaluated change of weight over the entire 2-yr period *(120)*. RIO-Lipids *(121)* and RIO-Diabetes evaluated the effect of rimonabant on the specific comorbidity factors, hyperlipidemia and diabetes, respectively.

There is an impressive consistency across all the studies that have been published to date. Subjects lose weight and have reduced waist circumference, and both the lipid profile and parameters of glucose homeostasis are improved. The effect is dose-dependent, and dropout rates were similar for placebo and drug conditions. In RIO-Lipids, 1036 obese patients with a body mass index (BMI) of 27 to 40 kg/m^2 and dyslipidemia were randomized in a double-blind trial to receive either rimonabant (5 or 20 mg/d) or placebo for 1 yr (Fig. 3) *(121)*. Patients treated with the larger dose (20 mg) lost a mean of 8.6 kg of body weight, which was significantly greater than the 2.3 kg lost by the placebo group following the run-in period. The percentage of patients who lost more than 10% of their body weight was significantly higher in the 20 mg rimonabant group than in the placebo group. Taking 20 mg rimonabant was also associated with a significant reduction in waist circumference, plasma triglycerides, and C-reactive protein, and an increase in HDL cholesterol and plasma adiponectin. There was also a shift to larger particle-sized LDLs in the rimonabant group. With regard to carbohydrate metabolism, patients receiving rimonabant had reduced plasma insulin and fasting glucose, and a reduced glucose area-under-the-curve during an oral glucose tolerance test. Finally, the number of patients in the 20 mg rimonabant group that were classified with metabolic syndrome was significantly reduced. The drug was generally well tolerated; the most frequently reported side effects of receiving 20 mg rimonabant were nausea, dizziness, and upper respiratory tract infections *(121)*.

Comparable results have recently been reported in the RIO-Europe study after 1 yr of treatment, although the subjects in that experiment did not have dyslipidemia *(120)*. Significantly more patients in the 20 mg rimonabant group achieved 5% or more weight loss as well as 10% or more weight loss. They also had sufficient reduction in waist circumference to be associated with a 30% decrease in intra-abdominal adiposity *(122)*. As was seen in RIO-Lipids, there was also a significant improvement in glycemic and

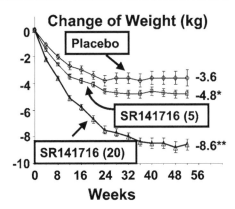

Fig. 3. SR141716 (rimonabant) decreases body weight in overweight and obese humans over the course of 1 yr. In RIO-Europe, a total of 1507 patients with body-mass index 30 kg/m² or greater, or body-mass index greater than 27 kg/m² with treated or untreated dyslipidemia, hypertension, or both, were randomized to receive double-blind treatment with placebo, 5 mg rimonabant, or 20 mg rimonabant once daily in addition to a mild hypocaloric diet (600 kcal/d deficit). ($*p < 0.05$; $** p < 0.01$; redrawn from ref. *120*).

lipid profiles *(120)*. There were no interactions among weight loss and sex, changes in metabolic parameters, or reduction in waist circumference. Importantly, analyses of both studies suggest that the improvement in the lipid and glycemic profiles is greater than could be explained by the decrease of body weight. Hence, as has also been observed in animal experiments, rimonabant causes improved metabolic parameters beyond its effects on food intake and body weight. In summary, the first data obtained from clinical trials indicate that the pharmacological blockade of CB1 has therapeutic potential for the treatment of obesity and its associated risk factors.

CONCLUSION

Endocannabinoids are fatty acid signals derived from cell membranes in the brain and many other tissues. Although they influence numerous systems and behaviors, this review has focused on their coordinated action at multiple tissues to act at CB1 receptors and promote increased food intake, lipogenesis, and the storage of fat. Within the brain, endocannabinoids interact with hypothalamic circuits as well as with reward areas to enhance intake of palatable foods. Within adipose tissue and liver, endocannabinoids increase expression of enzymes that remove fat from the blood and store it in cells, as well as enzymes that facilitate the *de novo* generation of fatty acids. There is also evidence that cannabinoid activity in the gastrointestinal tract and in skeletal muscle also contributes to the net anabolic action. Converging evidence indicates that activity of the endocannabinoid system is tonically increased in animal and human obesity, and that animals lacking cannabinoid receptors are resistant to becoming obese. Consistent with these findings, acute or chronic administration of selective synthetic CB1 antagonists to overweight or obese individuals results in weight loss, reduced waist circumference, and an improved lipid and glycemic profile. Developing ligands for endocannabinoid receptors is an important novel therapeutic strategy for the treatment of metabolic dysregulation.

REFERENCES

1. Seeley RJ,, Woods SC. Monitoring of stored and available fuel by the CNS: implications for obesity. Nat Rev Neurosci 2003;4(11):901–909.
2. Matsuda LA, et al. Structure of a cannabinoid receptor and functional expression of the cloned cDNA. Nature 1990;346(6284):561–564.
3. Piomelli D. The molecular logic of endocannabinoid signalling. Nat Rev Neurosci 2003;4(11):873–884.
4. Munro S, Thomas KL, Abu-Shaar M. Molecular characterization of a peripheral receptor for cannabinoids. Nature 1993;365(6441):61–65.
5. Freund TF, Katona I, Piomelli D. Role of endogenous cannabinoids in synaptic signaling. Physiol Rev 2003;83(3):1017–1066.
6. Howlett AC, et al. International Union of Pharmacology. XXVII. Classification of cannabinoid receptors. Pharmacol Rev 2002;54(2):161–202.
7. Howlett AC, et al. Cannabinoid physiology and pharmacology: 30 years of progress. Neuropharmacology 2004;47 Suppl 1:345–358.
8. Pertwee RG. Pharmacology of cannabinoid CB1 and CB2 receptors. Pharmacol Ther 1997;74(2):129–180.
9. Breivogel CS, Childers SR. The functional neuroanatomy of brain cannabinoid receptors. Neurobiol Dis 1998;5(6 Pt B):417–431.
10. Herkenham M, et al. Characterization and localization of cannabinoid receptors in rat brain: a quantitative in vitro autoradiographic study. J Neurosci 1991;11(2):563–583.
11. Stella N. Cannabinoid signaling in glial cells. Glia 2004;48(4):267–277.
12. Costa B, Colleoni M. Changes in rat brain energetic metabolism after exposure to anandamide or delta(9)-tetrahydrocannabinol. Eur J Pharmacol 2000;395(1):1–7.
13. Pertwee RG. Cannabinoids and the gastrointestinal tract. Gut 2001;48(6):859–867.
14. Gomez R, et al. A peripheral mechanism for CB1 cannabinoid receptor-dependent modulation of feeding. J Neurosci 2002;22(21):9612–9617.
15. Duncan M, Davison JS, Sharkey KA. Endocannabinoids and their receptors in the enteric nervous system. Aliment Pharmacol Therapeut 2005;22:667–683.
16. Cota D, et al. The endogenous cannabinoid system affects energy balance via central orexigenic drive and peripheral lipogenesis. J Clin Invest 2003;112(3):423–431.
17. Bensaid M, et al. The cannabinoid CB1 receptor antagonist SR141716 increases Acrp30 mRNA expression in adipose tissue of obese fa/fa rats and in cultured adipocyte cells. Mol Pharmacol 2003;63(4):908–914.
18. Osei-Hyiaman D, et al. Endocannabinoid activation at hepatic CB(1) receptors stimulates fatty acid synthesis and contributes to diet-induced obesity. J Clin Invest 2005;115(5):1298–1305.
19. Liu YL, et al. Effects of the cannabinoid CB1 receptor antagonist SR141716 on oxygen consumption and soleus muscle glucose uptake in Lep(ob)/Lep(ob) mice. Int J Obes Relat Metab Disord 2005;29(2):183–187.
20. Engeli S, et al. Activation of the peripheral endocannabinoid system in human obesity. Diabetes 2005;54:2838–2843.
21. Begg M, et al. Evidence for novel cannabinoid receptors. Pharmacol Therapeut 2005;106:133–145.
22. Klein TW, et al. The cannabinoid system and immune modulation. J Leucocyte Biol 2003;74:486–496.
23. Van Sickle MD, et al. Identification and functional characterization of brainstem cannabinoid CB2 receptors. Science 2005;310:329–332.
24. Devane WA, et al. Isolation and structure of a brain constituent that binds to the cannabinoid receptor. Science 1992;258(5090):1946–1949.
25. Mechoulam R, et al. Identification of an endogenous 2-monoglyceride, present in canine gut, that binds to cannabinoid receptors. Biochem Pharmacol 1995;50(1):83–90.
26. Sugiura T, et al. Biosynthesis and degradation of anandamide and 2-arachidonoylglycerol and their possible physiological significance. Prostaglandins Leukot Essent Fatty Acids 2002;66(2–3):173–192.
27. Bisogno T, Ligresti A, Di Marzo V. The endocannabinoid signalling system: biochemical aspects. Pharmacol Biochem Behav 2005;81:224–238.
28. Di Marzo ., Bifulco M, De Petrocellis L. The endocannabinoid system and its therapeutic exploitation. Nat Rev Drug Discov 2004;3(9):771–784.
29. Beltramo M, et al. Functional role of high-affinity anandamide transport, as revealed by selective inhibition. Science 1997;277(5329):1094–1097.

30. Hillard CJ, et al. Accumulation of N-arachidonoylethanolamine (anandamide) into cerebellar granule cells occurs via facilitated diffusion. J Neurochem 1997;69:631–638.

31. Hillard CJ, et al. Synthesis and characterization of potent and selective agonists of the neuronal cannabinoid receptor (CB1). J Pharmacol Exp Ther 1999;289(3):1427–1433.

32. Brown SP, Brenowitz SD, Regehr WG. Brief presynaptic bursts evoke synapse-specific retrograde inhibition mediated by endogenous cannabinoids. Nature Neurosci 2003;6:1048–1057.

33. Pazos MR, et al. Functional neuroanatomy of the endocannabinoid system. Pharmacol Biochem Behav 2005;81:239–247.

34. Bisogno T, et al. Brain regional distribution of endocannabinoids: implications for their biosynthesis and biological function. Biochem Biophys Res Commun 1999;256(2):377–380.

35. Bojesen IN, Hansen HS. Binding of anandamide to bovine serum albumin. J Lipid Res 2003;44(9): 1790–1794.

36. Sugiura T, et al. Evidence that the cannabinoid CB1 receptor is a 2-arachidonoylglycerol receptor. Structure-activity relationship of 2-arachidonoylglycerol, ether-linked analogues, and related compounds. J Biol Chem 1999;274(5):2794–2801.

37. Zygmunt PM, et al. Vanilloid receptors on sensory nerves mediate the vasodilator action of anandamide. Nature 1999;400:452–457.

38. Katona I, et al. Presynaptically located CB1 cannabinoid receptors regulate GABA release from axon terminals of specific hippocampal interneurons. J Neurosci 1999;19(11):4544–4558.

39. Alger BE. Retrograde signaling in the regulation of synaptic transmission: focus on endocannabinoids. Prog Neurobiol 2002;68:247–286.

40. Di Marzo V, et al. Formation and inactivation of endogenous cannabinoid anandamide in central neurons. Nature 1994;372:686–691.

41. Kim J, et al. Activation of muscarinic acetylcholine receptors enhances the release of endogenous endocannabinoids in the hippocampus. J Neurosci 2002;22:10,182–10,191.

42. Varma N, et al. Metabotropic glutamate receptors drive the endocannabinoid system in hippocampus. J Neurosci 2001;21:RC188(1–5).

43. Losonczy A, Biro AA, Nusser Z. Persistently active cannabinoid receptors mute a subpopulation of hippocampal interneurons. Proc Natl Acad Sci USA 2004;101:1362–1367.

44. Hentges NT, Low MJ, Williams JT. Differential regulation of synaptic inputs by constitutively released endocannabinoids and exogenous cannabinoids. J Neurosci 2005;25:9746–9751.

45. Xu AW, et al. PI3K integrates the action of insulin and leptin on hypothalamic neurons. J Clin Invest 2005;115:951–958.

46. Seeley R, et al. Melanocortin receptors in leptin effects. Nature 1997;390(Nov 27):349.

47. Di Marzo V, et al. Leptin-regulated endocannabinoids are involved in maintaining food intake. Nature 2001;410(6830):822–825.

48. Pagotto U, et al. The emerging role of the endocannabinoid system in endocrine regulation and energy balance. Endocr Rev 2006;27:73–100.

49. Wadman M, Appetite downer awaits approval. Nature 2005;437:618–619.

50. Fride E, et al. Critical role of the endogenous cannabinoid system in mouse pup suckling and growth. Eur J Pharmacol 2001;419(2–3):207–214.

51. Sipe JC, et al. Overweight and obesity associated with a missense polymorphism in fatty acid amide hydrolase (FAAH). Int J Obes Relat Metab Disord 2005.

52. Schwartz MW, et al. Central nervous system control of food intake. Nature 2000;404(6778):661–671.

53. Woods SC, et al. Signals that regulate food intake and energy homeostasis. Science 1998;280(5368): 1378–1383.

54. Flier JS. Obesity wars: molecular progress confronts an expanding epidemic. Cell 2004;116:337–350.

55. Woods SC, et al. Signals that regulate food intake and energy homeostasis. Science 1998;280:1378–1383.

56. Gamber KM, Macarthur H, Westfall TC. Cannabinoids augment the release of neuropeptide Y in the rat hypothalamus. Neuropharmacology 2005;49:646–652.

57. Hanus L, et al. Short-term fasting and prolonged semistarvation have opposite effects on 2-AG levels in mouse brain. Brain Res 2003;983(1–2):144–51.

58. Kirkham TC, et al. Endocannabinoid levels in rat limbic forebrain and hypothalamus in relation to fasting, feeding and satiation: stimulation of eating by 2-arachidonoyl glycerol. Br J Pharmacol 2002;136(4):550–557.

59. Horvath TL, Endocannabinoids and the regulation of body fat: the smoke is clearing. J Clin Invest 2003;112(3):323–326.

60. Anderson-Baker WC, McLaughlin CL, Baile CA. Oral and hypothalamic injections of barbiturates, benzodiazepines and cannabinoids and food intake in rats. Pharmacol Biochem Behav 1979;11(5):487–491.

61. Verty AN, McGregor IS, Mallet PE. Paraventricular hypothalamic CB(1) cannabinoid receptors are involved in the feeding stimulatory effects of Delta(9)-tetrahydrocannabinol. Neuropharmacology 2005;49:1101–1109.

62. Trojniar W, Wise RA. Facilitory effect of delta 9-tetrahydrocannabinol on hypothalamically induced feeding. Psychopharmacology (Berl) 1991;103(2):172–176.

63. Jamshidi N, Taylor DA. Anandamide administration into the ventromedial hypothalamus stimulates appetite in rats. Br J Pharmacol 2001;134(6):1151–1154.

64. Williams CM, Kirkham TC. Anandamide induces overeating: mediation by central cannabinoid (CB1) receptors. Psychopharmacology (Berl) 1999;143(3):315–317.

65. Hao S, et al. Low dose anandamide affects food intake, cognitive function, neurotransmitter and corticosterone levels in diet-restricted mice. Eur J Pharmacol 2000;392(3):147–156.

66. Ravinet Trillou C, et al. CB1 cannabinoid receptor knockout in mice leads to leanness, resistance to diet-induced obesity and enhanced leptin sensitivity. Int J Obes Relat Metab Disord 2004;28(4):640–648.

67. Wiley JL, et al. CB1 cannabinoid receptor-mediated modulation of food intake in mice. Br J Pharmacol 2005;145:293–300.

68. Poncelet M, et al. Overeating, alcohol and sucrose consumption decrease in CB1 receptor deleted mice. Neurosci Lett 2003;343(3):216–218.

69. Tucci SA, et al. The cannabinoid CB1 receptor antagonist SR141716 blocks the orexigenic effects of intrahypothalamic ghrelin. Br J Pharmacol 2004;143(5):520–523.

70. Hilairet S, et al. Hypersensitization of the orexin 1 receptor by the CB1 receptor: evidence for cross-talk blocked by the specific CB1 antagonist, SR141716. J Biol Chem 2003;278(26):23,731–23,737.

71. Haj-Dahmane S, Shen RY. The wake-promoting peptide orexin-B inhibits glutamatergic transmission to dorsal raphe nucleus serotonin neurons through retrograde endocannabinoid signaling. J Neurosci 2005;25(4):896–905.

72. Verty AN, et al. Evidence for an interaction between CB1 cannabinoid and melanocortin MCR-4 receptors in regulating food intake. Endocrinology 2004;145(7):3224–3231.

73. Berridge KC, Food reward: brain substrates of wanting and liking. Neurosci Biobehav Rev 1996;20(1):1–25.

74. Berthoud HR. Multiple neural systems controlling food intake and body weight. Neurosci Biobehav Rev 2002;26(4):393–428.

75. Kelley AE, et al. Corticostriatal-hypothalamic circuitry and food motivation: Integration of energy, action and reward. Physiol Behav 2005;86:773–795.

76. Abel EL, Cannabis: effects on hunger and thirst. Behav Biol 1975;15(3):255–281.

77. Brown JE, Kassouny M, Cross JK. Kinetic studies of food intake and sucrose solution preference by rats treated with low doses of delta9-tetrahydrocannabinol. Behav Biol 1977;20(1):104–110.

78. Williams CM, Rogers PJ, Kirkham TC. Hyperphagia in pre-fed rats following oral delta9-THC. Physiol Behav 1998;65(2):343–346.

79. Kirkham TC, Williams CM. Endogenous cannabinoids and appetite. Nutr Res Rev 2001;14:65–86.

80. Freedland CS, et al. Effects of SR141716A on ethanol and sucrose self-administration. Alcohol Clin Exper Res 2001;25(2):277–282.

81. Gallate JE, McGregor IS. The motivation for beer in rats: effects of ritanserin, naloxone and SR 141716. Psychopharmacology (Berl) 1999;142(3):302–308.

82. Simiand J, et al. SR 141716, a CB1 cannabinoid receptor antagonist, selectively reduces sweet food intake in marmoset. Behav Pharmacol 1998;9(2):179–181.

83. Colombo G, et al. Appetite suppression and weight loss after the cannabinoid antagonist SR 141716. Life Sci 1998;63(8):PL113–PL117.

84. Freedland CS, Poston JS, Porrino LJ. Effects of SR141716A, a central cannabinoid receptor antagonist, on food-maintained responding. Pharmacol Biochem Behav 2000;67(2):265–270.

85. Harrold JA, et al. Down-regulation of cannabinoid-1 (CB-1) receptors in specific extrahypothalamic regions of rats with dietary obesity: a role for endogenous cannabinoids in driving appetite for palatable food? Brain Res 2002;952(2):232–238.

86. Hermann H, Marsicano G, Lutz B. Coexpression of the cannabinoid receptor type 1 with dopamine and serotonin receptors in distinct neuronal subpopulations of the adult mouse forebrain. Neuroscience 2002;109(3):451–460.

87. Gardner EL, Vorel SR. Cannabinoid transmission and reward-related events. Neurobiol Dis 1998; 5(6 Pt B):502–533.

88. Tanda G, Goldberg SR. Cannabinoids: reward, dependence, and underlying neurochemical mechanisms—a review of recent preclinical data. Psychopharmacology (Berl) 2003169(2):115–134.

89. Rada P, Avena NM, Hoebel BG. Daily bingeing on sugar repeatedly releases dopamine in the accumbens shell. Neuroscience 2005;134:737–744.

90. Wurtman RJ, Wurtman JJ. Brain serotonin, carbohydrate-craving, obesity and depression. Obes Res 1995;3 Suppl 4:477S–480S.

91. Rowland NE, Mukherjee M, Robertson K. Effects of the cannabinoid receptor antagonist SR 141716, alone and in combination with dexfenfluramine or naloxone, on food intake in rats. Psychopharmacology (Berl) 2001;159(1):111–116.

92. Halford JC, et al. Serotonin (5HT) drugs: effects on appetite expression and use for the treatment of obesity. Curr Drug Targets 2005;6:201–213.

93. Fattore L, et al. Cannabinoids and reward: interactions with the opioid system. Crit Rev Neurobiol 2004;16(1–2):147–158.

94. Mansour A, et al. The cloned mu, delta and kappa receptors and their endogenous ligands: evidence for two opioid peptide recognition cores. Brain Res 1995;700(1–2):89–98.

95. Rodriguez JJ, Mackie K, Pickel VM. Ultrastructural localization of the CB1 cannabinoid receptor in mu-opioid receptor patches of the rat caudate putamen nucleus. J Neurosci 2001;21(3):823–833.

96. Corchero J, et al. delta-9-Tetrahydrocannabinol increases prodynorphin and proenkephalin gene expression in the spinal cord of the rat. Life Sci 1997;61(4):PL39–PL43.

97. Corchero J, Fuentes JA, Manzanares J. delta 9-Tetrahydrocannabinol increases proopiomelanocortin gene expression in the arcuate nucleus of the rat hypothalamus. Eur J Pharmacol 1997;323(2–3):193–195.

98. Vigano D, et al. Chronic morphine modulates the contents of the endocannabinoid, 2-arachidonoyl glycerol, in rat brain. Neuropsychopharmacology 2003;28(6):1160–1167.

99. Corchero J, Manzanares J, Fuentes JA. Cannabinoid/opioid crosstalk in the central nervous system. Crit Rev Neurobiol 2004;16(1–2):159–172.

100. Kirkham TC, Williams CM. Synergistic effects of opioid and cannabinoid antagonists on food intake. Psychopharmacology (Berl) 2001;153(2):267–270.

101. Chen RZ, et al. Synergistic effects of cannabinoid inverse agonist AM251 and opioid antagonist nalmefene on food intake in mice. Brain Res 2004;999(2):227–230.

102. Williams CM, Kirkham TC. Reversal of delta 9-THC hyperphagia by SR141716 and naloxone but not dexfenfluramine. Pharmacol Biochem Behav 2002;71(1–2):333–340.

103. Massa F, et al. The endogenous cannabinoid system protects against colonic inflammation. J Clin Invest 2004;113(8):1202–1209.

104. Hildebrandt AL, Kelly-Sullivan DM, Black SC. Antiobesity effects of chronic cannabinoid CB1 receptor antagonist treatment in diet-induced obese mice. Eur J Pharmacol 2003;462(1–3):125–132.

105. Ravinet Trillou C, et al. Anti-obesity effect of SR141716, a CB1 receptor antagonist, in diet-induced obese mice. Am J Physiol Regul Integr Comp Physiol 2003;284(2):R345–R353.

106. Jbilo O, et al. The CB1 receptor antagonist rimonabant reverses the diet-induced obesity phenotype through the regulation of lipolysis and energy balance. FASEB J 2005;19:1567–1569.

107. Poirier B, et al. The anti-obesity effect of rimonabant is associated with an improved serum lipid profile. Diabetes Obes Metab 2005;7(1):65–72.

108. Yamauchi T., et al. Adiponectin stimulates glucose utilization and fatty-acid oxidation by activating AMP-activated protein kinase. Nat Med 2002;8(11):1288–1295.

109. Moran TH, Kinzig, KP. Gastrointestinal satiety signals II. Cholecystokinin. Am J Physiol 2004;286:G183–G188.

110. Strader AD, Woods SC. Gastrointestinal hormones and food intake. Gastroenterology 2005;128(1):175–191.

111. Woods SC. Gastrointestinal satiety signals I. An overview of gastrointestinal signals that influence food intake. Am J Physiol 2004;286:G7–G13.

112. Burdyga G, et al. Expression of cannabinoid CB1 receptors by vagal afferent neurons is inhibited by cholecystokinin. J Neurosci 2004;24:2708–2715.

113. Van Sickle MD, et al. Delta9-tetrahydrocannabinol selectively acts on CB1 receptors in specific regions of dorsal vagal complex to inhibit emesis in ferrets. Am J Physiol 2003;285:G566–G576.
114. Derbenev AV, Stuart TC, Smith BN. Cannabinoids suppress synaptic input to neurones of the rat dorsal motor nucleus of the vagus nerve. J Physiol (Lond) 2004;559:923–938.
115. Batkai S, et al. Endocannabinoids acting at vascular CB1 receptors mediate the vasodilated state in advanced liver cirrhosis. Nat Med 2001;7(7):827–832.
116. Mukhopadhyay S, et al. The CB(1) cannabinoid receptor juxtamembrane C-terminal peptide confers activation to specific G proteins in brain. Mol Pharmacol 2000;57:162–170.
117. Bouaboula M, et al. A selective inverse agonist for central cannabinoid receptor inhibits mitogen-activated protein kinase activation stimulated by insulin or insuloin-like growth factor 1. Evidence for a new model of receptor/ligand interactions. J Biol Chem 1997;272:22,330–22,339.
118. Huestis MA, et al. Blockade of effects of smoked marijuana by the CB1-selective cannabinoid receptor antagonist SR141716. Arch Gen Psychiatry 2001;58(4):322–328.
119. Cleland JG, et al. Clinical trials update and cumulative meta-analyses from the American College of Cardiology: WATCH, SCD-HeFT, DINAMIT, CASINO, INSPIRE, STRATUS-US, RIO-Lipids and cardiac resynchronisation therapy in heart failure. Eur J Heart Fail 2004;6(4):501–508.
120. Van Gaal LF, et al. Effects of the cannabinoid-1 receptor blocker rimonabant on weight reduction and cardiovascular risk factors in overweight patients: 1-year experience from the RIO-Europe study. Lancet 2005;365(9468):1389–1397.
121. Després JP, Golay A, Sjöström L. Effects of rimonabant on metabolic risk factors in overweight patients with dyslipidemia. N Engl J Med 2005;353:2121–2134.
122. Despres JP, Lemieux I, Prud'homme D. Treatment of obesity: need to focus on high risk abdominally obese patients. Br Med J 2001;322(7288):716–720.

4

Obesity and Adipokines

Nicole H. Rogers, MS, Martin S. Obin, PhD, and Andrew S. Greenberg, MD

CONTENTS

INTRODUCTION TO ADIPOSE TISSUE
INFLAMMATORY ALTERATIONS IN ADIPOSE TISSUE WITH OBESITY
ROLE OF REGIONAL ADIPOSE TISSUE DEPOTS IN METABOLISM
PATHOLOGY-ASSOCIATED CHANGES IN ADIPOKINES
CONCLUSION
REFERENCES

Summary

Adipose tissue (AT) is composed of adipocytes and a diverse population of nonadipocytes that are commonly referred to as stromal–vascular cells. Adipose tissue has traditionally been considered a passive storage energy depot that, indeed, does serve as a long-term reservoir for fuel stored as triglyceride. However, laboratory, clinical, and epidemiological studies over the past decade have redefined and greatly expanded our understanding of the physiological role of AT. We now appreciate that AT is an endocrine organ with important roles in maintaining whole-body energy homeostasis and systemic metabolism. This appreciation derives in large part from the identification of multiple AT-secreted factors that modulate central and peripheral processes. These include free fatty acids, which have significant effects on glucose and insulin homeostasis, as well as bioactive peptides termed adipokines. Adipokines act in an autocrine, paracrine, and/or endocrine fashion to promote metabolic homeostasis, and integrate adipose tissue, liver, muscle, and CNS physiology.

There are currently more than 50 known adipokines, as well as locally generated hormones and metabolites that, together, affect multiple physiological functions including food intake, glucose homeostasis, lipid metabolism, inflammation, vascular tone, and angiogenesis. Because they affect such diverse and important processes, regulation of adipokine secretion from AT is critically important to regulating systemic metabolism. Notably, increased AT mass (as in obesity) induces characteristic qualitative and quantitative changes in adipose tissue metabolism and adipokine secretion. These changes are now implicated in the development of metabolic syndrome and its progression to more severe obesity-associated pathologies, including type 2 diabetes and cardiovascular disease.

Key Words: Adiponectin; leptin; adipose tissue; adipocyte; cytokine; tumor necrosis factor-α; adipokines; mononcyte-chemoattractant protein; interleukin-6; inflammation; plasminogen activator inhibitor-1; 11-β hydroxydehydrogenase-1.

From: *Contemporary Endocrinology: Treatment of the Obese Patient*
Edited by: R. F. Kushner and D. H. Bessesen © Humana Press Inc., Totowa, NJ

INTRODUCTION TO ADIPOSE TISSUE

Adipose tissue (AT) is composed of adipocytes and a diverse population of nonadipocytes that are commonly referred to as stromal–vascular cells (SVC). Adipose tissue has traditionally been considered a passive storage energy depot that serves as a long-term reservoir for fuel stored as triglyceride. However, laboratory, clinical, and epidemiological studies over the past decade have redefined and greatly expanded our understanding of the physiological role of AT. We now appreciate that AT is an endocrine organ with important roles in maintaining whole-body energy homeostasis and systemic metabolism. This appreciation derives in large part from the identification of multiple AT-secreted factors that modulate central and peripheral processes. These include free fatty acids (FFA), which have significant effects on glucose and insulin homeostasis, as well as bioactive peptides termed adipokines. Adipokines act in an autocrine, paracrine, and/or endocrine fashion to promote metabolic homeostasis, and integrate adipose tissue, liver, muscle, and CNS physiology.

There are currently more than 50 known adipokines, as well as locally generated hormones and metabolites that, together, affect multiple physiological functions including food intake, glucose homeostasis, lipid metabolism, inflammation, vascular tone, and angiogenesis (Fig. 1) (1). Because they affect such diverse and important processes, regulation of adipokine secretion from AT is critically important to regulating systemic metabolism. Notably, increased AT mass (as in obesity) induces characteristic qualitative and quantitative changes in adipose tissue metabolism and adipokine secretion. These changes are now implicated in the development of metabolic syndrome and its progression to more severe obesity-associated pathologies, including type 2 diabetes and cardiovascular disease.

The goal of this chapter is to provide the practicing physician with an overview of clinically relevant adipokines, the pathophysiological impacts of their dysregulation in obesity, and current therapies directed at ameliorating this dysregulation and/or its sequelae.

Before describing the specific actions of adipokines, it is important to understand that adipocytes have an active role in modulating normal health. Our understanding of the role of adipocytes in maintaining normal metabolism was enhanced by a series of elegant experiments that utilized mice that were genetically engineered to not express adipocytes. These fatless, or lipoatrophic, mice were found to have elevated circulating levels of fatty acids, hyperglycemia, and hypertriglyceridemia. Additional abnormalites included increased hyperglycemia and insulin resistance (2). Remarkably, transplantation of adipocytes back into the lipoatrophic mice normalized many of these metabolic parameters. These observations could be explained by the fact that adipocytes serve as a reservoir of fatty acids and/or secrete hormones that modulate systemic metabolism.

Leptin

The discovery that was perhaps the greatest catalyst in propelling understanding of adipokines was that of leptin. The discovery of this adipocyte hormone was revealed by the identification of a single gene and its protein product that was able to explain the phenotype of the *ob/ob* mouse, a recessive, genetic model of obesity (3). *Ob/ob* mice are extremely hyperphagic, obese, insulin-resistant, and infertile. By using genetic analysis, it was discovered that these mice produced a mutant RNA for the leptin protein. The product of the ob gene was termed leptin, which is both exclusively synthesized and

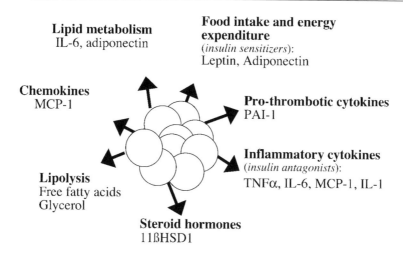

Fig. 1. Adipose tissue as an endocrine organ.

secreted by adipocytes and circulates in the blood. Possibly owing to an estrogen effect, serum levels are higher in females than males, even after correcting for body fat *(4)*. Administration of leptin to ob/ob mice demonstrated proof of the concept, as it significantly reduced food intake while ameliorating obesity, insulin resistance, hyperlipidemia, and abnormal glucose homeostasis *(5,6)*. Initial experiments demonstrated that ob/ob mice were extremely sensitive to leptin's ability to modulate food intake by acting on the hypothalamus. By crossing the blood–brain barrier and directly affecting hypothalamic pathways, leptin activates anorexigenic signals and suppresses orexigenic signals. Leptin thus controls appetite via the hypothalamic network, and the lack of leptin signaling to the hypothalamus sends a very strong message of hunger *(7)*. There are extremely rare obese individuals who, secondary to genetic abnormalities, do not express leptin and who, upon exogenous adminstration of leptin, will have a significant decrease in body weight, primarily by reducing appetite *(8)*.

Interestingly, leptin may act beyond the central nervous system and exert peripheral effects. In rodents leptin directly acts on muscle cells, adipocytes, and the β-cells of the pancreas to increase energy expenditure *(9)*. One of the most exciting observations was that leptin directly activates an intracellular signaling pathway resulting in activation of AMP-activated kinase (AMPK) in mouse skeletal muscle *(10)*. In animals as well as humans, AMPK, the metabolic sensor of the cell, is activated by both exercise and antidiabetic drugs such as thiazolidinediones (TZDs). One of the most significant effects of AMPK is its ability to increase fatty acid oxidation by promoting entry of fatty acids into mitochondria and inhibiting lipogenesis. In addition, AMPK, similar to insulin, increases glucose uptake in skeletal muscle *(11)*.

Leptin treatment of lipoatrophic mice was found to ameliorate the associated insulin resistance and diabetes *(12)*. These studies in rodents were followed by pioneering studies in lipoatrophic humans who lack fat. Lipoatrophic diabetes is an extremely rare condition in humans. In general, individuals with lipoatrophic diabetes have hypertriglyceridemia, sometimes reaching levels that require plasmapheresis. These individuals suffer from ectopic fat deposition in skeletal muscle and liver, the latter resulting in hepatomegaly and steatohepatitis. In addition, these individuals often are hyperglycemic to the point of requiring antidiabetic medicines. In a series of exciting studies, investigators at the NIH found that leptin administration in lipoatrophic individuals, in general, ameliorated the diabetes, steatohepatitis, and hypertriglyceridemia *(13,14)*. As far as the underlying mechanisms, although leptin significantly reduced food intake, there are also data from human studies to suggest that leptin may be acting on peripheral tissues to ameliorate this metabolic disorder *(14)*. In addition, although it is beyond the scope of this chapter, leptin has also been suggested to be important in modulating the neurohormonal regulation of puberty *(15)*.

Although initial hopes were raised that exogenous leptin administration might ameliorate human obesity, it soon become apparent that with increasing obesity, leptin levels actually go up. This observation suggested that obese humans develop resistance to the antiobesity effects of leptin. Consistent with this hypothesis, exogenous administration of supraphysiologic levels of leptin to obese individuals in general did not ameliorate obesity *(16)*. Investigations in animals revealed that leptin can increase an intracellular protein that blocks leptin effects on intracellular pathways, reducing its efficacy.

One possible therapeutic role for leptin in body weight regulation may be in maintaining long-term weight loss. Obese individuals who lose weight have a significantly reduced metabolic rate and reduced thyroid hormone levels *(17,18)*. Weight-reduced humans have decreased leptin levels. Administration of leptin to these individuals appears to maintain energy expenditure, skeletal muscle work efficiency, and thyroid hormone levels, thus enhancing the likelihood of maintaining weight loss. These and other studies have suggested that leptin, though increased in response to fasting, may act as a "thermostat" to maintain body weight at a certain set point. With weight loss in obese individuals, reduced leptin levels may act to reduce metabolic and hormonal pathways and increase appetite as a means to return to previous weight levels. Conversely, increases in obesity may result in leptin resistance.

In summary, leptin is an extremely important adipokine whose secretion and synthesis is increased with obesity. Leptin appears to regulate both central and peripheral pathways that modulate energy and metabolic homeostasis. Unfortunately, with obesity, individuals become resistant to these salutary benefits of leptin. Leptin—and understanding leptin physiology—may ultimately prove beneficial to the maintenance of lost weight. Additionally, the discovery of leptin was the initial, critical finding that has catalyzed the understanding of central pathways that regulate food intake.

Adiponectin

Adiponectin, also called gelatin-binding protein (GBP)28 *(19)*, adipocyte complement-related protein (Acrp30) *(20)*, AdipoQ *(21)*, and adipose most abundant gene transcript 1 (apMI) *(22)*, was discovered at approximately the same time as leptin, in 1995. Similar to leptin, adiponectin is expressed exclusively by mature adipocytes, and increases dramatically with differentiation of preadipocytes to adipocytes *(23)*. However, unlike leptin, its expression does not increase with obesity, but as will be discussed later, it decreases. Adiponectin circulates in plasma in the microgram-per-milliliter range, which is the highest plasma concentration of any of the adipose-secreted proteins, most of which are in the nanogram-per-milliliter range *(24)*. Production of both leptin and adiponectin production is higher in subcutaneous fat than the deeper visceral depots *(25)*, and similarly, the concentration of this hormone tends to be higher in females than in males *(26)*.

Interestingly, adiponectin proteins can bind to each other in varying numbers, and the resulting combinations appear to have differing levels of importance in terms of their effects on metabolic homeostasis. In particular, adiponectin circulates as low-molecular-weight (LMW) and high-molecular-weight (HMW) forms *(27)*. The HMW form has been shown to be the most metabolically active, with its primary effects thought to be on the liver *(28)*. Initially, a fragment of the adiponectin molecule lacking the N-terminus, referred to as the "globular domain," was thought to have significant metabolic effects, as suggested by animal studies *(29)*. However, its presence has not yet been confirmed and it most likely does not normally circulate in humans, leaving the physiological significance unclear *(30)*.

Adiponectin, like leptin, has a critical role in whole-body metabolism and insulin sensitivity. This adipocyte hormone appears to significantly affect liver metabolism, where it suppresses hepatic glucose output *(31)*. The antidiabetic drugs, TZDs, are known to increase adiponectin expression *(32)*. Like leptin and TZDs, adiponectin has been shown to activate AMPK. In fact, in adiponectin-deficient mice, TZDs cannot activate AMPK in liver and muscle *(33)*. Unlike leptin, adiponectin levels decrease with obesity *(34)*. Such reduced levels of adiponectin have been suggested to significantly increase the risk of developing metabolic disorders such as metabolic syndrome, diabetes, and atherosclerosis.

Studies of adiponectin polymorphisms pointed toward the importance of alterations in this protein in promoting deleterious metabolic disorders and obesity. Kissebah et al. used genetic mapping techniques to demonstrate that the chromosomal adiponectin gene location is strongly correlated with components of metabolic syndrome in patients *(35)*. Polymorphisms in the adiponectin gene have been linked with risk for diabetes *(36)*. Polymorphisms resulting in hypoadiponectinemia are additionally associated with insulin resistance, diabetes, and cardiovascular disease (CVD), and polymorphisms in the receptor have also been associated with diabetes *(37)*.

In addition, adiponectin gene polymorphisms have been associated with severe obesity in both children and adults *(38)*. Although adiponectin is the only known adipose-specific protein that declines with obesity *(39)*, weight loss significantly increases adiponectin levels *(40)*. Rimonabant, a drug recently developed to treat obesity and metabolic syndrome, significantly increased serum adiponectin levels in patients *(41)*.

Case-control studies have shown altered adiponectin levels to be an independent risk factor for the development of type 2 diabetes *(42,43)*. Increased plasma levels of this protein are associated with increased insulin sensitivity and glucose tolerance *(44)*. Decreased circulating adiponectin, as well as decreased adipose tissue concentrations, are associated with insulin resistance *(45,46)*. For example, in obese monkeys as well as humans that develop diabetes, the fall in adiponectin levels strongly correlates with the onset of insulin resistance *(47,48)*.

Mice lacking adiponectin have diet-induced insulin resistance *(49)*, and administration of adiponectin to rodent models of type 2 diabetes results in a very significant improvement in insulin resistance *(50)*. Full-length adiponectin has been demonstrated to increase AMPK activity in both liver and skeletal muscle *(51)*. Importantly, these insulin-sensitizing effects are seen even in normal animals *(52)*. Adiponectin administration also reverses the insulin resistance observed in lipoatrophic mice, known to have low adiponectin levels *(50)*.

Interestingly, it has been shown that even without a change in total serum adiponectin levels, increasing the proportion of complexes that are in the HMW form increases insulin sensitivity *(53)*. Intriguingly, TZDs increase the ratio of HMW multimers, which is thought to have greater ameliorative effects on metabolic abnormalities than total adiponectin *(54)*. Likewise, some patients with changes in total adiponectin values, but no difference in the proportion that are of the HMW form, fail to see improvement in insulin sensitivity *(53)*. As a result of these findings, the Scherer lab has coined the term "adiponectin sensitivity index" (S_A), which refers to the relative level of HMW form of adiponectin to total adiponectin in circulation *(53)*.

Adiponectin abnormalities have also been implicated in the development of atherosclerosis. Markers of dyslipidemia, including low HDL-C levels, hypertriglyceridemia, and smaller, denser LDL-C, have all been correlated with hypoadiponectinemia, independent of body fat *(55)*. Furthermore, higher serum triglycerides, apo B-48, and apo C-III levels are predicted by low serum adiponectin levels *(56)*. Hypoadiponectinemia is also an independent risk factor for developing hypertension *(57)* and heart disease *(58)*, and patients with coronary heart disease have lower concentrations of adiponectin than controls, even after controlling for body mass index (BMI) *(47,59)*.

Likewise, animal models demonstrate that exogenous administration of adiponectin protects against the development of diet-induced atherosclerosis *(60)*, as well as limiting damage in an experimental animal model of acute myocardial infarction *(61)*. Mechanistically, it seems that adiponectin can stimulate nitric oxide production in vascular endothelial cells, thus increasing vasodilation *(62)*. Furthermore, adiponectin is thought to stimulate angiogenesis. Accordingly, mice lacking adiponectin have decreased angiogenic activity following ischemia, and overexpression of adiponectin increases angiogenesis *(61)*.

Adiponectin also inhibits vascular smooth muscle cell proliferation, as well as inhibiting expression of scavenger receptor class A proteins *(58)*, which are thought to recruit atherogenic lipid particles into macrophages. The antiatherogenic capabilities of adiponectin may also be due in part to its anti-inflammatory properties. By inhibiting myocardial expression of tumor necrosis factor (TNF)-α, adiponectin decreases expression of monocyte adhesion molecules in the vascular wall and inhibits the transformation of macrophages to foam cells. Furthermore, adiponectin inhibits plaque formation by downregulating adhesion molecules such as vascular cell adhesion molecule (VCAM) *(63)*.

Very recently, a new family of highly conserved proteins, homologous to adiponectin, has been identified *(64)*. In vitro models suggest that some of these "adiponectin paralogs" may have metabolic effects similar to adiponectin, rendering them plausible pharmacological targets.

In summary, adiponectin blocks many key components of the atherogenic process, and is currently a very promising drug target for preventing atherosclerosis.

INFLAMMATORY ALTERATIONS IN ADIPOSE TISSUE WITH OBESITY

The profile of adipokines synthesized and secreted in adipose tissue changes dramatically as individuals become obese. One of the first clues that adiposity alters adipose tissue function was that adiposity was associated with increased expression of inflammatory cytokines, in particular TNF-α and interleukin (IL)-6 *(65)*. TNF-α is a member of a family of secreted proteins that are characteristically produced by immune cells. Cytokines can exert their effect locally via paracrine/autocrine signaling, as well as circulating in the blood to act on distal tissues. TNF-α was initially implicated in the pathogenesis of the cachexia associated with cancer and infectious diseases. In fact, one laboratory initially referred to TNF-α as cachetin (66). It was therefore an initial surprise to find that obese individuals had increased expression levels of TNF-α in their adipose tissue (67,68).

Subsequent studies demonstrated a second AT-derived cytokine, IL-6, to be elevated in the serum of obese individuals and significantly correlated with FFA levels (69). Interestingly, more than 90% of IL-6 in adipose tissue was produced by nonadipocyte cells. In 2003 two separate laboratories independently reported a key observation concerning the appearance of macrophages in obese adipose tissue (70,71). There was a strong correlation between macrophage numbers with increasing adipocyte cell size (essentially reflecting increasing amounts of adipocyte triglyceride) and obesity. Adipose tissue macrophages were found to secrete several cytokines, including TNF-α and IL-6, as well as bioactive mediators of nitric oxide. These cytokines and other inflammatory mediators produced by macrophages are thought to alter adipocyte metabolism and function, as well as adipokine profile (72,73), and are further discussed later in the "TFN-α" and "IL-6" sections.

Interestingly, macrophage infiltration in adipose tissue appeared to precede or coincide with significant insulin resistance in obese rodents. The underlying mechanism(s) of macrophage infiltration remains unclear. The immune factor, monocyte chemotactic protein (MCP)-1 is one factor that has been suggested to be involved in recruiting macrophages in adipose tissue (74). Macrophages in obese animals and humans have been described to predominantly localize and form granuloma-type structures around dead adipocytes (75). It remains unclear whether the necrotic adipocytes promote macrophage infiltration into adipose tissue or if the macrophages enter the adipose tissue and actually kill adipocytes. Regardless, the residual insoluble triglyceride droplet from dead adipocytes may be viewed by the body as analogous to a foreign body, as the macrophages appear to surround, sequester, and scavenge the residual lipid droplet in similar manner.

Future studies (including those in our own laboratory) are aimed at understanding the basis of macrophage infiltration, adipocyte cell death, and adipose tissue inflammation. New information regarding the inflammatory state in obese adipose tissue, as well as how inflammatory cells contribute to or are causal to obesity-related diseases, will be critical to future pharmacological intervention.

Obesity is associated with increased fatty acids, one of the products of adipocyte lipolysis. Fatty acids are released from adipose tissue and then enter the circulation. Increases in circulating levels of fatty acids have been demonstrated to promote insulin resistance in both skeletal muscle and liver, as well as increase hepatic gluconeogenesis (76,77). The role and regulation of fatty acids in metabolism and obesity are discussed in detail in Chapter 5 of this book.

ROLE OF REGIONAL ADIPOSE TISSUE DEPOTS IN METABOLISM

In discussing the role of adipose tissue in modulating systemic metabolism, although controversial to some, we will now address the growing evidence suggesting that different adipose tissue depots may each have distinct influences on metabolism. It has been observed that insulin-resistant individuals often have increased central or visceral fat, or more specifically, increased fat accumulation in omental and mesenteric anatomic regions. Fatty acids and cytokines secreted from omental and mesenteric fat empty into the portal vein, directly exposing the liver to these factors. As the liver is important in regulating glucose and very-low-density lipoprotein (VLDL) production, these factors may influence hepatic metabolism. Recent reports also suggest that visceral adiposity, but not total adiposity, is a better determinant of metabolic disturbance such as insulin resistance *(78,79)*. Finally, antidiabetic drugs such as TZDs have been shown to differentially affect the various fat depots—for example, reducing central fat accumulation while increasing subcutaneous fat *(80)*. It seems that as active investigation of this area continues, accumulating evidence may point to a potential differential role for the various AT depots in promoting abnormalities such as insulin resistance.

PATHOLOGY-ASSOCIATED CHANGES IN ADIPOKINES

Tumor Necrosis Factor-α

Of recent intense study, TNF-α has been at the center of attention as a mediator of obesity. Earlier observations in the literature revealed that adipose tissue expression of TNF-α was positively correlated with insulin resistance in humans *(67–69)* and that as humans became obese, adipose tissue expression of TNF-α increased *(67)*. It is now known that the vast majority, approx 95%, of TNF-α in adipose tissue of obese individuals is synthesized by macrophages, with only a small percentage released from adipocytes *(81)*. Nonetheless, it is not well understood how these two sources of TNF-α, from both the adipocytes themselves and the infiltrated macrophages, contribute to obesity-associated disease etiology.

In general, plasma levels of TNF-α are low and do not correlate with obesity or insulin resistance *(69)*. It is known that one role for TNF-α is for it to stimulate an increase in expression of other proinflammatory molecules, such as IL-6 and MCP-1 *(82)*, as well as to positively feed back on its own expression *(73)*. Thus, it is currently believed that circulating TNF-α is likely to be contributing to the chronic inflammation accompanying obesity through this cytokine amplification cascade.

Animal data indicate that this cytokine, when found in increased amounts in plasma, does promote insulin resistance in peripheral tissues. When rats are chronically administered TNF-α, skeletal muscle is less able to utilize glucose in response to insulin *(83)*. Incubation of adipocytes with TNF-α increases lipolysis *(84,85)*, downregulates glucose transporter type 4 (GLUT4) receptors in adipose tissue *(83)*, and interferes with the insulin signaling cascade *(86)*. Mice that lack TNF-α receptors and TNF-α protein are protected from obesity-induced insulin resistance. These animals also display decreased circulating FFA, as well as protection from obesity-induced defects in insulin signaling in both muscle and adipose tissue *(87)*.

Unfortunately, in vivo human research is less conclusive. In obesity, adipose tissue TNF-α does not appear to be secreted into the bloodstream; however, adipose tissue TNF-α does correlate with insulin resistance *(69,88)*. Presumably the cytokine influences systemic metabolism by altering adipocyte gene and protein expression as well as metabolism. Along these lines, cellular studies indicate that TNF-α may reduce the mRNA and protein expression of adiponectin *(73)*.

Treatment of obese humans with TZDs reduces adipose tissue production of TNF-α and adipose tissue inflammation. However, treatment of obese patients and type 2 diabetics with neutralizing TNF-α antibodies did not improve insulin sensitivity *(89)*. Interpretation of these antibody studies is confounded, however, by whether the administered antibodies actually have access to the TNF-α within the different adipose depots. Interestingly, TNF-α may contribute to the development of obesity-associated sleep apnea. Administration of anti-TNF-α appears to improve sleep apnea *(90)*.

In summary, with obesity, adipose tissue produces increased amounts of TNF-α. The primary source of this cytokine appears to be macrophages. The cytokine is not secreted by adipose tissue in significant amounts. However, it appears to alter systemic metabolism by increasing adipocyte lipolysis, releasing fatty acids into the circulation, and reducing adipocyte production of adiponectin.

Interleukin-6

IL-6 is a pleiotropic cytokine produced by adipose tissue, immune cells *(91)*, and contracting muscle fibers *(92)*. It functions by activating various signaling cascades via binding to receptors, which exist in both membrane-bound and soluble forms. It has been shown to have multiple, sometimes contradictory, physiological effects on the periphery, particularly muscle, liver, and endothelium.

Visceral depots release two to three times as much IL-6 as subcutaneous adipocytes *(93)*, and high levels of this cytokine are found circulating in the serum. It has been estimated that up to 35% comes from adipose tissue *(88)*; thus, the majority of circulating IL-6 is derived from nonadipose sources.

As an inflammatory molecule, IL-6 is involved in the immune system's host defense to tissue injury. As mentioned earlier, it is thought that IL-6 expression in adipose tissue is induced in a paracrine fashion by other proinflammatory molecules, such as TNF-α *(94)*, though whether IL-6 itself is proinflammatory or anti-inflammatory in adipose tissue is still unclear *(95)*. Both higher circulating levels of IL-6 and increased adipose tissue concentrations are associated with obesity. Furthermore, weight loss results in a decrease in IL-6 serum concentrations *(96)*. Importantly, in obesity, unlike other situations, IL-6 is chronically elevated, and this chronic elevation may result in detrimental alterations in systemic metabolism.

Higher concentrations of adipose tissue IL-6 are associated with insulin resistance *(96)*. In a study that carefully examined adipose tissue and systemic insulin sensitivity, including measures of serum fatty acids, IL-6, and TNF-α in the lean and obese, insulin resistance was most highly correlated with serum measures of IL-6. Additionally, serum IL-6 correlated with serum measurements of fatty acids *(69)*. However, it is currently unclear as to whether this is merely a reflection of the correlation between insulin resistance and inflammation, or is in fact a causal relationship. One possible effect of IL-6 may be indirect in the sense that IL-6 has been reported to decrease adiponectin levels *(96)*. Additionally, IL-6 can increase lipolysis *(97)*. Another possibility is that IL-6 can inhibit insulin by increasing the cellular expression of suppressor of cytokine signaling (SOCS)-3, a negative regulator of both leptin and insulin signaling. IL-6-induced SOCS-3 expression has been demonstrated in skeletal muscle, adipocytes *(98)*, and hepatocytes *(99)*. In vivo experiments further confirm that IL-6 decreases insulin sensitivity in the liver *(100)*.

As with type 2 diabetes, there is some evidence that IL-6 has a role in the early pathogenesis of cardiovascular disease. This inflammatory cytokine is reported to be an independent marker of increased mortality in patients with unstable coronary artery disease (101). Furthermore, increased serum IL-6 concentrations tend to parallel dyslipidemia (102). A partial explanation may be the increase in adipocyte lipolysis, as noted above. It is known that IL-6 infusion in humans results in higher serum FFA (103). However, the exact role that the cytokine plays, and whether it is more than simply a reflection of the correlation between atherosclerosis and inflammation, is still to be determined.

Similar to observations for TNF-α, serum levels of IL-6 are also correlated with obesity-associated sleep apnea and have been implicated in its pathogenesis (104–107). Increased cytokine levels and associated sleep disturbances have been proposed to be consequences of metabolic syndrome (108).

In summary, adipose tissue and serum levels of IL-6 increase with obesity. There is evidence that IL-6 has some anti-inflammatory actions, perhaps as a brake to inflammatory states. In certain situations, IL-6 has been suggested to have beneficial effects on systemic metabolism. However, obesity is associated with chronic elevations of IL-6 that may promote adipocyte lipolysis, insulin resistance, and other metabolic alterations.

Monocyte Chemoattractant Protein-1

The primary function of MCP-1, a proinflammatory chemokine, is thought to be the mediation of monocyte trafficking (109). In adipose tissue, adipocytes, stromal–vascular cells, and macrophages probably all contribute to adipose secretion of this protein (110,111). MCP-1 has both local and systemic effects, with all effects mediated by its receptor, the CCR2 receptor (74).

As an adipokine with very low basal expression, normal plasma levels of MCP-1 are virtually undetectable. However, MCP-1 is significantly induced by inflammatory molecules such as TNF-α and IL-1 (112). Its expression is also induced by insulin, even in insulin-resistant cells (113).

MCP-1 is hyperexpressed in adipose tissue from obese mice compared with control animals (114). Plasma and adipose tissue levels of this protein are also increased with increasing adiposity/BMI (115). Likewise, levels are decreased after weight reduction (115). MCP-1 has also been implicated in type 2 diabetes: patients with type 2 diabetes have higher circulating levels of MCP-1 (116).

Chronic incubation of adipocytes with insulin results in the synthesis and secretion of MCP-1. This occurs even though certain other actions of insulin are blocked with chronic incubation. Interestingly, incubation of adipocytes with MCP-1 in vitro results in decreased insulin-stimulated glucose uptake (113).

Animal studies suggest that MCP-1 could contribute negatively to cardiovascular disease. Blocking the MCP-1 pathway with gene therapy can prevent atheroma formation (117), as well as slow the progression of established lesions (111). The jury is still out, however, as to whether this adipokine contributes to the pathogenesis of atherosclerosis, or is merely a marker (115).

In summary, MCP-1 is a cytokine that is thought to promote macrophage recruitment into AT. The chronically elevated levels of insulin that are often seen with obesity may promote the synthesis and secretion of MCP-1 from adipocytes. Though more research is needed, these higher levels of MCP-1 may then have distinct metabolic effects, possibly contributing to the development of metabolic disease.

Plasminogen Activator Inhibitor-1

Plasminogen activator inhibitor (PAI)-1 is released by adipocytes, as well as other adipose tissue constituents, with visceral fat contributing higher amounts compared to subcutaneous depots *(81)*. This adipokine acts as an inhibitor of fibrinolysis and proteinolysis *(118)*, thereby helping to maintain vascular homeostasis. Higher levels of this protein promote increased susceptibility to clotting, a critical event in the pathogenesis of such conditions as myocardial infarction and stroke. Its release is also induced by the proinflammatory cytokine TNF-α *(119)*.

Plasma levels of PAI-1 are elevated with obesity and strongly correlated with visceral adiposity *(120)*. It appears that secretion from AT is increased in obese individuals *(121)*. Interestingly, mice that lack PAI-1 are completely protected against high-fat diet-induced obesity *(122)*. Even *ob/ob* mice, as a model of genetic morbid obesity, are protected *(123)*. This suggests that PAI-1 effects are not limited to clotting but may have other systemic effects.

Interestingly, plasma levels of PAI-1 are predictive of type 2 diabetes, independent of insulin resistance *(124)*. TZD treatment results in a decrease in plasma levels *(125)*. As with MCP-1, even insulin-resistant cells can continue to produce PAI-1 when exposed to insulin, suggesting that this protein may be regulated by a pathway that does not become resistant to the effects of insulin *(126)*.

The primary role of PAI-1 is to help maintain vascular homeostasis *(127)*. This protein is actually implicated in the pathogenesis of cardiovascular disease, with plasma levels being a strong predictor of future cardiovascular disease development *(128)*. It will be interesting to follow the results of future studies when it might be determined how PAI-1 contributes to obesity-related pathologies.

11β Hydroxydehydrogenase-1

Cushing's disease or administration of exogenous glucocorticoids such as prednisone are often associated with increased weight gain, central adiposity, increased food intake, insulin resistance, and in certain individuals, increased likelihood of developing diabetes. However, in general, obese individuals do not have increased circulating levels of cortisol. Interestingly, over the past few years, research has demonstrated that certain enzymes can actually convert inactive cortisol metabolites into active cortisol. One of the first hints that AT was in fact an endocrine organ was its identification as a major site for steroid hormone metabolism *(129)*.

11βHydroxydehydrogenase (11βHSD)-1 is an enzyme that converts circulating inactive metabolites of glucortiocoids into the active hormone, cortisol. This enzyme has been detected in liver, lung, brain, vasculature, and adipose tissue *(130)*. 11βHSD-1 increases local adipose tissue cortisol levels by converting local inactive cortisol metabolites, although it does not alter serum levels *(131)*. In the strictest sense, 11βHSD-1 is not a true adipokine, as it is not a secreted protein. However, because expression and local effects of this enzyme are manifest as elevated cortisol levels, 11βHSD-1 can be considered an adipokine.

Animal experiments have provided insight into the role of 11βHSD-1 in obesity and obesity complications. Adipocyte-specific overexpression of 11βHSD-1 in mice results in increased visceral adiposity and hyperphagia. In addition, these animals develop insulin resistance *(132)*. Interestingly, mice that do not express 11βHSD-1 are resistant to high fat diet-induced obesity *(133,134)*. Interestingly, obese humans appear to have increased adipose tissue concentrations of the enzyme *(131)*, possibly contributing to the development of central adiposity. Furthermore, healthy volunteers given an 11βHSD-1 inhibitor called carbenoxolone showed increased insulin sensitivity *(135)*.

In summary, adipocytes from obese individuals appear to express increased levels of 11βHSD-1, which converts inactive cortisol metabolites into cortisol. In rodents, adipocyte-specific overexpression of this enzyme mimics many attributes of metabolic syndrome. While the exact mechanisms are not yet clear, increased local levels of 11βHSD-1 in adipose tissue may promote metabolic syndrome. The identification of inhibitors of 11βHSD-1 is currently a research focus of pharmaceutical companies.

CONCLUSION

Although historically adipocytes have been thought of basically as a reservoir of triglyceride, it is clear that AT can synthesize and secrete local as well as systemic mediators of metabolism. Thus, AT can be viewed as an endocrine organ. In lean individuals small adipocytes secrete adipokines, such as leptin and adiponectin, which promote healthy metabolic homeostasis. However, with the onset of obesity, a macrophage-mediated profile is observed in AT. Multiple cytokines, such as TNF-α and IL-6, are secreted, with some acting locally in AT and some being released into the circulation to act at distal sites. In addition, these cytokines can act locally to increase adipocyte release of fatty acids and to reduce adiponectin levels. Chronically, this altered adipokine secretion that accompanies obesity significantly contributes to the development of insulin resistance, metabolic syndrome, atherosclerosis, and diabetes.

REFERENCES

1. Trayhurn P, Wood IS. Adipokines: inflammation and the pleiotropic role of white adipose tissue. Br J Nutr 2004;92(3):347–355.
2. Gavrilova O, Marcus-Samuels B, Graham D, et al. Surgical implantation of adipose tissue reverses diabetes in lipoatrophic mice. J Clin Invest 2000;105:271–278.
3. Zhang Y, Proenca R, Maffei M, et al. Positional cloning of the mouse obese gene and its human homologue. Nature 1994;372(6505):425–432.
4. Havel P, Kasim-Karakas S, Dubuc G, et al. Gender differences in plasma leptin concentrations. Nat Med 1996;2:949–950.
5. Halaas J, Gajiwala K, Maffei M, et al. Weight-reducing effects of the plasma protein encoded by the obese gene. Science 1995;269:543–546.
6. Pelleymounter MA, Cullen MJ, Baker MB, et al. Effects of the obese gene product on body weight regulation in ob/ob mice. Science 1995;269(5223):540–543.
7. Friedman JM, Halaas JL. Leptin and the regulation of body weight in mammals. Nature 1998;395(6704):763–770.
8. Farooqi IS, Matarese G, Lord GM, et al. Beneficial effects of leptin on obesity, T cell hyporesponsiveness, and neuroendocrine/metabolic dysfunction of human congenital leptin deficiency. J Clin Invest 2002;110(8):1093–1103.
9. Bjorbaek C, Kahn BB. Leptin signaling in the central nervous system and the periphery. Recent Prog Horm Res 2004;59:305–331.
10. Minokoshi Y, Kim YB, Peroni OD, et al. Leptin stimulates fatty-acid oxidation by activating AMP-activated protein kinase. Nature 2002;415(6869):339–343.
11. Iglesias MA, Ye JM, Frangioudakis G, et al. AICAR administration causes an apparent enhancement of muscle and liver insulin action in insulin-resistant high-fat-fed rats. Diabetes 2002;51(10):2886–2894.
12. Shimomura I, Hammer R, Ikemoto S, et al. Leptin reverses insulin resistance and diabetes mellitus in mice with congenital lipodystrophy. Nature 1999;401:73–76.

13. Oral E, Simha V, Ruiz E, et al. Leptin-replacement therapy for lipodystrophy. N Engl J Med 2002;346:570–578.
14. Javor ED, Cochran EK, Musso C, et al. Long-term efficacy of leptin replacement in patients with generalized lipodystrophy. Diabetes 2005;54(7):1994–2002.
15. Farooqi IS. Leptin and the onset of puberty: insights from rodent and human genetics. Semin Reprod Med 2002;20(2):139–144.
16. Heymsfield S, Greenberg A, Fujoka K, et al. Recombinant leptin for weight loss in obese and lean adults: a randomized, controlled, dose escalation trial. JAMA 1999;282:1568–1575.
17. Rosenbaum M, Goldsmith R, Bloomfield D, et al. Low-dose leptin reverses skeletal muscle, autonomic, and neuroendocrine adaptations to maintenance of reduced weight. J Clin Invest 2005;115(12): 3579–3586.
18. Rosenbaum M, Murphy EM, Heymsfield SB, et al. Low dose leptin administration reverses effects of sustained weight-reduction on energy expenditure and circulating concentrations of thyroid hormones. J Clin Endocrinol Metab 2002;87(5):2391–2394.
19. Nakano Y, Tobe T, Choi-Miura NH, et al. Isolation and characterization of GBP28, a novel gelatin-binding protein purified from human plasma. J Biochem (Tokyo) 1996;120(4):803–812.
20. Scherer PE, Williams S, Fogliano M, et al. A novel serum protein similar to C1q, produced exclusively in adipocytes. J Biol Chem 1995;270(45):26,746–26,749.
21. Hu E, Liang P, Spiegelman BM. AdipoQ is a novel adipose-specific gene dysregulated in obesity. J Biol Chem 1996;271(18):10,697–10,703.
22. Maeda K, Okubo K, Shimomura I, et al. cDNA cloning and expression of a novel adipose specific collagen-like factor, apM1 (AdiPose Most abundant Gene transcript 1). Biochem Biophys Res Commun 1996;221(2):286–289.
23. Chandran M, Phillips SA, Ciaraldi T, et al. Adiponectin: more than just another fat cell hormone? Diabetes Care 2003;26(8):2442–2450.
24. Fantuzzi G. Adipose tissue, adipokines, and inflammation. J Allergy Clin Immunol 2005;115(5):911–919; quiz 920.
25. Matsuzawa Y, Funahashi T, Kihara S, et al. Adiponectin and metabolic syndrome. Arterioscler Thromb Vasc Biol 2004;24(1):29–33.
26. Bottner A, Kratzsch J, Muller G, et al. Gender differences of adiponectin levels develop during the progression of puberty and are related to serum androgen levels. J Clin Endocrinol Metab 2004;89(8):4053–4061.
27. Trujillo ME, Scherer PE. Adiponectin—journey from an adipocyte secretory protein to biomarker of the metabolic syndrome. J Intern Med 2005;257(2):167–175.
28. Fisher FF, Trujillo ME, Hanif W, et al. Serum high molecular weight complex of adiponectin correlates better with glucose tolerance than total serum adiponectin in Indo-Asian males. Diabetologia 2005;48(6):1084–1087.
29. Freubis J, Tsao T-S, Javorschi S, et al. Proteolytic cleavage product of 30-kDa aidpocyte complement-related protein increases in fatty acid oxidation in muscle and causes weight loss in mice. Proc Natl Acad Sci USA 2001;98:2005–2010.
30. Tomas E, Tsao T-S, Saha AK, et al. Enhanced muscle fat oxidation and glucose transport by ACRP30 globular domain: Acetyl-CoA carboxylase inhibition and AMP-activated protein kinase activation. PNAS 2002;99(25):16,309–16,313.
31. Combs TP, Berg AH, Obici S, et al. Endogenous glucose production is inhibited by the adipose-derived protein Acrp30. J Clin Invest 2001;108(12):1875–1881.
32. Bouskila M, Pajvani UB, Scherer PE. Adiponectin: a relevant player in PPARgamma-agonist-mediated improvements in hepatic insulin sensitivity? Int J Obes (Lond) 2005;29 Suppl 1:S17–S23.
33. Nawrocki AR, Rajala MW, Tomas E, et al. Mice lacking adiponectin show decreased hepatic insulin sensitivity and reduced responsiveness to peroxisome proliferator-activated receptor gamma agonists. J Biol Chem 2006;281(5):2654–2660.
34. Arita Y, Kihara S, Ouchi N, et al. Paradoxical decrease of an adipose-specific protein, adiponectin, in obesity. Bioc Biophys Res Commun 1999;2:79–83.
35. Kissebah AH, Sonnenberg GE, Myklebust J, et al. Quantitative trait loci on chromosomes 3 and 17 influence phenotypes of the metabolic syndrome. Proc Natl Acad Sci USA 2000;97(26):14,478–14,483.
36. Hara K, Boutin P, Mori Y, et al. Genetic variation in the gene encoding adiponectin is associated with an increased risk of type 2 diabetes in the Japanese population. Diabetes 2002;51(2):536–540.

37. Wang H, Zhang H, Jia Y, et al. Adiponectin receptor 1 gene (ADIPOR1) as a candidate for type 2 diabetes and insulin resistance. Diabetes 2004;53(8):2132–2136.
38. Bouatia-Naji N, Meyre D, Lobbens S, et al. ACDC/adiponectin polymorphisms are associated with severe childhood and adult obesity. Diabetes 2006;55(2):545–550.
39. Diez JJ, Iglesias P. The role of the novel adipocyte-derived hormone adiponectin in human disease. Eur J Endocrinol 2003;148(3):293–300.
40. Yang WS, Lee WJ, Funahashi T, et al. Weight reduction increases plasma levels of an adipose-derived anti-inflammatory protein, adiponectin. J Clin Endocrinol Metab 2001;86(8):3815–3819.
41. Despres JP, Golay A, Sjostrom L. Effects of rimonabant on metabolic risk factors in overweight patients with dyslipidemia. N Engl J Med 2005;353(20):2121–2134.
42. Lindsay RS, Funahashi T, Hanson RL, et al. Adiponectin and development of type 2 diabetes in the Pima Indian population. Lancet 2002;360(9326):57–58.
43. Spranger J, Kroke A, Mohlig M, et al. Adiponectin and protection against type 2 diabetes mellitus. Lancet 2003;361(9353):226–228.
44. Yamauchi T, Oike Y, Kamon J, et al. Increased insulin sensitivity despite lipodystrophy in Crebbp heterozygous mice. Nat Genet 2002;30(2):221–226.
45. Pellme F, Smith U, Funahashi T, et al. Circulating adiponectin levels are reduced in nonobese but insulin-resistant first-degree relatives of type 2 diabetic patients. Diabetes 2003;52(5):1182–1186.
46. Kern PA, Di Gregorio GB, Lu T, et al. Adiponectin expression from human adipose tissue: relation to obesity, insulin resistance, and tumor necrosis factor-alpha expression. Diabetes 2003;52(7):1779–1785.
47. Hotta K, Funahashi T, Bodkin NL, et al. Circulating concentrations of the adipocyte protein adiponectin are decreased in parallel with reduced insulin sensitivity during the progression to type 2 diabetes in rhesus monkeys. Diabetes 2001;50(5):1126–1133.
48. Yamamoto Y, Hirose H, Saito I, et al. Adiponectin, an adipocyte-derived protein, predicts future insulin resistance: two-year follow-up study in Japanese population. J Clin Endocrinol Metab 2004;89(1):87–90.
49. Maeda N, Shimomura I, Kishida K, et al. Diet-induced insulin resistance in mice lacking adiponectin/ACRP30. Nat Med 2002;8(7):731–737.
50. Yamauchi T, Kamon J, Waki H, et al. The fat-derived hormone adiponectin reverses insulin resistance associated with both lipoatrophy and obesity. Nat Med 2001;7(8):941–946.
51. Yamauchi T, Kamon J, Minokoshi Y, et al. Adiponectin stimulates glucose utilization and fatty-acid oxidation by activating AMP-activated protein kinase. Nat Med 2002;8(11):1288–1295.
52. Berg AH, Combs TP, Du X, et al. The adipocyte-secreted protein Acrp30 enhances hepatic insulin action. Nat Med 2001;7(8):947–953.
53. Pajvani UB, Hawkins M, Combs TP, et al. Complex distribution, not absolute amount of adiponectin, correlates with thiazolidinedione-mediated improvement in insulin sensitivity. J Biol Chem 2004;279(13):12,152–12,162.
54. Tsuchida A, Yamauchi T, Takekawa S, et al. Peroxisome proliferator-activated receptor (PPAR) α activation increases adiponectin receptors and reduces obesity-related inflammation in adipose tissue: comparison of activation of PPARα, PPARγ, and their combination. Diabetes 2005;54(12):3358–3370.
55. Cnop M, Havel PJ, Utzschneider KM, et al. Relationship of adiponectin to body fat distribution, insulin sensitivity and plasma lipoproteins: evidence for independent roles of age and sex. Diabetologia 2003;46(4):459–469.
56. Chan DC, Watts GF, Ng TW, et al. Adiponectin and other adipocytokines as predictors of markers of triglyceride-rich lipoprotein metabolism. Clin Chem 2005;51(3):578–585.
57. Iwashima Y, Katsuya T, Ishikawa K, et al. Hypoadiponectinemia is an independent risk factor for hypertension. Hypertension 2004;43(6):1318–1323.
58. Kumada M, Kihara S, Sumitsuji S, et al. Association of hypoadiponectinemia with coronary artery disease in men. Arterioscler Thromb Vasc Biol 2003;23(1):85–89.
59. Ouchi N, Kihara S, Arita Y, et al. Novel modulator for endothelial adhesion molecules: adipocyte-derived plasma protein adiponectin. Circulation 1999;100(25):2473–2476.
60. Okamoto Y, Kihara S, Ouchi N, et al. Adiponectin reduces atherosclerosis in apolipoprotein E-deficient mice. Circulation 2002;106(22):2767–2770.
61. Shibata R, Sato K, Pimentel DR, et al. Adiponectin protects against myocardial ischemia-reperfusion injury through AMPK- and COX-2-dependent mechanisms. Nat Med 2005;11(10):1096–1103.

62. Chen H, Montagnani M, Funahashi T, et al. Adiponectin stimulates production of nitric oxide in vascular endothelial cells. J Biol Chem 2003;278(45):45,021–45,026.
63. Goldstein BJ, Scalia R. Adiponectin: a novel adipokine linking adipocytes and vascular function. J Clin Endocrinol Metab 2004;89(6):2563–2568.
64. Wong GW, Wang J, Hug C, et al. A family of Acrp30/adiponectin structural and functional paralogs. Proc Natl Acad Sci USA 2004;101(28):10,302–10,307.
65. Hotamisligil GS, Spiegelman BM. Tumor necrosis factor a: A key component of the obesity-diabetes link. Diabetes 1994;43:1271–1278.
66. Beutler B, Greenwald D, Hulmes J, et al. Identifty of tumor necrosis factor and the macrophage-secreted factor cachetin. Nature 1985;316:552–554.
67. Hotamisligil GS, Arner P, Caro JF, et al. Increased adipose tissue expression of tumor necrosis factor-alpha in human obesity and insulin resistance. J Clin Invest 1995;95(5):2409–2415.
68. Kern PA, Saghizadeh M, Ong JM, et al. The expression of tumor necrosis factor in human adipose tissue: regulation by obesity, weight loss, and relationship to lipoprotein lipase. J Clin Invest 1995;95:2111–2119.
69. Kern PA, Ranganathan S, Li C, et al. Adipose tissue tumor necrosis factor and interleukin-6 expression in human obesity and insulin resistance. Am J Physiol Endocrinol Metab 2001;280(5):E745–E751.
70. Weisberg SP, McCann D, Desai M, et al. Obesity is associated with macrophage accumulation in adipose tissue. J Clin Invest 2003;112(12):1796–1808.
71. Xu H, Barnes G, Yang Q, et al. Chronic inflammation in fat plays a crucial role in the development of obesity-related insulin resistance. J Clin Invest 2003;112:1821–30.
72. Fasshauer M, Kralisch S, Klier M, et al. Adiponectin gene expression and secretion is inhibited by interleukin-6 in 3T3-L1 adipocytes. Biochem Biophys Res Commun 2003;301(4):1045–1050.
73. Wang B, Jenkins JR, Trayhurn P. Expression and secretion of inflammation-related adipokines by human adipocytes differentiated in culture: integrated response to TNF-alpha. Am J Physiol Endocrinol Metab 2005;288(4):E731–E740.
74. Weisberg SP, Hunter D, Huber R, et al. CCR2 modulates inflammatory and metabolic effects of high-fat feeding. J Clin Invest 2006;116(1):115–124.
75. Cinti S, Mitchell G, Barbatelli G, et al. Adipocyte death defines macrophage localization and function in adipose tissue of obese mice and humans. J Lipid Res 2005;46(11):2347–2355.
76. Boden G. Role of fatty acids in the pathogenesis of insulin resistance and NIDDM. Diabetes 1997;46:3–10.
77. Shulman G. Cellular mechanism of insulin resistance. J Clin Invest 2000;196:171–176.
78. Carr DB, Utzschneider KM, Hull RL, et al. Intra-abdominal fat is a major determinant of the National Cholesterol Education Program Adult Treatment Panel III criteria for the metabolic syndrome. Diabetes 2004;53(8):2087–2094.
79. Gastaldelli A, Miyazaki Y, Pettiti M, et al. Metabolic effects of visceral fat accumulation in type 2 diabetes. J Clin Endocrinol Metab 2002;87:5098–5103.
80. Miyazaki Y, Mahankali A, Matsuda M, et al. Effect of pioglitazone on abdominal fat distribution and insulin sensitivity in type 2 diabetic patients. J Clin Endocrinol Metab 2002;87(6):2784–2791.
81. Fain J, Bahouth S, Madan A. TNF-alpha release by the nonfat cells of human adipose tissue. Int J Obes Relat Metab Discord 2004;28:616–622.
82. Gerhardt CC, Romero IA, Cancello R, et al. Chemokines control fat accumulation and leptin secretion by cultured human adipocytes. Mol Cell Endocrinol 2001;175(1–2):81–92.
83. Moller DE. Potential role of TNF-alpha in the pathogenesis of insulin resistance and type 2 diabetes. Trends Endocrinol Metab 2000;11(6):212–217.
84. Souza SC, Yamamoto M, Franciosa M, et al. BRL blocks the lipolytic actions of tumor necrosis factor-alpha (TNF-a): a potential new insulin-sensitizing mechanism for the thiazolidinediones. Diabetes 1998;47:691–695.
85. Zhang H, Halbleib M, Ahmed F, et al. Tumor necrosis factor-alpha stimulates lipolysis in differentiated human adipocytes through activation of extracellular signal related kinase and elevated extracelular related kinase and elevation of intracellular cAMP. Diabetes 2002;51:2929–2935.
86. Hotamisligil GS, Murray DL, Choy LN, et al. TNF-a inhibits signaling from insulin receptor. Proc Natl Acad Sci USA 1994;91:4854–4858.
87. Uysal K, Wiesbrock S, Marino M, et al. Protection from obesity-linked insulin resistance in mice lacking TNF-a function. Nature 1997;389:610–614.

88. Mohamed-Ali V, Goodrick S, Rawesh A, et al. Subcutaneous adipose tissue releases interleukin-6, but not tumor necrosis factor-alpha, in vivo. J Clin Endocrinol Metab 1997;82(12):4196–4200.

89. Ofei F, Hurel S, Newkirk J, et al. Effects of an engineered human anti-TNF-alpha antibody (CDP571) on insulin sensitivity and glycemic control in patients with NIDDM. Diabetes 1996;45(7):881–885.

90. Vgontzas A, Zoumakies E, Lin H, et al. Marked decrease in sleepiness in patients with sleep apnez by etanercept, a tumor necrosis factor-alpha antagonist. J Clin Endocrinol Metab 2004;89:4409–4412.

91. van Hall G, Steensberg A, Sacchetti M, et al. Interleukin-6 stimulates lipolysis and fat oxidation in humans. J Clin Endocrinol Metab 2003;88(7):3005–3010.

92. Steensberg A, van Hall G, Osada T, et al. Production of interleukin-6 in contracting human skeletal muscles can account for the exercise-induced increase in plasma interleukin-6. J Physiol 2000;529 Pt 1:237–242.

93. Fried SK, Bunkin DA, Greenberg AS. Omental and subcutaneous adipose tissues of obese subjects release interleukin-6: depot difference and regulation by glucocorticoid. J Clin Endocrinol Metab 1998;83(3):847–850.

94. Rotter V, Nagaev I, Smith U. Interleukin-6 (IL-6) induces insulin resistance in 3T3-L1 adipocytes and is, like IL-8 and tumor necrosis factor-alpha, overexpressed in human fat cells from insulin-resistant subjects. J Biol Chem 2003;278(46):45,777–45,784.

95. Kristiansen OP, Mandrup-Poulsen T. Interleukin-6 and diabetes: the good, the bad, or the indifferent? Diabetes 2005;54 Suppl 2:S114–S124.

96. Fernandez-Real JM, Ricart W. Insulin resistance and chronic cardiovascular inflammatory syndrome. Endocr Rev 2003;24(3):278–301.

97. Trujillo ME, Sullivan S, Harten I, et al. Interleukin-6 regulates human adipose tissue lipid metabolism and leptin production in vitro. J Clin Endocrinol Metab 2004;89(11):5577–5582.

98. Rieusset J, Bouzakri K, Chevillotte E, et al. Suppressor of cytokine signaling 3 expression and insulin resistance in skeletal muscle of obese and type 2 diabetic patients. Diabetes 2004;53(9):2232–2241.

99. Senn JJ, Klover PJ, Nowak IA, et al. Suppressor of cytokine signaling-3 (SOCS-3), a potential mediator of interleukin-6-dependent insulin resistance in hepatocytes. J Biol Chem 2003;278(16): 13740–13746.

100. Kim HJ, Higashimori T, Park SY, et al. Differential effects of interleukin-6 and -10 on skeletal muscle and liver insulin action in vivo. Diabetes 2004;53(4):1060–1067.

101. Lindmark E, Diderholm E, Wallentin L, et al. Relationship between interleukin 6 and mortality in patients with unstable coronary artery disease: effects of an early invasive or noninvasive strategy. JAMA 2001;286(17):2107–2113.

102. Pickup JC, Mattock MB, Chusney GD, et al. NIDDM as a disease of the innate immune system: association of acute-phase reactants and interleukin-6 with metabolic syndrome X. Diabetologia 1997;40(11):1286–1292.

103. Stouthard JM, Romijn JA, Van der Poll T, et al. Endocrinologic and metabolic effects of interleukin-6 in humans. Am J Physiol 1995;268(5 Pt 1):E813–E819.

104. Vgontzas A, Papanicolaou D, Bixler E, et al. Sleep apnea and daytime sleepiness and fatigue: relation to visceral obesity, insulin resistance, and hypercytokinemia. J Clin Endocrinol Metab 2000;85:1151–1158.

105. Vgontzas A, Papnicoaou D, Bixler E, et al. Elevation of plasma cytokines in disorders of excessive daytime sleepiness: role of sleep disturbance and obesity. J Clin Endocrinol Metab 1997;82:1313–1316.

106. Vgontzas A, Papanicolaou D, Bixler E, et al. Circadian interleukin-6 secretion and quantity and depth of sleep. J Clin Endocrinol Metab 2000;84:2603–2607.

107. Vgontzas AN, Papanicolaou DA, Bixler EO, et al. Sleep apnea and daytime sleepiness and fatigue: relation to visceral obesity, insulin resistance, and hypercytokinemia. J Clin Endocrinol Metab 2000;85(3):1151–1158.

108. Vgontzas AN, Bixler EO, Chrousos GP. Sleep apnea is a manifestation of the metabolic syndrome. Sleep Med Rev 2005;9(3):211–224.

109. Boisvert WA. Modulation of atherogenesis by chemokines. Trends Cardiovasc Med 2004;14(4):161–165.

110. Wellen KE, Hotamisligil GS. Obesity-induced inflammatory changes in adipose tissue. J Clin Invest 2003;112(12):1785–1788.

111. Inoue S, Egashira K, Ni W, et al. Anti-monocyte chemoattractant protein-1 gene therapy limits progression and destabilization of established atherosclerosis in apolipoprotein E-knockout mice. Circulation 2002;106(21):2700–2706.

112. Juge-Aubry CE, Henrichot E, Meier CA. Adipose tissue: a regulator of inflammation. Best Pract Res Clin Endocrinol Metab 2005;19(4):547–566.
113. Sartipy P, Loskutoff DJ. Expression profiling identifies genes that continue to respond to insulin in adipocytes made insulin-resistant by treatment with TNF-alpha. J Biol Chem 2003;278(52):52,298–52,306.
114. Sartipy P, Loskutoff DJ. Monocyte chemoattractant protein 1 in obesity and insulin resistance. Proc Natl Acad Sci USA 2003;100(12):7265–7270.
115. Christiansen T, Richelsen B, Bruun JM. Monocyte chemoattractant protein-1 is produced in isolated adipocytes, associated with adiposity and reduced after weight loss in morbid obese subjects. Int J Obes (Lond) 2005;29(1):146–150.
116. Nomura S, Shouzu A, Omoto S, et al. Significance of chemokines and activated platelets in patients with diabetes. Clin Exp Immunol 2000;121:437–443.
117. Ni W, Egashira K, Kitamoto S, et al. New anti-monocyte chemoattractant protein-1 gene therapy attenuates atherosclerosis in apolipoprotein E-knockout mice. Circulation 2001;103(16):2096–2101.
118. Kershaw EE, Flier JS. Adipose tissue as an endocrine organ. J Clin Endocrinol Metab 2004;89(6):2548–2556.
119. Samad F, Uysal KT, Wiesbrock SM, et al. Tumor necrosis factor alpha is a key component in the obesity-linked elevation of plasminogen activator inhibitor 1. Proc Natl Acad Sci USA 1999;96(12):6902–6907.
120. Wajchenberg BL. Subcutaneous and visceral adipose tissue: their relation to the metabolic syndrome. Endocr Rev 2000;21(6):697–738.
121. Alessi MC, Bastelica D, Morange P, et al. Plasminogen activator inhibitor 1, transforming growth factor-beta1, and BMI are closely associated in human adipose tissue during morbid obesity. Diabetes 2000;49(8):1374–1380.
122. Ma LJ, Mao SL, Taylor KL, et al. Prevention of obesity and insulin resistance in mice lacking plasminogen activator inhibitor 1. Diabetes 2004;53(2):336–346.
123. Schafer K, Fujisawa K, Konstantinides S, et al. Disruption of the plasminogen activator inhibitor 1 gene reduces the adiposity and improves the metabolic profile of genetically obese and diabetic ob/ob mice. FASEB J 2001;15(10):1840–1842.
124. Festa A, D'Agostino RJ, Haffner S, The Insulin Resistance Atherosclerosis Study. Elevated levels of acute-phase proteins and plasminogen activator inhibitor-I predict the development of type 2 diabetes; the insulin resistance atherosclerosis study. Diabetes 2002;51:1131–1137.
125. Mertens I, Van Gaal LF. Obesity, haemostasis and the fibrinolytic system. Obes Rev 2002;3(2):85–101.
126. Samad F, Pandey M, Bell PA, Loskutoff DJ. Insulin continues to induce plasminogen activator inhibitor 1 gene expression in insulin-resistant mice and adipocytes. Mol Med 2000;6(8):680–692.
127. Skurk T, Hauner H. Obesity and impaired fibrinolysis: role of adipose production of plasminogen activator inhibitor-1. Int J Obes Relat Metab Disord 2004;28(11):1357–1364.
128. Juhan-Vague I, Alessi M-C, Mavri A, et al. Plasminogen activator inhibitor-1, inflammation, obesity, insulin resistance and vascular risk. J Thromb Haemost 2003;1(7):1575–1579.
129. Siiteri PK. Adipose tissue as a source of hormones. Am J Clin Nutr 1987;45(1 Suppl):277–282.
130. Seckl JR, Walker BR. Minireview: 11beta-hydroxysteroid dehydrogenase type 1- a tissue-specific amplifier of glucocorticoid action. Endocrinology 2001;142(4):1371–1376.
131. Rask E, Olsson T, Soderberg S, et al. Tissue-specific dysregulation of cortisol metabolism in human obesity. J Clin Endocrinol Metab 2001;86(3):1418–1421.
132. Masuzaki H, Paterson j, Shiyama H, et al. A transgenic model of visceral obesity and the metabolic syndrome. Science 2001;294:2166–2170.
133. Kershaw EE, Morton NM, Dhillon H, et al. Adipocyte specific glucocorticoid inactivation protects against diet-induced obesity. Diabetes 2005;54:1023–1031.
134. Morton N, Paterson J, Masuzaki H, et al. Novel adipose tissue-mediated resistance to diet-induced visceral obesity in 11 beta-hydroxysteroid dehydrogenase type 1-deficient mice. Diabetes 2004;53:931–938.
135. Walker BR, Connacher AA, Lindsay RM, et al. Carbenoxolone increases hepatic insulin sensitivity in man: a novel role for 11-oxosteroid reductase in enhancing glucocorticoid receptor activation. J Clin Endocrinol Metab 1995;80(11):3155–3159.

5

Free Fatty Acids, Insulin Resistance, and Ectopic Fat

David E. Kelley, MD

CONTENTS

INTRODUCTION
HISTORY OF CONCEPT OF INSULIN RESISTANCE
GLUCOSE–FFA SUBSTRATE COMPETITION
THE GOOD SIDE OF GLUCOSE–FFA SUBSTRATE COMPETITION
METABOLIC CHALLENGE OF MAINTAINING MACRONUTRIENT BALANCE
POOR TIMING OF FAT OXIDATION IN OBESITY
BIOCHEMICAL DETERMINANTS OF METABOLIC INFLEXIBILITY
ECTOPIC FAT IN LIVER AND MUSCLE
CONCLUSIONS
REFERENCES

Summary

The development of obesity induces resistance to the effect of insulin to stimulate uptake of glucose and suppress release of fatty acids. These metabolic impairments are inter-related and competition between glucose and fatty acids is a key aspect of the pathogenesis of insulin resistance. Another important factor is that fat calories accumulate within muscle and liver and the presence of an increased fat content in these organs correlates with severity of insulin resistance. This chapter reviews recent findings and background concepts regarding "ectopic fat" and substrate competition and how these contribute to obesity induced insulin resistance.

Key Words: Free fatty acids; insulin resistance; ectopic fat; macronutrients.

INTRODUCTION

Insulin resistance (IR) occurs commonly in obesity and is closely related to the increase in adiposity. There are a number of aspects of adiposity that contribute to the pathogenesis of IR. One is the distribution of adipose tissue, notably within intra-abdominal depots, whereas another aspect of fat distribution concerns that located with liver and muscle. In this book, intra-abdominal adiposity is discussed in a separate chapter; this chapter will focus on ectopic fat and on the topic of substrate competition between glucose and fatty acids, which is also regarded as strongly influencing IR in obesity.

From: *Contemporary Endocrinology: Treatment of the Obese Patient*
Edited by: R. F. Kushner and D. H. Bessesen © Humana Press Inc., Totowa, NJ

Ectopic fat is a term that refers to the accumulation of stored fat within muscle, liver, and potentially other tissues important for the pathogenesis of complications of IR, such as myocardium and pancreatic β-cells. However, it is normal for myocytes and hepatocytes to contain stored triglyceride, which, like glycogen, is a depot of readily available substrate. Therefore, the term "ectopic fat" is a misnomer, but this limitation aside, the term has value for descriptive purposes. One of the axioms that will be explored in this chapter is that myocytes and hepatocytes with ectopic fat can be viewed as a recapitulation at a cellular level the systemic pathophysiology that characterizes obesity. Ectopic fat derives from perturbations in the balance between storage and oxidation of fat, obviously, but also in interaction with carbohydrate availability.

With regard to "substrate competition" between free fatty acids (FFA) and glucose, it is most common to frame this as pathophysiology rather than physiology, and to posit that FFA is the "culprit" substrate. This perception certainly resonates with much that is understood about the pathogenesis of IR in obesity, yet is only part of the story. With substrates, as with much else, competition is more often healthy than unhealthy. In fact, competition between glucose and FFA is an essential part of the ebb and flow of daily life in the transitions between fed and fasted conditions. Moreover, in obesity, recent work indicates that glucose competitively inhibits oxidation of fat and that this may be as important in generating metabolic problems as the converse, which is FFA inhibition of glucose utilization.

HISTORY OF CONCEPT OF INSULIN RESISTANCE

If it can be argued that there is ambiguity concerning whether substrate competition is always adverse for metabolism or whether it is glucose or FFA that causes problems, then this note of ambiguity might also be extended to a consideration of IR itself. Insulin resistance has been an enigma since it was initially described 75 yr ago (1). It is customary that a pathophysiological process like IR is regarded as a mechanism of disease. But there is another perspective. There is an emerging body of evidence that IR is a highly regulated adaptation that protects, or at least partially protects, the very organ systems (muscle, adipocytes, and liver) that are pivotal in generating IR. This latter perspective has relevance to the discussion of both substrate competition and ectopic fat.

Even at the inception of the concept of IR, it was recognized to be a process that did not fit into established paradigms for categorizing endocrine disorders. Endocrine disorders, then as now, can nearly always be categorized into those of hormone deficiency and those of hormone excess. Insulin resistance is a chimera of these. It is a manifestation of deficient hormone action but one that is not accounted for by insulin deficiency.

Insulin resistance was initially described by Himsworth in the 1930s (1–3). Himsworth, a physician then beginning to implement treatment with insulin, the "wonder drug" of that age, was perceptive in noticing that some diabetic patients appeared refractory to this treatment. To test this concept, he gave research volunteers, nondiabetics and diabetics, injections of glucose, alone and with insulin injections, and noted the effect on the glycemic responses. This procedure revealed "responders" and "nonresponders." The descriptions of the respective clinical characteristics that were made by Himsworth foreshadowed clinical criteria that remain effective for distinguishing between individuals with type 1 compared with type 2 diabetes. Yet despite these provocative and seminal observations, the concept of IR did not take firm root in the contemporary sensibilities of the pathogenesis of diabetes mellitus; that was to come years later, and the current public health implications were not then anticipated.

Thirty years following the seminal work of Himsworth, the development of the radioimmunoassay to measure plasma insulin revealed hyperinsulinemia in many with glucose intolerance (4) and in obesity, even in the absence of glucose intolerance. Development of clinical investigation techniques to quantify insulin action in humans demonstrated that insulin resistance is almost always present in glucose intolerance and type 2 diabetes. An association between hypertriglyceridemia and insulin resistance began to be recognized in the 1970s, and later a connection with essential hypertension was also perceived (5). Insulin resistance is now perceived as a major metabolic risk factor and a target for intervention. Indeed, interventions that ameliorate insulin resistance, notably by weight loss and physical activity, commonly yield multifactorial risk reductions across these domains of glucose homeostasis, hyperlipidemia, and hypertension.

In the past seven decades much about insulin resistance has been delineated, yet some fundamental issues remain enigmatic. Is insulin resistance truly a disease, or is it a physiological adaptation that like most yields a mixed bag of beneficial compensation and other unfavorable consequences? It is little debated that as a consequence of IR, much of the body—the vasculature in particular—suffers unfavorable effects. Yet it can be postulated that at a cellular level, in particular that of a fat-laden hepatocyte or a fat-laden myocyte, insulin resistance is a defensive posture evoked to protect the cell (and the organ) against further excesses of substrate. This ambiguity as to whether insulin resistance is a disease or a regulated adaptation with some redeeming features will resurface at several junctures in this chapter in discussing substrate competition and ectopic fat.

GLUCOSE–FFA SUBSTRATE COMPETITION

In the early 1960s, Randle and colleagues established the principle that glucose–FFA substrate competition can contribute to the pathophysiology of IR in diabetes mellitus (DM) and obesity (6). In a series of biochemical studies, it was demonstrated that provision of FFA reduced glucose utilization by skeletal muscle, especially oxidative muscle. The studies by Randle were performed with in vitro preparations of muscle, yet highly analogous findings can be demonstrated in vivo both in animals and in human studies. Indeed, it is quite remarkable and has been repeatedly demonstrated in clinical investigations that a lipid infusion can acutely induce IR even in healthy, normal-weight individuals. Several hours of infusion of a lipid emulsion (of a composition as is used for parenteral nutrition) is not only sufficient to induce IR, but does so with a consequent metabolic profile that is nearly identical to that observed in type 2 DM and obesity (7,8).

Effect of FFA Infusion

In the author's laboratory, the effect of FFA infusion to induce IR was examined using the paradigm of a lipid emulsion infused only at a rate that maintained plasma FFA at the usual fasting (postabsorptive) levels despite insulin infusion (9). In these studies, insulin was infused to achieve steady-state levels in the upper physiological range for insulin, 500 to 600 pmol. Each of the participants, lean, healthy young men, had two studies, one being an insulin infusion/glucose clamp with concomitant lipid emulsion infusion and the other without the lipid emulsion. As is typical in individuals with normal insulin sensitivity, this rate of insulin infusion dramatically suppressed plasma FFA to approximately one-tenth the fasting level. The lipid emulsion infusion was sufficient to sustain plasma FFA at the fasting level. Otherwise, the study conditions were similar with matched concentrations for glucose and insulin. The infusion of lipid emulsions induced insulin resistance; it required approximately one-third less glucose to maintain euglycemia than in studies without the infusion of the lipid emulsion.

Metabolic profiles of glucose metabolism were measured by assessing rates of glucose oxidation, release of lactate, and glycogen formation *(9)*. FFA induced a substantial impairment in glycogen formation as well as a significant, though less dramatic, inhibition of glucose oxidation. As a proportion of glucose uptake, the release of lactate was increased. A key conclusion that can be drawn from these studies is that the effect of insulin to stimulate increased glucose uptake into skeletal muscle is contingent on the effectiveness with which insulin suppresses plasma fatty acids. This is a point to which we will later return in discussing the importance of IR in the suppression of lipolysis as central to the pathogenesis of IR in obesity. The second main point to be made concerning these data is that this profile of reduced glucose uptake, markedly suppressed glycogen formation, impaired glucose oxidation, and a relative increase in the proportion of glucose uptake accounted for by lactate release from muscle is precisely the pattern observed in obesity and type 2 diabetes *(10)*. This remarkable similarity in metabolic profiles infers the importance of FFA in the pathogenesis of IR.

Fasting plasma concentrations of FFA are only modestly increased in most glucose-tolerant obese men and women. This is interesting, as by definition, the mass of adipose tissue is greatly increased. Thus rates of appearance of FFA (FFA flux) are actually decreased if expressed per kilogram of fat mass and, as mentioned previously, only modestly increased when expressed on the basis of fat-free mass, the tissues of FFA consumption. Fasting plasma concentrations of FFA are generally increased in most patients with type 2 diabetes, by approx 10 to 20% above values in normal-weight or overweight glucose tolerant individuals. In cross-sectional studies, fasting levels of plasma FFA are often observed to correlate negatively with insulin-stimulated rates of glucose metabolism (i.e., insulin sensitivity) *(11)*. Nonetheless, there is not major decompensation with regard to fasting conditions of fatty acids. Typically, stronger correlations are observed for insulin-suppressed levels of plasma FFA in relation to insulin sensitivity *(11)*. Clinical investigations have revealed that overnight lowering of FFA in patients with type 2 diabetes improves IR *(12)*.

In obesity and in type 2 diabetes, the effect of insulin to suppress plasma FFA is blunted; this impairment is, in certain respects, more evident than are fasting abnormalities. Levels of plasma FFA during insulin infusion have repeatedly been shown to correlate in a robust manner with the severity of IR. Following weight loss there is improved insulin suppression of lipolysis and plasma FFA; this is a key metabolic aspect that contributes to improvement of IR *(13)*.

Regional Patterns of Adiposity

Resistance to insulin suppression of plasma FFA is influenced by regional patterns of adiposity, by a predominance of large adipocytes, and by altered endocrine and adipokine activity of adipose tissue. Insulin resistance of adipose tissue tends to be more pronounced, with an upper body predominance of adiposity as compared to lower body, or gluteal–femoral, predominance of adiposity. There are regional differences across depots of adipose tissue in responsiveness to insulin in suppressing lipolysis. Adipocytes from omentum and mesenteric adipose tissue have higher basal rates of lipolysis and suppress less in response to insulin than adipocytes from gluteal femoral adipose tissue (14). Thus, regional differences in adipocyte metabolism with regard to insulin sensitivity of lipolysis may be an important mechanism accounting for differing relationships of these depots with systemic insulin sensitivity. The majority of systemic fatty acid flux derives from abdominal subcutaneous adipose tissue (15). This reflects both the greater absolute amount of adiposity in this depot than in visceral AT (VAT), and the regional differences in adipocyte metabolism mentioned above. Preceding the contemporary emphasis on characterizing obesity by assessing patterns of adipose tissue distribution, obesity research centered on assessments of adipocyte size and number. Obesity is associated with larger adipocytes (16). Adipocyte size in abdominal subcutaneous adipose tissue is a risk factor for type 2 diabetes independent of overall obesity and central adiposity (17). Large adipocytes have higher rates of lipolysis and may have altered patterns of adipokine secretion that contribute to insulin resistance.

THE GOOD SIDE OF FFA–GLUCOSE SUBSTRATE COMPETITION

The experiments performed by Randle and colleagues provided a basis for scientists to think about the adverse aspects of substrate competition, but a series of equally important studies, performed in the 1950s and 1960s by Andres and colleagues at Johns Hopkins, delineated healthy or positive aspects of glucose–FFA substrate competition (18). In clinical investigations, Andres and colleagues showed that during fasting conditions, FFA is the predominant oxidative substrate for skeletal muscle (18). The respiratory quotient (RQ)—the quotient of carbon dioxide release to oxygen consumption—across the forearm during fasting conditions was approx 0.80, denoting that lipid oxidation accounted for the majority of energy expenditure. The RQ reflects the chemical composition of the substrate being oxidized and is 1.0 for purely glucose oxidation and 0.70 for purely lipid oxidation. The low RQ by skeletal muscle during fasting conditions indicates low reliance on glucose oxidation and only minor glucose uptake, with a fractional extraction of 1 to 2%. This contrasts markedly with the 40% or more extraction of plasma FFA by muscle during fasting conditions. There are several implications for metabolic health from these findings. First, in this context of fasting metabolism, use of FFA rather than glucose by muscle spares glucose for the CNS. From the perspective of obesity, these studies demonstrate the importance of skeletal muscle as a site for disposal of FFA and oxidation of fat calories.

In the sections that follow, three metabolically adverse aspects of glucose–FFA substrate competition will be discussed. The first, which has already been described, is the adverse effect of FFA that impairs the effect of insulin to stimulate glucose utilization by muscle. The second concept that will be addressed is the adverse effect of hyperglycemia to inhibit utilization of FFA, even in the setting of fasting concentrations of insulin. The third concept that will be presented is "metabolic inflexibility," an aspect of the pathophysiology of obesity that is characterized by diminished capacity of muscle to switch between glucose and FFA in the transition from fed to fasted conditions. However, before addressing these, it is worthwhile to frame out the macronutrient challenges of glucose and lipid oxidation at a whole body level and as these pertain to weight regulation.

METABOLIC CHALLENGE OF MAINTAINING MACRONUTRIENT BALANCE

Macronutrient Balance

One way to frame a discussion of substrate competition is to consider what is required to maintain macronutrient balance in a normal-weight, weight-stable individual. To maintain macronutrient balance, the amounts of carbohydrate and fat that are consumed daily must be oxidized. Intake of calories in excess of the amounts oxidized leads of course to weight gain, whereas negative energy balance must be achieved to accomplish weight loss. Carbohydrates typically comprise 40 to 50% of daily caloric intake in an average American diet. For this discussion, this will be assumed to be approx 1,000 kcal (or 250 g). Daily ingestion of carbohydrate is considerable as compared with systemic glycogen. Stores of glycogen are relatively small at approx 500 g, just twice the amount of daily consumption. It is interesting to consider that a 75-kg man or woman can be estimated to consume his or her body weight in carbohydrates annually. Most of this glycogen, 400 g, is contained in skeletal muscle. In muscle, glycogen stores are kept remarkably stable, and seldom is expanded above this; indeed, increases of muscle glycogen induce IR *(19)*. A point that can be taken from this is that there is a metabolic priority placed on carbohydrate oxidation given the rather small and tightly regulated capacity for glycogen storage.

In accord with this principle, it is estimated that following meal ingestion, approximately one-third of the carbohydrate content of the meal is oxidized promptly by the CNS, and the other two-thirds, divided approximately equally between liver and muscle with minor fractions into other organ systems, is split between oxidization and glycogen. Maintaining normal insulin sensitivity is based in large measure on maintaining capacity to readily activate glucose oxidation in response to meal ingestion and to readily activate glycogen storage.

With regard to achieving a balance among amounts consumed, oxidized, and stored for fat, the considerations are quite different from glucose. Daily consumption of approx 40% of calories as fat is now common, meaning that about 1,000 kcal of fat are ingested per day and must be oxidized to maintain a zero net balance. A 75-kg man can be estimated to have 10 kg of fat mass, or 90,000 stored kcal. Thus, oxidizing 1,000 kcal of fat per day is less than 1% of lipid reserves, whereas the proportion for glucose was that daily oxidation of dietary carbohydrate was equivalent to approx 50% of stored glycogen. In obesity, by definition, the calories stored as fat are greatly increased, by a factor of at least two even for Class I obesity.

Arguably, one of the greatest metabolic challenges individuals face in the context of modern lifestyles is to create opportunities that favor fat oxidation. Fasting or undernourishment creates this opportunity, but happens rarely in modern life. Indeed, with a schedule of three meals daily, a majority of the 24 h is spent in postprandial metabolism. The other physiological circumstance for promoting fat oxidation is low- to moderate-intensity physical activity, especially sustained duration of physical activity. For many in modern society, careful scheduling and a commitment to undertake daily exercise are required as work and daily living no longer require manual labor. Thus, the structure of modern life impedes the physiology of fat oxidation and disposes instead to fat storage.

Physiological Effects of Insulin

There is a second point that can be taken from this review of daily partitioning of ingested fat between oxidation and storage: because of the quite small fractional turnover of the pool of stored fat, there is implicitly a strong metabolic primacy for tightly regulating fractional release of stored FFA. Insulin is crucial in regulating this process, normally having potent effects to govern rates of lipolysis. In normal-weight individuals, it is estimated that a circulating insulin concentration of ~15 μU/mL, or only twice normal fasting levels of insulin, is sufficient to achieve 50% suppression of fasting rates of lipolysis. This is of higher sensitivity than the effect of insulin to control hepatic production of glucose and far more sensitive than the levels of insulin that are needed to achieve robust stimulation of glucose uptake into skeletal muscle. Therefore, one summation of normal insulin action is that this promotes glucose oxidation rather than that of fat, along with maintenance of quite small storage depots of glycogen, and tightly conserves fat storage, parsimoniously releasing a minute fraction of this depot even when levels of insulin are near physiological nadir.

There is an intrinsic priority in carbohydrate metabolism to oxidize glucose and thereby not overload the relatively modest capacities that exist for glucose storage. For fatty acid metabolism, there is not a prominent limitation on the capacity to store fat, and the priority to oxidize fat is conditional on circumstances of fasting or exercise. Rather, a key priority is to control fractional release of FFA. The dysfunction of substrate competition that underlies the pathophysiology of IR in obesity represents the collision of these two metabolic priorities; one of the main consequences of this collision is the accumulation of ectopic fat. Thus, the stage and conditions for substrate competition are set.

POOR TIMING OF FAT OXIDATION IN OBESITY

Glucose-Induced Fat Inhibition

More than a decade ago, the author's laboratory began to assess substrate competition in type 2 diabetes and obesity from the perspective of whether fat oxidation is appropriately regulated during fasting conditions. Using arteriovenous limb balance methods to assess oxygen and carbon dioxide exchange across the leg, we observed an elevated RQ across the leg after an overnight fast in type 2 DM (20), which denoted a decreased reliance on fat oxidation. Furthermore, there was reduced fractional extraction of fatty acids across the leg in type 2 DM (21). Experimentally, in lean, healthy volunteers, an increase in RQ across the leg was induced by hyperglycemia, even without elevation of insulin or marked suppression of plasma fatty acids; an even more pronounced effect was observed in obese, nondiabetic individuals (22). Thus, increased glucose availability was associated with depressed reliance on fat oxidation during fasting conditions. The elevated RQ response was associated with activation of pyruvate dehydrogenase (PDH) in muscle (22), the outer mitochondrial membrane enzyme complex controlling entry of glycolytic flux into the Krebs cycle for oxidation.

Thus, the pattern of glucose induced inhibition of fat oxidation in many respects is a mirror image of the opposite pattern of perturbations induced by elevating fatty acids, in which a blunting of the normal rise in RQ stimulated by insulin, and impaired activation of PDH are among key physiological alterations caused by elevated plasma fatty acids (9).

Metabolic Inflexibility

These clinical investigations began to outline aspects of "insulin resistance" in skeletal muscle in obesity and type 2 diabetes that were manifest during fasting conditions. Studies performed in obesity provided a more complete picture, one that integrated the perturbations previously well described during insulin-stimulated conditions with the fasting phenotype. Amongst a group of forty obese but nondiabetic volunteers, equally divided between men and women, an elevated RQ across the leg was observed compared with the RQ of lean men and women during fasting conditions *(23)*. During insulin-stimulated conditions, using the glucose clamp method, the RQ across the leg increased in lean volunteers, to a value that denoted nearly complete reliance on glucose oxidation. However, in the obese volunteers, the values for RQ across the leg remained unchanged from the basal value obtained after an overnight fast *(23)*. The failure to increase RQ across the leg under insulin stimulation was clearly a manifestation of IR, but what was equally striking were the findings that values for RQ by muscle remained simply remained static and inappropriate to the physiological context of either fasting or insulin-stimulated conditions. This "metabolic inflexibility" appears to represent a detachment of muscle to respond to normal homeostatic cues of either fasting or insulin. Furthermore, the concept of metabolic inflexibility as a phenotype of IR in muscle raised the idea that perhaps this might be a target for intervention, perhaps one that is in certain respects separate from that of rectifying diminished insulin-stimulated glucose metabolism *(24)*.

BIOCHEMICAL DETERMINANTS OF METABOLIC INFLEXIBILITY

Delineating a physiological phenotype of metabolic inflexibility, a term we have used to describe the failure of oxidative metabolism in skeletal muscle in IR to fully adapt to either fat oxidation during fasting conditions or glucose oxidation during insulin-stimulated conditions, raised questions concerning the biochemical basis of this impairment. In collaboration with Jean-Aime Simoneau, an examination of potential factors intrinsic to muscle was begun; from the beginning, this work focused on mitochondria. It was observed that muscle from obese individuals and from those with type 2 DM had reduced activity of oxidative enzymes, such as those of the Krebs cycle and the fatty acid β-oxidation pathway, as well as reduction in activity of carnitine-palmitoyl transferase (CPT) *(25–27)*. Using single-fiber histochemical methods, He et al. *(28)* found that muscle oxidative enzyme activity was lower in obesity and in type 2 DM regardless of fiber type. More specific studies of mitochondria in the biopsy samples of human skeletal muscle, by Ritov et al. *(29)*, were used to assess activity of NADH-oxidase, the activity of complexes I through IV of the electron transport chain (ETC) in muscle from lean and obese nondiabetic volunteers and from those with type 2 DM. Conjunctive studies of mitochondrial morphology were carried out using transmission electron microscopy (TEM). NADH-oxidase activity was significantly lower in skeletal muscle in obesity compared with lean volunteers, and lower still in type 2 DM; overall, a reduction by approx 40% was noted compared with ETC activity in muscle from lean volunteers *(30)*. Mitochondria were smaller in obesity and type 2 DM *(30)*. Both of these parameters—ETC activity and mitochondrial size—correlated with systemic insulin sensitivity, indicating that mitochondrial dysfunction was a cell biology component of IR. Subsequently, gene array studies of skeletal muscle have found that decreased expression of nuclear genes encoding mitochondrial proteins, including constituents of the

ETC, occurs in type 2 DM and in those at risk for type 2 DM *(31,32)*. Also, noninvasive imaging of oxidative phosphorylation, using nuclear magnetic resonance spectroscopy, indicated impaired mitochondrial function in association with the IR in those at high risk for developing type 2 DM *(33)*. Additionally, whereas insulin infusion was found to induce expression of genes encoding mitochondrial proteins in muscle of lean, healthy volunteers, this effect is blunted in type 2 DM *(34)*.

ECTOPIC FAT IN LIVER AND MUSCLE

For at least a decade, it has been recognized that the intramyocellular content of lipids (IMCL) can be strongly associated with IR *(35)*. During the past several years, similar findings with regard to hepatic steatosis have also emerged from a number of investigators. Thus, increases of IMCL and hepatic steatosis are two aspects of body composition that are now perceived to be closely related to the pathogenesis of IR in obesity and type 2 DM.

Skeletal muscle and liver normally contain small amounts of triglyceride, far smaller than that contained in adipose tissue. In obesity, these repositories can be greatly increased. Hepatic steatosis occurs commonly in obesity, especially in visceral obesity and especially in type 2 DM *(36)*, and is strongly correlated with IR. In patients with type 2 DM, the amount of insulin required to achieve glycemic control is correlated to the amount of hepatic steatosis *(37)*, indicating the importance of this depot to the pathogenesis of hepatic insulin resistance. Hepatic steatosis is also correlated with the severity of dyslipidemia *(36)*.

IMCL is increased in obesity, in type 2 DM, and in first-degree relatives of those with type 2 DM. A strong possibility is that mitochondrial dysfunction limits capacity for fat oxidation, which contributes to accumulation of IMCL. Elevated fatty acid delivery is also a key factor leading to hepatic steatosis and increased muscle lipid content. There are emerging data that FFA uptake into muscle, mediated by fatty acid transporters, is increased in obesity and type 2 DM. Thus, increases of uptake in the face of reduced or at least finite capacity for fat oxidation and energy expenditure during sedentary conditions leads to triglyceride accumulation. In addition, part of the pathophysiology may entail increases in malonyl CoA that inhibit CPT I, and thus, fat oxidation.

Although IMCL has served as a useful marker for IR in muscle, it is not clear, however, that it is specifically the accumulation of triglyceride that mediates IR. There is uncertainty as to which aspect of IMCL induces IR. It is postulated that other lipid moieties may actually induce signaling that mediates IR. One candidate is diacyl glycerol (DAG), which is often increased in conjunction with IMCL and can activate protein kinase C (PKC), certain isoforms of which lead to serine phosphorylation and impede insulin signaling *(35)*. Other candidate lipids include long-chain acylCoA and ceramides. Unfortunately, at this juncture, there are conflicting results in the literature, and a consensus as to how the connection between IMCL and IR is mediated remains somewhat uncertain. One concept is that the IMCL induces a low-grade inflammatory condition within myocytes, and a similar postulate has gained considerable acceptance with regard to the metabolic repercussions of hepatic steatosis as well. Part of this conundrum as to whether IMCL is causative for IR in muscle is that IMCL is increased not only in sedentary obese individuals but also in lean, endurance-trained athletes *(38)*. The latter group maintains very high levels of insulin sensitivity despite levels of IMCL that are similar to those found in obesity. A key difference is that in muscle of lean, endurance-trained athletes, there is a heightened oxidative capacity and a high reliance on fat oxidation during fasting conditions and during physical activity. This, as earlier described, contrasts quite vividly with the suppressed oxidative capacity of skeletal muscle in obese, sedentary individuals and with the concomitant reduced reliance on fat oxidation. So, it is also speculated that an aspect of IMCL that triggers IR is its relationship to rates of fat oxidation and the turnover time of lipid droplets. In athletes, the pool of IMCL would be continually depleted by exercise and then refilled, as occurs for glycogen, whereas in obese, sedentary individuals the pool of IMCL may stay more stagnant, perhaps vulnerable to peroxidation and more susceptible to the generation of lipids that directly signal IR.

CONCLUSIONS

In metabolism of fatty acids, as in other domains of life, location and timing prove to be quite crucial. Certainly one perspective concerning the pathogenesis of IR is that accumulation of fat in the wrong locations and inopportune timing in the patterns of reliance on fat oxidation can lead to IR and disorders of glucose homeostasis. Ironically, one of the best therapeutic approaches to alleviate the metabolic complications of induced by glucose–FFA substrate competition and ectopic fat is to promote physical activity. Physical activity, by enhancing oxidative capacity of muscle, does help to restore as well a greater reliance on fat oxidation during fasting conditions and restore metabolic flexibility in suppressing fat oxidation during insulin-stimulated conditions.

REFERENCES

1. Himsworth H, Kerr R. Insulin-sensitive and insulin-insensitive types of diabetes mellitus. Clin Sci 1939;4:119–152.
2. Himsworth H. The mechanism of diabetes mellitus. I. Lancet 1939;2:1–6.
3. Himsworth H. The mechanism of diabetes mellitus. II. The control of the blood sugar level. Lancet 1939;2:65–68.
4. Yalow RS, Berson SA. Immunoassay of endogenous plasma insulin in man. J Clin Invest 1960;39:1157–1175.
5. Ferrannini E, Buzzigoli G, Bonadonna R, et al. Insulin resistance in essential hypertension. N Engl J Med 1987;317:350–357.
6. Randle P, Garland P, Hales C, et al. The glucose fatty acid cycle. Its role in insulin sensitivity and the metabolic disturbances of diabetes mellitus. Lancet 1963;1:785–789.
7. Boden G. Role of fatty acids in the pathogenesis of insulin resistance in NIDDM. Diabetes 1997;46:3–10.
8. Boden G, Chen X. Effects of fat on glucose uptake and utilization in patients with non-insulin-dependent diabetes mellitus. J Clin Invest 1995;96:1261–1268.
9. Kelley D, Mokan M, Simoneau J-A, et al. Interaction between glucose and free fatty acid metabolism in human skeletal muscle. J Clin Invest 1993;92:93–98.
10. Kelley D, Mokan M, Mandarino L. Intracellular defects in glucose metabolism in obese patients with noninsulin-dependent diabetes mellitus. Diabetes 1992;41:698–706.
11. Kelley D, Williams K, Price J, et al. Plasma fatty acids, adiposity, and variance of skeletal muscle insulin resistance in type 2 diabetes mellitus. J Clin Endocrinol Metab 2001;86:5412–5419.
12. Santomauro A, Boden G, Silva M, et al. Overnight lowering of free fatty acids with Acipimox improves insulin resistance and glucose tolerance in obese diabetic and nondiabetic subjects. Diabetes 1999;48:1836–1841.
13. Goodpaster BH, Thaete FL, Simoneau JA, et al. Subcutaneous abdominal fat and thigh muscle composition predict insulin sensitivity independently of visceral fat. Diabetes 1997;46:1579–1585.
14. Kirtland J, Gurr MI. Adipose tissue cellularity: a review. 2. The relationship between cellularity and obesity. Int J Obes 1979;3:15–55.

15. Basu A, Basu R, Shah P, et al. Systemic and regional free fatty acid metabolism in type 2 diabetes. Am J Physiol Endocrinol Metab 2001;280:E1000–E1006.
16. Salans LB, Cushman SW, Weismann RE. Studies of human adipose tissue. Adipose cell size and number in nonobese and obese patients. J Clin Invest 1973;52:929–941.
17. Weyer C, Wolford JK, Hanson RL, et al. Subcutaneous abdominal adipocyte size, a predictor of type 2 diabetes, is linked to chromosome 1q21–q23 and is associated with a common polymorphism in LMNA in Pima Indians. Mol Genet Metab 2001;72:231–238.
18. Andres R, Cader G, Zierler K. The quantitatively minor role of carbohydrate in oxidative metabolism by skeletal muscle in intact man in the basal state. Measurement of oxygen and glucose uptake and carbon dioxide and lactate production in the forearm. J Clin Invest 1956;35:671-682.
19. Mott D, Lillioja S, Bogardus C. Overnutrition induced decrease in insulin action for glucose storage: in vivo and in vitro in man. Metabolism 1986;35:160–165.
20. Kelley DE, Mandarino LJ. Hyperglycemia normalizes insulin-stimulated skeletal muscle glucose oxidation and storage in noninsulin-dependent diabetes mellitus. J Clin Invest 1990;86:1999–2007.
21. Kelley D, Simoneau J: Impaired free fatty acid utilization by skeletal muscle in non-insulin-dependent diabetes mellitus. J Clin Invest 1994;94:2349–2356.
22. Mandarino LJ, Consoli A, Jain A, et al. Differential regulation of intracellular glucose metabolism by glucose and insulin in human muscle. Am J Physiol 1993;265:E898–E905.
23. Kelley D, Goodpaster B, Wing R, et al. Skeletal muscle fatty acid metabolism in association with insulin resistance, obesity and weight loss. Am J Physiol 1999;277:E1130–E1141.
24. Kelley D, Mandarino L. Fuel selection in human skeletal muscle in insulin resistance: a reexamination. Diabetes 2000;49:677–683.
25. Simoneau J, Colberg S, Thaete F, et al. Skeletal muscle glycolytic and oxidative enzyme capacities are determinants of insulin sensitivity and muscle composition in obese women. FASEB J 1995;9:273–278.
26. Simoneau J, Kelley D. Altered glycolytic and oxidative capacities of skeletal muscle contribute to insulin resistance in NIDDM. J Appl Physiol 1997;83:166–171.
27. Colberg S, Simoneau J-A, Thaete F, et al. Impaired FFA utilization by skeletal muscle in women with visceral obesity. J Clin Invest 1995;95:1846–1853.
28. He J, Watkins S, Kelley D. Skeletal muscle lipid content and oxidative enzyme activity in relation to muscle fiber type in type 2 diabetes and obesity. Diabetes 2001;50: 817–823.
29. Ritov VB, Menshikova EV, Kelley DE. High-performance liquid chromatography-based methods of enzymatic analysis: electron transport chain activity in mitochondria from human skeletal muscle. Anal Biochem 2004;333:27–38.
30. Kelley D, He J, Menshikova E, Ritov V. Dysfunction of mitochondria in human skeletal muscle in type 2 diabetes mellitus. Diabetes 2002;51:2944–2950.
31. Mootha VK, Bunkenborg J, Olsen JV, et al. Integrated analysis of protein composition, tissue diversity, and gene regulation in mouse mitochondria. Cell 2003;115:629–640.
32. Patti M, Butte A, Crunkhorn S, et al. Coordinated reduction in genes of oxidative metabolism in humans with insulin resistance and diabetes: potential roles of PGC1 and NRF-1. Proc Natl Acad Sci USA 2003;100:8466–8471.
33. Petersen K, Dufour S, Befoy D, et al. Impaired mitochondrial activity in the insulin-resistant offspring of patients with type 2 diabetes. N Engl J Med 2004;350:664–671.
34. Stump C, Short K, Bigelow M, et al. Effect of insulin on human skeletal muscle mitochondrial ATP production, protein synthesis and mRNA transcripts. Proc Natl Acad Science USA 2003;100:7996–8001.
35. Shulman G. Cellular mechanisms of insulin resistance. J Clin Invest 2000;106:171–176.
36. Kelley D, McKolanis T, Hegazi R, et al. Fatty liver in type 2 diabetes mellitus: relation to regional adiposity, fatty acids, and insulin resistance. Am J Physiol (Endocrinol Metab) 2003;285:E906–E916.
37. Seppala-Lindroos A, Vehkavaara S, Hakkinen AM, et al. Fat accumulation in the liver is associated with defects in insulin suppression of glucose production and serum free fatty acids independent of obesity in normal men. J Clin Endocrinol Metab 2002;87:3023–3028.
38. Goodpaster BH, He J, Watkins S, et al. Skeletal muscle lipid content and insulin resistance: evidence for a paradox in endurance-trained athletes. J Clin Endocrinol Metab 2001;86:5755–5761.

6

Critical Importance of the Perinatal Period in the Development of Obesity

Barry E. Levin, MD

CONTENTS

INTRODUCTION
GESTATION, LACTATION, AND MATERNAL ENVIRONMENT
PERINATAL ENVIRONMENT AND BRAIN DEVELOPMENT
CONCLUSIONS
REFERENCES

Summary

Epidemiological studies suggest that maternal undernutrition, obesity, and diabetes during gestation and lactation can all produce obesity in offspring. Animal models provide a means of assessing the independent consequences of altering the pre- versus postnatal environments on a variety of metabolic, physiologic, and neuroendocrine functions that lead to the development of offspring obesity, diabetes, hypertension, and hyperlipidemia. During the gestational period, maternal malnutrition, obesity, type 1 and type 2 diabetes, and psychological, immunological, and pharmacological stressors can all promote offspring obesity. Normal postnatal nutrition can sometimes reduce the adverse impact of some of these prenatal factors but may also exacerbate the development of obesity and diabetes in offspring of dams that were malnourished during gestation. The genetic background of the individual is also an important determinant of outcome when the perinatal environment is perturbed. Individuals with an obesity-prone genotype are more likely to be adversely affected by factors such as maternal obesity and high-fat diets. Many perinatal manipulations are associated with reorganization of the central neural pathways that regulate food intake, energy expenditure, and storage in ways that enhance the development of obesity and diabetes in offspring. Both leptin and insulin have strong neurotrophic properties so that either an excess or an absence of either during the perinatal period may underlie some of these adverse developmental changes. Because perinatal manipulations can permanently and adversely alter the systems that regulate energy homeostasis, it behooves us to gain a better understanding of the factors during this period that promote the development of offspring obesity as a means of stemming the tide of the emerging worldwide obesity epidemic.

Key Words: Obesity; diabetes; development; gestation; lactation; hypothalamus; neuropeptide Y; POMC; arcuate nucleus; genotype; high-fat diet; leptin; insulin.

From: *Contemporary Endocrinology: Treatment of the Obese Patient*
Edited by: R. F. Kushner and D. H. Bessesen © Humana Press Inc., Totowa, NJ

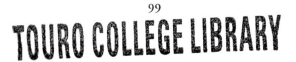

INTRODUCTION

An epidemic of obesity of unprecedented magnitude is sweeping the world without apparent regard for geographic boundaries, socioeconomic status, or degree of technological advancement *(1–7)*. This is of particular concern because of the associated metabolic syndrome (hypertension, dyslipidemia, diabetes), which raises the morbidity and mortality of obesity *(8–12)*. The obesity epidemic has become particularly problematic in the United States *(13–15)*. The prevalence of obesity has significantly increased among the US population over the past 30 yr; data from 1999 to 2002 estimated that almost a third of adults were obese and that this increased prevalence crossed all age, gender, and racial/ethnic groups *(16)*. Of even greater concern is the increasing prevalence of childhood obesity, which was estimated to be one in six US children from 1999 to 2002 *(14–17)*. This is an ominous sign for the future, as maternal obesity is associated with reduced offspring energy expenditure *(18)* and an increased risk of obesity *(19,20)*. Although most obesity follows a polygenic mode of inheritance *(21–24)*, it is clear that the current epidemic of obesity cannot be caused by alterations in genotype because of the very short interval over which it has occurred. This makes it likely that environmental factors have provided the impetus for the current epidemic.

Throughout human history there have been cycles of famine interspersed with periods of plenty *(25)*. Although it is controversial, the "thrifty gene" hypothesis posits that these cycles have selected for individuals who can withstand periods of famine by being able to ingest and store as many calories as possible during times of plenty as a buffer against times of famine *(26)*. The problem with such individuals comes when food is readily obtainable at low financial and energetic cost *(27)*. Add to this the logarithmic increase in "supersized" portions of highly palatable, high-fat foods and the result is the recipe for an obesity epidemic, particularly in genetically predisposed individuals.

However, the epidemic of obesity has also struck in underdeveloped countries where periods of famine still occur. Studies of individuals who were *in utero* during the European famine that followed World War II suggest that maternal undernutrition during the first two trimesters was associated with an increased risk of obesity and/or type 2 diabetes mellitus (T2DM) in their offspring *(28–30)*. This led Barker *(31)* to postulate that human fetuses in such circumstances adapt to a limited supply of nutrients by permanently changing their physiology to become more metabolically efficient. These metabolically programmed changes underlie the development of a number of diseases in later life, including obesity, T2DM, coronary heart disease, stroke, and hypertension *(29, 31–34)*. Besides maternal obesity and undernutrition, both T2DM or type 1 diabetes (T1DM) during pregnancy and lactation can also predispose offspring to develop obesity and T2DM *(35–37)*. Based on such human epidemiological data and animal studies reviewed below, Waterland and Garza *(38)* proposed the concept of "metabolic imprinting" by which a variety of perturbations that occur during a critical developmental window will have a persistent effect that lasts into adulthood. Because most human studies are retrospective and therefore uncontrolled, a number of investigators have turned to animal models to test hypotheses about the effects of perturbing the perinatal environment on the development of obesity and metabolic syndrome in offspring. Animal models allow us to control for the independent effects of the pre- versus postnatal environment. They also allow us to assess the effect of perturbations of the perinatal environment on the function of neural pathways that are critical regulators of energy homeostasis. These studies can be generally grouped into those in which the entire perinatal period is manipulated or where either the pre- or postnatal environment is specifically altered to affect the offspring.

GESTATION, LACTATION, AND MATERNAL ENVIRONMENT

The majority of human beings are raised with their biological mothers. This means that they are exposed to the maternal environment throughout gestation and lactation, as well as through the rest of their formative years. Thus, outcome in humans is dependent not only on the biological effects of the perinatal maternal environment but also on a number of psychosocial and socioeconomic variables. Because these variables are not major factors in animal models, these models are best suited for investigating the effects of altering the metabolic perinatal environment on offspring outcome. Rodent models also have the advantage that lifelong patterns of food intake and body weight are generally established by the second week of life as long as dietary content is held constant thereafter *(39,40)*. Whereas human studies can only suggest a relationship, it is clear that maternal obesity throughout gestation and lactation in rats leads to the development of obesity and metabolic syndrome in offspring *(41–48)*. The one caveat is that the diets required to produce maternal obesity may themselves have an effect that is independent of the presence of obesity and a genetic predisposition to become obese. For example, feeding dams high-fat diets throughout the perinatal period produces obesity in all offspring in certain rat strains *(44,49)*, whereas it is clear that genetic predisposition is a critical determinant of the way in which such maternal diets affect the development of offspring obesity *(41,42)*.

To separate out the independent effects of genotype, obesity, and diet on offspring, we used rats that were selectively bred from the outbred Sprague-Dawley strain to be either prone or resistant to the development of diet-induced obesity (DIO) on a moderate (high-energy [HE]) fat diet *(50)*. Similar to the inheritance of much human obesity *(21)*, the DIO and diet-resistant (DR) phenotypes are also inherited as polygenic traits *(43,50,51)*. On a low-fat diet, DIO and DR rats are both lean. However, when the caloric density and fat content of the diet are increased, only DIO rats become obese, hyperinsulinemic, glucose-intolerant, hypertensive, and hyperlipidemic on the HE diet *(50,52–55)*. The phenotype of the DIO and DR rats has remained stable for more than 35 generations *(50,55)*, making these rats ideal for the separating the genetic from dietary factors influencing the development of obesity in offspring. When DIO dams were made obese on an HE diet throughout gestation and lactation, their offspring became more obese than those of DIO dams fed a low-fat diet. But dietary fat was not the critical determinant of this obesity, as offspring of DR dams fed an HE diet became no more obese than those of dams fed a low-fat diet *(41,42)*. Furthermore, the presence of maternal obesity also had no impact on offspring of DR dams. Offspring of DR dams made obese during gestation and lactation on a highly palatable diet became no more obese than those whose dams remained lean on either a low-fat or an HE diet. These studies demonstrate how important the interactions among genotype, diet, and the metabolic state of the dam are on the development of offspring obesity. They also strongly suggest that an obesity-prone genotype is a critical determinant of the outcome of manipulations of the perinatal environment.

Besides genetic background, the macronutrient composition of the maternal diet has important independent effects on the development of offspring obesity. Although maternal high-fat diets generally promote offspring obesity *(44,49)*, this effect is dependent on the type of fats in the diet. Diets with high omega-6 fatty acid contents produce obese offspring with increased hepatic lipid content and hepatic insulin resistance *(56)*. On the other hand, diets high in essential fatty acids fed to dams throughout late gestation and lactation have the opposite effect: they appear to protect against offspring obesity and insulin resistance *(57–59)*. Maternal diets high in carbohydrate content can have a similar protective effect on offspring *(60)* and can actually alter the preference for carbohydrates in offspring when fed to dams throughout gestation and lactation *(61)*. Protein content of the maternal diet is also important. When dams are fed a severely protein-restricted diet throughout gestation and lactation, their offspring become obese, insulin-resistant, hyperlipidemic, and hypertensive as adults. These adverse outcomes are magnified even more when the protein-restricted diet is replaced by a highly palat-able one at weaning *(62,63)*. This outcome is also dependent on gender. Female offspring of dams that are protein-restricted throughout gestation and lactation actually have lower body weights, food intake, and increased insulin sensitivity as adults *(64)*.

Finally, maternal diabetes also has a deleterious effect on offspring. Mothers with T2DM produce offspring that become obese and have abnormalities of insulin secretion *(65)*, whereas T1DM during pregnancy produces both cardiovascular dysfunction *(66)* and accelerated growth through the first 6 to 10 wk of adult life *(67)*.

Prenatal Influences on Offspring

It is not surprising that major alterations in the metabolic milieu in which a fetus grows can markedly affect its development. Cross-fostering studies in which pups are placed with surrogate dams shortly after birth suggest that prenatal factors account for 61 to 96% of the variance in body weight gain in male and 35 to 92% in female offspring *(68)*. Offspring of dams fed a high-fat diet during gestation became more obese than those whose dams were fed a low-fat diet, even if the high-fat offspring were fostered with dams on a low-fat diet throughout lactation *(49,69)*. As suggested by human epidemio-logical studies, malnutrition during gestation can also result in obese offspring. To model these studies, Jones and colleagues *(70,71)* restricted the caloric intake of dams by up to 50% during the first two trimesters of pregnancy. Male (but not female) off-spring of these calorically restricted dams became hyperphagic, gained more weight beginning at weaning *(71)*, and became obese as adults *(70,71)*. This finding may be dependent on the specific rat strain used, as others found that gestational undernutrition produced obese female but lean male offspring *(72)*. The timing of caloric restriction during gestation in rats may also not be as critical as it appears to be in humans, as 30% caloric restriction during the last trimester produced obesity in offspring of dams with an obesity-prone, insulin-resistant genotype *(43)*. Also, severe maternal undernutrition (70% caloric restriction) throughout the entire pregnancy produced low-birthweight offspring that had stunted linear growth but then became hyperphagic, obese, hyperinsulinemic, hypertensive, and hypoactive as adults *(73,74)*.

Maternal exposure to a variety of stressors during gestation can also affect offspring development. Administration of endotoxin *(75)*, tumor necrosis factor-α, or interleukin-6 *(76)* to dams during the first two trimesters of gestation produces offspring that become obese as adults. Somewhat paradoxically, immunosuppressant corticosteroid (dexam-ethasone) injections of dams during the first two trimesters produced effects on offspring that were virtually identical to those seen in offspring of dams injected with

Table 1
Prenatal Factors That Influence Body Weight of Offspring

Factors That Promote Obesity in Offspring
– Maternal dietary factors
  • High-fat diets *(49,69)*
  • Diets high in omega-6 fatty acids *(56)*
  • Protein-restricted diets *(62–64)*
  • Energy-restricted diets *(28–30,43,70,71–74)*
– Maternal type 1 or 2 diabetes *(35–37,65,86)*
– Maternal insulin treatment *(82,83)*
– Maternal stress hormones and cytokines
  • Endotoxin *(75)*
  • Tumor necrosis factor-α *(76)*
  • Interleukin-6 *(76)*
  • Dexamethasone *(43,76)*
Factors That Protect Against Development of Obesity in Offspring
– Maternal dietary factors
  • Diets high in essential fatty acids *(57–59)*
  • Diets high in carbohydrate *(60)*

proinflammatory agents over this same period *(76)*. However, dexamethasone injections during the third trimester can also produce obesity and insulin resistance in offspring of dams with a genetic predisposition to develop insulin resistance and DIO *(43)*. Thus, depending on the type and timing, a variety of maternal stressors during gestation can promote obesity and insulin resistance in adult offspring.

The hormonal milieu to which the fetus is exposed during gestation can also have a major impact on its development. Both insulin and leptin are important in this regard. Aside from its role in glucose homeostasis, insulin has important trophic properties on neural development *(77–79)*. Although not all studies agree *(80)*, maternal insulin may actually cross the placenta and enter the fetal circulation *(81)*. This could explain why offspring of rat dams injected daily with insulin during the last trimester develop obesity as adults *(82)*. In keeping with its neurotrophic properties, such gestational insulin injections lead to major alterations in the development of hypothalamic norepinephrine circuits *(82,83)*. Maternal hyperinsulinemia and hyperglycemia, such as that which occurs in gestational diabetes, can increase glucose transport across the placenta *(84)*, leading to fetal hyperglycemia and hyperinsulinemia *(85)*. This prenatal environment is associated with increased fetal weight *(86)*. On the other hand, the low birthweight of offspring of mothers with T2DM might be caused by insulin resistance that develops in the fetus, causing reduced effectiveness of insulin as a trophic factor and resultant *in utero* growth retardation *(87)*. As with exogenous administration of insulin *(82,83)*, offspring of dams with hyperinsulinemia during gestation have abnormal hypothalamic norepinephrine (NE) circuitry in association with adult obesity *(41,42)*. However, this outcome is dependent on genotype, as it occurs in offspring of hyperinsulinemic DIO but not DR dams.

Leptin also significantly affects the developing fetus and its nervous system *(88–93)*. Leptin also plays a role in embryo implantation *(94)*. A significant amount of leptin is produced by the placenta *(95,96)* and cord blood leptin levels correlate positively with birth weight and body mass index *(97)*. Insulin treatment of T1DM mothers increases placental leptin production *(98)*, leading to increased cord-blood leptin levels *(99)*. In normal pregnancies, maternal leptin levels increase progressively during gestation and are higher at term than in nonpregnant women *(100)*. Besides being produced by the placenta, leptin undergoes transplacental transport. In keeping with rising maternal leptin levels, placental transport and the resultant fetal plasma leptin levels are increased 10-fold during the last trimester of gestation *(101)*. Thus, both maternal obesity and hyperinsulinemia can produce fetal hyperleptinemia. Since leptin has neurotrophic properties, such hyperleptinemia might have a major impact on brain development and the central pathways involved in energy homeostasis *(93,102,103)*.

Postnatal Influences on Offspring

Although the prenatal environment has a major impact on the developing fetus, a number of postnatal factors can alter the development of ingestive behavior in neonates and predispose them to develop obesity and metabolic syndrome as adults. Metabolic, hormonal, and behavioral interactions of pups with their dams are critical factors in this regard. Maternal milk is composed primarily of fatty acids *(104–106)* and the composition of milk understandably has a major impact on the developing neonate. Because maternal milk contains more fat than carbohydrate, neonates utilize fatty acids and ketone bodies as their primary energy substrates. During suckling, neonates transport ketone bodies preferentially over carbohydrates across the blood–brain barrier, and ketone bodies serve as the primary energy substrate for neuronal and glial metabolism *(107,108)*. Blockade of both fatty acid oxidation (lipoprivation) *(109)* and glucose oxidation (glucoprivation) *(110)* increase food intake in adults. But, despite the high lipid content of their diets, feeding in response to such lipoprivation does not develop in rat pups until 12 d of age, and glucoprivic feeding does not occur at any time during suckling *(111–113)*. Nor are gastric filling or postaborptive metabolic signals major determinants of intake in neonates as they are in adults. Rather, osmotic load appears to be the most important regulator of feeding *(113,114)*. This osmoregulatory effect may be mediated by cholecystokinin (CCK), which can cause satiety in neonates as early as the second week of life *(115)*.

As would be expected, maternal diet is a primary determinant of milk composition. "Cafeteria diets" composed of highly palatable junk foods increase the long-chain and decrease the medium-chain fatty acid content of maternal milk and have an additive effect to the presence of maternal obesity in lowering the protein and raising the long-chain fatty acid content of milk *(104)*. Diets high in polyunsaturated fatty acids have the effect of lowering pup body weight and adiposity and leptin levels *(58)*. Feeding dams a high-fat diet also accelerates the onset of independent feeding in neonates by 1 to 2 days *(116)* in association with increased weight gain *(117)* and the development of hypertension and abnormal glucose homeostasis as adults *(118)*. Furthermore, feeding successive generations of dams a high-fat diet leads to progressive increases the level of obesity of their offspring *(119)*. This feed-forward effect may have important relevance to the increasing incidence of obesity in the developed world.

Under conditions somewhat comparable to bottle-feeding, high-carbohydrate diets can produce obesity in pups. When pups are artificially raised away from their dams and fed a high-carbohydrate diet by gastric tube, they develop obesity and insulin resistance

Table 2
Postnatal Factors That Affect the Risk of Developing Obesity

Factors That Promote Obesity in the Pup
- Maternal high-fat diet *(117–119)*
- Maternal high-carbohydrate diets *(120–124)*
- Small litter size *(39,40,128–132,136)*
- Being raised by an obese dam *(137,138)*
- Hypothalamic Insulin administration *(150)*

Factors That Protect Against the Development of Obesity in the Pup
- High polyunsaturated fat diet *(58)*
- Being raised by an obesity-resistant dam *(137,138)*
- Being raised by a diabetic dam *(140)*
- Large litter size *(39,128–131)*
- Leptin administration *(90,1443,144)*

---

as compared to those fed either a low-fat, low-carbohydrate, or high-fat diet *(120–123)*. This effect is most marked in female offspring *(123,124)*; therefore their obesity carries forward to their offspring, even when those offspring are raised under normal perinatal conditions *(123)*. Finally, whereas maternal protein malnutrition during pregnancy lowers offspring birthweight, this effect can be overcome by fostering those offspring with dams fed a normal diet postnatally. Unfortunately, such "recuperated" offspring become more obesity-prone and develop hypertension when subsequently fed a cafeteria diet *(62,125,126)*, suggesting that the increased metabolic efficiency developed by the fetuses *in utero* predisposed them to become obese as adults *(127)*. As with artificial rearing on high-carbohydrate diets, this effect of gestational protein malnutrition carries over into subsequent generations *(64)*. Again, these feed-forward effects might be an important contributor to the upward spiral of obesity incidence in our society.

The quantity of food available during suckling is also a determinant of the development of obesity in pups. Kennedy first used large and small litter sizes as a strategy to alter the intake of neonates *(39)*. He, and later others, showed that rat pups raised in small litters were heavier at weaning and gained more weight as adults, whereas those raised in large litters gained less weight than pups raised in normal-size litters *(39,40,128–130)*. These differences in weight gain appeared to be due to early differences in milk availability and intake *(39,130)*. The increased weight gain of adult rats raised in small litters is associated with the development of obesity *(128,129,131,132)*, hyperleptinemia *(133)*, abnormal insulin secretion *(134)*, insulin resistance *(132)*, and dyslipidemia *(135)*. Interestingly, the postweaning weight gain seen in the original Kennedy study was not associated with increased intake as a function of body weight *(39)*, suggesting that reduced energy expenditure rather than actual hyperphagia was responsible for the subsequent development of obesity *(136)*. Thus, the amount of milk consumed during the suckling period and the content of that milk, as determined by maternal diet and metabolic status, can have an enormous impact on the subsequent development of obesity.

Although maternal obesity and gestational diabetes promote the development of obesity and insulin resistance in offspring, cross-fostering studies demonstrate that altering the postnatal maternal environment can overcome even genetic predispositions to become obese or lean. Raising pups with an obesity-prone genotype with an obesity-resistant dam can attenuate their development of insulin resistance and/or obesity, whereas raising obesity-resistant pups with genetically obese dams causes them to develop obesity and insulin resistance *(137,138)*. Also, pups born to mothers made diabetic during gestation are heavier and hyperinsulinemic at weaning *(65,139)*, whereas offspring of normal dams fostered to diabetic dams develop early postnatal growth delay and decreased body weight gain *(140)*. Whereas stressing the dam during the last trimester of gestation produces smaller, obese offspring *(43)*, this effect can be reversed by handling the pups repeatedly during the postnatal period *(141)*.

Both leptin and insulin can affect development during the postnatal period. Rat pups are born relatively undeveloped as compared with human infants. They have little body fat and produce very little leptin over the first 7 to 10 d of life *(142)*. Depending on the doses given, pups may *(90,143,144)* or may not *(89)* respond to exogenous leptin administration by reducing their weight gain or adiposity during this period. It is likely that leptin given during this early postnatal period primarily increases metabolic rate rather than reducing food intake *(145)*. Elevated leptin levels in the milk of obese dams might alter the metabolism of their pups through a similar mechanism, as leptin can be absorbed from the milk and enter the circulation of the pup during this early postnatal period *(146–149)*. When leptin is administered orally to pups at 4 d of age, it not only reduces their adiposity and brown adipose tissue thermogenic capacity but also decreases their endogenous production of leptin *(149)*. Aside from altering metabolic rate, leptin also acts on the developing neonatal nervous system through its neurotrophic properties *(102,103)*. For example, the hypothalamic pathways that are critical regulators of energy homeostasis do not develop normally in the absence of leptin or intact leptin signaling *(91,93)*. Exogenous leptin administration during the first 2 wk of life to normal animals can also affect the development of these pathways *(90)*. Insulin may also play an important neurotrophic role during this critical period. Direct injections into the rat hypothalamus on the eighth day of life significantly alter the development of hypothalamic areas involved in the control of energy homeostasis in normal rats *(150)*.

PERINATAL ENVIRONMENT AND BRAIN DEVELOPMENT

The brain is undoubtedly the master controller of energy homeostasis, but it requires neural, hormonal, and metabolic signals from the body and external environment to perform this task. Mammals have evolved a unique set of "metabolic sensing" neurons to receive these multiple inputs from the periphery. These neurons are arrayed in multiple interconnected sites throughout the brain *(151–154)*. These neurons were originally recognized as "glucose-sensing" because, unlike most neurons that use glucose only to fuel their metabolic needs, these neurons utilize glucose as a signaling molecule to alter their firing rate when ambient glucose levels change *(155,156)*. It is now clear that many of these same glucose-sensing neurons also utilize metabolites such as lactate *(157–159)*, ketone bodies *(160)*, and fatty acids *(161)* as signaling molecules. They also have receptors for and respond to hormones such as leptin and insulin *(162–166)*. Because of their ability to use metabolic substrates, as well as hormones and peptides associated with adiposity, gut function, and feeding, we have called them "metabolic-sensing" neurons *(153,167)*. Hindbrain areas such as the nucleus tractus solitarius, area postrema, raphe pallidus and obscurus, and A2/C2 areas contain such metabolic sensing neurons

(168–174). Some of these receive direct neural inputs from sensors in peripheral organs such as the gastrointestinal tract and hepatic portal vein *(169,175–177)*. Metabolic sensing neurons within the hindbrain express the monoamines NE, epinephrine (Epi), and serotonin (5HT) *(168,170,172)* and neuropeptides such as neuropeptide Y (NPY) and pro-opiomelanocortin (POMC) *(178,179)*. These hindbrain neurons relay information from the periphery to hypothalamic areas that mediate feeding behavior and metabolic processes involved in the control of energy homeostasis *(179–184)*, as well as to limbic and forebrain structures involved in the affective and rewarding properties of food *(185,186)*. Metabolic sensing neurons also reside in the hypothalamus. Neurons expressing NPY and POMC in the hypothalamic arcuate nucleus (ARC) receive inputs from hindbrain metabolic sensing neurons, as do several neuropeptide and neurotransmitter expressing neurons within the paraventricular nucleus (PVN) and lateral hypothalamus (LH). The PVN and LH are major effector areas involved in neuroendocrine function, food intake, energy assimilation, and energy expenditure *(180–183,187–190)*.

Although much more of brain development occurs postnatally in rodents than it does in primates *(92,191–194)*, there are enough similarities that we can learn a great deal from developmental studies in rodents. Neuropeptides and neurotransmitters affecting various aspects of energy homeostasis can be grouped according to their predominantly catabolic, anabolic, or reward-related properties. Many neuropeptide and transmitter systems also serve other functions besides the regulation of energy homeostasis. However, regulation of energy homeostasis seems to be the primary role of ARC and hindbrain NPY and POMC neurons *(92,195–202)*. Neuropeptide Y is a prototypic anabolic neuropeptide that increases food intake and decreases energy expenditure when injected into areas around the hypothalamus *(195–197,203)*. POMC is the precursor of α-melanocyte-stimulating hormone (α-MSH), which is a prototypic catabolic peptide that acts on melanocortin 3 and 4 receptors (MC3/4R) to inhibit intake and increase energy expenditure *(198,204–207)*. The ARC NPY neurons also produce agouti-related peptide (AgRP), which is a unique neuropeptide as it is the only known example of an endogenous inverse agonist (functional antagonist) of the MC3/4Rs *(208–210)*. Thus, activation of ARC NPY neurons leads to the release of both a potent anabolic peptide and a potent inhibitor of the catabolic melanocortin system. The anabolic NPY and catabolic POMC neuron projections from the ARC to the neurohumoral output neurons in the PVN and LH overlap almost completely. In rats, these projections from the ARC do not reach their targets until the eighth to tenth day of life *(92,191,192)*. Hindbrain NE and Epi neurons also project to hypothalamic targets, where they modulate the expression and release of NPY, AgRP and α-MSH *(182,183,211)*. But these catecholamine neurons do not fully innervate their hypothalamic targets until the end of the third postnatal week in rats *(193)*.

Although human and rodent brains develop at different pre- and postnatal stages, the same general principles apply. The development of a coherent, distributed network of metabolic sensing neurons and their efferent pathways is dependent on the preprogrammed arrival of afferents, which then determine the function of target neurons *(212)*. This programming is dependent on an number of trophic factors, which include leptin and insulin *(91–93,102,213–216)*. Because the development of critical pathways involved in energy homeostasis in rodents continues well into the postnatal period, it can be influenced by both pre- and postnatal environmental conditions. It is likely that similar principles hold for human beings, although the timing of pathway development occurs earlier than in rodents. In rats, maternal obesity throughout gestation and weaning has a major impact on the development of monoamine pathways from the hindbrain to the hypothalamus. Offspring of obese dams with a genetic predisposition to develop DIO have abnormal development of both NE and 5HT projections to the hypothalamus *(42)*. These offspring become more obese as adults in association with a reduced complement of NE reuptake transporters in the PVN as compared to that seen in offspring of either lean or obese obesity-resistant dams or lean DIO dams *(41,42)*. Because NE is removed from the synapse after release primarily by reuptake into NE axon terminals, reduction of reuptake transporters would increase synaptic NE availability at receptors. This should predispose such animals to become obese, as acute injections of NE into the PVN increase food intake and chronic administration causes hyperphagia and obesity *(217,218)*. Thus, the reduced complement of NE transporters in the PVN of offspring of obese DIO dams may explain why they become obese and hyperinsulinemic as adults, even when fed low-fat diets from weaning *(41)*.

Obese DIO dams are hyperinsulinemic during gestation and lactation *(41)*. Maternal hyperinsulinemia may promote offspring obesity. Injection of insulin into nonobese dams during the last trimester is produces obese offspring that have increased PVN NE innervation and release *(82,83)*. This similarity to the offspring of obese DIO dams suggests that gestational hyperinsulinemia leading to increased PVN synaptic NE levels may be a common factor promoting offspring hyperphagia and obesity. Because leptin also has trophic effects on neural pathways, hyperleptinemia associated with maternal obesity might also play a role in promoting offspring obesity. Leptin is secreted into the milk and can elevate plasma leptin levels in pups that ingest it *(146,149)*. Thus, maternal hyperleptinemia might alter development of pathways in the pups by direct transfer from the dams' milk to the pups' bloodstream *(90)*.

Once obesity develops, it effectively becomes a permanent condition, particularly in genetically predisposed individuals *(219–223)*. This appears to be due to a neural set point that resides in the network of metabolic sensing neurons involved in energy homeostasis and is determined by a host of factors including genetic predisposition, diet composition, sex, and environmental conditions *(220,221,224–231)*. Regardless of the starting point, the brain and periphery interact to preserve adipose stores when food supply is limited. Thus, during prolonged periods of caloric restriction, rats and humans maintain a reduced level of energy expenditure *(219,222,223,232)*. When allowed *ad libitum* access to food, they increase their intake and maintain a reduced level of energy expenditure until they regain their previous level of obesity *(220–223)*. This protective mechanism undoubtedly underlies the high recidivism rate in the treatment of human obesity *(233,234)*. Thus, the best "treatment" for obesity is probably primary prevention. This is particularly the case in certain individuals who appear to have their neural circuitry wired in such a way as to promote the development of obesity when they are presented with a diet relatively high in calories and fat content. For example, rats that express the DIO genotype have a number of inborn abnormalities of oxidative metabolism *(235)*, leptin *(236,237)* and insulin sensitivity *(238)*, glucose-sensing *(187,239–241)*, and neuropeptide *(242,243)* and neurotransmitter function *(244–249)* that predispose them to become obese when fed a high-fat diet. In many cases, development of obesity on such diets in adult rats is associated with actual normalization of these neural functions, suggesting that obesity might be the "normal" physiologic state of these animals *(225,240,244,246,249–251)*. Whereas the function and anatomy of these pathways can be altered in adults, the developmental period is the most important time for intervening in obesity-prone individuals. Injection of dams and the injection of dams *(82,83)* and neonates with insulin *(252)* alters development of several neural pathways involved in the regulation of energy homeostasis. So does raising rats in large or small litters *(253–256)*, feeding dams either a high-fat or high-carbohydrate diet *(60,257–259)*, gestational diabetes *(260)* and maternal undernutrition *(261)*. The majority of changes in neural function induced by these manipulations promote the development of obesity and/or insulin resistance, especially when the individual is exposed to high-fat diets later in life.

CONCLUSIONS

A variety of perturbations of both the pre- and postnatal environments can alter ingestive behavior and energy expenditure and storage in offspring. The outcome of such perturbations is dependent on both the genetic background and gender of the offspring. Many of these manipulations permanently alter the development of neural pathways involved in the regulation of energy homeostasis, leaving the individual with a raised body weight set point that predisposes them to become obese when food is abundant and the energy expenditure required to attain food is minimized. Given the worldwide obesity epidemic and the particularly high rate of obesity in children, it is likely that initial prevention will be the most effective way to stem the tide of this epidemic. Thus, it is imperative that we gain better insights into the conditions that promote or ameliorate the development of obesity during the perinatal period.

REFERENCES

1. Popkin BM, Doak CM. The obesity epidemic is a worldwide phenomenon. Nutr Rev 1999;56:106–114.
2. Keinan-Boker L, Noyman N, Chinich A, et al. Overweight and obesity prevalence in Israel: findings of the first national health and nutrition survey (MABAT). Isr Med Assoc J 2005;7:219–223.
3. Al-Almaie SM. Prevalence of obesity and overweight among Saudi adolescents in Eastern Saudi Arabia. Saudi Med J 2005;26:607–611.
4. Kim DM, Ahn CW, Nam SY. Prevalence of obesity in Korea. Obes Rev 2005;6:117–121.
5. Andersen LF, Lillegaard IT, Overby N, et al. Overweight and obesity among Norwegian schoolchildren: changes from 1993 to 2000. Scand J Public Health 2005;33:99–106.
6. Sanchez-Castillo CP, Velasquez-Monroy O, Lara-Esqueda A, et al. Diabetes and hypertension increases in a society with abdominal obesity: results of the Mexican National Health Survey 2000. Public Health Nutr 2005;8:53–60.
7. Allison DB, Edlen-Nezin L, Clay-Williams G. Obesity among African American women: prevalence, consequences, causes, and developing research. Women's Health 1997;3:243–274.
8. Reaven GM. Banting Lecture 1988: role of insulin resistance in human disease. Diabetes 1988;37:1595–1607.
9. Bjorntorp P. Abdominal obesity and the metabolic syndrome. Ann Med 1992;24:465–468.
10. Ford ES, Giles WH, Mokdad AH. Increasing prevalence of the metabolic syndrome among US adults. Diabetes Care 2004;27:2444–2449.
11. Allison DB, Zannolli R, Faith MS, et al. Weight loss increases and fat loss decreases all-cause mortality rate: results from two independent cohort studies. Int J Obes Relat Metab Disord 1999;23:603–611.
12. Allison DB, Fontaine KR, Manson JE, et al. Annual deaths attributable to obesity in the United States. JAMA 1999;282:1530–1538.
13. Must A, Spadano J, Coakley EH, et al. The disease burden associated with overweight and obesity. JAMA 1999;282:1523–1529.

14. Wang Y. Cross-national comparison of childhood obesity: the epidemic and the relationship between obesity and socioeconomic status. Int J Epidemiol 2001;30:1129–1136.
15. Ogden CL, Flegal KM, Carroll MD, et al. Prevalence and trends in overweight among US children and adolescents, 1999-2000. JAMA 2002;288:1728–1732.
16. Baskin ML, Ard J, Franklin F, et al. Prevalence of obesity in the United States. Obes Rev 2005;6:5–7.
17. Rosenbloom AL, Joe JR, Young RS, et al. Emerging epidemic of type 2 diabetes in youth. Diabetes Care 1999;22:345–354,
18. Roberts SB, Savage J, Coward WA, et al. Energy expenditure and intake in infants born to lean and overweight mothers. N Engl J Med 1988;318:461–466.
19. Plagemann A, Harder T, Kohlhoff R, et al. Overweight and obesity in infants of mothers with long-term insulin-dependent diabetes or gestational diabetes. Int J Obes Relat Metab Disord 1997;21:451–456.
20. Whitaker RC. Predicting preschooler obesity at birth: the role of maternal obesity in early pregnancy. Pediatrics 2004;114:e29–e36.
21. Bouchard C, Perusse L. Genetics of obesity. Ann Rev Nutr 1993;13:337–354.
22. Stunkard AJ, Harris JR, Pedersen NL, et al. The body-mass index of twins who have been reared apart. N Eng J Med 1990;322:1483–1487.
23. Allison DB, Kaprio J, Korkeila M, et al. The heritability of body mass index among an international sample of monozygotic twins reared apart. Int J Obes Relat Metab Disord 1996;20:501–506.
24. Comuzzie AG, Allison DB. The search for human obesity genes. Science 1998;280:1374–1377.
25. Diamond J. Guns, Germs and Steel. W. W. Norton, New York, London: 1997.
26. Neel V. In diabetes mellitus: a "thrifty" genotype rendered detrimental by progress. Am J Hum Genet 1962;14:353–362.
27. Drewnowski A, Darmon N. The economics of obesity: dietary energy density and energy cost. Am J Clin Nutr 2005;82:265S–273S.
28. Dorner G, Mohnike A, Thoelke H. Further evidence for the dependence of diabetes prevalence on nutrition in perinatal life. Exp Clin Endocrinol 1984;84:129–133.
29. Ravelli GP, Stein ZA, Susser MW. Obesity in young men after famine exposure in utero and early infancy. N Engl J Med 1976;295:349–353.
30. Phipps K, Barker DJ, Hales CN, et al. Fetal growth and impaired glucose tolerance in men and women. Diabetologia 1993;36:225–228.
31. Barker DJ. The Wellcome Foundation Lecture, 1994. The fetal origins of adult disease. Proc Royal Soc Lond 1995;262:37–43.
32. Hales CN, Barker DJ. The thrifty phenotype hypothesis. Br Med Bull 2001;60:5–20.
33. Ravelli AC, Der Meulen JH, Osmond C, et al. Obesity at the age of 50 years in men and women exposed to famine prenatally. Am J Clin Nutr 1999;70:811–816.
34. Hoet JJ, Hanson MA. Intrauterine nutrition: its importance during critical periods for cardiovascular and endocrine development. J Physiol 1999;514:617–627.
35. Silverman BL, Metzger BE, Cho NH, et al. Impaired glucose tolerance in adolescent offspring of diabetic mothers. Relationship to fetal hyperinsulinism. Diabetes Care 1995;18:611–617.
36. Berenson GS, Bao W, Srinivasan SR. Abnormal characteristics of young offspring of parents with non-insulin-dependent diabetes mellitus. The Bogalusa Heart Study. Am J Epidemiol 1997;144:962–967.
37. Pettitt DJ, Aleck KA, Baird HR, et al. Congenital susceptibility to NIDDM. Role of intrauterine environment. Diabetes 1988;37:622–628.
38. Waterland RA, Garza C. Potential mechanisms of metabolic imprinting that lead to chronic disease. Am J Clin Nutr 1999;69:179–197.
39. Kennedy GC. The development with age of hypothalamic restraint upon the appetite of the rat. J Endocrinol 1957;16:9–17.
40. Widdowson EM, McCance RA. Some effects of accelerating growth. I. General somatic development. Proc R Soc Lond B Biol Sci 1960;152:188–206.
41. Levin BE, Govek E. Gestational obesity accentuates obesity in obesity-prone progeny. Am J Physiol 1998;275:R1374–R1379.
42. Levin BE, Dunn-Meynell AA. Maternal obesity alters adiposity and monoamine function in genetically predisposed offspring. Am J Physiol 2002;283:R1087–R1093.
43. Levin BE, Magnan C, Migrenne S, et al. The F-DIO obesity-prone rat is insulin resistant prior to obesity onset. Am J Physiol 2005;289:R704–R711.
44. Guo F, Jen K-L. High-fat feeding during pregnancy and lactation affects offspring metabolism in rats. Physiol Behav 1995;57:681–686.

45. Langley-Evans SC, Gardner DS, Jackson AA. Maternal protein restriction influences the programming of the rat hypothalamic-pituitary-adrenal axis. J Nutr 1996;126:1578–1585.
46. Khan IY, Taylor PD, Dekou V, et al. Gender-linked hypertension in offspring of lard-fed pregnant rats. Hypertension 2003;41:168–175.
47. Palinski W, D'Armiento FP, Witztum JL, et al. Maternal hypercholesterolemia and treatment during pregnancy influence the long-term progression of atherosclerosis in offspring of rabbits. Circ Res 2001;89:991–996.
48. Taylor PD, McConnell J, Khan IY, et al. Impaired glucose homeostasis and mitochondrial abnormalities in offspring of rats fed a fat-rich diet in pregnancy. Am J Physiol Regul Integr Comp Physiol 2005;288:R134–139.
49. Wu Q, Mizushima Y, Komiya M, et al. Body fat accumulation in the male offspring of rats fed high-fat diets. J Clin Biochem Nutr 1998;25:71–79.
50. Levin BE, Dunn-Meynell AA, Balkan B, et al. Selective breeding for diet-induced obesity and resistance in Sprague-Dawley rats. Am J Physiol 1997;273:R725–R730.
51. Levin BE, Dunn-Meynell AA, McMinn JE, et al. A new obesity-prone, glucose intolerant rat strain (F.DIO). Am J Physiol 2003;285:R1184–R1191.
52. Levin BE, Dunn-Meynell AA, Ricci MR, et al. Abnormalities of leptin and ghrelin regulation in obesity-prone juvenile rats. Am J Physiol 2003;285:E949–E957.
53. Dobrian AD, Davies MJ, Prewitt RL, et al. Development of hypertension in a rat model of diet-induced obesity. Hypertension 2000;35:1009–1015.
54. Weigle DS, Levin BE. Defective dietary induction of uncoupling protein 3 in skeletal muscle of obesity-prone rats. Obes Res 2000;8:385–391.
55. Ricci MR, Levin BE. Ontogeny of diet-induced obesity in selectively-bred Sprague-Dawley rats. Am J Physiol 2003;285:R610–R618.
56. Buckley AJ, Keseru B, Briody J, et al. Altered body composition and metabolism in the male offspring of high fat-fed rats. Metabolism 2005;54:500–507.
57. Korotkova M, Gabrielsson B, Hanson LA, et al. Maternal dietary intake of essential fatty acids affects adipose tissue growth and leptin mRNA expression in suckling rat pups. Pediatr Res 2002;52:78–84.
58. Korotkova M, Gabrielsson B, Lonn M, et al. Leptin levels in rat offspring are modified by the ratio of linoleic to alpha-linolenic acid in the maternal diet. J Lipid Res 2002;43:1743–1749.
59. Korotkova M, Gabrielsson B, Hanson LA, et al. Maternal essential fatty acid deficiency depresses serum leptin levels in suckling rat pups. J Lipid Res 2001;42:359–365.
60. Kozak R, Burlet A, Burlet C, et al. Dietary composition during fetal and neonatal life affects neuropeptide Y functioning in adult offspring. Brain Res Devel Brain Res 2000;125:75–82.
61. Kozak R, Richy S, Beck B. Persistent alterations in neuropeptide Y release in the paraventricular nucleus of rats subjected to dietary manipulation during early life. Eur J Neurosci 2005;21:2887–2892.
62. Petry CJ, Ozanne SE, Wang CL, et al. Early protein restriction and obesity independently induce hypertension in 1-year-old rats. Clin Sci 1997;93:147–152.
63. Fernandez-Twinn DS, Wayman A, Ekizoglou S, et al. Maternal protein restriction leads to hyperinsulinemia and reduced insulin signalling protein expression in 21 month-old female rat offspring. Am J Physiol Regul Integr Comp Physiol 2004;288:R368–R373.
64. Zambrano E, Martinez-Samayoa PM, et al. Sex differences in transgenerational alterations of growth and metabolism in progeny (F2) of female offspring (F1) of rats fed a low protein diet during pregnancy and lactation. J Physiol 2005;566:225–236.
65. Boloker J, Gertz SJ, Simmons RA. Gestational diabetes leads to the development of diabetes in adulthood in the rat. Diabetes 2002;51:1499–1506.
66. Holemans K, Gerber RT, Meurrens K, et al. Streptozotocin diabetes in the pregnant rat induces cardiovascular dysfunction in adult offspring. Diabetologia 1999;42:81–89.
67. Oh W, Gelardi NL, Cha CJ. Maternal hyperglycemia in pregnant rats: its effect on growth and carbohydrate metabolism in the offspring. Metabolism 1988;37:1146–1151.
68. Kurniato E, Shinjo A, Suga D. Prenatal and postnatal maternal effects on body weight in cross-fostering experiment on two subspecies of mice. Exp Anim 1998;47:97–103.
69. Wu Q, Mizushima Y, Komiya M, et al. The effects of high-fat diet feeding over generations on body fat accumulation associated with lipoprotein lipase and leptin in rat adipose tissues. Asia Pacific J Clin Nutr 1999;8:46–52.
70. Jones AP, Simson EL, Friedman MI. Gestational undernutrition and the development of obesity in rats. J Nutr 1984;114:1484–1492.

71. Jones AP, Assimon SA, Friedman MI. The effect of diet on food intake and adiposity in rats made obese by gestational undernutrition. Physiol Behav 1986;37:381–386.
72. Anguita RM, Sigulem DM, Sawaya AL. Intrauterine food restriction is associated with obesity in young rats. J Nutr 1993;123:1421–1428.
73. Vickers MH, Breier BH, Cutfield WS, et al. Fetal origins of hyperphagia, obesity, and hypertension and postnatal amplification by hypercaloric nutrition. Am J Physiol Endocrinol Metab 2000;279:E83–87.
74. Vickers MH, Breier BH, McCarthy D, et al. Sedentary behavior during postnatal life is determined by the prenatal environment and exacerbated by postnatal hypercaloric nutrition. Am J Physiol Regul Integr Comp Physiol 2003;285:R271–R273.
75. Nilsson C, Larsson BM, Jennische E, et al. Maternal endotoxemia results in obesity and insulin resistance in adult male offspring. Endocrinology 2001;142:2622–2630.
76. Dahlgren J, Nilsson C, Jennische E, et al. Prenatal cytokine exposure results in obesity and gender-specific programming. Am J Physiol 2001;281:E326–E334.
77. Puro DG, Agardh E. Insulin-mediated regulation of neuronal maturation. Science 1984;225:1170–1172.
78. Recio-Pinto E, Ishii DN. Effects of insulin, insulin-like growth factor-II and nerve growth factor on neurite outgrowth in cultured human neuroblastoma cells. Brain Res 1984;302:323–334.
79. Heidenreich KA, Toledo SP. Insulin receptors mediate growth effects in cultured fetal neurons. I. Rapid stimulation of protein synthesis. Endocrinology 1989;125:1451–1457.
80. Freinkel N. Banting Lecture 1980. Of pregnancy and progeny. Diabetes 1980;29:1023–1035.
81. Menon RK, Cohen RM, Sperling MA, et al. Transplacental passage of insulin in pregnant women with insulin-dependent diabetes mellitus. Its role in fetal macrosomia. N Engl J Med 1990;323:309–315.
82. Jones AP, Olster DH, States B. Maternal insulin manipulations in rats organize body weight and noradrenergic innervation of the hypothalamus in gonadally intact male offspring. Dev Brain Res1996; 97:16–21.
83. Jones AP, Pothos EN, Rada P, et al. Maternal hormonal manipulations in rats cause obesity and increase medial hypothalamic norepinephrine release in male offspring. Brain Res Devel Brain Res 1995;88:127–131.
84. Osmond DT, King RG, Brennecke SP, et al. Placental glucose transport and utilisation is altered at term in insulin-treated, gestational-diabetic patients. Diabetologia 2001;44:1133–1139.
85. Kainer F, Weiss PA, Huttner U, et al. Levels of amniotic fluid insulin and profiles of maternal blood glucose in pregnant women with diabetes type-I. Early Hum Devel 1997;49:97–105.
86. Taricco E, Radaelli T, Nobile de Santis MS, et al. Foetal and placental weights in relation to maternal characteristics in gestational diabetes. Placenta 2003;24:343–347.
87. Hattersley AT, Tooke JE. The fetal insulin hypothesis: an alternative explanation of the association of low birthweight with diabetes and vascular disease. Lancet 1999;353:1789–1792.
88. Steppan CM, Swick AG. A role for leptin in brain development. Biochem Biophys Res Commun 1999;256:600–602.
89. Ahima RS, Hileman SM. Postnatal regulation of hypothalamic neuropeptide expression by leptin: implications for energy balance and body weight regulation. Regul Pept 2000;92:1–7.
90. Proulx K, Richard D, Walker CD. Leptin regulates appetite-related neuropeptides in the hypothalamus of developing rats without affecting food intake. Endocrinology 2002;143:4683–4692.
91. Bouret SG, Simerly RB. Minireview: leptin and development of hypothalamic feeding circuits. Endocrinology 2004;145:2621–2626.
92. Bouret SG, Draper SJ, Simerly RB. Formation of projection pathways from the arcuate nucleus of the hypothalamus to hypothalamic regions implicated in the neural control of feeding behavior in mice. J Neurosci 2004;24:2797–2805.
93. Bouret SG, Draper SJ, Simerly RB. Trophic action of leptin on hypothalamic neurons that regulate feeding. Science 2004;304:108–110.
94. Ramos MP, Rueda BR, Leavis PC, et al. Leptin serves as an upstream activator of an obligatory signaling cascade in the embryo-implantation process. Endocrinology 2005;146:694–701.
95. Hoggard N, Hunter L, Duncan JS, et al. Leptin and leptin receptor mRNA and protein expression in the murine fetus and placenta. Proc Natl Acad Sci USA 1997;94:11,073–11,078.
96. Senaris R, Garcia-Caballero T, Casabiell X, et al. Synthesis of leptin in human placenta. Endocrinology 1997;138:4501–4504.
97. Shekhawat PS, Garland JS, Shivpuri C, et al. Neonatal cord blood leptin: its relationship to birth weight, body mass index, maternal diabetes, and steroids. Pediatr Res 1998;43:338–343.

98. Lepercq J, Cauzac M, Lahlou N, et al. Overexpression of placental leptin in diabetic pregnancy: a critical role for insulin. Diabetes 1998;47:847–850.

99. Persson B, Westgren M, Celsi G, et al. Leptin concentrations in cord blood in normal newborn infants and offspring of diabetic mothers. Horm Metab Res 1999;31:467–471.

100. Matsuda J, Yokota I, Iida M, et al. Dynamic changes in serum leptin concentrations during the fetal and neonatal periods. Pediatr Res 1999;45:71–75.

101. Smith JT, Waddell BJ. Leptin distribution and metabolism in the pregnant rat: transplacental leptin passage increases in late gestation but is reduced by excess glucocorticoids. Endocrinology 2003;144:3024–3030.

102. Ahima RS, Bjorbaek C, Osei S, et al. Regulation of neuronal and glial proteins by leptin: implications for brain development. Endocrinology 1999;140:2755–2762.

103. Pinto S, Roseberry AG, Liu H, et al. Rapid rewiring of arcuate nucleus feeding circuits by leptin. Science 2004;304:110–115.

104. Rolls BA, Gurr MI, van Duijvenvoorde PM, et al. Lactation in lean and obese rats: effect of cafeteria feeding and of dietary obesity on milk composition. Physiol Behav 1986;38:185–190.

105. Grigor MR, Allan J, Carne A, et al. Milk composition of rats feeding restricted litters. Biochem J 1986;233:917–919.

106. Del Prado M, Delgado G, Villalpando S. Maternal lipid intake during pregnancy and lactation alters milk composition and production and litter growth in rats. J Nutr 1997;127:458–462.

107. Vannucci SJ, Maher F, Simpson IA. Glucose transporter proteins in brain: delivery of glucose to neurons and glia. Glia 1991;21:2–21.

108. Pellerin L, Pellegri G, Martin JL, et al. Expression of monocarboxylate transporter mRNAs in mouse brain: support for a distinct role of lactate as an energy substrate for the neonatal vs. adult brain. Proc Natl Acad Sci 1998;95:3990–3995.

109. Horn CC, Friedman MI. Methyl palmoxirate increases eating behavior and brain Fos-like immunoreactivity in rats. Brain Res 1998;781:8–14.

110. Smith GP, Epstein AN. Increased feeding in response to decreased glucose utilization in the rat and monkey. Am J Physiol 1969;217:1083–1087.

111. Swithers SE. Development of independent ingestive responding to blockade of fatty acid oxidation in rats. Am J Physiol 1997;273:R1649–R1656.

112. Swithers SE. Effects of metabolic inhibitors on ingestive behavior and physiology in preweanling rat pups. Appetite 2000;35:9–25.

113. Weller A, Tsitolovskya L, Smith GP. Hypertonic glucose preloads act preabsorptively to decrease intake in rats on postnatal day 18. Physiol Behav 2001;72:199–203.

114. Davis RJ, Doerflinger A, McCurley M, et al. Gastric emptying and control of ingestion in preweanling rat pups. Nutr Neurosci 2003;6:81–91.

115. Weller A, Smith GP, Gibbs J. Endogenous cholecystokinin reduces feeding in young rats. Science 1990;247:1589–1591.

116. Doerflinger A, Swithers SE. Effects of diet and handling on initiation of independent ingestion in rats. Dev Psychobiol 2004;45:72–82.

117. Swithers SE, Melendez RI, Watkins BA, et al. Metabolic and behavioral responses in pre-weaning rats following alteration of maternal diet. Physiol Behav 2001;72:147–157.

118. Khan IY, Dekou V, Douglas G, et al. A high-fat diet during rat pregnancy or suckling induces cardiovascular dysfunction in adult offspring. Am J Physiol Regul Integr Comp Physiol 2005;288: R127–R133.

119. Lim K, Shimomura Y, Suzuki M. Effect of high-fat diet feeding over generations on body fat accretion. In: Romsos DR, Himms-Hagen J, Suzuki M, eds. Obesity: Dietary Factors and Control. Japan Sci Soc Press, Karger, Tokyo, Basel:1991, pp. 181–190.

120. West DB, Diaz J, Woods SC. Infant gastrostomy and chronic formula infusion as a technique to overfeed and accelerate weight gain of neonatal rats. J Nutr 1982;112:1339–1343.

121. West DB, Diaz J, Roddy S, et al. Long-term effects on adiposity after preweaning nutritional manipulations in the gastrostomy-reared rat. J Nutr 1987;117:1259–1264.

122. Hiremagalur BK, Vadlamudi S, Johanning GL, et al. Long-term effects of feeding high carbohydrate diet in pre-weaning period by gastrostomy: a new rat model for obesity. Int J Obes 1993;17:495–502.

123. Vadlamudi S, Kalhan SC, Patel MS. Persistence of metabolic consequences in the progeny of rats fed a HC formula in their early postnatal life. Am J Physiol 1995;269:E731–E738.

124. Diaz J, Taylor EM. Abnormally high nourishment during sensitive periods results in body weight changes across generations. Obes Res 1998;6:368–374.
125. Ozanne SE, Lewis R, Jennings BJ, et al. Early programming of weight gain in mice prevents the induction of obesity by a highly palatable diet. Clin Sci (Lond) 2004;106:141–145.
126. Desai M, Hales CN. Role of fetal and infant growth in programming metabolism in later life. Biol Rev Cambridge Philosoph Soc 1997;72:329–348.
127. Hales CN, Barker DJ. Type 2 (non-insulin-dependent) diabetes mellitus: the thrifty phenotype hypothesis. Diabetologia 1992;35:595–601.
128. Johnson PR, Stern JS, Greenwood MR, et al. Effect of early nutrition on adipose cellularity and pancreatic insulin release in the Zucker rat. J Nutr 1973;103:738–743.
129. Faust IM, Johnson PR, Hirsch J. Long-term effects of early nutritional experience on the development of obesity in the rat. J Nutr 1980;110:2027–2034.
130. Oscai LB, McGarr JA. Evidence that the amount of food consumed in early life fixes appetite in the rat. Am J Physiol 1978;235:R141–R144.
131. Knittle JL, Hirsch J. Effect of early nutrition on the development of rat epididymal fat pads: cellularity and metabolism. J Clin Invest 1968;47:2091–2098,
132. Levin BE, Triscari J, Marquet E, et al. Dietary obesity and neonatal sympathectomy I. Effects on body composition and brown adipose. Am J Physiol 1984;247:R979–R987.
133. Schmidt I, Fritz A, Scholch C, et al. The effect of leptin treatment on the development of obesity in overfed suckling Wistar rats. Int J Obes 2001;25:1168–1174.
134. Waterland RA, Garza C. Early postnatal nutrition determines adult pancreatic glucose-responsive insulin secretion and islet gene expression in rats. J Nutr 2002;132:357–364.
135. Hahn P. Effect of litter size on plasma cholesterol and insulin and some liver and adipose tissue enzymes in adult rodents. J Nutr 1984;114:1231–1234.
136. Wiedmer P, Klaus S, Ortmann S. Energy metabolism of young rats after early postnatal overnutrition. Br J Nutr 2002;88:301–306.
137. Gorski J, Dunn-Meynell AA, Hartman TG, and Levin BE. Postnatal environment overrides genetic and prenatal factors influencing offspring obesity and insulin resistance. Am J Physiol 2006;291: R768–R778.
138. Reifsnyder PC, Churchill G, Leiter EH. Maternal environment and genotype interact to establish diabesity in mice. Genome Res 2000;10:1568–1578.
139. Plagemann A, Harder T, Janert U, et al. Malformations of hypothalamic nuclei in hyperinsulinemic offspring of rats with gestational diabetes. Dev Neurosci 1999;21:58–67.
140. Fahrenkrog S, Harder T, Stolaczyk E, et al. Cross-fostering to diabetic rat dams affects early development of mediobasal hypothalamic nuclei regulating food intake, body weight, and metabolism. J Nutr 2004;134:648–654,
141. Vallee M, Mayo W, Maccari S, et al. Long-term effects of prenatal stress and handling on metabolic parameters: relationship to corticosterone secretion response. Brain Res 1996;712:287–292.
142. Ahima RS, Prabakaran D, Flier JS. Postnatal leptin surge and regulation of circadian rhythm of leptin by feeding. Implications for energy homeostasis and neuroendocrine function. J Clin Invest 1998;101:1020–1027.
143. Yuan CS, Attele AS, Zhang L, et al. Leptin reduces body weight gain in neonatal rats. Pediatr Res 2000;48:380–383.
144. Kraeft S, Schwarzer K, Eiden S, et al. Leptin responsiveness and gene dosage for leptin receptor mutation (fa) in newborn rats. Am J Physiol 1999;276:E836–E842.
145. Mistry AM, Swick A, Romsos DR. Leptin alters metabolic rates before acquisition of its anorectic effect in developing neonatal mice. Am J Physiol 1999;277:R742–R747.
146. Casabiell X, Pineiro V, Tome MA, et al. Presence of leptin in colostrum and/or breast milk from lactating mothers: a potential role in the regulation of neonatal food intake. J Clin Endocrinol Metab 1997;82:4270–4273.
147. Stehling O, Doring H, Ertl J, et al. Leptin reduces juvenile fat stores by altering the circadian cycle of energy expenditure. Am J Physiol 1996;271:R1770–R1774.
148. Lyle RE, Kincaid SC, Bryant JC, et al. Human milk contains detectable levels of immunoreactive leptin. Adv Exp Med Biol 2001;501:87–92.
149. Sanchez J, Oliver P, Miralles O, et al. Leptin orally supplied to neonate rats is directly uptaken by the immature stomach and may regulate short-term feeding. Endocrinology 2005;146:2575–2582.

150. Plagemann A, Harder T, Rake A, et al. Morphological alterations of hypothalamic nuclei due to intrahypothalamic hyperinsulinemia in newborn rats. Int J Dev Neurosci 1999;17:37–44.

151. Levin BE. Glucosensing neurons do more than just sense glucose. Int J Obes Relat Metab Disord 2001;25:S68–S72.

152. Levin BE. Metabolic sensors: viewing glucosensing neurons from a broader perspective. Physiol Behav 2002;76:397–401.

153. Levin BE. Glucosensing neurons: the metabolic sensors of the brain? Diab Nutr Metab 2002;15:274–280.

154. Berthoud HR. Multiple neural systems controlling food intake and body weight. Neurosci Biobehav Rev 2002;26:393–428.

155. Anand BK, Chhina GS, Sharma KN, et al. Activity of single neurons in the hypothalamus feeding centers: effect of glucose. Am J Physiol 1964;207:1146–1154.

156. Oomura Y, Kimura K, Ooyama H, et al. Reciprocal activities of the ventromedial and lateral hypothalamic area of cats. Science 1964;143:484–485.

157. Song Z, Routh VH. Differential effects of glucose and lactate on glucosensing neurons in the ventromedial hypothalamic nucleus. Diabetes 2005;54:15–22.

158. Yang X, Kow L-M, Funabashi T, et al. Hypothalamic glucose sensor. Similarities to and differences from pancreatic β-cell mechanisms. Diabetes 1999;48:1763–1772.

159. Yang XJ, Kow LM, Pfaff DW, et al. Metabolic pathways that mediate inhibition of hypothalamic neurons by glucose. Diabetes 2004;53:67–73.

160. Minami T, Shimizu N, Duan S, et al. Hypothalamic neuronal activity responses to 3-hydroxybutyric acid, an endogenous organic acid. Brain Res 1990;509:351–354.

161. Oomura Y, Nakamura T, Sugimori M, et al. Effect of free fatty acid on the rat lateral hypothalamic neurons. Physiol Behav 1975;14:483–486.

162. Kang L, Routh VH, Kuzhikandathil EV, et al. Physiological and molecular characteristics of rat hypothalamic ventromedial nucleus glucosensing neurons. Diabetes 2004;53:549–559.

163. Spanswick D, Smith MA, Groppi VE, et al. Leptin inhibits hypothalamic neurons by activation of ATP- sensitive potassium channels. Nature 1997;390:521–525.

164. Routh VH, McArdle JJ, Spanswick DC, et al. Insulin modulates the activity of glucose responsive neurons in the ventromedial hypothalamic nucleus (VMN). Abst Soc Neurosci 1997;23:577A.

165. Harvey J, McKenna F, Herson PS, et al. Leptin activates ATP-sensitive potassium channels in the rat insulin-secreting cell line, CRI-G1. J Physiol (Lond) 1997;504:527–535.

166. Cowley MA, Smart JL, Rubinstein M, et al. Leptin activates anorexigenic POMC neurons through a neural network in the arcuate nucleus. Nature 2001;411:480–484.

167. Levin BE, Routh VH, Kang L, et al. Neuronal glucosensing: what do we know after 50 Years? Diabetes 2004;53:2521–2528.

168. Ritter S, Dinh TT, Zhang Y. Localization of hindbrain glucoreceptive sites controlling food intake and blood glucose. Brain Res 2000;856:37–47.

169. Adachi A, Shimizu N, Oomura Y, et al. Convergence of heptoportal glucose-sensitive afferent signals to glucose-sensitive units within the nucleus of the solitary tract. Neurosci Lett 1984;46:215–218.

170. Moriyama R, Reyes BA, Tsukamura H, et al. Glucoprivation-induced Fos expression in the hypothalamus and medulla oblongata in female rats. J Reprod Dev 2003;49:151–157.

171. Dallaporta M, Himmi T, Perrin J, et al. Solitary tract nucleus sensitivity to moderate changes in glucose level. NeuroReport 1999;10:2657–2660.

172. Sanders NM, Ritter S. Repeated 2-deoxy-D-glucose-induced glucoprivation attenuates Fos expression and glucoregulatory responses during subsequent glucoprivation. Diabetes 2000;49:1865–1874.

173. Sanders NM, Dunn-Meynell AA, Levin BE. Third ventricular alloxan reversibly impairs glucose counterregulatory responses. Diabetes 2004;53:1230–1236.

174. Levin BE, Routh VH, Sanders NM, et al. Anatomy, physiology and regulation of glucokinase as a brain glucosensor. In: Matschinsky FM, Magnuson MA, eds. Glucokinase and Glycemic Disease: From Basics to Normal Therapeutics. Karger, Basel: 2004, pp. 301–312.

175. Niijima A. Afferent impulse discharges from glucoreceptors in the liver of the guinea pig. Ann NY Acad Sci 1969;157:690–700.

176. Niijima A. Glucose-sensitive afferent nerve fibres in the hepatic branch of the vagus nerve in the guinea-pig. J Physiol 1982;332:315–323.

177. Hevener AL, Bergman RN, Donovan CM. Novel glucosensor for hypoglycemic detection localized to the portal vein. Diabetes 1997;46:1521–1525.

178. Li AJ, Ritter S. Glucoprivation increases expression of neuropeptide Y mRNA in hindbrain neurons that innervate the hypothalamus. Eur J Neurosci 2004;19:2147–2154.
179. Bugarith K, Dinh TT, Li AJ, et al. Basomedial hypothalamic injections of neuropeptide Y conjugated to saporin selectively disrupt hypothalamic controls of food intake. Endocrinology 2005;146:1179–1191.
180. Ritter S, Bugarith K, Dinh TT. Immunotoxic destruction of distinct catecholamine subgroups produces selective impairment of glucoregulatory responses and neuronal activation. J Comp Neurol 2001;432:197–216.
181. Watts AG, Sanchez-Watts G, Dinh TT, et al. Immunotoxic lesions of ascending catecholaminergic. Soc Neurosci Abst 2002;Abst# 865.861.
182. Fraley GS, Dinh TT, Ritter S. Immunotoxic catecholamine lesions attenuate 2DG-induced increase of AGRP mRNA. Peptides 2002;23:1093–1099.
183. Fraley GS, Ritter S. Immunolesion of norepinephrine and epinephrine afferents to medial hypothalamus alters basal and 2-deoxy-D-glucose-induced neuropeptide Y and agouti gene-related protein messenger ribonucleic acid expression in the arcuate nucleus. Endocrinology 2003;144:75–83.
184. Tang-Christensen M, Larsen PJ, Thulesen J, et al. The proglucagon-derived peptide, glucagon-like peptide-2, is a neurotransmitter involved in the regulation of food intake. Nat Med 2000;6:802–807.
185. Ricardo JA, Koh ET. Anatomical evidence of direct projections from the nucleus of the solitary tract to the hypothalamus, amygdala, and other forebrain structures in the rat. Brain Res 1978;153:1–26.
186. Gallagher M, Graham PW, Holland PC. The amygdala central nucleus and appetitive Pavlovian conditioning: Lesions impair one class of conditioned behavior. J Neurosci 1990;10:1906–1911.
187. Dunn-Meynell AA, Routh VH, Kang L, et al. Glucokinase is the likely mediator of glucosensing in both glucose excited and glucose inhibited central neurons. Diabetes 2002;51:2056–2065.
188. Muroya S, Yada T, Shioda S, et al. Glucose-sensitive neurons in the rat arcuate nucleus contain neuropeptide Y. Neurosci Lett 1999;264:113–116.
189. Ibrahim N, Bosch MA, Smart JL, et al. Hypothalamic proopiomelanocortin neurons are glucose responsive and express K(ATP) channels. Endocrinology 2003;144:1331–1340.
190. Ritter S, Watts AG, Dinh TT, et al. Immunotoxin lesion of hypothalamically projecting norepinephrine and epinephrine neurons differentially affects circadian and stressor-stimulated corticosterone secretion. Endocrinology 2003;144:1357–1367.
191. Grove KL, Smith MS. Ontogeny of the hypothalamic neuropeptide Y system. Physiol Behav 2003;79:47–63.
192. Grove KL, Allen S, Grayson BE, et al. Postnatal development of the hypothalamic neuropeptide Y system. Neuroscience 2003;116:393–406.
193. Rinaman L. Postnatal development of catecholamine inputs to the paraventricular nucleus of the hypothalamus in rats. J Comp Neurol 2001;438:411–422.
194. Rinaman L. Postnatal development of hypothalamic inputs to the dorsal vagal complex in rats. Physiol Behav 2003;79:65–70.
195. Levine AS, Morley JE. Neuropeptide Y: a potent inducer of consumatory behavior in rats. Peptides 1984;5:1025–1029.
196. Stanley BG, Leibowitz SF. Neuropeptide Y injected in the paraventricular hypothalamus: a powerful stimulant of feeding behavior. Proc Natl Acad Sci USA 1985;82:3940–3943.
197. Stanley BG, Kyrkouli SE, Lampert S, et al. Neuropeptide Y chronically injected into the hypothalamus: A powerful neurochemical inducer of hyperphagia and obesity. Peptides 1986;7:1189–1192.
198. Shimizu H, Shargill NS, Bray GA, et al. Effects of MSH on food intake, body weight and coat color of the yellow obese mouse. Life Sci 1989;45:543–552.
199. Yoshida M, Taniguchi Y. Projection of pro-opiomelanocortin neurons from the rat arcuate nucleus to the midbrain central gray as demonstrated by double staining with retrograde labeling and immunocytochemistry. Arch Histol Cytol 1988;51:175–183.
200. Brady LS, Smith MA, Gold PW, et al. Altered expression of hypothalamic neuropeptide mRNAs in food-restricted and food-deprived rats. Neuroendocrinology 1990;52:441–447.
201. Bergendahl M, Wiemann JN, Clifton DK, et al. Short-term starvation decreases POMC mRNA but does not alter GnRH mRNA in the brain of adult male rats. Neuroendocrinology 1992;56:913–920.
202. Grill HJ, Ginsberg AB, Seeley RJ, et al. Brainstem application of melanocortin receptor ligands produces long-lasting effects on feeding and body weight. J Neurosci 1998;18:10,128–10,135.
203. Billington CJ, Briggs JE, Grace M, et al. Effects of intracerebroventricular injection of neuropeptide Y on energy metabolism. Am J Physiol 1991;260:R321–R327.

204. Kask A, Mutulis F, Muceniece R, et al. Discovery of a novel superpotent and selective melanocortin-4 receptor antagonist (HS024): evaluation in vitro and in vivo. Endocrinology 1998;139:5006–5014.
205. Chen AS, Marsh DJ, Trumbauer ME, et al. Inactivation of the mouse melanocortin-3 receptor results in increased fat mass and reduced lean body mass. Nat Genet 2000;26:97–102.
206. Butler AA, Marks DL, Fan W, et al. Melanocortin-4 receptor is required for acute homeostatic responses to increased dietary fat. Nat Neurosci 2001;4:605–611.
207. Williams DL, Bowers RR, Bartness TJ, et al. Brainstem melanocortin 3/4 receptor stimulation increases uncoupling protein gene expression in brown fat. Endocrinology 2003;144:4692–4697.
208. Ollmann MM, Wilson BD, Yang YK, et al. Antagonism of central melanocortin receptors in vitro and in vivo by agouti-related protein. Science 1997;278:135–138.
209. Wilson BD, Bagnol D, Kaelin CB, et al. Physiological and anatomical circuitry between agouti-related peptide and leptin signaling. Endocrinology 1999;140:2387–2397.
210. Marsh DJ, Miura GI, Yagaloff KA, et al. Effects of neuropeptide Y deficiency on hypothalamic agouti-related protein expression and responsiveness to melanocortin analogues. Brain Res 1999;848:66–77.
211. Baker RA, Herkenham M, Brady LS. Effects of long-term treatment with antidepressant drugs on proopiomelanocortin and neuropeptide Y mRNA expression in the hypothalamic arcuate nucleus in rats. J Neuroendocrinol 1996;8:337–343.
212. Hebb DO. Organization of Behavior. John Wiley, New York: 1949.
213. Schechter R, Yanovitch T, Abboud M, et al. Effects of brain endogenous insulin on neurofilament and MAPK in fetal rat neuron cell culture. Brain Res 1998;808:270–278.
214. Hong M, Lee VM. Insulin and insulin-like growth factor-1 regulate tau phosphorylation in cultured human neurons. J Biol Chem 1997;272:19,547–19,553.
215. Folli F, Ghidella S, Bonfanti L, et al. The early intracellular signaling pathway for the insulin/insulin-like growth factor receptor family in the mammalian central nervous system. Mol Neurobiol 1996;13:155–183.
216. Tanaka M, Sawada M, Yoshida S, et al. Insulin prevents apoptosis of external granular layer neurons in rat cerebellar slice cultures. Neurosci Lett 1995;199:37–40.
217. Leibowitz SF. Adrenergic stimulation of the paraventricular nucleus and its effects on ingestive behavior as a function of drug dose and time of injection in the light-dark cycle. Brain Res Bull 1978;3:357–363.
218. Leibowitz SF, Roissin P, Rosenn M. Chronic norepinephrine injection into the hypothalamic paraventricular nucleus produces hyperphagia and increased body weight in the rat. Pharmacol Biochem Behav 1984;21:801–808.
219. Leibel RL, Hirsch J. Diminished energy requirements in reduced-obese patients. Metabolism 1984;33:164–170.
220. Levin BE, Keesey RE. Defense of differing body weight set-points in diet-induced obese and resistant rats. Am J Physiol 1998;274:R412–R419.
221. Levin BE, Dunn-Meynell AA. Defense of body weight against chronic caloric restriction in obesity-prone and -resistant rats. Am J Physiol 2000;278:R231–R237.
222. MacLean PS, Higgins JA, Johnson GC, et al. Metabolic adjustments with the development, treatment, and recurrence of obesity in obesity-prone rats. Am J Physiol Regul Integr Comp Physiol 2004;287:R288–R297.
223. MacLean PS, Higgins JA, Johnson GC, et al. Enhanced metabolic efficiency contributes to weight regain after weight loss in obesity-prone rats. Am J Physiol 2004;287:R1306–R1315.
224. Corbett SW, Wilterdink EJ, Keesey RE. Resting oxygen consumption in over- and underfed rats with lateral hypothalamic lesions. Physiol Behav 1985;35:971–977.
225. Levin BE, Dunn-Meynell AA. Defense of body weight depends on dietary composition and palatability in rats with diet-induced obesity. Am J Physiol 2002;282:R46–R54.
226. Levin BE. Metabolic imprinting on genetically predisposed neural circuits perpetuates obesity. Nutrition 2000;16:909–915.
227. Hoebel BG, Teitelbaum P. Weight regulation in normal and hypothalamic hyperphagic rats. J Comp Physiol Psychol 1966;61:189–193.
228. Sims EA, Horton ES. Endocrine and metabolic adaptation to obesity and starvation. Am J Clin Nutr 1968;21:1455–1470.

229. Beatty WW, O'Briant DA, Vilberg TR. Effects of ovariectomy and estradiol injections on food intake and body weight in rats with ventromedial hypothalamic lesions. Pharmacol Biochem Behav 1975;3:539–544.

230. Wirtshafter D, Davis JD. Set points, settling points, and the control of body weight. Physiol Behav 1977;19:75–78.

231. Fantino M, Cabanac M. Body weight regulation with a proportional hoarding response in the rat. Physiol Behav 1980;24:939–942.

232. Leibel RL, Berry EM, Hirsch J. Metabolic and hemodynamic responses to endogenous catecholamines in formerly obese subjects. Am J Physiol 1991;260:R785–R791.

233. Stunkard A, McLaren-Hume M. The results of treatment for obesity: a review of the literature and report of a series. AMA Arch Intern Med 1959;103:79–85.

234. Stallone DD, Stunkard AJ. Long-term use of appetite suppressant medication: rationale and recommendations. Drug Devel Res 1992;26:1–20.

235. Chang S, Graham B, Yakubu F, et al. Metabolic differences between obesity-prone and obesity-resistant rats. Am J Physiol Regul Integr Comp Physiol 1990;259:R1103–R1110.

236. Levin BE, Dunn-Meynell AA. Reduced central leptin sensitivity in rats with diet-induced obesity. Am J Physiol 2002;283:R941–R948.

237. Levin BE, Dunn-Meynell AA, Banks WA. Obesity-prone rats have normal blood-brain barrier transport but defective central leptin signaling prior to obesity onset. Am J Physiol 2003;286:R143–R150.

238. Clegg DJ, Benoit SC, Reed JA, et al. Reduced anorexic effects of insulin in obesity-prone rats and rats fed a moderate fat diet. Am J Physiol 2005;288:R981–R986.

239. Levin BE, Sullivan AC. Glucose-induced sympathetic activation in obesity-prone and resistant rats. Int J Obes 1989;13:235–246.

240. Levin BE, Brown KL, Dunn-Meynell AA. Differential effects of diet and obesity on high and low affinity sulfonylurea binding sites in the rat brain. Brain Res 1996;739:293–300.

241. Tkacs NC, Levin BE. Obesity-prone rats have pre-existing defects in their counterregulatory response to insulin-induced hypoglycemia. Am J Physiol 2004;287:R1110–R1115.

242. Levin BE, Dunn-Meynell AA. Dysregulation of arcuate nucleus preproneuropeptide Y mRNA in diet-induced obese rats. Am J Physiol 1997;272:R1365–R1370.

243. Levin BE. Arcuate NPY neurons and energy homeostasis in diet-induced obese and resistant rats. Am J Physiol 1999;276:R382–R387.

244. Wilmot CA, Sullivan AC, Levin BE. Effects of diet and obesity on brain α_1- and α_2-noradrenergic receptors in the rat. Brain Res 1988;453:157–166.

245. Levin BE. Obesity-prone and -resistant rats differ in their brain ^{3}H paraminoclonidine binding. Brain Res 1990;512:54–59.

246. Levin BE: Increased brain ^{3}H paraminoclonidine (α_2-adrenoceptor) binding associated with perpetuation of diet-induced obesity in rats. Int J Obes 1990;14:689–700.

247. Levin BE. Reduced norepinephrine turnover in organs and brains of obesity-prone rats. Am J Physiol 1995;268:R389–R394.

248. Levin BE. Reduced paraventricular nucleus norepinephrine responsiveness in obesity-prone rats. Am J Physiol 1996;270:R456–R461.

249. Hassanain M, Levin BE. Dysregulation of hypothalamic serotonin turnover in diet-induced obese rats. Brain Res 2002;929:175–180.

250. Levin BE. Diet cycling and age alter weight gain and insulin levels in rats. Am J Physiol 1994;267:R527–R535.

251. Levin BE, Hamm MW. Plasticity of brain α-adrenoceptors during the development of diet-induced obesity in the rat. Obes Res 1994;2:230–238.

252. Plagemann A, Heidrich I, Gotz F, et al. Lifelong enhanced diabetes susceptibility and obesity after temporary intrahypothalamic hyperinsulinism during brain organization. Exp Clin Endocrinol 1992;99:91–95.

253. Plagemann A, Harder T, Rake A, et al. Observations on the orexigenic hypothalamic neuropeptide Y-system in neonatally overfed weanling rat. J Neuroendocrinol 1999;11:541–546.

254. Davidowa H, Plagemann A. Inhibition by insulin of hypothalamic VMN neurons in rats overweight due to postnatal overfeeding. NeuroReport 2001;12:3201–3204.

255. Davidowa H, Plagemann A. Decreased inhibition by leptin of hypothalamic arcuate neurons in neonatally overfed young rats. NeuroReport 2000;11:2795–2798.

256. Plagemann A, Harder T, Rake A, et al. Increased number of galanin-neurons in the paraventricular hypothalamic nucleus of neonatally overfed weanling rats. Brain Res 1999;818:160–163.
257. Kozak R, Mercer JG, Burlet A, et al. Hypothalamic neuropeptide Y content and mRNA expression in weanling rats subjected to dietary manipulations during fetal and neonatal life. Regul Pept 1998;75-76:397–402.
258. Gao J, Ghibaudi L, Van Heek M, et al. Characterization of diet-induced obese rats that develop persistent obesity after 6 months of high-fat followed by 1 month of low-fat diet. Brain Res 2002;936:87–90.
259. Velkoska E, Cole TJ, Morris MJ. Early dietary intervention: long-term effects on blood pressure, brain neuropeptide Y, and adiposity markers. Am J Physiol Endocrinol Metab 2005;288:E1236–1243.
260. Plagemann A, Harder T, Lindner R, et al. Alterations of hypothalamic catecholamines in the newborn offspring of gestational diabetic mother rats. Brain Res 1998;109:201–209.
261. Plagemann A, Rittel F, Harder T, et al. Hypothalamic galanin levels in weanling rats exposed to maternal low-protein diet. Nutr Res 2001;20:977–983.

7 Measurement of Body Composition in Obesity

Jennifer L. Kuk, MSc, and Robert Ross, PhD

Contents

INTRODUCTION
ANTHROPOMETRY
BIOELECTRIC IMPEDANCE ANALYSIS
DUAL-ENERGY X-RAY ABSORPTIOMETRY
IMAGING METHODS OF BODY COMPOSITION IN OBESITY
MEASUREMENT OF SKELETAL MUSCLE AND LIVER FAT
OTHER NOVEL ECTOPIC FAT DEPOTS
CONCLUSIONS
REFERENCES

Summary

This chapter examines common methods for measuring body composition in obesity. These methods range from simple anthropometric measures that indirectly assess adiposity to more complex measures such as magnetic resonance imaging (MRI) and computed tomography (CT) that are able to directly measure numerous tissues in vivo. Anthropometric measurements are inexpensive, and are readily used in clinical settings and epidemiological studies, but lack precision to accurately quantify specific fat depots. On the other hand, imaging techniques such as MRI and CT are associated with high accuracy, but are limited by their availability and high cost. Application of other body composition measurement techniques such as dual-energy X-ray absorptiometry and magnetic resonance spectroscopy will also be considered. The focus of this review is on strengths and limitations of these body composition measurement techniques, and how they advance our understanding of how body composition influences the associations between obesity, morbidity, and mortality.

Key Words: Magnetic resonance imaging (MRI); magnetic resonance spectroscopy (MRS); computed tomography (CT); visceral adipose tissue; waist circumference; waist-hip ratio; fat distribution; liver fat.

INTRODUCTION

Interest in the measurement of body composition in obesity research is largely motivated by discovery of the underlying associations with morbidity and mortality. Obesity-related health risk is typically identified in large-scale, epidemiological studies that employ simple anthropometric methods (e.g., body mass index [BMI] and/or waist

From: *Contemporary Endocrinology: Treatment of the Obese Patient*
Edited by: R. F. Kushner and D. H. Bessesen © Humana Press Inc., Totowa, NJ

circumference) to identify the phenotypes associated with the greatest health risk. The findings from epidemiological studies identify targets for studies that use sophisticated methods such as magnetic resonance imaging and computerized tomography to measure body-composition components that help explain the associations between anthropometric measures and obesity-related health risk. In this chapter we examine the strengths and limitations of common methods for measuring body composition in obesity, and discuss how these measures advance understanding of the mechanisms that link obesity, morbidity, and mortality.

ANTHROPOMETRY

Anthropometry is the science of measuring the human body, and includes measures such as weight, stature, girth, skinfolds, and body diameters. Anthropometric measures have been employed extensively to determine the association between obesity and related morbidity *(1–6)* and mortality *(1,7–12)*. It is generally assumed that the associations between anthropometric measures and health risk are explained by the corresponding ability of anthropometry to predict body composition—in particular, body fat distribution independent of gender, age, and race. Although this may be true from a population perspective, the utility of anthropometric measures to determine human body composition on an individual basis is limited.

Body Mass Index

BMI is the measure commonly used in clinical settings for the identification of individuals at increased health risk. BMI is calculated using an individual's weight in kilograms divided by their height in meters squared. Height and weight are relatively simple measures, but in large studies they are often collected by self-report. Both men and women tend to overestimate their height and underestimate their weight, wherein the overestimation of height is increased with decreasing height, and the extent of the underestimation of weight is increased with increasing weight *(13)*. Accordingly, reports suggest that as many as 41% of men and 27% of women self-report as being overweight or normal weight *(13)*, when in fact they are obese.

BMI is positively associated with morbidity *(1,2)* and has a U- or J-shaped relationship with mortality *(1,7–9)*. Based on the associations among BMI, morbidity, and mortality, BMI categories for normal weight (18.5–24.9 kg/m^2), overweight (25.0–29.9 kg/m^2), and obese ($\geq$30.0 kg/m^2) have been established for the Caucasian population *(14)*.

It is commonly held that a high BMI is associated with increased health risk or mortality because of its association with adiposity. Indeed, within a given population, BMI is positively associated with adiposity (Fig. 1). It is noteworthy, however, that this relationship is altered by numerous factors such as age *(15)*, gender *(15)*, race *(16)*, and physical activity patterns *(17)*. For example, for a given age and BMI, women tend to have 12% more body fat than men *(15)*. Similarly, for a given BMI, white men aged 60 to 79 yr tend to have 4 to 5% more body fat than white men aged 20 to 39 years *(15)*.

It is important to appreciate that although there is a strong association between BMI and adiposity within a given population, BMI is a poor indicator of adiposity and/or lean mass on an individual basis. Indeed, despite presenting with a common BMI, adiposity levels between individuals may vary substantially (Fig. 1). Interestingly, it is reported

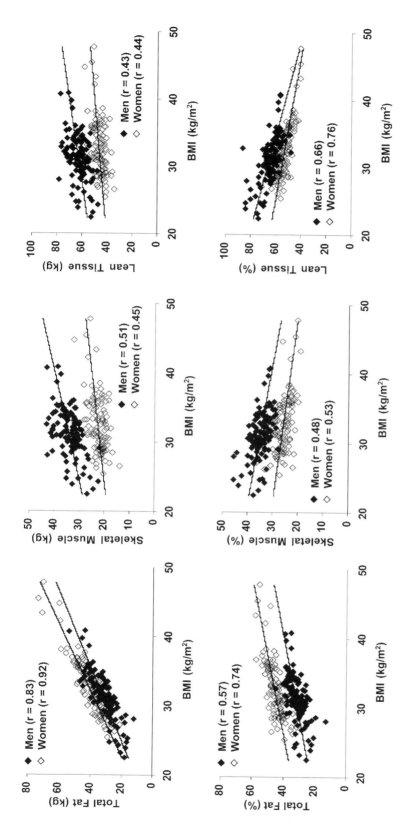

Fig. 1. Association between BMI and total body fat, skeletal muscle mass, and lean tissue mass in middle-aged men and women. Men (closed diamonds, $N = 110$), Women (open diamonds, $N = 111$). Data taken from refs. *42–45.*

123

that factors that influence the association between BMI and adiposity may also influence the association between BMI and health risk (8,16,18). For example, Stevens et al. (18) report that mortality risk at a given BMI decreases with age. In other words, having a BMI of 29 is associated with a greater relative risk of death in individuals 30 to 44 yr of age than individuals greater than 65 yr of age. Similarly, it has been proposed that the mortality rate associated with a given BMI is higher in men than in women (8).

Race also influences the level of adiposity for a given BMI (16) and may explain why observational studies report very high incidences of obesity-related metabolic disorders despite a very low obesity prevalence when using the Caucasian BMI cut-points in some Asian populations (16). Consequently, in 2004 the World Health Organization released revised BMI cut-points for certain Asian populations that were derived to reflect body fat values similar to Caucasian populations (19). However, mortality studies in Asian populations (20,21) show a similar J-shaped pattern with increasing BMI and mortality, wherein the nadir of the curve lies around 22 to 26 kg/m^2, a finding that is quite comparable to those in Caucasian populations (8,9). Thus, although it is clear that adiposity and health risk tend to increase with increasing BMI independent of age, gender, and race, the magnitude of the increment in adiposity and health risk with increasing BMI is influenced by these factors, and are therefore important to consider when examining these relationships.

There is also substantial evidence that a low body mass or BMI may also be associated with increased health risk and mortality (9). It is thought that a low BMI may be indicative of low lean mass representing a separate pathway linking BMI with disease (9). In fact, BMI is positively related to lean and skeletal muscle mass in both men and women, although there is a clear gender difference in this association (Fig. 1). However, the relationship between skeletal muscle mass and BMI is also influenced by age (22) and physical activity patterns (23). Further, as with total adiposity, substantial interindividual variation in lean and skeletal muscle mass exists for a given BMI. These observations confirm that determination of body composition using BMI on an individual basis is limited.

Waist Circumference

In 1947, Jean Vague (4) first recognized the importance of fat distribution in the assessment of health risk. Vague suggested that a preferential deposition of fat within the abdominal area, or an android body shape, may be associated with more deleterious outcomes than fat deposition in the lower body, or a gynoid fat distribution. Subsequent to this initial observation, a substantial amount of research has indicated that excess abdominal adiposity is associated with increased health risk. Abdominal obesity is commonly assessed using waist circumference, and it is now established that waist circumference is associated with morbidity and mortality independent of BMI (5).

Despite a growing literature establishing waist circumference as an independent predictor of morbidity and mortality (12), absent is a consensus as to the ideal placement of waist circumference when measuring abdominal obesity. Common landmarks include the visible narrowing of the waist, last rib, top of the iliac crest, or the midpoint between the last rib and the iliac crest. However, review of the literature reveals that waist circumference measures have been taken anywhere within a region bordered by the sternum to the iliac crest in the upright or supine position. Fortunately, waist circumferences at different measurement sites tend to be highly correlated, and

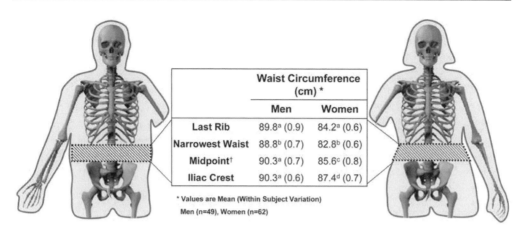

	Waist Circumference (cm) *	
	Men	Women
Last Rib	89.8[a] (0.9)	84.2[a] (0.6)
Narrowest Waist	88.8[b] (0.7)	82.8[b] (0.6)
Midpoint[†]	90.3[a] (0.7)	85.6[c] (0.8)
Iliac Crest	90.3[a] (0.6)	87.4[d] (0.7)

* Values are Mean (Within Subject Variation)

Men (n=49), Women (n=62)

Fig. 2. Comparisons among waist circumference measures at four different measurement sites in men and women. Within-subject variation based on repeat measurements on the same day in 49 men and 62 women. [†] Midpoint between the last rib and the iliac crest. Adapted from Table 3, ref. *24*.

Seidell et al. *(3)* report that the associations between waist circumferences and serum lipids were not significantly altered by measurement site. However, Wang et al. demonstrated that there is a substantial difference (~4.5 cm) in the absolute waist circumference measured at the minimal waist versus the iliac crest in 62 women with a wide range in age (36 ± 18, 7–76 yr) and adiposity (BMI: 26 ± 8, 9–43 kg/m^2) *(24)* (Fig. 2). Conversely, in a similar group of 49 men (age: 37 ± 16, range 10–83 yr; BMI: 25 ± 5, range 10–32 kg/m^2) this difference between measurements across the four sites was seen to be quite modest (~1.0 cm). Owing to these differences in measurement site and methodology, it is often difficult to compare waist circumference measures across studies or to create meaningful guidelines for clinicians or the general population.

The National Institutes of Health (NIH) has published sex-specific waist circumference cutoffs (men: 102 cm, women: 88 cm) to denote health risk in all individuals, regardless of their BMI *(25)*. However, unlike the BMI categories, these waist circumference cutoffs were not determined using the association with morbidity or mortality, but were derived by using the waist circumference values that corresponded to a BMI of 30 in Caucasian men and women, respectively. These waist circumference cut-points appear to be appropriate for non-Hispanic blacks and Mexican Americans *(26)*, but are likely too high for most Asian populations *(27)*. The appropriate cutoffs that should be employed to determine health risk in those populations remain the subject of investigation.

It is also important to note that men and women tend to underestimate their waist size when measured using a traditional measuring tape, wherein the underestimation increases with increasing waist size *(28)*. Consequently, only 35.5% of abdominally obese men (≥ 102 cm) and 44.9% of abdominally obese women (≥ 88 cm) correctly classified themselves into the highest health risk category. However, the good news is that when those same individuals used a tape measure with a spring mechanism, the error of measurement was reduced to 0.5 cm and 0.4 cm in men and women, respectively, and only 2% of the sample misclassified their waist circumference category. This suggests that spring-loaded tape measures may be a useful tool for minimizing the underestimation of waist circumference and may provide an accurate method for self-assessment of health risk.

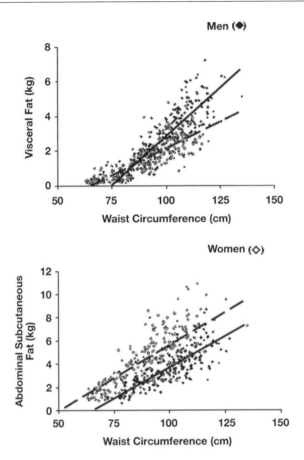

Fig. 3. Relationship between waist circumference and visceral and abdominal subcutaneous fat in men and women. Men (closed diamonds, solid line, $N = 230$), Women (open diamonds, dashed lines, $N = 251$). Adapted from ref. *40*.

The association between waist circumference and health risk may be explained by its corresponding association with abdominal subcutaneous and/or visceral fat (Fig. 3). Indeed, waist circumference is a strong predictor of both visceral fat ($r = 0.64$–0.89) *(29–35)* and abdominal subcutaneous fat ($r = 0.53$–0.98) *(30–35)*. Because visceral fat is a strong correlate of morbidity *(36–39)* and mortality *(12)*, considerable attention has been given to the ability of waist circumference to predict visceral fat. Although it is clear that waist circumference is the single best anthropometric predictor of visceral fat, substantial interindividual variation in visceral fat deposition exists for a given waist circumference. Previous studies report that the error associated with estimates for visceral fat using waist circumference is approx 25 to 35% *(29,31–33)*. The substantial interindividual variation is explained in large measure by corresponding variation in the relationship between visceral and subcutaneous fat. In other words, the relationship between visceral and subcutaneous fat varies substantially among individuals *(33,35)*.

There are also many factors such as age, gender, and fitness that influence the relationship between waist circumference and visceral fat and abdominal subcutaneous fat *(17,40,41)*. For a given waist circumference, the amount of visceral fat would be expected to be greater in an older individual than in a younger individual, and for a given age, men would be expected to have a greater amount of visceral fat than women. For example, an older man (>50 yr of age) with a waist circumference of 102 cm would be expected to have 70% more visceral fat than would a 25-yr-old man with the same waist circumference, and 140% more visceral fat than a 25-yr-old woman *(40)*. It is unclear whether race influences the quantity of visceral fat for a given waist circumference, but it may explain why waist circumference cut-points sometimes differ between races.

Although often overlooked, BMI is also a significant predictor of regional fat depots such as visceral or abdominal subcutaneous fat. Studies generally report weaker correlation coefficients for BMI and visceral fat ($r = 0.41$–0.85) *(29–35)*, but similar correlation coefficients for abdominal subcutaneous fat and BMI ($r = 0.52$–0.94) *(29–35)* as compared to waist circumference. Furthermore, BMI is a significant predictor of regional fat depots such as visceral or abdominal subcutaneous fat, independent of waist circumference *(30)*.

It is interesting to note that in our study sample *(42–45)* waist circumference is also positively associated with whole body skeletal muscle mass and lean mass with associations that are quite comparable to those observed using BMI (Fig. 4). However, similar to BMI, there is substantial interindividual variation in lean and skeletal muscle mass for a given waist circumference.

Waist-to-Hip Ratio

Another anthropometric measure used for characterizing obesity phenotype is the waist-to-hip ratio (WHR). Several prospective epidemiological studies in the 1980s reported that WHR was a significant predictor of type 2 diabetes *(6)*, coronary heart disease *(46)*, cardiovascular disease, and death *(10,11)* in both men and women. Subsequently a plethora of studies have confirmed these initial observations. In particular, a recent large epidemiological study reported that WHR was a significant predictor of myocardial infarction in a sample of 27,000 men and women with a large range in age and adiposity from 52 countries. In fact it was reported that WHR was a stronger predictor myocardial infarction than BMI or waist circumference alone *(47)*.

Similar to waist circumference, WHR is a significant correlate of visceral fat in men ($r = 0.56$–0.90) *(32–35,48–50)* and women ($r = 0.31$–0.68) *(29,32,35,48–50)*. Similarly, WHR is a significant correlate of abdominal subcutaneous fat ($r = 0.42$–0.76) *(33–35,51)*. Although these associations are generally similar to those observed for waist circumference and BMI, a WHR score can be difficult to interpret, as an elevated waist circumference or a low hip circumference may be responsible for an elevated WHR. As mentioned above, waist circumference is positively related with whole-body skeletal muscle mass. However, waist circumference is more strongly associated with abdominal and total adiposity than skeletal muscle, especially in women (Fig. 4).

As assessed by a single abdominal magnetic resonance imaging (MRI) image at the L4–L5 intervertebral space, there is 1.6 to 4.8 times more fat than skeletal muscle in obese men and 2.1 to 7.3 more times more fat than skeletal muscle in obese women (unpublished data). Thus, differences in waist circumference are more influenced by adiposity as opposed to skeletal muscle. This is not true for hip circumferences, as the ratio of subcutaneous fat to skeletal muscle area is much more variable. For example, as assessed by a single MRI image at the hip, the ratio of fat to skeletal muscle can range from 0.3 to 1.7 in men and 0.7 to 5.0 in women. In other words, two men with the same

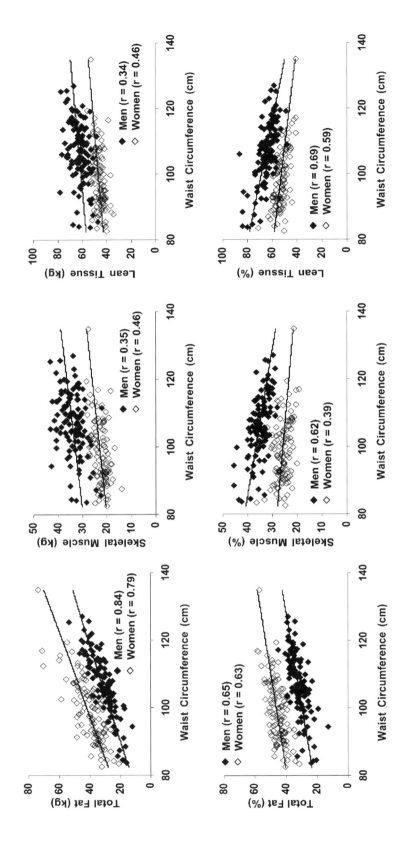

Fig. 4. Association between waist circumference and total body fat, skeletal muscle mass, and lean tissue mass in middle aged men and women. Men (closed diamonds, $N = 95$). Women (open diamonds, $N = 77$). Data taken from refs. *42–45*.

hip circumference can have nearly two times as much fat as muscle in the thigh or more than two times as much muscle as fat. Thus, using a hip circumference alone, it is unclear whether the tissue composition is predominantly fat or skeletal muscle. Consequently, a small hip circumference could indicate low muscle mass, and may be associated with elevated health risk through decreased functionality or underlying disease. Conversely, a small hip circumference may also reflect low levels of lower body fat. Thus, interpretation of the WHR becomes even more complicated, as an elevated WHR could be the result of elevated abdominal fat (high waist circumference), low levels of lower body lean mass, low levels of lower body fat mass, or a combination (low hip circumference).

Another issue when trying to interpret WHR and health risk is that there is no universally accepted landmark for measurement of hip circumference. Common measurement sites for hip circumference range from the iliac crest to the greatest protrusion of the buttocks, and thus the range of landmarks employed for waist and hip circumference across studies may confound interpretation of WHR. For example, Ross et al. *(32)* report that WHR using waist circumference measured at the last rib, but not the umbilicus, was associated with visceral fat in obese women. Conversely, in that study waist circumference alone at both landmarks was significantly associated with visceral fat.

Anthropometry and Change in Body Composition in Obesity

Waist circumference is commonly used to assess change in abdominal obesity. Changes in waist circumference are associated with changes in visceral fat in response to diet and/or exercise weight loss (Fig. 5) *(35,50,52)*. It is reported that a 1-cm reduction in waist circumference corresponds to a 4% reduction in visceral fat; however, there was a substantial amount of variance (standard deviation = 4%) in this relationship. The variation in this association is in part due to changes in subcutaneous fat and/or lean mass that mask the ability of waist circumference to accurately distinguish changes in abdominal tissues.

When examining the utility of WHR to estimate changes in body composition, a principal limitation of a ratio score becomes clear. Owing to the nature of ratio scores, changes in the ratio could be due to alterations in the numerator (waist) or the denominator (hip). For example, a reduction in the WHR after an exercise intervention could be due to reductions in the waist circumference or increases in the hip circumference due to increases in lower body muscle mass. Similarly, larger reductions in the hip circumference relative to the waist could result in no change or even an increase in the WHR despite significant diet- and/or exercise-induced weight loss. Furthermore, as mentioned before, reductions in waist or hip circumference with weight loss could be a consequence of reductions in fat or lean mass. Thus, a change or lack of change in the ratio score is difficult to interpret. Therefore, changes in WHR may not necessarily reflect changes in abdominal adiposity. This is reinforced when examining the relationship between corresponding changes in WHR and visceral fat. Unlike waist circumference, changes in WHR are not consistently associated with corresponding changes in visceral fat (Fig. 6) *(35,50,52)*. A primary example of the limits inherent to the interpretation of WHR when trying to assess body composition change in obesity studies is reflected in Fig. 7. In response to weight loss due to a negative energy balance, the mobilization of fat is rarely restricted to the abdomen. In fact, two-thirds of the fat loss in our studies *(42–45)* was seen to be from sites outside of the abdominal region (Fig. 8).

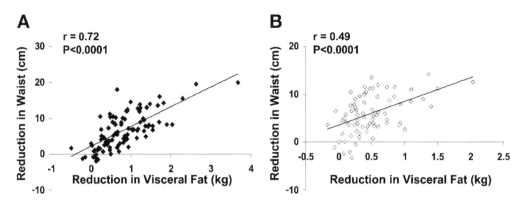

Fig. 5. Relationship between visceral fat and waist circumference, and changes in visceral fat and waist circumference in men and women. Panel A: Men (closed diamonds, $N = 96$), Panel B: Women (open diamonds, $N = 77$). Data taken from refs. *42–45.*

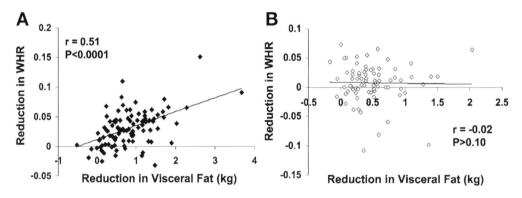

Fig. 6. Association between reductions in waist-to-hip ratio and visceral fat in men and women. Panel A: Men (closed diamonds, $N = 96$), Panel B: Women (open diamonds, $N = 77$). Data taken from refs. *42–45.*

Body Diameters

Selected body diameters, commonly taken in the sagittal plane in the abdominal area, are associated with cardiovascular disease *(53)* and mortality *(54)*. As with waist circumference and WHR, abdominal sagittal diameters are associated with visceral *(29,31,32, 34,55,56)* and abdominal subcutaneous fat *(34,55)*. Although there is some variability in the literature, waist circumference and abdominal sagittal diameters generally show similar associations with visceral fat (sagittal diameters: $r = 0.60–0.95$, waist circumference: $r = 0.66–0.97$) *(29,31,32,34,55,56)*, and abdominal subcutaneous fat (sagittal diameters: $r = 0.92–0.95$, waist circumference: $r = 0.91$) *(34,55)*. Perhaps owing to simplicity of measurement, waist circumference is a more common measure of abdominal obesity in clinical settings. To date there are no established values for sagittal diameter that denote health risk and/or abdominal obesity for a given individual or population.

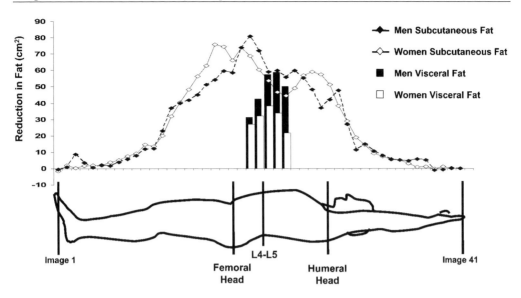

Fig. 7. Absolute fat loss across the body as measured using 45 MRI images in obese men and women in response to a diet- and/or exercise-induced 10% reduction in body weight. The line graph represents the mean subcutaneous fat loss (cm^2) at a given image (men: closed diamonds and solid line; women: open diamonds and dashed line). The bar graph represents visceral fat loss (cm^2) at a given image (men: black bars; women: white bars). Men ($N = 61$), Women ($N = 72$). Data taken from refs. *42–45.*

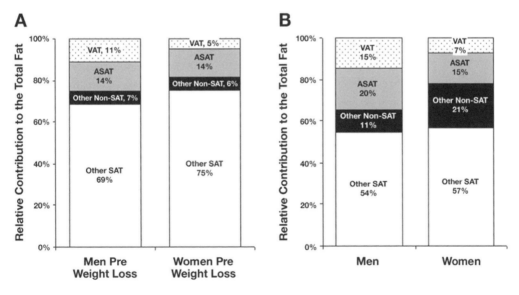

Fig. 8. Fat distribution in men and women (**A**), and the relative contribution of each fat depot to the total fat loss after a diet- and/or exercise-induced 10% reduction in body weight (**B**). Panel A: Men ($N = 236$), Women ($N = 229$). Mean age = 45 yr; BMI = 29 kg/m^2. Panel B: Men ($N = 61$), Women ($N = 72$). VAT, visceral fat; ASAT, abdominal subcutaneous fat; SAT, subcutaneous fat. Other non-SAT (intermuscular AT, intrapelvic AT and intrathoracis AT); other SAT (i.e., thigh, arm, chest SAT, etc). Data taken from refs. *42–45.*

Skinfolds

Detailed descriptions of skinfolds and their utility for measuring total and regional adiposity in vivo are provided elsewhere *(57–62)*. Briefly, skinfold calipers are used to measure the thickness of a double layer of folded skin and fat at various anatomical locations such in the arms, legs, and torso *(57,59–61)*. Skinfold measures are useful for estimating total adiposity, but are unable to directly measure visceral fat. There are several published equations that use various skinfold combinations to estimate total body fat with various degrees of accuracy (standard error of estimate [SEE]: 3–7%) *(59)*. Triceps and subscapular skinfolds are the most commonly acquired skinfolds *(59)*, and are obtained in large epidemiological studies such as the National Health and Nutrition Examination Study (NHANES) *(63)* and the Fels Longitudinal Study *(58)*. The acquisition of these measures require expertise and are subject to higher inter- and intraobserver error than circumferences *(62)*. It is generally reported that skinfold equations tend to overestimate total fat in extremely lean and underestimate total fat in extremely obese individuals *(58,64)*.

BIOELECTRIC IMPEDANCE ANALYSIS

The use of bioelectric impedance analysis (BIA) as a method of body composition in obesity has been the subject of several excellent reviews *(60,61,65)*. BIA uses the conductivity of the body to estimate fat-free mass and fat mass *(60,61,65)*. Conductivity is based on the presence of free ions or electrolytes in body water. As the highest concentrations of body water are in skeletal muscle or fat-free mass, measures of electrical conductivity are proportional to total body water and fat-free mass. However, conductivity is also affected by many other factors such as temperature, distribution of fluid within the intra- and extracellular compartments, the cross-sectional area of the limbs, and the length of the body *(60,61,65)*. Further studies comparing BIA with other measures have reported contrasting results. Depending on the model and equation, BIA has been reported to overestimate and underestimate fat mass in obese individuals *(66)*.

DUAL-ENERGY X-RAY ABSORPTIOMETRY

Although originally designed for the measurement of bone mineral content, dual-energy X-ray absorptiometry (DEXA) is commonly used to assess total and regional fat and fat-free mass in vivo *(60,61)*. DEXA assesses body composition by measuring the attenuation of X-rays emitted using pencil- or fan-beam technology at two energy levels as it traverses the body *(60,61)*. Measures of total and regional skeletal muscle (CV = 1–7%) *(67–69)* and fat mass (CV = 1–7%) *(68)* using either pencil- or fan-beam technology are highly repeatable, but results may differ between the two methods or model types (e.g., Lunar, Holigic, etc.) *(70)*. In addition to the scanner type (pencil- or fan-beam), measures of fat and fat-free mass using DEXA are affected by the software used (algorithms), and the sagittal diameter and hydration status of the individual *(71)*. Application of DEXA is also limited in obesity studies by the size of the subject, as obese individuals may exceed the weight (250 to 350 lb) and size (193–197 cm by 58–65 cm) limits of the machine *(71)*. In addition, increased tissue thickness, such as that found in obese individuals, is associated with a phenomenon called beam hardening that may result in an underestimation of the true fat content *(68,72)*. A whole-body scan using DEXA requires 15 to 35 min, depending on the scanner, and is relatively easy to use in most populations,

as it requires very little effort from the participant *(71)*. In addition, the radiation exposure associated with DEXA is less than that for computed tomography (CT), and is
readily available at a significantly lower cost.

DEXA measures of appendicular or total skeletal muscle mass are highly associated
with corresponding values obtained by CT or MRI ($r = 0.86–0.98$) *(67,69,72–74)*. Similarly, DEXA measures of appendicular fat mass are strongly associated with CT-fat mass
($r = 0.91–0.99$) *(72,74)*. There is also a tight association between total fat mass, as
measured by the four-compartment model, and fan-beam DEXA ($r = 0.98$) *(72)*.

DEXA has also been used to measure abdominal adiposity. Within the abdominal
region, DEXA measures of total abdominal fat correlate very well to measures by CT
($r = 0.87–0.98$) *(75,76)* in both black and Caucasian men and women *(75)*. However,
DEXA can assess body composition only two-dimensionally. Thus, it is unable to differentiate subcutaneous fat from visceral fat. Accordingly, the association between
DEXA measures of abdominal fat ($r = 0.51–0.90$) *(48,75–77)* and CT- or MRI-measured
visceral fat tend to be weaker than with total abdominal fat. In fact, some have argued
that the associations between visceral fat and DEXA-measured abdominal fat is no better
than those observed with simple anthropometry such as waist circumference ($r = 0.61–$
0.89) *(75,76)* and sagittal diameter ($r = 0.68–0.93$) *(48,75,76)*. In a study by Snijder et
al. *(75)*, DEXA-measured trunk fat explained only an additional 1 to 4% of the variance
in visceral fat beyond sagittal diameter or waist circumference alone, in Caucasian men
and black women. In that study none of the models that included DEXA trunk fat were
significantly better than the estimates derived from sagittal diameter in combination with
waist circumference *(75)*. There is some evidence that DEXA may be more useful for
predicting visceral adiposity beyond anthropometry alone in black men *(75)* and Caucasian women *(48,75)*; however, in those studies; models with DEXA and anthropometry accounted for only 60 to 80% of the total variance *(75)*.

There are very few studies in obese humans that have examined the ability of DEXA
to detect changes in fat mass or skeletal muscle as compared to criterion methods such
as the four-compartment model or CT, and none as compared with whole-body MRI.
Some researchers have examined the ability of DEXA to measure changes in fat by
adding pads of lard to the abdomen of a given individual. Two studies have reported that
DEXA underestimates the fat content in the lard pads when placed in the trunk region
by 40 to 50%, but accurately detected more than 90% of the fat content from the same
lard pads when placed in the thigh region *(72,78)*. It has been suggested that this may
have been due to a limitation of older software to accurately assess body composition
(79). However, this is unlikely to be the sole explanation, as this observation was also
reported in one of the aforementioned studies *(72)* that used a more recent software
version. More likely, this is probably due to the increased sagittal thickness of the
individual with the addition of the fat pads. As mentioned previously, it is documented
that high tissue thicknesses can cause beam hardening and an underestimation of fat
mass *(68,72)*.

Results from studies wherein DEXA is employed to measure change in body composition in obese persons suggest that DEXA underestimates changes in lean tissue mass
and overestimates changes in fat mass compared with criterion measures, such as the
four-compartment model or CT *(64,80,81)*. Further, it is reported that the change in
scores derived using DEXA tend to be no better than those derived using simpler mea-

sures such as BMI or BIA *(64,80)*. For example, in obese premenopausal women, although DEXA consistently overestimated fat mass (~10%) and underestimated fat-free mass (~7%) before and after a 14% diet-induced weight loss intervention, it did report comparable mean decreases in fat (11.5 vs 10.9 kg) and fat-free mass (1.6 vs 2.0 kg) as compared with the four-compartment model *(64)*. The authors concluded that DEXA provides unbiased estimates of fat loss in response to caloric restriction; however, those estimates were also no better than those derived using a simple equation with BMI (mean difference vs four-compartment model: 0.6 ± 2.1 vs -0.3 ± 2.1, DEXA vs BMI, respectively). Similarly, a study by Tylavsky et al. *(81)* reported that in response to a 7% weight loss in women, changes in the thigh fat mass and lean mass as measured by CT were correlated with changes as measured by fan-beam (fat: $r = 0.67$, lean mass: $r = 0.55$) and pencil-beam (fat: $r = 0.66$, lean mass: $r = 0.60$) DEXA *(81)*. However, again both fan- and pencil-beam DEXA tended to underestimate changes in lean tissue mass (–24.9 g and –11.8 g vs –44.7 g) and overestimate changes in fat mass (–112.1 g and –48.5 g vs –45.7 g) in the thigh as compared with CT.

The accuracy of DEXA to measure changes in fat-free mass in response to a resistance training program is also unclear, as studies using DEXA have reported differing results from other criterion measures such as CT and the four-compartment model *(82–84)*. For example, Nelson et al. *(82)* report that DEXA did not detect small changes in appendicular fat-free (skeletal muscle) mass that were identified using a single CT image in the mid-thigh, in response to a 1-yr resistance training program in postmenopausal women. On the other hand, Houtkooper et al. *(83)* suggest that DEXA may be a more sensitive measure of changes in fat-free mass than the four-compartment model or underwater weighing. In response to a different 1-yr resistance exercise regimen in postmenopausal women, DEXA identified significant increases in fat-free mass, which was not reported with the four-compartment model or underwater weighing. We would suggest that the opposite may also be true. That DEXA identified significant increases in fat-free mass that was not evident using the four-compartment model which is arguably a criterion measure, may indicate that the results using DEXA was a spurious observation, and that DEXA is not a good measure of changes in fat-free mass. Clearly, more research is needed in order to validate DEXA as a reliable measure of fat and fat-free changes before DEXA can truly be called a "gold standard" measure for body composition assessment *(84)*.

IMAGING METHODS OF BODY COMPOSITION IN OBESITY

Imaging methods are considered the most accurate available for in vivo quantification of body composition at the tissue level. CT and MRI can be used to measure fat and skeletal muscle in vivo, and are the only methods available for measurement of internal tissues and organs *(60,61,85)*. Although access and cost remain obstacles to routine use, these imaging approaches are increasingly available, and are now used extensively in body composition research.

Computed Tomography: Quantification of Tissue Size

CT uses ionizing radiation and differences in tissue X-ray attenuation characteristics to construct cross-sectional images of the body *(60,61)*. The X-ray attenuation is determined mainly by the density of the matter, and is expressed as an attenuation coefficient or more commonly, in Hounsfield units (HU), which is a linear scale relative to air and water (−1000 and 0 HU, respectively). Cross-sectional CT images are composed of picture elements or pixels, each of which has a CT number or HU value on a gray scale that reflects the molecular composition of the tissue. Although CT is more assessable than MRI, exposure to radiation precludes its use for multiple-image whole-body tissue quantification, and limits applicability in children and premenopausal women.

Magnetic Resonance Imaging: Quantification of Tissue Size

MRI does not employ ionizing radiation, but rather is based on the interaction between strong magnetic fields and hydrogen nuclei (protons), which are abundant in all biological tissues, and form the basis for generation of fat and muscle images (60,86). As MRI is not associated with any known adverse side effects, it is the method of choice for assessing whole-body tissue composition. However, the image acquisition time for MRI is significantly longer than CT and image analysis is more complex and time-consuming. Using multiple-image protocols acquired with standard clinical magnets (e.g., 1.5 Tesla), acquisition of whole-body MRI data for fat and lean mass can be acquired in about 45 min (42,87,88).

Determination of Tissue Area

CT and MRI images are normally analyzed using a similar approach. The perimeter of the tissue of interest can be traced using a light pen, trackball, or mouse-controlled pointer (89); the area within the perimeter can be calculated by multiplying the number of pixels in the region of interest by their known area. Alternatively, image segmentation algorithms can be used that identify all pixels within a selected range of intensities (e.g., HU for CT) believed to be representative of a specific tissue (90). The latter approach, however, is considered more problematic when applied to MRI than to CT images for three reasons: (1) the distributions of pixel intensity (gray-scale) values for different tissues overlap more for MRI than for CT images; (2) noise from respiratory motion blurs the borders between tissues in the abdomen to a greater extent in MRI than in CT; and (3) inhomogeneity in the magnetic field can produce "shading" at the peripheries of MRI images (33).

Determination of Tissue Volume and Mass

If multiple CT or MRI images are obtained, tissue volumes can be calculated by integrating the cross-sectional area data from consecutive images. Because the acquisition and analysis of contiguous images over the whole body or a given region is very time-consuming and expensive, axial images are typically collected with gaps between images (e.g., space between the top of one image and the bottom of the next image), usually ranging from 20 to 40 mm. Volumes are then calculated using various geometric models based on the tissue areas in the images and the distance between adjacent images (42,87,91,92). Because tissue densities for adipose tissue, skeletal muscle, and organs are fairly constant from person to person, CT and MRI volume measures for these tissues can be converted to mass units by multiplying the volume by the assumed density values for that tissue. For example, the constant densities for adipose tissue and skeletal muscle are 0.92 g/cm^3 and 1.04 g/cm^3, respectively (93). Density values are also available for the brain and visceral organs, although these vary from organ to organ (94).

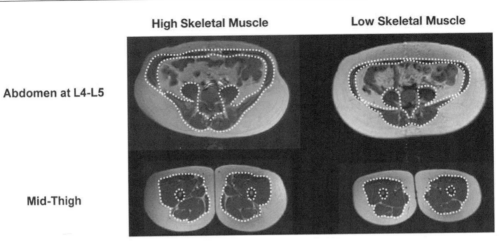

Age	39 years	38 years
Body Mass Index	33.2 kg/m^2	32.0 kg/m^2
Skeletal Muscle at L4-L5	160.2 cm^2	97.6 cm^2
Skeletal Muscle at Mid-Thigh	433.3 cm^2	374.6 cm^2
Whole Body Skeletal Muscle	31.3 kg	17.6 kg

Fig. 9. Differences in abdominal muscle at L4–L5 and thigh muscle in two obese premenopausal women with high and low levels of whole-body skeletal muscle mass as measured by magnetic resonance imaging.The skeletal muscle is outlined by the white dotted line.

Measurement of Skeletal Muscle Mass

MRI and CT are the only measures available for in vivo quantification of body composition at the tissue level; accordingly, they are commonly used to measure skeletal muscle mass. Measures of skeletal muscle by a single CT and MRI image have been reported to be strongly correlated with results from cadaver sections across a wide range of values ($r = 0.97$, SEE = 10%), with a low coefficient of variation (CV ~2%) (85). By comparison with cadaver values, the error associated with MRI was further improved to <1% when volume measures were acquired using multiple images. However, this is a very time-consuming and expensive process. Consequently, a single image at the mid-thigh is commonly used as a proxy measure of whole-body skeletal muscle in both men and women ($R^2 = 0.77$–0.79) (95). Interestingly, Lee et al. (95) have also reported that abdominal muscle measured using a single image at L4–L5 is a significant predictor of whole-body muscle mass in a cohort of middle-aged men ($R^2 = 0.63$) and women ($R^2 = 0.58$) across a wide range of adiposity (Fig. 9). As abdominal obesity is also an important predictor of future morbidity and mortality, measurement of skeletal muscle in addition to abdominal adiposity using the same image may be of clinical importance. However, the utility of this measure to predict total muscle mass in the elderly population, where muscle mass may be of greater concern, is unclear and warrants further investigation.

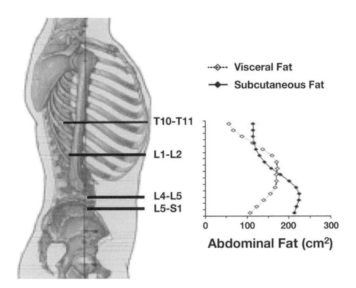

Fig. 10. Visceral fat and abdominal subcutaneous fat deposition at various measurement sites across the abdomen in men. Each data point represents the mean visceral or abdominal subcutaneous fat at each intervertebral space and midpoint of each vertebral body between L5–S1 and T10–T11 in 85 Caucasian men. Adapted from ref. *96.*

Measurement of Visceral Fat

Radiographic imaging is the only in vivo method available to quantify visceral fat. Measurement of visceral fat in vivo has stimulated great interest because a plethora of data consistently demonstrates that visceral fat is an independent predictor of both morbidity *(36–39)* and mortality *(12).* In this way it is important to note that similar to waist circumference, there is no consensus as to the optimal location for measurement of visceral fat. It has been suggested that T10–T11 and L5–S1 may represent the anatomical boundaries for portally drained visceral fat, and that a contiguous image protocol within this region may represent the gold-standard measure. However, this approach is labor-intensive and, in the case of CT, would be associated with substantial radiation exposure. Consequently, visceral fat is normally assessed using a single MRI or CT image. Visceral fat measures at any given anatomical level using a single image are highly correlated with mass measures using multiple image protocols, and also tend to be highly intercorrelated, although there may be a substantial difference in the absolute amount of visceral fat measured (Fig. 10) *(96).* Historically, visceral fat is measured using a single image at L4–L5. However, Kuk et al. *(96)* report that visceral fat at the L1–L2 level may be a stronger predictor of the total visceral fat mass and metabolic syndrome (Fig. 11) than visceral fat measured at the commonly used L4–L5 level in Caucasian men. Because visceral fat distribution is influenced by sex and race, it is unclear whether measurement site also influences the association with metabolic risk in non-Caucasian populations.

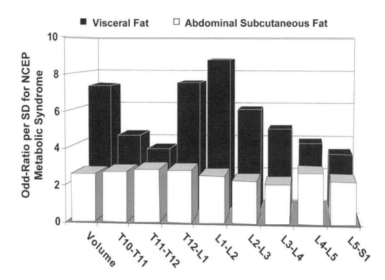

Fig. 11. Odds ratios for prevalent metabolic syndrome using National Cholesterol Education Program (NCEP) criteria according to measurement location for visceral fat and abdominal subcutaneous fat in men. All odds ratios significant at $p < 0.05$. $N = 85$. Adapted from ref. *96*.

Measurement of Abdominal Subcutaneous Fat

Consensus is also lacking with respect to the ideal measurement protocol for abdominal subcutaneous fat. Although it is reported that there are metabolic differences in subcutaneous adipocytes within various regions within the abdomen *(97)*, or between the upper and lower body *(98)*, the anatomical borders that distinguish these different regions is unclear. It is not surprising that traditionally, abdominal subcutaneous fat is measured on the single image acquired to measure visceral fat. In a manner similar to visceral fat distribution, it is reported that substantial differences exist in the absolute amount of abdominal subcutaneous fat measured across the abdomen (Fig. 10). However, unlike visceral fat, the association between metabolic syndrome and abdominal subcutaneous fat appears to be similar across all measurement sites (Fig. 11) *(96)*.

MEASUREMENT OF SKELETAL MUSCLE AND LIVER FAT

Emerging evidence suggests that excess fat deposition in regions other than the abdomen may carry independent health risk *(99–101)*. Perhaps the two most studied examples of these ectopic depots include skeletal muscle and liver. Traditionally, fat accumulation within the muscle and liver has been measured by biopsy. However, biopsy acquisition may be painful, provides a limited amount of tissue for analysis, and in the case of the liver, there is the added risk of bleeding and other complications that may result in hospitilization and possible mortality *(102)*. Further, there are other ectopic fat depots such as those within or around the heart, kidneys, pancreas, or blood vessels that are difficult, if not impossible, to assess using biopsy in humans, which may also be important fat depots in the characterization of obesity and obesity-related metabolic disease *(103)*. Consequently, it is important to develop accurate noninvasive measures such as CT, MRI, or magnetic resonance spectroscopy (MRS) for the quantification of these ectopic fat depots.

Computed Tomography: Quantification of Ectopic Fat

Although CT was originally employed in body composition research for assessing tissue size, it has also recently been used to measure skeletal muscle tissue composition. In addition, the average HU or mean attenuation value for adipose tissue-free skeletal muscle voxels can be used as an index of skeletal muscle lipid content. Thus, the lower the skeletal muscle mean attenuation value, or the greater the number of low-density skeletal muscle voxels (e.g., 0–30 HU), the higher the skeletal muscle lipid content. However, it is important to note that muscle attenuation values by CT are a reflection of both intramyocellular and extramyocellular lipid content, and are not analogous to intramyocellular lipid values obtained by skeletal muscle biopsy or proton MRS.

In a manner similar to that used to determine skeletal muscle density, CT has also been employed to determine the density of liver tissue (104–106). In obesity research, this approach has been used to identify fatty liver, which is an emerging predictor of metabolic abnormalities such as insulin resistance (100) and dyslipidemia (99). As with skeletal muscle, lower mean liver attenuation values are indicative of greater fatty infiltration or steatosis in the liver. In other words, CT-measured liver attenuation can be used as a surrogate measure of liver steatosis, as liver density is inversely related to liver fat (105). Unlike in the skeletal muscle, fat in the liver resides solely inside the hepatocytes; thus there is no extracellular lipid component. However, it has been reported that although extremely low HU values have been measured in biopsy-diagnosed fatty livers, an overlap exists between normal and abnormal liver HU values (107). Therefore, the absolute liver density determined by CT may not be sensitive for predicting fatty liver. Because a constant relationship exists between liver and spleen attenuation in individuals with normal livers, the ratio of mean liver to spleen attenuation values is used as an index of liver fat, as originally described by Piekarski et al. (107). This method has been verified against histological methods (108) and is commonly used in obesity research. Normally, the liver and spleen mean attenuation values are derived from two or three regions of interest within the liver and spleen. However, owing to the small area of interest, and subjectivity involved in placing the regions of interest, we have recently suggested that the whole liver and spleen surface areas should be used to derive the respective mean attenuation values (Fig. 12). Contrary to previous reports (109), we demonstrate that the attenuation values within the liver and spleen are fairly homogeneous throughout, and by using the whole surface area the interobserver coefficient of variation in the analyses is slightly reduced, from 5.1% (99) to 2.9% (109).

Obtaining a CT image that contains both liver and spleen presents a challenge; variation exists not only in the vertical positioning of the spleen relative to the liver, but also in positioning of both organs within the abdominal cavity. As a multi-image approach is not feasible because of excess exposure (110), Davidson et al. proposed that a single axial image at the T12–L1 intervertebral space may provide the most optimal landmark for assessing both liver and spleen attenuation, as liver and spleen were identified at that level in approx 90% of the men and women studied (Fig. 13) (109). Interestingly, T12–L1 is also a good predictor of visceral fat volume and metabolic syndrome that was in a similar order of magnitude of L1–L2. As such, there is evidence that a single image in the abdomen could be used to accurately quantify liver fat, visceral fat, abdominal subcutaneous fat, and skeletal muscle. These studies are cross-sectional in nature, but provide very important insight into measuring body composition in obesity.

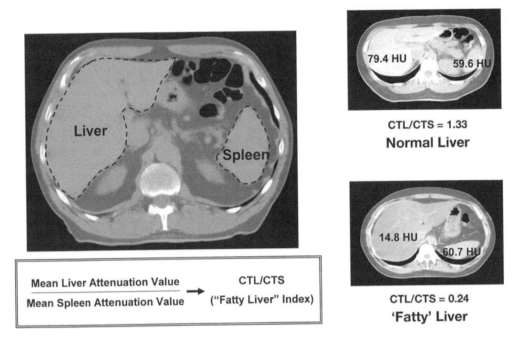

Fig. 12. An example of a normal and a "fatty" liver as measured using the ratio of liver-to-spleen attenuation.

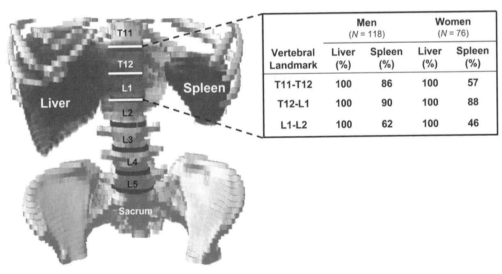

Fig. 13. Likelihood of simultaneous visualization of liver and spleen at three anatomical locations in men and women. Men ($N = 118$), Women ($N = 76$). Adapted from Table 1 and Figure 1 from ref. *109.*

Magnetic Resonance Imaging: Quantification of Ectopic Fat

MRI may also be employed to measure the fatty infiltration within tissues such as skeletal muscle and liver *(111)*. Because fat and water have different characteristics, the water and fat signals within a region of interest can be separated using "chemical shift" techniques such as the Dixon method. Using a similar method, Marks et al. have described another method using MRI *(112)* to create a liver fat index by examining the signal intensity in a region of interest within the right lobe of the liver and comparing this to the signal intensity of an identically sized region of interest within the adjacent sub-cutaneous fat (e.g., liver fat index = signal intensity of liver expressed as a percentage of the intentiy of subcutaneous fat). Both these methods are highly correlated with surrogate measures by biopsy *(112)* or MRS *(113,114)*; however, as with CT, neither of these methods can be used to separate the lipid into intra- and extracellular lipid compartments.

Magnetic Resonance Spectroscopy: Quantification of Ectopic Fat

Unlike CT or MRI, proton magnetic resonance spectroscopy (H^1 MRS) is able to partition the lipid signal into separate intra- and extramyocellular lipid (IMCL and EMCL) components within the skeletal muscle. As it has been suggested that IMCL is an important fat depot that is associated with deleterious effects on insulin sensitivity, it may be important to accurately quantify this depot. Briefly, the principles of MRS are very similar to those of MRI, and in many cases MRS can be acquired using the same machine, and is used in conjunction with MRI in order to carefully landmark and place the region of interest or voxel in a location that is free from visible macroscopic fat depots. This voxel is generally 2 to 3 cm^2, and it is important that the voxel contain as little visible interstitial tissue or fat as possible, as the presence of large fat deposits such as subcutaneous fat or large quantities of EMCL will obscure the relatively smaller IMCL signal. Similar to MRI, H^1 MRS uses magnetic fields to deviate hydrogen protons from their normal orbits. When the protons relax back to the normal orbit, there is an energy release and the generation of radio-frequency signals. Instead of using these signals to generate cross-sectional images as with MRI, H^1 MRS uses the differing proton resonance signals from the fatty acyl groups within the muscle to quantify IMCL *(115–118)*. MRS tends to be highly repeatable (CV ~6%) *(115–117)* and is more sensitive to small changes in IMCL than muscle biopsies.

Schick et al. *(118)* were the first to identify two compartments of triglycerides in muscle that have resonant frequencies separated by 0.02 ppm. The two compartments were identified to represent the lipid located inside (IMCL) and outside (EMCL) the muscle cell. IMCL droplets are spherical with a relatively homogenous distribution, and as such, are independent of muscle orientation relative to the magnetic field *(115–117,119)*. On the other hand, EMCL lies outside the muscle fiber, and appears in plate-like structures *(115–117,120)* that have a highly variable distribution throughout the muscle. Due to the varying orientations and patterns of EMCL, misalignment of the muscle fibers relative to the magnetic field will cause the EMCL line to broaden, and potentially overlap the IMCL resonance peak *(117)*. Further, Boesch et al. demonstrated that IMCL, and not EMCL, signals scale linearly with voxel size, water, and creatine signals, which are used to quantify and scale the IMCL spectra *(115,116)*. Thus, H^1 MRS is typically used only for quantifying IMCL content within muscle, such as the tibialis anterior muscle, which has an easily assessable fiber orientation, and cannot be used to accurately quantify EMCL. Presently there is no available method for quantifying EMCL. Consequently, the metabolic significance of EMCL has yet to be clearly demonstrated in a well-controlled study. Nevertheless, it is generally thought to be a metabolically inert lipid depot *(120)*.

When assessing IMCL, it is important to also consider the muscle fiber type used to quantify IMCL, as IMCL content within a muscle fiber correlates with the oxidative capacity of the fiber *(115,121–123)*. For example, the soleus is composed mainly of type I fibers (slow twitch), and has two to three times the amount of IMCL as the tibialis anterior, which is mainly type II fibers (fast twitch) *(120)*. As mentioned previously, MRS is normally measured in the tibialis anterior, and is used to reflect whole-body IMCL values. However, this clearly has limitations due to the heterogeneity of the lipid distribution between muscle groups.

Measurement of liver fat using H^1 MRS tends to be much simpler than in muscle, as the liver is devoid of extracellular lipid. Consequently, placement of the region of interest or voxel is much simpler, as there will be no macroscopic extracellular lipid depots to contaminate the spectra. The region of interest is generally placed in the parenchyma of the right lobe, while the subjects lie supine to minimize motion artifacts. This process is facilitated by MRI to ensure accurate and consistent landmarking, and in order to avoid major blood vessels and areas of inhomogeneity within the liver. Liver spectra will have only one peak that will reflect the IMCL component (methelyene signal) measured at 0 to 3.0 ppm, and another larger peak from the water signal between 3.0 and 7.8 ppm (108). As with skeletal muscle, the percentage of liver fat is derived from the ratio of the area under the curve for fat and then compared with the area under the curve for water *(100,108,124)*. This method has been validated against histological samples from human liver biopsies *(125)*.

OTHER NOVEL ECTOPIC FAT DEPOTS

As mentioned above, the advent of CT and MRI has allowed recent investigation into other smaller ectopic fat depots such as those within or around the heart, kidneys, pancreas, or blood vessels that are not measurable by biopsy. Most of this literature has focused on the use of CT, as it has a much shorter acquisition time, resulting in a much clearer image. Further, CT provides an attenuation score that may reflect fatty infiltration within the tissue.

Pericardial Fat

Another emerging depot of potential interest is pericardial fat, the fat depot that lies within the pericardial sac surrounding the heart. In human studies this fat depot is associated with increased risk for coronary artery disease *(126,127)*, and may be a source of production for several inflammatory cytokines, which themselves are established antecedents for disease *(128)*. In animal models, increases in the size of the fat pads around the heart have been shown to increase ventricular stiffness and impair cardiac function through physical alterations such as limiting ventricular expansion, impairing venous return, and increasing atrial pressure, which may ultimately lead to heart failure. The extent to which this ectopic fat store is responsible for the alterations in cardiac function

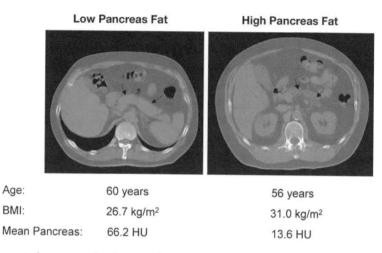

	Low Pancreas Fat	High Pancreas Fat
Age:	60 years	56 years
BMI:	26.7 kg/m²	31.0 kg/m²
Mean Pancreas:	66.2 HU	13.6 HU

Fig. 14. Computed tomography image of a man with high and low pancreas fat. Pancreas is indicated by black arrows.

is still unclear, as these changes may also be due to cardiac hypertrophy related to the increased cardiac work demand or even hemodynamic changes such as hypertension that are also associated with obesity and an increased body mass. The independent contribution of the pericardial fat depot to obesity-related morbidity and mortality is unknown.

Perivascular Fat

Increases in ectopic fat around the blood vessels or perivascular fat may be associated with an increased risk of cardiovascular disease (103). Nearly all blood vessels in the body are surrounded by perivascular fat, which is thought to serve as structural support. However, large amounts of perivascular fat could serve as a mechanical restraint, resulting in reduced vascular distensibility or increased vascular stiffness. It is unclear whether perivascular fat has an independent contribution to vascular stiffness because obesity-induced hypertension, endothelial dysfunction, insulin resistance, inflammation, or even lipid accumulation within the vascular smooth muscle cell are also plausible candidates. Because of the small size of this fat depot, this depot is difficult to quantify, and as such, the present data are derived from animal models and await confirmation in humans.

Pancreas Fat

Fatty infiltration within the pancreas is the most common histological change in the pancreas (129). Pancreas fat infiltration in vivo, commonly measured using CT (Fig. 14), is thought to be associated with β-cell hyperfunction, dysfunction, or apoptosis (111,130–132). It is hypothesized that in the pre-diabetes stage, insulin secretion increases to compensate for insulin resistance (133). However, when the increased pancreatic fat accumulation reaches a critical point, lipoapoptosis ensues, and insulin secretion is reduced, resulting in diabetes and hyperglycemia. This theory has been difficult to confirm in humans owing to the challenges inherent to the measure of fat within this relatively small organ. Thus, the majority of data suggesting the metabolic importance of pancreas fat derive from animal models.

Kidney Fat

Ectopic fat storage in the kidney is another depot reported to be associated with sodium retention and hypertension in animal models *(128)*. In obese rabbits, lipid accumulation occurs in the renal sinus and may compress the renal vasculature and other structures, impeding sodium excretion. Further, increases in visceral adiposity may also increase intra-abdominal pressure *(134)* and further exaggerate the compression associated with renal sinus lipomatosis by preventing the kidneys from expanding, thereby exacerbating the restriction in renal vascularization and sodium excretion.

CONCLUSIONS

Understanding of the complex relationships between various components of human-body composition and disease have advanced through the use of both simple and complex methods. Anthropometry represents a straightforward and inexpensive set of tools that can be used in the clinic to identify individuals at increased risk for obesity related metabolic disorders. The extent to which these anthropometric measures are linked to disease via their utility to measure body composition components relies on studies that employ research-based imaging methods such as CT and MRI that quantify the major body composition components at the tissue-system level. Indeed, these imaging techniques allow for the quantification of several novel depots such as liver, skeletal muscle, pericardial, perivascular, pancreatic, and kidney ectopic fat depots—fat depots that may also have independent associations with morbidity and mortality. Further, novel applications of MRS are useful for assessing ectopic fat deposition within the cells of various tissues in the body. In many ways the study of the associations between body composition in obesity and related comorbidities is in its infancy. Advances in our understanding of these complex relationships will doubtless follow corresponding advances in technology. However, the use of both simple and complex methods will be required to identify the targets for obesity reduction and hence, the reduction of obesity related morbidity and mortality.

REFERENCES

1. Folsom AR, Kushi LH, Anderson KE, et al. Associations of general and abdominal obesity with multiple health outcomes in older women: the Iowa Women's Health Study. Arch Intern Med 2000;160:2117–2128.
2. Ho SC, Chen YM, Woo JL, et al. Association between simple anthropometric indices and cardiovascular risk factors. Int J Obes Relat Metab Disord 2001;25:1689–1697.
3. Seidell JC, Cigolini M, Charzewska J, et al. Regional obesity and serum lipids in European women born in 1948. A multicenter study. Acta Med Scand Suppl 1988;723:189–197.
4. Vague J. La differenciation sexuelle, facteur determinant des formes de l'obesité. La Presse Medicale 1947;30:339–340.
5. Janssen I, Katzmarzyk PT, Ross R. Waist circumference and not body mass index explains obesity-related health risk. Am J Clin Nutr 2004;79:379–384.
6. Ohlson LO, Larsson B, Svardsudd K, et al. The influence of body fat distribution on the incidence of diabetes mellitus. 13.5 years of follow-up of the participants in the study of men born in 1913. Diabetes 1985;34:1055–1058.
7. Allison DB, Gallagher D, Heo M, et al. Body mass index and all-cause mortality among people age 70 and over: the Longitudinal Study of Aging. Int J Obes Relat Metab Disord 1997;21:424–431.
8. Calle EE, Thun MJ, Petrelli JM, et al. Body-mass index and mortality in a prospective cohort of U.S. adults. N Engl J Med 1999; 41:1097–1105.

9. Bigaard J, Tjonneland A, Thomsen BL, et al. Waist circumference, BMI, smoking, and mortality in middle-aged men and women. Obes Res 2003;11:895–903.
10. Lapidus L, Bengtsson C, Lissner L. Distribution of adipose tissue in relation to cardiovascular and total mortality as observed during 20 years in a prospective population study of women in Gothenburg, Sweden. Diabetes Res Clin Pract 1990;10 Suppl 1:S185–S189.
11. Larsson B, Svardsudd K, Welin L, et al. Abdominal adipose tissue distribution, obesity, and risk of cardiovascular disease and death: 13 year follow up of participants in the study of men born in 1913. Br Med J (Clin Res Ed) 1984;288:1401–1404.
12. Kuk JL, Katzmarzyk PT, Nichaman MZ, et al. Visceral fat is an independent predictor of all-cause mortality in men. Obes Res 2006;14:336–341.
13. Spencer EA, Appleby PN, Davey GK, et al. Validity of self-reported height and weight in 4808 EPIC-Oxford participants. Public Health Nutr 2002;5:561–565.
14. Executive summary of the clinical guidelines on the identification, evaluation, and treatment of overweight and obesity in adults. Arch Intern Med 1998;158:1855–1867.
15. Gallagher D, Heymsfield SB, Heo M,et al. Healthy percentage body fat ranges: an approach for developing guidelines based on body mass index. Am J Clin Nutr 2000;72:694–701.
16. Deurenberg-Yap M, Chew SK, Deurenberg P. Elevated body fat percentage and cardiovascular risks at low body mass index levels among Singaporean Chinese, Malays and Indians. Obes Rev 2002;3:209–215.
17. Janssen I, Katzmarzyk PT, Ross R, et al. Fitness alters the associations of BMI and waist circumference with total and abdominal fat. Obes Res 2004;12:525–537.
18. Stevens J, Cai J, Pamuk ER, et al. The effect of age on the association between body-mass index and mortality. N Engl J Med 1998;338:1–7.
19. Appropriate body-mass index for Asian populations and its implications for policy and intervention strategies. Lancet 2004;363:157–163.
20. Stevens J, Nowicki EM. Body mass index and mortality in asian populations: implications for obesity cut-points. Nutr Rev 2003;61:104–107.
21. Song YM, Sung J. Body mass index and mortality: a twelve-year prospective study in Korea. Epidemiology 2001;12:173–179.
22. Lee RC, Wang Z, Heo M, et al. Total-body skeletal muscle mass: development and cross-validation of anthropometric prediction models. Am J Clin Nutr 2000;72:796–803.
23. Rice B, Janssen I, Hudson R, et al. Effects of aerobic or resistance exercise and/or diet on glucose tolerance and plasma insulin levels in obese men. Diabetes Care 1999;22:684–691.
24. Wang J, Thornton JC, Bari S, et al. Comparisons of waist circumferences measured at 4 sites. Am J Clin Nutr 2003;77:379–384.
25. Clinical Guidelines on the Identification, Evaluation, and Treatment of Overweight and Obesity in Adults—The Evidence Report. National Institutes of Health. Obes Res 1998;6 Suppl 2:51S–209S.
26. Zhu S, Heymsfield SB, Toyoshima H, et al. Race-ethnicity-specific waist circumference cutoffs for identifying cardiovascular disease risk factors. Am J Clin Nutr 2005;81:409–415.
27. The IDF consensus worldwide definition of the metabolic syndrome: International Diabetes Federation, 2005.
28. Han TS, Lean ME. Self-reported waist circumference compared with the 'Waist Watcher' tape-measure to identify individuals at increased health risk through intra-abdominal fat accumulation. Br J Nutr 1998;80:81–88.
29. Han TS, McNeill G, Seidell JC, et al. Predicting intra-abdominal fatness from anthropometric measures: the influence of stature. Int J Obes Relat Metab Disord 1997;21:587–593.
30. Janssen I, Heymsfield SB, Allison DB, et al. Body mass index and waist circumference independently contribute to the prediction of nonabdominal, abdominal subcutaneous, and visceral fat. Am J Clin Nutr 2002;75:683–688.
31. Despres JP, Prud'homme D, Pouliot MC, et al. Estimation of deep abdominal adipose-tissue accumulation from simple anthropometric measurements in men. Am J Clin Nutr 1991;54:471–477.
32. Ross R, Shaw KD, Rissanen J, et al. Sex differences in lean and adipose tissue distribution by magnetic resonance imaging: anthropometric relationships. Am J Clin Nutr 1994;59:1277–1285.
33. Ross R, Leger L, Morris D, et al. Quantification of adipose tissue by MRI: relationship with anthropometric variables. J Appl Physiol 1992;72:787–795.
34. Seidell JC, Bjorntorp P, Sjostrom L, et al. Regional distribution of muscle and fat mass in men—new insight into the risk of abdominal obesity using computed tomography. Int J Obes 1989;13:289–303.

35. van der Kooy K, Leenen R, Seidell JC, et al. Waist-hip ratio is a poor predictor of changes in visceral fat. Am J Clin Nutr 1993;57:327–333.
36. Carr DB, Utzschneider KM, Hull RL, et al. Intra-abdominal fat is a major determinant of the National Cholesterol Education Program Adult Treatment Panel III criteria for the metabolic syndrome. Diabetes 2004;53:2087–2094.
37. Kuk JL, Nichaman MZ, Church TS, et al. Liver fat is not a marker of metabolic risk in lean premenopausal women. Metabolism 2004;53:1066–1071.
38. Goodpaster BH, Krishnaswami S, Harris TB, et al. Obesity, regional body fat distribution, and the metabolic syndrome in older men and women. Arch Intern Med 2005;165:777–783.
39. Boyko EJ, Fujimoto WY, Leonetti DL, et al. Visceral adiposity and risk of type 2 diabetes: a prospective study among Japanese Americans. Diabetes Care 2000;23:465–471.
40. Kuk JL, Lee S, Heymsfield SB, et al. Waist circumference and abdominal adipose tissue distribution: influence of age and sex. Am J Clin Nutr 2005;81:1330–1334.
41. Wong SL, Katzmarzyk P, Nichaman MZ, et al. Cardiorespiratory fitness is associated with lower abdominal fat independent of body mass index. Med Sci Sports Exerc 2004;36:286–291.
42. Ross R, Rissanen J, Pedwell H, et al. Influence of diet and exercise on skeletal muscle and visceral adipose tissue in men. J Appl Physiol 1996;81:2445–2455.
43. Ross R, Pedwell H, Rissanen J. Effects of energy restriction and exercise on skeletal muscle and adipose tissue in women as measured by magnetic resonance imaging. Am J Clin Nutr 1995;61:1179–1185.
44. Ross R, Janssen I, Dawson J, et al. Exercise-induced reduction in obesity and insulin resistance in women: a randomized controlled trial. Obes Res 2004;12:789–798.
45. Ross R, Dagnone D, Jones PJ, et al. Reduction in obesity and related comorbid conditions after diet-induced weight loss or exercise-induced weight loss in men. A randomized, controlled trial. Ann Intern Med 2000;133:92–103.
46. Ducimetiere P, Richard JL. The relationship between subsets of anthropometric upper versus lower body measurements and coronary heart disease risk in middle-aged men. The Paris Prospective Study. I. Int J Obes 1989;13:111–121.
47. Yusuf S, Hawken S, Ounpuu S, et al. Obesity and the risk of myocardial infarction in 27,000 participants from 52 countries: a case-control study. Lancet 2005;366:1640–1649.
48. Kamel EG, McNeill G, Han TS, et al. Measurement of abdominal fat by magnetic resonance imaging, dual-energy X-ray absorptiometry and anthropometry in non-obese men and women. Int J Obes Relat Metab Disord 1999;23:686–692.
49. Bonora E, Micciolo R, Ghiatas AA, et al. Is it possible to derive a reliable estimate of human visceral and subcutaneous abdominal adipose tissue from simple anthropometric measurements? Metabolism 1995;44:1617–1625.
50. Ross R, Rissanen J, Hudson R. Sensitivity associated with the identification of visceral adipose tissue levels using waist circumference in men and women: effects of weight loss. Int J Obes Relat Metab Disord 1996;20:533–538.
51. Ross R, Shaw KD, Martel Y, et al. Adipose tissue distribution measured by magnetic resonance imaging in obese women. Am J Clin Nutr 1993;57:470–475.
52. Kamel EG, McNeill G, Van Wijk MC. Change in intra-abdominal adipose tissue volume during weight loss in obese men and women: correlation between magnetic resonance imaging and anthropometric measurements. Int J Obes Relat Metab Disord 2000;24:607–613.
53. Empana JP, Ducimetiere P, Charles MA, et al. Sagittal abdominal diameter and risk of sudden death in asymptomatic middle-aged men: the Paris Prospective Study I. Circulation 2004;110:2781–2785.
54. Ohrvall M, Berglund L, Vessby B. Sagittal abdominal diameter compared with other anthropometric measurements in relation to cardiovascular risk. Int J Obes Relat Metab Disord 2000;24:497–501.
55. Pouliot MC, Despres JP, Lemieux S, et al. Waist circumference and abdominal sagittal diameter: best simple anthropometric indexes of abdominal visceral adipose tissue accumulation and related cardiovascular risk in men and women. Am J Cardiol 1994;73:460–468.
56. Onat A, Avci GS, Barlan MM, et al. Measures of abdominal obesity assessed for visceral adiposity and relation to coronary risk. Int J Obes Relat Metab Disord 2004;28:1018–1025.
57. Lohman TG, Roche AF, Martello R. Anthropometric Standardization Reference Manual. Human Kinetics, Champaign, IL: 1988.
58. Peterson MJ, Czerwinski SA, Siervogel RM. Development and validation of skinfold-thickness prediction equations with a 4-compartment model. Am J Clin Nutr 2003;77:1186–1191.

59. Wang J, Thornton JC, Kolesnik S, et al. Anthropometry in body composition. An overview. Ann NY Acad Sci 2000;904:317–326.

60. Heymsfield SB, Lohman TG, Wang Z, et al. Human Body Composition. Human Kinetics, Windsor, ON: 2005.

61. Bray GA, Bouchard C, James WPT. Handbook of Obesity. Marcel Dekker, New York:1998.

62. Mueller WH, Malina RM. Relative reliability of circumferences and skinfolds as measures of body fat distribution. Am J Phys Anthropol 1987;72:437–439.

63. Cronk CE, Roche AF. Race- and sex-specific reference data for triceps and subscapular skinfolds and weight/stature. Am J Clin Nutr 1982;35:347–354.

64. Fogelholm GM, Sievanen HT, van Marken Lichtenbelt WD, et al. Assessment of fat-mass loss during weight reduction in obese women. Metabolism 1997;46:968–975.

65. Ellis KJ, Bell SJ, Chertow GM, et al. Bioelectrical impedance methods in clinical research: a follow-up to the NIH Technology Assessment Conference. Nutrition 1999;15:874–880.

66. Fogelholm M, van Marken Lichtenbelt W. Comparison of body composition methods: a literature analysis. Eur J Clin Nutr 1997;51:495–503.

67. Kim J, Wang Z, Heymsfield SB, Baumgartner RN, et al. Total-body skeletal muscle mass: estimation by a new dual-energy X-ray absorptiometry method. Am J Clin Nutr 2002;76:378–383.

68. Genton L, Hans D, Kyle UG, et al. Dual-energy X-ray absorptiometry and body composition: differences between devices and comparison with reference methods. Nutrition 2002;18:66–70.

69. Visser M, Fuerst T, Lang T, et al. Validity of fan-beam dual-energy X-ray absorptiometry for measuring fat-free mass and leg muscle mass. Health, Aging, and Body Composition Study—Dual-Energy X-ray Absorptiometry and Body Composition Working Group. J Appl Physiol 1999;87:1513–1520.

70. Tylavsky F, Lohman T, Blunt BA, et al. QDR 4500A DXA overestimates fat-free mass compared with criterion methods. J Appl Physiol 2003;94:959–965.

71. Brownbill RA, Ilich JZ. Measuring body composition in overweight individuals by dual energy X-ray absorptiometry. BMC Med Imaging 2005;5:1.

72. Salamone LM, Fuerst T, Visser M, et al. Measurement of fat mass using DEXA: a validation study in elderly adults. J Appl Physiol 2000;89:345–352.

73. Wang W, Wang Z, Faith MS, et al. Regional skeletal muscle measurement: evaluation of new dual-energy X-ray absorptiometry model. J Appl Physiol 1999;87:1163–1171.

74. Levine JA, Abboud L, Barry M, et al. Measuring leg muscle and fat mass in humans: comparison of CT and dual-energy X-ray absorptiometry. J Appl Physiol 2000;88:452–456.

75. Snijder MB, Visser M, Dekker JM, et al. The prediction of visceral fat by dual-energy X-ray absorptiometry in the elderly: a comparison with computed tomography and anthropometry. Int J Obes Relat Metab Disord 2002;26:984–993.

76. Clasey JL, Bouchard C, Teates CD, et al. The use of anthropometric and dual-energy X-ray absorptiometry (DXA) measures to estimate total abdominal and abdominal visceral fat in men and women. Obes Res 1999;7:256–264.

77. Park YW, Heymsfield SB, Gallagher D. Are dual-energy X-ray absorptiometry regional estimates associated with visceral adipose tissue mass? Int J Obes Relat Metab Disord 2002;26:978–983.

78. Snead DB, Birge SJ, Kohrt WM. Age-related differences in body composition by hydrodensitometry and dual-energy X-ray absorptiometry. J Appl Physiol 1993;74:770–775.

79. Kohrt WM. Preliminary evidence that DEXA provides an accurate assessment of body composition. J Appl Physiol 1998;84:372–377.

80. Evans EM, Saunders MJ, Spano MA, et al. Body-composition changes with diet and exercise in obese women: a comparison of estimates from clinical methods and a 4-component model. Am J Clin Nutr 1999;70:5–12.

81. Tylavsky FA, Lohman TG, Docktrell M, et al. Comparison of the effectiveness of 2 dual-energy X-ray absorptiometers with that of total body water and computed tomography in assessing changes in body composition during weight change. Am J Clin Nutr 2003;77:356–363.

82. Nelson ME, Fiatarone MA, Layne JE, et al. Analysis of body-composition techniques and models for detecting change in soft tissue with strength training. Am J Clin Nutr 1996;63:678-86.

83. Houtkooper LB, Going SB, Sproul J, et al. Comparison of methods for assessing body-composition changes over 1 y in postmenopausal women. Am J Clin Nutr 2000;72:401–406.

84. Roubenoff R, Kehayias JJ, Dawson-Hughes B, et al. Use of dual-energy X-ray absorptiometry in body-composition studies: not yet a "gold standard." Am J Clin Nutr 1993;58:589–591.

85. Mitsiopoulos N, Baumgartner RN, Heymsfield SB, et al. Cadaver validation of skeletal muscle measurement by magnetic resonance imaging and computerized tomography. J Appl Physiol 1998;85:115–122.

86. Ross R, Goodpaster B, Kelley D, et al. Magnetic resonance imaging in human body composition research. From quantitative to qualitative tissue measurement. Ann NY Acad Sci 2000;904:12–17.

87. Ross R. Magnetic resonance imaging provides new insights into the characterization of adipose and lean tissue distribution. Can J Physiol Pharmacol 1996;74:778–785.

88. Thomas EL, Saeed N, Hajnal JV, et al. Magnetic resonance imaging of total body fat. J Appl Physiol 1998;85:1778–1785.

89. Abate N, Burns D, Peshock RM, et al. Estimation of adipose tissue mass by magnetic resonance imaging: validation against dissection in human cadavers. J Lipid Res 1994;35:1490–1496.

90. Mourier A, Gautier JF, De Kerviler E, et al. Mobilization of visceral adipose tissue related to the improvement in insulin sensitivity in response to physical training in NIDDM. Effects of branched-chain amino acid supplements. Diabetes Care 1997;20:385–391.

91. Kvist H, Sjostrom L, Tylen U. Adipose tissue volume determinations in women by computed tomography: technical considerations. Int J Obes 1986;10:53–67.

92. Shen W, Wang Z, Tang H, et al. Volume estimates by imaging methods: model comparisons with visible women as the reference. Obes Res 2003;11:217–225.

93. Snyder WS, Cooke MJ, Manssett ES, et al. Report of the Task Group on Reference Man. Pergamon, Oxford: 1975.

94. Gallagher D, Belmonte D, Deurenberg P, et al. Organ-tissue mass measurement allows modeling of REE and metabolically active tissue mass. Am J Physiol 1998;275:E249–E258.

95. Lee SJ, Janssen I, Heymsfield SB, et al. Relation between whole-body and regional measures of human skeletal muscle. Am J Clin Nutr 2004;80:1215–1221.

96. Kuk JL, Church TS, Blair SN, et al. Does the measurement site for visceral and abdominal subcutaneous adipose tissue alter the associations with the metabolic syndrome? Diabetes Care 2006;29:679–684.

97. Monzon JR, Basile R, Heneghan S, et al. Lipolysis in adipocytes isolated from deep and superficial subcutaneous adipose tissue. Obes Res 2002;10:266–269.

98. Jansson PA, Smith U, Lonnroth P. Interstitial glycerol concentration measured by microdialysis in two subcutaneous regions in humans. Am J Physiol 1990;258:E918–E922.

99. Nguyen-Duy TB, Nichaman MZ, Church TS, et al. Visceral fat and liver fat are independent predictors of metabolic risk factors in men. Am J Physiol Endocrinol Metab 2003;284:E1065–E1071.

100. Tiikkainen M, Tamminen M, Hakkinen AM, et al. Liver-fat accumulation and insulin resistance in obese women with previous gestational diabetes. Obes Res 2002;10:859–867.

101. Boden G, Lebed B, Schatz M, et al. Effects of acute changes of plasma free fatty acids on intramyocellular fat content and insulin resistance in healthy subjects. Diabetes 2001;50:1612–1617.

102. Laurin J. Motion—All patients with NASH need to have a liver biopsy: Arguments against the motion. Can J Gastroenterol 2002;16:722–726.

103. Montani JP, Carroll JF, Dwyer TM, et al. Ectopic fat storage in heart, blood vessels and kidneys in the pathogenesis of cardiovascular diseases. Int J Obes Relat Metab Disord 2004;28 Suppl 4:S58–S65.

104. Banerji MA, Buckley MC, Chaiken RL, et al. Liver fat, serum triglycerides and visceral adipose tissue in insulin-sensitive and insulin-resistant black men with NIDDM. Int J Obes Relat Metab Disord 1995;19:846–850.

105. Ricci C, Longo R, Gioulis E, et al. Noninvasive in vivo quantitative assessment of fat content in human liver. J Hepatol 1997;27:108–113.

106. Goto T, Onuma T, Takebe K, et al. The influence of fatty liver on insulin clearance and insulin resistance in non-diabetic Japanese subjects. Int J Obes Relat Metab Disord 1995;19:841–845.

107. Piekarski J, Goldberg HI, Royal SA, et al. Difference between liver and spleen CT numbers in the normal adult: its usefulness in predicting the presence of diffuse liver disease. Radiology 1980;137:727–729.

108. Longo R, Ricci C, Masutti F, et al. Fatty infiltration of the liver. Quantification by 1H localized magnetic resonance spectroscopy and comparison with computed tomography. Invest Radiol 1993;28:297–302.

109. Davidson LE, Kuk JL, Church TS, et al. Protocol for measurement of liver fat by computedtomography. J Appl Physiol 2006;100:864–868.

110. Joy D, Thava VR, Scott BB. Diagnosis of fatty liver disease: is biopsy necessary? Eur J Gastroenterol Hepatol 2003;15:539-43.
111. Kovanlikaya A, Mittelman SD, Ward A, et al. Obesity and fat quantification in lean tissues using three-point Dixon MR imaging. Pediatr Radiol 2005;35:601–607.
112. Marks SJ, Moore NR, Ryley NG, et al. Measurement of liver fat by MRI and its reduction by dexfenfluramine in NIDDM. Int J Obes Relat Metab Disord 1997;21:274–279.
113. Schick F, Machann J, Brechtel K, et al. MRI of muscular fat. Magnet Reson Med 2002;47:720–727.
114. Fishbein M, Castro F, Cheruku S, et al. Hepatic MRI for fat quantitation: its relationship to fat morphology, diagnosis, and ultrasound. J Clin Gastroenterol 2005;39:619–625.
115. Boesch C, Decombaz J, Slotboom J, et al. Observation of intramyocellular lipids by means of 1H magnetic resonance spectroscopy. Proc Nutr Soc 1999;58:841–850.
116. Boesch C, Kreis R. Observation of intramyocellular lipids by 1H-magnetic resonance spectroscopy. Ann NY Acad Sci 2000;904:25–31.
117. Szczepaniak LS, Babcock EE, Schick F, et al. Measurement of intracellular triglyceride stores by H spectroscopy: validation in vivo. Am J Physiol 1999;276:E977–E989.
118. Schick F, Eismann B, Jung WI, et al. Comparison of localized proton NMR signals of skeletal muscle and fat tissue in vivo: two lipid compartments in muscle tissue. Magn Reson Med 1993;29:158–167.
119. Steidle G, Machann J, Claussen CD, et al. Separation of intra- and extramyocellular lipid signals in proton MR spectra by determination of their magnetic field distribution. J Magn Reson 2002;154:228–235.
120. Hwang JH, Pan JW, Heydari S, et al. Regional differences in intramyocellular lipids in humans observed by in vivo 1H-MR spectroscopic imaging. J Appl Physiol 2001;90:1267–1274.
121. Essen B, Jansson E, Henriksson J, et al. Metabolic characteristics of fiber types in human skeletal muscle. Acta Physiol Scand 1975;95:153–165.
122. Larson-Meyer DE, Newcomer BR, Hunter GR. Influence of endurance running and recovery diet on intramyocellular lipid content in women: a 1H NMR study. Am J Physiol Endocrinol Metab 2002;282:E95–E106.
123. Malenfant P, Joanisse DR, Theriault R, et al. Fat content in individual muscle fibers of lean and obese subjects. Int J Obes Relat Metab Disord 2001;25:1316–1321.
124. Szczepaniak LS, Nurenberg P, Leonard D, et al. Magnetic resonance spectroscopy to measure hepatic triglyceride content: prevalence of hepatic steatosis in the general population. Am J Physiol Endocrinol Metab 2005;288:E462–E468.
125. Thomsen C, Becker U, Winkler K, et al. Quantification of liver fat using magnetic resonance spectroscopy. Magn Reson Imaging 1994;12:487–495.
126. Iacobellis G, Ribaudo MC, Zappaterreno A, et al. Relation between epicardial adipose tissue and left ventricular mass. Am J Cardiol 2004;94:1084–1087.
127. Taguchi R, Takasu J, Itani Y, et al. Pericardial fat accumulation in men as a risk factor for coronary artery disease. Atherosclerosis 2001;157:203–209.
128. Mazurek T, Zhang L, Zalewski A, et al. Human epicardial adipose tissue is a source of inflammatory mediators. Circulation 2003;108:2460–2466.
129. Olsen TS. Lipomatosis of the pancreas in autopsy material and its relation to age and overweight. Acta Pathol Microbiol Scand [A] 1978;86A:367–373.
130. Lewis GF, Carpentier A, Adeli K, et al. Disordered fat storage and mobilization in the pathogenesis of insulin resistance and type 2 diabetes. Endocr Rev 2002;23:201–229.
131. Raz I, Eldor R, Cernea S, et al. Diabetes: insulin resistance and derangements in lipid metabolism. Cure through intervention in fat transport and storage. Diabetes Metab Res Rev 2004;21:3–14.
132. Koyama K, Chen G, Lee Y, et al. Tissue triglycerides, insulin resistance, and insulin production: implications for hyperinsulinemia of obesity. Am J Physiol 1997;273:E708–E713.
133. Unger RH. Longevity, lipotoxicity and leptin: the adipocyte defense against feasting and famine. Biochimie 2005;87:57–64.
134. Sugerman HJ, DeMaria EJ, Felton WL 3rd, et al. Increased intra-abdominal pressure and cardiac filling pressures in obesity-associated pseudotumor cerebri. Neurology 1997;49:507–511.

8 Energy Expenditure in Obesity

Leanne M. Redman, PhD,
and Eric Ravussin, PhD

CONTENTS

METHODS OF MEASURING ENERGY EXPENDITURE
COMPONENTS OF ENERGY EXPENDITURE AND THEIR RELEVANCE
    TO OBESITY
ENERGY EXPENDITURE IN THE ETIOLOGY OF OBESITY
ENERGY EXPENDITURE IN CHILDREN
MOLECULAR MECHANISMS OF ENERGY EXPENDITURE VARIABILITY
CONCLUSION
REFERENCES

Summary

Body weight is dependent on an intricate balance between energy intake and energy expenditure. When energy intake exceeds energy expenditure weight is gained, and the majority of this excess energy is stored as body fat. Whether the culprit of weight gain is increased food intake or reduced energy expenditure is generally unknown but it is most likely to be both, with proportions varying from case to case. An accurate assessment of dietary energy intake is difficult and precise only under laboratory conditions, but then the dietary intake tends not to accurately represent everyday life. Measurements of food intake in free-living conditions are, however, weakened by poor accuracy and precision. Scientists, therefore, have concentrated on the energy expenditure side of the energy balance equation. This chapter will review the methods by which energy expenditure can be measured in humans, the components of daily energy expenditure, their inherent interindividual variability, and their contribution to weight gain in adults and children. Finally, recent advances in our understanding of some of the molecular mechanisms underlying the regulation of energy expenditure will be discussed.

Key Words: Energy balance; 24-h energy expenditure; resting metabolic rate; spontaneous physical activity; diet-induced thermogenesis.

METHODS OF MEASURING ENERGY EXPENDITURE

Several methods have been developed to measure daily energy expenditure in humans (Fig. 1). The most accurate methods involve continuous measurements of heat output (direct calorimetry) or gas exchange (indirect calorimetry) in individuals confined within a metabolic chamber. Confined individuals, however, are unable to pursue habitual

From: *Contemporary Endocrinology: Treatment of the Obese Patient*
Edited by: R. F. Kushner and D. H. Bessesen © Humana Press Inc., Totowa, NJ

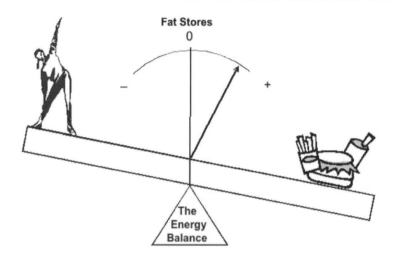

Fig. 1. Body weight is dependent on an intricate balance between energy intake and energy expenditure. When energy intake exceeds energy expenditure, weight is gained; the majority of this excess energy is stored as body fat. Whether the culprit of weight gain is increased food intake or reduced energy expenditure is generally unknown but it is most likely to be both, with proportions varying from case to case.

activities; therefore, several field methods have been developed to measure energy expenditure in free-living conditions. These include doubly labeled water, self-reports, and portable monitors.

Direct Calorimetry

Heat is the ultimate fate of all the body's metabolic processes; energy expenditure can, therefore, be measured directly as heat loss. Direct calorimetry, first described by Zuntz and Hagerman in the late 1800s, involves placing an individual in a small insulated chamber in which all the heat released in the form of dry heat (representing heat dissipated by convection and radiation) or evaporative heat (representing heat loss in the evaporation of water from the lungs and skin) is measured. This method has been applied to various animal and human studies *(1–3)*, but has become largely obsolete because these studies are very expensive to conduct and require individuals to be confined in a very small room. Despite their limited use today, direct calorimeters have played an important role for validating indirect calorimetry methods.

Indirect Calorimetry

The term "indirect calorimetry" arises from the premise that heat released from the metabolic processes in the body can be measured indirectly from oxygen consumption. Under normal physiological conditions, neither oxygen nor carbon dioxide is stored within the body. Therefore, an indirect method of assessing energy expenditure is to measure oxygen consumption, carbon dioxide production, and nitrogen excretion. The use of indirect calorimetry in the study of energy expenditure dates back to the end of the 19th century. Indirect calorimetry has proved useful for the study of energy expenditure and/or substrate oxidation in normal and diseased states. Indirect calorimetry can be measured using both open-circuit and closed-circuit systems.

Closed-circuit spirometry, developed in the late 1800s, involves rebreathing 100% oxygen from a prefilled spirometer while the exhaled carbon dioxide is absorbed by a canister of soda lime in the breathing circuit. The change in the volume of the circuit is used to measure the rate of oxygen removal from the system and corresponds to an individual's oxygen consumption. This method has almost been abandoned by most hospitals and research laboratories.

Open-circuit spirometry provides a relatively simple way to measure oxygen consumption at rest and during exercise. The individual inhales ambient air with a constant composition. Changes in oxygen and carbon dioxide percentages in the expired air compared with percentages in inspired ambient air reflect ongoing energy metabolism. With the addition of the volume of air breathed during a specific time period, respiratory gas exchange can be measured and energy expenditure calculated indirectly. Early measurements of resting metabolic rate were performed using mouthpieces or face masks, but these have now been replaced by ventilated hood systems to improve the comfort for the individual. During the past three decades, the indirect calorimetry method has been applied to confined rooms called respiratory or metabolic chambers *(4–16)*. These chambers are large enough (12,000–40,000 L) for an individual to live in comfortably for several days. Respiratory chambers enable the measurement of various components of daily energy expenditure, including sleeping metabolic rate, the energy cost of arousal, the thermic effect of food, and the energy cost of spontaneous physical activity (Fig. 2). The measurement of energy expenditure in the chamber is accurate and is used extensively to assess the determinants of daily sedentary energy expenditure in humans.

Doubly Labeled Water

The doubly labeled water (DLW) method was first developed in animals by Lifson in 1966 *(17)* and its first use in humans was reported by Schoeller and Van Santen *(18)*. The method is based on indirect calorimetry assumptions and on the differential elimination of two nonradioactive isotopes, deuterium (^{2}H) and ^{18}oxygen (^{18}O) from body water following a single oral dose of the two isotopes. Oxygen tagged with the ^{18}O tracer will equilibrate not only in body water but also in circulating bicarbonate and expired carbon dioxide. Over time the ^{18}O tracer in body water will decrease as CO_2 is expired and water is lost in respiration, perspiration, and urine. The hydrogen molecule tagged with the ^{2}H tracer will distribute only in the circulating water and bicarbonate and over time will decrease as water is lost. The elimination rates of the two isotopes from the body are measured by mass spectroscopy in blood, saliva, or, most commonly, urine. The difference between the elimination rates of the two isotopes therefore provides a measurement of carbon dioxide production from which energy expenditure is then calculated from classical indirect calorimetric equations. The major advantage of the DLW method is that it provides an integrated measure of total carbon dioxide production over periods of 1 to 2 wk, requiring only periodic sampling of urine for measurements of ^{2}H and ^{18}O enrichments. The DLW method allows individuals to be studied in the free-living state, without being influenced or limited in their activity by wearing cumbersome monitors. The DLW method has been validated repeatedly with excellent accuracy (1–3%) and precision (2–8%) against the gold-standard indirect calorimetry. The method is noninvasive, and can be used for measuring energy expenditure in various populations, such as pregnant women, infants, children, and the elderly *(19–21)*, where other assessments of energy expenditure are problematic. In conjunction with other determinations

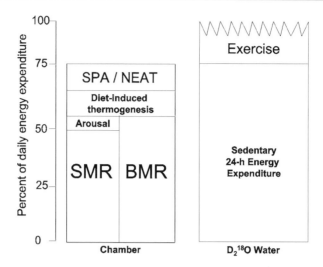

Fig. 2. The components of daily energy expenditure. Daily energy is expended in three major physiological components: resting (basal) metabolic rate (BMR), which includes the energy cost of maintaining the integrated systems of the body and the homeothermic temperature at rest and can be divided into sleeping metabolic rate (SMR) and the energy cost of arousal; the thermic effect of food or diet-induced thermogenesis, reflecting the surplus energy expended after the administration of a meal related to absorption, digestion, and storage of the energy; and the energy cost of physical activity, being the energy expended during both volitional (exercise) and nonvolitional activities. These nonvolitional activities include the energy cost of sitting, fidgeting, maintaining posture, muscle tone, and performing leisure activities such as playing guitar, shopping, etc. It has been named spontaneous physical activity (SPA) or nonexercise activity thermogenesis (NEAT). The primary determinants of total daily energy expenditure are weight, height, age, and gender. Total daily energy expenditure and its components can be measured in the laboratory under standard conditions and in free-living situations. The left panel illustrates the measurement of 24-h energy expenditure by indirect calorimetry in a metabolic chamber, and the right shows the total energy expenditure measured over 7 to 10 d using the doubly labeled water method.

of resting energy expenditure using indirect calorimetry, DLW is the best and most accurate way of assessing the energy cost of physical activity in humans. The major drawbacks of the method are the high costs of the ^{18}O isotope for large clinical trials and of the mass spectrometer necessary to determine the isotopic enrichments of ^2H and ^{18}O.

Self-Reported Assessments

An individual's habitual and occupational physical activity can also be captured with the use of activity diaries, questionnaires, interviews, or time-and-motion studies, with the energy cost of the activities estimated from energy expenditure tables. This method is called the factorial method. Factorial assessments of energy expenditure require that the type and duration of physical activities be recorded across several days. The energy cost of each activity is then estimated from energy-equivalent tables and multiplied by the time spent in any given activity. This method therefore is extremely time-consuming for individuals and investigators. Substantial variability with the technique has been reported, which is owed to poor and inaccurate recall by individuals, as well as the availability of numerous energy coefficients that can be applied to determine the energy cost of the activities. Although factorial methods have been criticized *(22)*, when compared with other field assessments they provide reasonably good agreement for groups, but not for individuals *(23–28)*.

Portable Devices

Pedometers and accelerometers are devices worn by an individual to quantify movement. Pedometers assess displacement of the body with a single stride, and the output represents steps taken or steps/d. Because they are relatively cheap, pedometers are commonly used by individuals, researchers, and practitioners to monitor physical activity *(29)*. Pedometers are not designed to quantify stride length or the amount of body displacement and hence cannot discriminate between different activities or intensities of effort and do not provide any quantification of energy expenditure *per se*. Accelerometers, on the other hand, are devices that detect body displacement in terms of acceleration. Accelerometers can assess movements via piezoelectric sensors in a single plane, usually vertical (uniaxial accelerometer) or within three planes, anterior–posterior, mediolateral, and vertical (triaxial accelerometer). Accelerometers are worn on the wrist or, more commonly, on the hip or waist; they capture the duration and intensity of activities and can provide data storage for a number of days, which can be downloaded directly to a computer *(30)*. The triaxial devices tend to provide the best precision *(31)* and correlation with activity energy expenditure measured by indirect calorimetry and DLW *(32)*. With the inability of the free-living assessments of energy expenditure to differentiate between the type, intensity, and duration of activities, several laboratories have begun to incorporate the use of multiple accelerometers on various body parts *(33–39)*. These studies have proven that multiple accelerometers can quantify varying activities and posture allocations. Recently, a single device incorporating these concepts has been developed and made commercially available *(40)*. The Intelligent Device for Energy Expenditure and Activity (IDEEA; MiniSun LLC, Fresno, CA) system monitors body and limb movements constantly via five sensors positioned to the chest, thighs, and feet. Combinations of signals from the five sensors represent different physical activities, which were coded as 32 different movements. The IDEEA device provides data not only on the specific type of activity (e.g., sitting, climbing stairs, jumping) but also the duration, and estimated intensity on second-by-second basis (ranging from milliseconds to hours). The ability of IDEEA to quantify type, duration, and intensity of various activities has been validated *(40)*. In terms of energy expenditure, IDEEA shows accuracy against both portable and chamber indirect calorimetry techniques *(41)*.

COMPONENTS OF ENERGY EXPENDITURE AND THEIR RELEVANCE TO OBESITY

Total daily energy expenditure (TDEE) varies substantially in humans *(42)* such that two adults of the same size could have an EE that varies by 1500 kcal/d. The largest determinants of TDEE are weight, height, age, and gender *(42)*. Whereas both weight and height are positive determinants of TDEE, age is a negative predictor in adults. Across all ages, TDEE is approx 11% higher in males, after adjustments for body size *(42)*. With the increasing prevalence of obesity, understanding the inherent interindividual variation in TDEE is important. The variability in daily energy requirements is related to the variability in the energy expended in its three major components: resting metabolic rate, diet-induced thermogenesis, and activity thermogenesis (Fig. 2).

Resting Metabolic Rate

The resting metabolic rate (RMR) is the energy expended by an individual who is resting but awake and fasted in comfortable ambient conditions. RMR, which includes the energy cost of maintaining the integrated systems of the body and the homeothermic temperature at rest, accounts for approx 60 to 70% of daily energy expenditure in sedentary adults *(8)* and is therefore the largest component of TDEE. There is a close relationship between RMR and body size; this association has led to the development of widely used equations to predict RMR from height and weight *(43–47)*. Three-quarters of the variation in RMR is determined by fat-free mass *(48)* and, to a lesser extent, by fat mass, gender, and age. Together, these four components explain 80 to 85% of the interindividual variance in RMR. Some of the remaining variance can be further explained by family membership; therefore, genetic factors probably contribute *(48,49)*.

Interestingly, RMR adjusted for differences in fat-free mass, fat mass, and age is related to variability in body temperature *(50)*. Such results indicate that body temperature could be a marker for a high or low relative metabolic rate. It is not clear whether the heat production in the body—i.e., the metabolic rate—is regulated to maintain a given "preset" temperature or whether the temperature is simply a reflection of the equilibrium between the heat-producing and heat-losing mechanisms that are controlled by other factors. Some of the variability in RMR has also been shown to be related to be variability in muscle sympathetic nerve activity *(51)*. Resting skeletal muscle metabolism seems also to be a significant determinant of whole-body metabolism *(52,53)*, and studies suggest that uncoupling protein (UCP)-3 expression *(54)* and UCP-2 polymorphisms *(55,56)* appear to underlie some of this variability. Finally, whether the level of physical activity and training are determinants of the RMR remains controversial *(57–60)*.

Diet-Induced Thermogenesis

Diet-induced thermogenesis, or the thermic effect of food (TEF), is the increase in energy expenditure observed after the administration of a meal; therefore, it corresponds to the energy cost of chewing, digestion, and absorption of food. The TEF is the smallest component of daily energy expenditure, accounting for approx 10% of TDEE *(61,62)*. The TEF is, however, the most difficult and least reproducible component of energy expenditure to measure, and for these reasons its role in the etiology of obesity is controversial. A comprehensive review of 49 studies that compared TEF in lean and obese individuals suggested that obesity may be associated with an impaired TEF *(63)*; however, a recent paper *(64)* identified substantial shortcomings in the methods used to calculate TEF, questioning the role of low TEF in the development of obesity. The methods for assessing diet-induced thermogenesis are cumbersome; in addition, the energy expended following a meal is influenced by meal size and nutrient composition, palatability of the food, and time of the meal, as well as the individual's genetic background, age, physical fitness, and sensitivity to insulin. Importantly, prospective studies have not identified a relationship between the TEF and weight change *(61,65)*. It is safe to say that a decrease in the TEF amounts to only a small number of calories and, therefore, is very unlikely to explain significant degrees of obesity.

Activity Thermogenesis

Activity thermogenesis, the most variable component of TDEE, can account for a significant amount of calories in very active people. However, sedentary adult individuals exhibit a range of physical activity, which represents only 20 to 30% of total energy expenditure. Reduced physical activity as a cause of obesity is an obvious and attractive hypothesis. The energy expended in physical activity is quite variable, and the world-wide increase in obesity parallels the increase in sedentary lifestyles *(66)*. However, until the introduction of the DLW method for measuring energy expenditure in free-living conditions *(18,67)*, there has been no satisfactory method by which to assess the impact of physical activity on TDEE in humans. An increasing database of DLW in more than 1000 individuals confirms the wide variability in total energy expenditure in adults and children alike and, therefore, in physical activity *(42,68–70)*. In a review of 574 DLW measurements, Black et al. compiled data to: (1) establish the extremes of sustainable human energy expenditure; (2) establish the average and range of habitual energy expenditure in relationship to age and sex and; (3) describe the lifestyles and activity patterns associated with different levels of physical activity *(42)*. Prentice et al. described the relationship between graded levels of obesity and free-living energy expenditure in men and women of affluent societies and confirmed that habitual total energy expenditure is increased with obesity because of concomitant increase in fat-free mass *(68)*. They also suggest that except in massive obesity, the energy cost of physical activity is quite similar at different levels of body weight and BMI. Using the ratio between total energy expenditure and resting metabolic rate as an index of the level of physical activity, they have also shown that physical activity is decreased in heavier or fatter individuals. This, however, does not exclude the possibility that an inactive lifestyle may be an important risk factor for the development of obesity. Whether a low level of physical activity is a cause or a consequence of obesity can be tested only in prospective studies. Recent data in pairs of twin children suggest that despite the high heritability of BMI, physical activity was explained predominantly by shared environmental factors and not by genetic variability *(71)*.

There are two distinct types of activity thermogenesis—that is, the energy expended during exercise or structured physical activity (normally planned activities) and the energy expended in all other nonexercise activities (usually unplanned activities). The latter activities include the energy cost of sitting, fidgeting, maintaining posture and muscle tone, and performing leisure activities such as playing guitar, shopping, and the like. The unplanned activity energy expenditure, also termed spontaneous physical activity (SPA) or, more recently, nonexercise activity thermogenesis (NEAT), is quite variable between individuals *(72)*. Prospective studies are providing initial evidence that differences in this nonvolitional muscle activity may be important in determining predisposition to obesity and/or resistance to diet-induced weight gain *(73,74)*. Levine et al found that resistance to the development of obesity might be caused by the ability of an individual to increase NEAT *(73)*. In response to overfeeding (1000 kcal/d), fat gain varied 10-fold within the group; the individuals who gained the least amount of weight had the greatest increase in unplanned activities. In a follow-up study, Levine and colleagues published some intriguing findings that suggests that some of the interindividual variation in NEAT could be explained by a genetic component *(37)*, therefore confirming our initial observation *(74)*. In Levine's latest study *(37)*, NEAT measured by posture allocation and ambulation remained unchanged before and after weight gain (~8 kg) or weight loss (~4 kg), in lean and obese individuals, respectively. Obese individuals spent significantly more time seated compared with their lean counterparts, resulting in an energy surplus of 350 kcal/d. Put another way, if the obese individuals assumed the same posture allocation as their lean counterparts, they would accrue a daily energy deficit of 269 to 477 kcal/d that, if maintained, could result in substantial weight loss. Clearly there is a need for more prospective studies in which free-living physical activity is measured to assess if the level of unplanned physical activities is a major predisposing factor for weight gain *(75)*.

ENERGY EXPENDITURE IN THE ETIOLOGY OF OBESITY

Cross-sectional studies that compare lean and obese individuals have added little to our understanding of the physiological mechanisms predisposing to weight gain *(76)*. An understanding of the etiology of human obesity demands longitudinal studies to reveal predictors or risk factors. Several studies have prospectively examined these predictors in the Pima Indian population in southwestern Arizona, a population where obesity is extremely prevalent *(77)* and, therefore, weight gain is common in young adults. In these individuals at least six metabolic parameters have been found to be predictive of weight gain. In particular, related to energy expenditure and relevant to understanding the etiology of obesity, are low metabolic rate, low activity thermogenesis, low sympathetic nervous system activity, and low fat oxidation.

Low Metabolic Rate

Obesity is associated with a high absolute metabolic rate, both in resting conditions and over 24 h *(8,78)*, and therefore, cannot be caused by a low absolute metabolic rate, as is often proposed. Many investigators who have studied energy expenditure in humans have suggested that when a clear defect in energy expenditure is lacking in obese individuals, obesity can be only the result of excessive energy intake. It is important to note, however, that there is wide variability in the relationship between metabolic rate and body size, suggesting that, at any given body size, individuals can have "high," "normal," or "low" relative metabolic rates. Studies in adult nondiabetic Pima Indians found that a low relative metabolic rate (resting and 24-h) adjusted for differences in fat-free mass, fat mass, age, and sex was a risk factor for body weight gain *(79)*. Specifically, 4 yr of follow-up in the same individuals identified that the risk of gaining 10 kg in body weight was approx 8 times greater in those individuals within the lowest tertile of RMR compared with those within the highest tertile of RMR. These findings were later confirmed in an independent group of nondiabetic Pima Indians where weight change (–9 to 26 kg) with 4 yr of follow-up was negatively associated with RMR independent of body size and body composition *(80)*. Moreover, a meta-analysis of 12 published studies identified high rates of weight regain in formerly obese individuals related to a 3 to 5% lower mean relative RMR in these individuals compared with control individuals *(81)*. In contrast, relative low energy expenditure does not seem to be a predictor of weight gain in other adult populations *(82,83)*. In studies of the Pima Indians, it is important to note that weight gain in most individuals could not be accounted for entirely by lower rates of energy expenditure. Furthermore, theoretical estimates suggest that only 30 to 40% of the increase in body energy stores in people who gained weight can be attributed to the baseline deficit in energy expenditure. These results could indicate that energy intake as well as a low physical activity could also contribute to the observed variability in weight gain. It is also interesting to note, however, that in response to weight gain, the new metabolic rate (adjusted) increases to "normal" levels and is com-

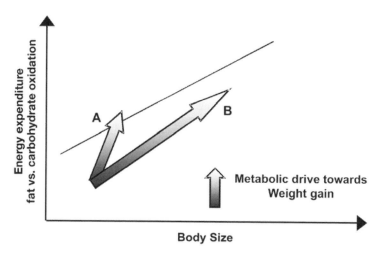

Fig. 3. Weight gain is the price to pay to counteract low energy expenditure or low fat oxidation. The role of energy metabolism in metabolic adaptation and the long-term regulation of body weight has been described by Weyer et al. *(156)*. Cross-sectional studies show that energy expenditure and fat oxidation increase with increasing body size, but for any given body size both parameters vary substantially. Prospective studies demonstrated the relevance of this variation, in that low rates of energy expenditure and fat oxidation predispose individuals to body weight gain. Longitudinal studies suggest that upon gaining weight, the low rates of energy expenditure and fat oxidation are increased on average and restored to normal levels and may oppose further weight gain. The arrows in the figure represent this metabolic drive toward weight gain, which probably diminishes at some point in some individuals, thereby limiting the amount of weight gain (metabolic adaptation, arrow A), whereas it may be sustained in others, who will thus be predisposed to further increases in weight (arrow B).

parable to the metabolic rates of individuals who remained weight-stable (Fig. 3). This explains why it is so difficult to identify impairment in energy metabolism in obese compared with lean individuals. Weight gain seems to be the price to pay to "normalize" energy metabolism (metabolic rate and fat oxidation).

Low-Activity Thermogenesis

Another component of 24-h energy expenditure is the energy cost of spontaneous physical activity, which accounts for 8 to 15% of total daily expenditure *(8)*. Consistent with the cross-sectional observation of decreased spontaneous physical activity in obese individuals, longitudinal studies in the Pima Indians showed that even in the confined environment of a respiratory chamber, spontaneous physical activity is a familial trait accounting for 57% of its variance. After 33 mo of follow-up, the level of spontaneous physical activity was inversely correlated with weight change (–16 to 28 kg) and fat mass change in males but despite significant weight change, these relationships were not evident in females *(74)*. Even though it could be argued that spontaneous physical activity during a respiratory chamber study is limited, spontaneous physical activity is highly correlated with habitual physical activity (measured by DLW) whether it is expressed as the energy cost of physical activity (activity energy expenditure, AEE), physical activity level (PAL), or body-size independent activity units *(84)*. Prospective studies in which free-living physical activity is measured (by the DLW technique) provide conflicting evidence for the hypothesis that a low level of physical activity is a major predisposing factor for weight gain in individuals and in populations. In a longitudinal study of 92 nondiabetic Pima Indians (80), AEE or PAL (measured by DLW) was not associated with changes in body weight (9 to 26 kg).

Low SNS Activity

Studies in Caucasians indicate that the activity of the sympathetic nervous system (SNS) is related to each of the major components of energy expenditure — RMR (51), TEF (85), and SPA (86). SNS activity is also negatively correlated with the 24-h respiratory quotient (87). Cross-sectional studies indicate that Pima Indians, who are prone to obesity, have lower rates of muscle sympathetic nerve activity compared with weight-matched Caucasians (51). The role of impaired SNS and/or adrenal medullary function in the etiology of human obesity was prospectively studied in 64 Pima Indian men. At baseline and follow-up (~3 yr), sympathoadrenal function (estimated by 24-h urinary norepinephrine and epinephrine excretion rates) was measured. At follow-up, body weight increased (8.4 ± 9.5 kg) and the gain in weight was negatively correlated with baseline urinary norepinephrine excretion rate ($r = -0.38$; $p = 0.009$), adjusted for its determinants (i.e., fat-free mass, fat mass, and waist-to-thigh circumference ratio). Baseline epinephrine excretion rate was correlated negatively with changes in waist-to-thigh circumference ratio ($r = -0.44$; $p = 0.003$). These results demonstrate that sympathetic nervous system activity is associated with body weight gain in humans and that a low activity of the adrenal medulla is associated with the development of central adiposity. Further indications of the possible role of SNS activity in the regulation of energy balance in humans comes from a study showing that low SNS activity was associated with poor weight loss outcomes in obese individuals treated with a dietary restriction intervention (88).

Low Fat Oxidation

The composition of nutrient intake has been shown to be an important factor in the development of obesity, and consequently, one might expect that the composition of nutrient oxidation would also play a role in its etiology. The nonprotein respiratory quotient is an index of the ratio of carbohydrate to fat oxidation. Values ranges from approx 0.80 after an overnight fast when fat is the primary oxidative substrate (89) to values approaching 1.00 following ingestion of a large carbohydrate meal when glucose is the major substrate (90). Apart from the obvious impact of diet composition, the respiratory quotient is also influenced by recent energy balance (negative balance causing more fat oxidation), sex (females tend to have reduced fat oxidation), adiposity (higher fat mass leads to higher fat oxidation), and family membership, suggesting genetic determinants (91). Toubro et al. confirmed that substrate oxidation rates, measured by respiratory quotient, exhibit familial aggregation after adjustment for energy balance, sex, and age (92).

A longitudinal study of Pima Indians showed that a high 24-h respiratory quotient predicted weight gain (91). Individuals in the 90th percentile for respiratory quotient — i.e., "low fat oxidizers" — had a 2.5 times greater risk of gaining 5 kg or more body weight than those individuals in the 10th percentile — i.e. "high fat oxidizers." This effect was independent of a relatively low or high 24-h metabolic rate. Similar results have been also reported in Caucasians (93). In support of these observations, others have demonstrated that postobese volunteers have high respiratory quotients—i.e., low rates of fat oxidation *(94,95)*—and those who are able to maintain weight loss have lower respiratory quotients compared with those experiencing weight relapse *(96)*.

ENERGY EXPENDITURE IN CHILDREN

One of the most troubling aspects of the current epidemic of obesity is the increasing prevalence of obesity and type 2 diabetes among children *(97)*. Childhood obesity is a very serious problem because tracking of adiposity is observed between childhood and adulthood *(98)* and children with one or two obese parents are at a higher risk of weight gain during childhood and adolescence than children with both parents of normal weight. Furthermore, duration of obesity is an independent predictor of health outcomes *(99)*. The risk of developing obesity seems to be especially elevated during early infancy, the adiposity rebound period during prepubertal growth, and the adolescent growth phase *(100)*.

The observation that obesity occurs more frequently in children of obese parents led to a variety of studies to determine how much of the genetic predisposition to obesity is related to energy metabolism. Stunkard et al. reported data on energy intake and energy expenditure in infants born to lean and overweight mothers and concluded that excessive energy intake, rather than low energy expenditure, is the cause of obesity in infants at high risk of obesity *(101)*. Childhood obesity is a vastly unexplored area and more studies are needed to understand how eating behavior forms and solidifies in conjunction with the final maturation of the human brain from childhood to adulthood. A hallmark study *(102)* found that infants who were overweight at 12 mo of age had a 20% lower TDEE (measured by DLW) compared with normal-weight infants when measured 9 mo earlier (i.e., 3 mo of age). Similarly, low energy expenditure in 5-yr-old girls was negatively correlated with BMI at adolescence *(103)*. In girls, reduction in TEE as a result of a marked reduction in physical activity during prepubertal growth has been reported *(104)*. However, other studies *(105,106)* have failed to confirm that resting energy expenditure, TDEE, or AEE measured in early childhood are inversely related to the development of obesity. Despite these large inconsistencies in the literature and because low levels of aerobic fitness *(107)*, excessive TV viewing *(108,109)*, and limited playing time *(109)* have all been associated with increased risk of weight gain, it seems reasonable to conclude that a sedentary lifestyle in early childhood should be discouraged.

A recent study in 100 twin pairs provides some intriguing data on the role of genetics and environment on the potential development of obesity *(71)*. In monozygotic and dizygotic twins aged 4 to 10 yr, physical activity energy expenditure (adjusted for weight, age, sex, season, ethnicity, and study date) was not at all explained by genetic influences, whereas environmental factors were the most significant determinants. These data suggest that genetics play a small role in the tendency for children to be physically active and that the environment shared by siblings is far more important for the variation in activity levels among children and possibly later in life. This also provides a basis to expose children to physical activity early in life.

Despite the attractiveness of prevention strategies aimed at children, which could be based on correcting some of these early risk factors for obesity, caution should be exercised. Until we fully comprehend the interplay among variability of energy metabolism, growth, and obesity, we must be concerned about the risk of unforeseen adverse consequences, particularly in respect to interruption of the normal growth pattern in

Table 1
Gene Disruption Leading to Alteration of Energy Metabolism

Genetic disruption	Phenotype	Effect on energy balance metabolism
ob/ ob	Obese	↓Activity, ↓fat oxidation
MC3R KO	Obese	↓Activity, ↓fat oxidation
MC4R KO	Obese	↓Activity, ↓energy expenditure
MCH KO	Lean	↑Activity, ↑energy expenditure
DGAT1 KO	Lean	↑Energy expenditure, ↑activity
ACC2 KO	Lean	↓Fat acid synthesis, ↑fat oxidation
VGF KO	Lean	↑Activity, ↑energy expenditure
PKA RIIbB KO	Lean	↑Energy expenditure
PTP1B KO	Lean	↑Energy expenditure, (↑leptin signaling)
Mahogany	Suppress obesity	↑Activity, ↑energy expenditure
Mohoganoid	Suppress obesity	↑Activity (?), ↑energy expenditure

Abbreviations and references: ob/ob (123); MC3R, melanocortin receptor 3 (157); MC4R, melanocortin receptor 4 (158); MCH, melaninconcentrating hormone (159); DGAT1, diacylglycerol transferase (120); ACC2, Acetyl CoA carboxylase (151); VGF (160); PKARIIβ, protein kinase A RII regulatory unit (161); PTP1B, protein tyrosine phosphatase (162); mahogany (163); mahoganoid (163).

early childhood and distorted body image, excessive dieting, and anorexia in adolescence. Taken together, these results suggest that a reduced physical activity-related energy expenditure constitutes an important factor in the etiology of subsequent weight gain and although genetics may be important for the development of this disease, lifestyle and environmental factors deserve significant attention to reduce its prevalence in society.

MOLECULAR MECHANISMS OF ENERGY EXPENDITURE VARIABILITY

The study of obesity in human individuals is inherently difficult. This is because of factors related to the disease itself, including heterogeneity, age-dependent penetrance, uncontrollable gene-environment interactions, and gene–gene interactions. Ultimately, proof that a putative mechanism of energy expenditure actually has a role in maintaining caloric homeostasis must come through genetic studies in animal models and then through the discovery of genetic variability for these mechanisms in humans. It is likely that further gene discoveries in animal models will add to this knowledge and continue to identify novel pathways that are important in nutrient partitioning and energy balance in humans. Evidence that these mechanisms actually promote or limit the development of obesity by stimulating or decreasing energy expenditure or nutrient partitioning must be demonstrated. Some of the significant advances in our understanding of the regulation of energy balance have stemmed from work in animal models; some of this work is discussed below and summarized in Table 1. Genetic engineering of mice (knockout or transgenic) has yielded many unexpected phenotypes, including obesity or resistance to high-fat diets. When further refined phenotyping was obtained, it became clearer that some of these mice were lean or obese not only because of hypo- or hyperphagia but also because of an impact on energy metabolism.

β3-*Adrenergic Receptors*

β3-adrenergic receptors (β3-ARs), which are located in skeletal muscle (88) and both white *(110)* and brown *(111)* adipocytes, have been demonstrated to significantly regulate antiobesity and insulinsensitizing actions in rodents (*see*, e.g., refs. *112,113*). Mice lacking β3-ARs have a modest increase in body fat, indicating that β3-ARs play a role in regulating energy balance. Acute treatment of normal animals with β3-selective agonists leads to increased serum FFA and insulin levels, increased whole-body energy expenditure, and decreased food intake, whereas when administered to β3-AR$^{-/-}$ mice, each of these effects was completely absent, indicating that these responses are mediated exclusively by β3-ARs *(114)*. Indeed, testing in humans of the first generation of β3-AR agonists, such as BRL 26830A *(115,116)* and CL 316243 *(117)*, revealed encouraging antidiabetic and antiobesity characteristics including energy metabolism. However, some of these compounds shared substantial selectivity with the β1- and β2-AR subtypes, inducing many undesired effects such as accelerated heart rate *(118)*, hand tremors *(119,120)*, and hypokalemia *(121)*. A novel generation of β3-AR agonists proved more potent in rodents *(122)* by increasing the expression of UCP-1 in adipose tissue and simultaneous conversion of large adipocytes into smaller ones. The effect of this novel generation of β3-AR agonists in humans has yet to be reported.

Leptin

In 1994, the genetic mutation causing massive obesity in *ob/ob* mice was described *(123)*. The gene encodes an adipocyte-derived hormone known as leptin, which acts primarily on the hypothalamus as a " lipostat," thus tending to adjust the size of the body's energy stores. Mice homozygous for the *ob* mutation completely lack the presence of circulating leptin; these animals develop severe, early-onset obesity, with many associated metabolic and hormonal abnormalities including hyperphagia, defective thermogenesis, infertility, and type 2 diabetes. The next experiments demonstrated that these metabolic and physiologic abnormalities were rapidly corrected by leptin administration, which caused significant reductions in food intake and increased energy expenditure; resulting in weight loss after only a few days of leptin administration *(124–126)*. These findings led to optimism that leptin therapy might be important for treating human obesity. The human gene encoding leptin has been screened in a large number of obese individuals, and only two families have been shown to have mutations resulting in complete leptin deficiency *(127,128)*. Treatment of three known leptin-deficient adults with a functional recessive mutation in the leptin gene with recombinant human leptin for 3 mo resulted in drastic changes in energy metabolism, with normalization of energy expenditure and large increases in fat oxidation *(129)*. Leptin was extremely potent in causing weight loss (especially fat loss; 85% on average, by dual-energy X-ray absorptiometry [DEXA]) resulting mostly from a drastic reduction in food intake and increasing fat oxidation. By 18 mo the BMI had decreased by an astonishing 50% and the individuals had a complete restoration of type 2 diabetes and hypogonadism *(130)*. Although the discovery of leptin and its receptor may ultimately facilitate the development of new obesity treatments acting through this pathway, clinical trials in humans have indicated that only some obese individuals may be sensitive to the weight-loss effect of exogenous leptin administration *(131)*. However, leptin may prove to be very efficacious for weight-loss maintenance *(132,133)*.

Uncoupling Protein

UCP-3 is abundantly expressed in skeletal muscle, an important tissue for thermogenesis *(53)*. Phenotypes of mice in which UCP-3 genes have been inactivated do not indicate that these homologs have a function in regulating either body temperature or body weight *(134–137)*. In one study in which UCP-3 was overexpressed in skeletal muscle of transgenic mice, mice showed a resistance to diet-induced obesity and an improvement in insulin sensitivity *(138)*. As the amount of UCP-3 in the muscle of the transgenic mice was at a level that had been shown previously, by the same group of investigators, to be toxic to the mitochondria of mammalian cells, it is possible that the mitochondria of the transgenic mice were leaky owing to toxicity from the high levels of UCP-3 *(139)*. Consequently, the effects of the UCP-3 transgene expression were not indicative of normal physiological function. A recent study, in which UCP-3 was induced in human muscle by a high-fat diet and then the rate of recovery of energy stores (i.e., creatine phosphate) was determined, failed to find an effect, suggesting that UCP-3 in humans does not uncouple muscle mitochondria *(140)*. It is interesting to note that a genetic variation at UCP-2–UCP-3 is associated with low metabolic rate in Pima Indians *(54,141)*. However, whether UCPs play a significant role in human obesity remain to be established.

Diacylglycerol Transferase

Triglyceride synthesis has been implicated to occur through the acyl CoA: diacylglycerol transferases (DGATs), enzymes that catalyze the final reaction in the glycerol phosphate pathway. DGAT enzymes are highly expressed in tissues associated with triglyceride synthesis. In humans, an abundant expression of DGAT enzymes has been observed in adipose tissue and liver *(142,143)*. Dgat1$^{-/-}$ mice are leaner than wild-type mice and have smaller adipocytes *(120,144)*. When fed a high-fat diet, Dgat1$^{-/-}$ mice are resistant to obesity and are protected from diet-induced hepatic steatosis *(120)*. These effects are likely caused in part by increased energy expenditure. Moreover, Dgat$^{-/-}$ mice demonstrate an increase in spontaneous physical activity *(145)*, increased expression of UCP-1 *(144,146)*, and increased leptin sensitivity *(144)*. An intact leptin pathway appears to be required for the effects of DGAT deficiency on energy metabolism. Although DGAT1 deficiency reverses obesity and insulin resistance in yellow agouti mice, it has no impact on the leptin-deficient *ob/ob* mice *(144)*. In general, the expression profile of DGAT1 is similar in mice and humans but the mechanism of increased energy expenditure in mice partially involves the increased expression of UCP-1 in brown adipose tissue. Therefore, pharmacological inhibition of DGAT1 in humans may not work in humans. Although genetic mutations leading to the complete inactivation of the protein have not yet been identified in humans, a polymorphism in the promoter of the DGAT1 gene was discovered and shown to be associated with body mass index in a Turkish population *(147)*. Because of the profound effects of DGAT deficiency on energy metabolism, studies are under way to identify suitable natural and synthetic compounds that can specifically inhibit its action.

Acetyl CoA Carboxylase 2

Acetyl CoA carboxylase (ACC), which exists in at least two isoforms in humans, is responsible for synthesizing malonyl coenzyme A, a potent inhibitor of fatty acid oxidation. ACC1 is expressed mainly in lipogenic tissue such as liver and adipose, and ACC2 in the heart and skeletal muscle *(148)*. In humans both isoforms have central roles in fatty acid biosynthesis and oxidation *(149)*. Although mice lacking ACC1 die young, the ACC2-null mice have a normal life span and, compared with wild-type animals, demonstrate continuous oxidation of fatty acid and therefore have substantial reductions in fat stores and body weight *(150,151)*. When fed a high-fat/high-carbohydrate diet, the ACC2$^{-/-}$ mice demonstrate a resistance to obesity and the development of diabetes *(150)*. Primary adipocyte cells cultured from the ACC2-null mice fed either a normal or high-fat/high-carbohydrate diet suggested that higher levels of fatty acid oxidation and lipolysis are major factors contributing to leaner ACC2$^{-/-}$ mice *(152)*. These findings indicate that pharmaceutical targets that inhibit ACC2 may prove to be important for the treatment of obesity and diabetes *(149)*. An isoform-nonselective inhibitor of ACC has recently been identified and tested in mice, rodents, and monkeys *(153)*. Pharmacological inhibition of ACC in experimental animals resulted in a reduction of malonyl-CoA concentration in both lipogenic (liver and adipose) and oxidative (liver and muscle) tissues, a consequential reduction in liver and adipose tissue fatty acid synthesis, and increased whole-body fatty acid oxidation. Together these findings provide convincing evidence that ACC inhibitors may serve as therapeutic targets in the treatment of obesity.

To date more than 600 genetic markers and chromosomal regions have been associated or linked with human obesity phenotypes *(154)*. These have been identified from human obesity cases owing to single-gene mutations, Mendelian disorders, transgenic and knockout models relevant to obesity, quantitative trait loci from animal crossbreeding, association studies with candidate genes, and linkages from genome scans. Future studies will no doubt report that additional genetic loci will prove to affect energy metabolism.

CONCLUSION

In summary, energy expenditure includes many components, such as physical activity, fidgeting, the thermic effect of food, ambient temperature, fever, shivering, and the efficiency of basal metabolism. The effects of some of these factors, such as physical exercise and ambient temperature, are obvious; however, what determines "metabolic efficiency" is extremely complex. All components of energy expenditure, whether simple or complex, are most likely influenced by variations in the genetic constitution of an individual. Based on the "thrifty gene" hypothesis *(155)*, one would predict that mutations changing the efficiency of energy metabolism should exist. Yet biochemical spontaneous or induced mutations in mice or humans that can cause obesity without increased food consumption are rare. Recent studies in animal models have contributed greatly to our understanding of the regulation of energy balance. New peptides and pathways have been discovered that could potentially lead to new therapies for the treatment of human obesity.

REFERENCES

1. Benzinger T, Kitzinger G. Gradient layer calorimetry and human calorimetry. In: Hardy, ed. Temperature: Its Measurement and Control in Science and Industry. Reinhold, New York: 1963, pp. 87–109.
2. Spinnler G, Jequier E, Favre R, et al. Human calorimeter with a new type of gradient layer. J Appl Physiol 1973;35(1):158–165.

3. Webb P. Human calorimeters. In: Endocrinology and Metabolism. Praeger Publishers, Westwood, CT: 1985, pp 53–55.
4. Dauncey MJ, Murgatroyd PR, Cole TJ. A human calorimeter for the direct and indirect measurement of 24 h energy expenditure. Br J Nutr 1978;39(3):557–566.
5. Dullo A, Ismail M, Ryall M, et al. A low budget easy-to-operate room respirometer for measuring daily energy expenditure in man. Am J Clin Nutr 1988;48:1267–1274.
6. Jequier E, Schutz Y. Long-term measurements of energy expenditure in humans using a respiration chamber. Am J Clin Nutr 1983;38(6):989–998.
7. Minghelli G, Schutz Y, Charbonnier A, et al. Twenty-four-hour energy expenditure and basal metabolic rate measured in a whole-body indirect calorimeter in Gambian men. Am J Clin Nutr 1990;51(4):563–570.
8. Ravussin E, Lillioja S, Anderson TE, et al. Determinants of 24-hour energy expenditure in man. Methods and results using a respiratory chamber. J Clin Invest 1986;78(6):1568–1578.
9. Rumpler WV, Seale JL, Conway JM, et al. Repeatability of 24-h energy expenditure measurements in humans by indirect calorimetry. Am J Clin Nutr 1990;51(2):147–152.
10. Van Es AJ, Vogt JE, Niessen C, et al. Human energy metabolism below, near and above energy equilibrium. Br J Nutr 1984;52(3):429–442.
11. Heymsfield SB, Allison DB, Pi-Sunyer FX, Sun Y. Columbia respiratory-chamber indirect calorimeter: a new approach to air-flow modelling. Med Biol Eng Comput 1994;32(4):406–410.
12. Kriketos AD, Sharp TA, Seagle HM, et al. Effects of aerobic fitness on fat oxidation and body fatness. Med Sci Sports Exerc 2000;32(4):805–811.
13. Nguyen T, de Jonge L, Smith SR, et al. Chamber for indirect calorimetry with accurate measurement and time discrimination of metabolic plateaus of over 20 min. Med Biol Eng Comput 2003;41(5):572–578.
14. Schoffelen PF, Westerterp KR, Saris WH, et al. A dual-respiration chamber system with automated calibration. J Appl Physiol 1997;83(6):2064–2072.
15. Sun M, Reed GW, Hill JO. Modification of a whole room indirect calorimeter for measurement of rapid changes in energy expenditure. J Appl Physiol 1994;76(6):2686–2691.
16. White MD, Bouchard G, Buemann B, et al. Energy and macronutrient balances for humans in a whole body metabolic chamber without control of preceding diet and activity level. Int J Obes Relat Metab Disord 1997;21(2):135–140.
17. Lifson N. Theory of use of the turnover rates of body water for measuring energy and material balance. J Theor Biol 1966;12(1):46–74.
18. Schoeller DA, van Santen E. Measurement of energy expenditure in humans by doubly labeled water method. J Appl Physiol 1982;53(4):955–959.
19. Coward W, Prentice A, Murgatroyd P. Measurement of CO_2 and water production rates in man using ^2H, ^{18}O-labelled H_2O; comparisons between calorimeter and isotope values. In: van Es WA, ed. Human energy metabolism: physical activity and energy expenditure measurements in epidemiological research based upon direct and indirect calorimetry (European Nutrition Report): Stichting Netherlands Instituut voor de Voeding: 1984; pp. 126–128.
20. Klein PD, James WP, Wong WW, et al. Calorimetric validation of the doubly-labelled water method for determination of energy expenditure in man. Hum Nutr Clin Nutr 1984;38(2):95–106.
21. Schoeller DA, Webb P. Five-day comparison of the doubly labeled water method with respiratory gas exchange. Am J Clin Nutr 1984;40(1):153–158.
22. Garrow J. Energy Balance and Obesity in Man. 1st ed. North-Holland, Amsterdam: 1974.
23. Acheson KJ, Campbell IT, Edholm OG, et al. The measurement of daily energy expenditure—an evaluation of some techniques. Am J Clin Nutr 1980;33(5):1155–1164.
24. Borel MJ, Riley RE, Snook JT. Estimation of energy expenditure and maintenance energy requirements of college-age men and women. Am J Clin Nutr 1984;40(6):1264–1272.
25. Bradfield RB, Huntzicker PB, Fruehan GJ. Simultaneous comparison of respirometer and heart-rate telemetry techniques as measures of human energy expenditure. Am J Clin Nutr 1969;22(6):696–700.
26. Durnin JV, Brockway JM. Determination of the total daily energy expenditure in man by indirect calorimetry: assessment of the accuracy of a modern technique. Br J Nutr 1959;13(1):41–53.
27. Edholm O. Energy expenditure and food intake. In: Apfelbaum M, ed. Energy Balance in Man. Masson, Paris: 1973; pp. 51–60.
28. Geissler CA, Dzumbira TM, Noor MI. Validation of a field technique for the measurement of energy expenditure: factorial method versus continuous respirometry. Am J Clin Nutr 1986;44(5):596–602.

29. Tudor-Locke CE, Myers AM. Challenges and opportunities for measuring physical activity in sedentary adults. Sports Med 2001;31(2):91–100.
30. Westerterp KR, Plasqui G. Physical activity and human energy expenditure. Curr Opin Clin Nutr Metab Care 2004;7(6):607–613.
31. Bouten CV, Westerterp KR, Verduin M, et al. Assessment of energy expenditure for physical activity using a triaxial accelerometer. Med Sci Sports Exerc 1994;26(12):1516–1523.
32. Bouten CV, Verboeket-van de Venne WP, et al. Daily physical activity assessment: comparison between movement registration and doubly labeled water. J Appl Physiol 1996;81(2):1019–1026.
33. Busser HJ, Ott J, van Lummel RC, et al. Ambulatory monitoring of children's activity. Med Eng Phys 1997;19(5):440–445.
34. Foerster F, Fahrenberg J. Motion pattern and posture: correctly assessed by calibrated accelerometers. Behav Res Methods Instrum Comput 2000;32(3):450–457.
35. Kiani K, Snijders CJ, Gelsema ES. Computerized analysis of daily life motor activity for ambulatory monitoring. Technol Health Care 1997;5(4):307–318.
36. Kiani K, Snijders CJ, Gelsema ES. Recognition of daily life motor activity classes using an artificial neural network. Arch Phys Med Rehabil 1998;79(2):147–154.
37. Levine JA, Lanningham-Foster LM, McCrady SK, et al. Interindividual variation in posture allocation: possible role in human obesity. Science 2005;307(5709):584–586.
38. Uiterwaal M, Glerum EB, Busser HJ, et al. Ambulatory monitoring of physical activity in working situations, a validation study. J Med Eng Technol 1998;22(4):168–172.
39. Walker DJ, Heslop PS, Plummer CJ, et al. A continuous patient activity monitor: validation and relation to disability. Physiol Meas 1997;18(1):49–59.
40. Zhang K, Werner P, Sun M, et al. Measurement of human daily physical activity. Obes Res 2003;11(1):33–40.
41. Zhang K, Pi-Sunyer FX, Boozer CN. Improving energy expenditure estimation for physical activity. Med Sci Sports Exerc 2004;36(5):883–889.
42. Black AE, Coward WA, Cole TJ, et al. Human energy expenditure in affluent societies: an analysis of 574 doubly-labelled water measurements. Eur J Clin Nutr 1996;50(2):72–92.
43. Boothby W, Sandiford I. Summary of the basal metabolism data on 8,614 subjects with special reference to the normal standards for the estimation of the basal metabolic rate. J Biol Chem 1922;54:783–803.
44. Cunningham JJ. Body composition as a determinant of energy expenditure: a synthetic review and a proposed general prediction equation. Am J Clin Nutr 1991;54(6):963–969.
45. Harris J, Benedict F. A Biometric Study of Basal Metabolism in Man. The Carnegie Institute, Washington, DC: 1919.
46. Roza AM, Shizgal HM. The Harris Benedict equation reevaluated: resting energy requirements and the body cell mass. Am J Clin Nutr 1984;40(1):168–182.
47. Schofield WN. Predicting basal metabolic rate, new standards and review of previous work. Hum Nutr Clin Nutr 1985;39 Suppl 1:5–41.
48. Bogardus C, Lillioja S, Ravussin E, et al. Familial dependence of the resting metabolic rate. N Engl J Med 1986;315(2):96–100.
49. Bouchard C, Tremblay A, Nadeau A, et al. Genetic effect in resting and exercise metabolic rates. Metabolism 1989;38(4):364–370.
50. Rising R, Keys A, Ravussin E, et al. Concomitant interindividual variation in body temperature and metabolic rate. Am J Physiol 1992;263(4 Pt 1):E730–E734.
51. Spraul M, Ravussin E, Fontvieille AM, et al. Reduced sympathetic nervous activity. A potential mechanism predisposing to body weight gain. J Clin Invest 1993;92(4):1730–1735.
52. Kirkwood SP, Zurlo F, Larson K, et al. Muscle mitochondrial morphology, body composition, and energy expenditure in sedentary individuals. Am J Physiol 1991;260(1 Pt 1):E89–E94.
53. Zurlo F, Larson K, Bogardus C, et al. Skeletal muscle metabolism is a major determinant of resting energy expenditure. J Clin Invest 1990;86(5):1423–1427.
54. Schrauwen P, Xia J, Walder K,et al. A novel polymorphism in the proximal UCP3 promoter region: effect on skeletal muscle UCP3 mRNA expression and obesity in male non-diabetic Pima Indians. Int J Obes Relat Metab Disord 1999;23(12):1242–1245.
55. Bouchard C, Perusse L, Chagnon YC, et al. Linkage between markers in the vicinity of the uncoupling protein 2 gene and resting metabolic rate in humans. Hum Mol Genet 1997;6(11):1887–1889.

56. Kovacs P, Ma L, Hanson RL, et al. Genetic variation in UCP2 (uncoupling protein-2) is associated with energy metabolism in Pima Indians. Diabetologia 2005;48(11):2292–2295.

57. Hill JO, Sparling PB, Shields TW, et al. Effects of exercise and food restriction on body composition and metabolic rate in obese women. Am J Clin Nutr 1987;46(4):622–630.

58. Poehlman ET, Melby CL, Badylak SF. Resting metabolic rate and postprandial thermogenesis in highly trained and untrained males. Am J Clin Nutr 1988;47(5):793–798.

59. Schulz LO, Nyomba BL, Alger S, et al. Effect of endurance training on sedentary energy expenditure measured in a respiratory chamber. Am J Physiol 1991;260(2 Pt 1):E257–E261.

60. Tremblay A, Fontaine E, Poehlman ET, et al. The effect of exercise-training on resting metabolic rate in lean and moderately obese individuals. Int J Obes 1986;10(6):511–517.

61. Tataranni PA, Larson DE, Snitker S, et al. Thermic effect of food in humans: methods and results from use of a respiratory chamber. Am J Clin Nutr 1995;61(5):1013–1019.

62. Weststrate JA. Resting metabolic rate and diet-induced thermogenesis: a methodological reappraisal. Am J Clin Nutr 1993;58(5):592–601.

63. de Jonge L, Bray GA. The thermic effect of food and obesity: a critical review. Obes Res 1997;5(6): 622–631.

64. Granata GP, Brandon LJ. The thermic effect of food and obesity: discrepant results and methodological variations. Nutr Rev 2002;60(8):223–233.

65. Riumallo JA, Schoeller D, Barrera G, et al. Energy expenditure in underweight free-living adults: impact of energy supplementation as determined by doubly labeled water and indirect calorimetry. Am J Clin Nutr 1989;49(2):239–246.

66. Prentice AM, Jebb SA. Obesity in Britain: gluttony or sloth? BMJ 1995;311(7002):437–439.

67. Schoeller DA, Fjeld CR. Human energy metabolism: what have we learned from the doubly labeled water method? Annu Rev Nutr 1991;11:355–373.

68. Prentice AM, Black AE, Coward WA, et al. Energy expenditure in overweight and obese adults in affluent societies: an analysis of 319 doubly-labelled water measurements. Eur J Clin Nutr 1996;50(2):93–97.

69. Schulz LO, Schoeller DA. A compilation of total daily energy expenditures and body weights in healthy adults. Am J Clin Nutr 1994;60(5):676–681.

70. Swinburn BA, Jolley D, Kremer PJ, et al. Estimating the effects of energy imbalance on changes in body weight in children. Am J Clin Nutr 2006;83:859–863.

71. Franks PW, Ravussin E, Hanson RL, et al. Habitual physical activity in children: the role of genes and the environment. Am J Clin Nutr 2005;82:901–908.

72. Levine JA. Non-exercise activity thermogenesis (NEAT). Best Pract Res Clin Endocrinol Metab 2002;16(4):679–702.

73. Levine JA, Eberhardt NL, Jensen MD. Role of nonexercise activity thermogenesis in resistance to fat gain in humans. Science 1999;283(5399):212–214.

74. Zurlo F, Ferraro RT, Fontvielle AM, et al. Spontaneous physical activity and obesity: cross-sectional and longitudinal studies in Pima Indians. Am J Physiol 1992;263(2 Pt 1):E296–E300.

75. Ravussin E. Physiology. A NEAT way to control weight? Science 2005;307(5709):530–531.

76. Ravussin E, Swinburn BA. Metabolic predictors of obesity: cross-sectional versus longitudinal data. Int J Obes Relat Metab Disord 1993;17 Suppl 3:S28–S31; discussion S41–S42.

77. Knowler WC, Pettitt DJ, Saad MF, et al. Obesity in the Pima Indians: its magnitude and relationship with diabetes. Am J Clin Nutr 1991;53(6 Suppl):1543S–1551S.

78. Weyer C, Snitker S, Rising R, et al. Determinants of energy expenditure and fuel utilization in man: effects of body composition, age, sex, ethnicity and glucose tolerance in 916 subjects. Int J Obes Relat Metab Disord 1999;23(7):715–722.

79. Ravussin E, Lillioja S, Knowler WC, et al. Reduced rate of energy expenditure as a risk factor for body-weight gain. N Engl J Med 1988;318(8):467–472.

80. Tataranni PA, Harper IT, Snitker S, et al. Body weight gain in free-living Pima Indians: effect of energy intake vs expenditure. Int J Obes Relat Metab Disord 2003;27(12):1578–1583.

81. Astrup A, Gotzsche PC, van de Werken K, et al. Meta-analysis of resting metabolic rate in formerly obese subjects. Am J Clin Nutr 1999;69(6):1117–1122.

82. Amatruda JM, Statt MC, Welle SL. Total and resting energy expenditure in obese women reduced to ideal body weight. J Clin Invest 1993;92(3):1236–1242.

83. Weinsier RL, Nelson KM, Hensrud DD, et al. Metabolic predictors of obesity. Contribution of resting energy expenditure, thermic effect of food, and fuel utilization to four-year weight gain of post-obese and never-obese women. J Clin Invest 1995;95(3):980–985.

84. Snitker S, Tataranni PA, Ravussin E. Spontaneous physical activity in a respiratory chamber is correlated to habitual physical activity. Int J Obes Relat Metab Disord 2001;25(10):1481–1486.
85. Schwartz RS, Jaeger LF, Veith RC. Effect of clonidine on the thermic effect of feeding in humans. Am J Physiol 1988;254(1 Pt 2):R90–R94.
86. Christin L, O'Connell M, Bogardus C, et al. Norepinephrine turnover and energy expenditure in Pima Indian and white men. Metabolism 1993;42(6):723–729.
87. Snitker S, Tataranni PA, Ravussin E. Respiratory quotient is inversely associated with muscle sympathetic nerve activity. J Clin Endocrinol Metab 1998;83(11):3977–3979.
88. Astrup A, Bulow J, Madsen J, et al. Contribution of BAT and skeletal muscle to thermogenesis induced by ephedrine in man. Am J Physiol 1985;248(5 Pt 1):E507–E515.
89. McNeill G, Bruce AC, Ralph A, et al. Inter-individual differences in fasting nutrient oxidation and the influence of diet composition. Int J Obes 1988;12(5):455–463.
90. Flatt JP, Ravussin E, Acheson KJ, et al. Effects of dietary fat on postprandial substrate oxidation and on carbohydrate and fat balances. J Clin Invest 1985;76(3):1019–1024.
91. Zurlo F, Lillioja S, Esposito-Del Puente A, et al. Low ratio of fat to carbohydrate oxidation as predictor of weight gain: study of 24-h RQ. Am J Physiol 1990;259(5 Pt 1):E650–E657.
92. Toubro S, Sorensen TI, Hindsberger C, et al. Twenty-four-hour respiratory quotient: the role of diet and familial resemblance. J Clin Endocrinol Metab 1998;83(8):2758–2764.
93. Seidell JC, Muller DC, Sorkin JD, et al. Fasting respiratory exchange ratio and resting metabolic rate as predictors of weight gain: the Baltimore Longitudinal Study on Aging. Int J Obes Relat Metab Disord 1992;16(9):667–674.
94. Astrup A, Buemann B, Christensen NJ, et al. Failure to increase lipid oxidation in response to increasing dietary fat content in formerly obese women. Am J Physiol 1994;266(4 Pt 1):E592–E599.
95. Larson DE, Ferraro RT, Robertson DS, et al. Energy metabolism in weight-stable postobese individuals. Am J Clin Nutr 1995;62(4):735–739.
96. Froidevaux F, Schutz Y, Christin L, et al. Energy expenditure in obese women before and during weight loss, after refeeding, and in the weight-relapse period. Am J Clin Nutr 1993;57(1):35–42.
97. Mokdad AH, Serdula MK, Dietz WH, et al. The spread of the obesity epidemic in the United States, 1991–1998. JAMA 1999;282(16):1519–1522.
98. Serdula MK, Ivery D, Coates RJ, et al. Do obese children become obese adults? A review of the literature. Prev Med 1993;22(2):167–177.
99. McCance DR, Pettitt DJ, Hanson RL, et al. Glucose, insulin concentrations and obesity in childhood and adolescence as predictors of NIDDM. Diabetologia 1994;37(6):617–623.
100. Dietz WH. Critical periods in childhood for the development of obesity. Am J Clin Nutr 1994;59(5):955–959.
101. Stunkard AJ, Berkowitz RI, Stallings VA, et al. Energy intake, not energy output, is a determinant of body size in infants. Am J Clin Nutr 1999;69(3):524-30.
102. Roberts SB, Savage J, Coward WA, et al. Energy expenditure and intake in infants born to lean and overweight mothers. N Engl J Med 1988;318(8):461–466.
103. Griffiths M, Payne PR, Stunkard AJ, et al. Metabolic rate and physical development in children at risk of obesity. Lancet 1990;336(8707):76–78.
104. Goran MI, Gower BA, Nagy TR, et al. Developmental changes in energy expenditure and physical activity in children: evidence for a decline in physical activity in girls before puberty. Pediatrics 1998;101(5):887–891.
105. Goran MI, Hunter G, Nagy TR, et al. Physical activity related energy expenditure and fat mass in young children. Int J Obes Relat Metab Disord 1997;21(3):171–178.
106. Goran MI, Shewchuk R, Gower BA, et al. Longitudinal changes in fatness in white children: no effect of childhood energy expenditure. Am J Clin Nutr 1998;67(2):309–316.
107. Johnson MS, Figueroa-Colon R, Herd SL, et al. Aerobic fitness, not energy expenditure, influences subsequent increase in adiposity in black and white children. Pediatrics 2000;106(4):E50.
108. Robinson TN. Reducing children's television viewing to prevent obesity: a randomized controlled trial. JAMA 1999;282(16):1561–1567.
109. Salbe A, Weyer C, Fontvieille A, et al. Low levels of physical activity and time spent viewing television at 9 years of age predict weight gain 8 years later in Pima Indian children. Int J Obes 1998;22(Suppl 4):S10.
110. Foster DO, Frydman ML. Brown adipose tissue: the dominant site of nonshivering thermogenesis in the rat. Experientia Suppl 1978;32:147–151.

111. Schiffelers SL, Brouwer EM, Saris WH, et al. Inhibition of lipolysis reduces beta1-adrenoceptor-mediated thermogenesis in man. Metabolism 1998;47(12):1462–1467.

112. Arch JR, Ainsworth AT, Ellis RD, et al. Treatment of obesity with thermogenic beta-adrenoceptor agonists: studies on BRL 26830A in rodents. Int J Obes 1984;8 Suppl 1:1–11.

113. Cawthorne MA, Carroll MJ, Levy AL, et al. Effects of novel beta-adrenoceptor agonists on carbohydrate metabolism: relevance for the treatment of non-insulin-dependent diabetes. Int J Obes 1984;8 Suppl 1:93–102.

114. Susulic VS, Frederich RC, Lawitts J, et al. Targeted disruption of the beta 3-adrenergic receptor gene. J Biol Chem 1995;270(49):29,483–29,492.

115. Connacher AA, Jung RT, Mitchell PE. Weight loss in obese subjects on a restricted diet given BRL 26830A, a new atypical beta adrenoceptor agonist. Br Med J (Clin Res Ed) 1988;296(6631):1217–1220.

116. Zed CA, Harris GS, Harrison PJ, et al. Anti-obesity activity of a novel b-adrenoreceptor agonist (BLR 26830A) in diet-restricted obese animals. Int J Obes 1985;9:231.

117. Weyer C, Tataranni PA, Snitker S, et al. Increase in insulin action and fat oxidation after treatment with CL 316,243, a highly selective beta3-adrenoceptor agonist in humans. Diabetes 1998;47(10):1555–1561.

118. Henny C, Buckert A, Schutz Y, et al. Comparison of thermogenic activity induced by the new sympathomimetic Ro 16-8714 between normal and obese subjects. Int J Obes 1988;12(3):227–236.

119. Connacher AA, Lakie M, Powers N, et al. Tremor and the anti-obesity drug BRL 26830A. Br J Clin Pharmacol 1990;30(4):613–615.

120. Smith SJ, Cases S, Jensen DR, et al. Obesity resistance and multiple mechanisms of triglyceride synthesis in mice lacking DGAT. Nat Genet 2000;25(1):87–90.

121. Wheeldon NM, McDevitt DG, McFarlane LC, et al. Beta-adrenoceptor subtypes mediating the metabolic effects of BRL 35135 in man. Clin Sci (Lond) 1994;86(3):331–337.

122. Francke S. TAK-677 (Dainippon/Takeda). Curr Opin Investig Drugs 2002;3(11):1624–1628.

123. Zhang Y, Proenca R, Maffei M, et al. Positional cloning of the mouse obese gene and its human homologue. Nature 1994;372(6505):425–432.

124. Campfield LA, Smith FJ, Guisez Y, et al. Recombinant mouse OB protein: evidence for a peripheral signal linking adiposity and central neural networks. Science 1995;269(5223):546–549.

125. Halaas JL, Gajiwala KS, Maffei M, et al. Weight-reducing effects of the plasma protein encoded by the obese gene. Science 1995;269(5223):543–546.

126. Pelleymounter MA, Cullen MJ, Baker MB, et al. Effects of the obese gene product on body weight regulation in ob/ob mice. Science 1995;269(5223):540–543.

127. Montague CT, Farooqi IS, Whitehead JP, et al. Congenital leptin deficiency is associated with severe early-onset obesity in humans. Nature 1997;387(6636):903–908.

128. Strobel A, Issad T, Camoin L, et al. A leptin missense mutation associated with hypogonadism and morbid obesity. Nat Genet 1998;18(3):213–215.

129. Ravussin E, Caglayan S, Williamson DF, et al. Effects of human leptin replacement on food intake and energy metabolism in 3 leptin-deficient adults. Int J Obes 2002;26(S1):S136.

130. Licinio J, Caglayan S, Ozata M, et al. Phenotypic effects of leptin replacement on morbid obesity, diabetes mellitus, hypogonadism, and behavior in leptin-deficient adults. Proc Natl Acad Sci USA 2004;101(13):4531–4536.

131. Heymsfield SB, Greenberg AS, Fujioka K, et al. Recombinant leptin for weight loss in obese and lean adults: a randomized, controlled, dose-escalation trial. JAMA 1999;282(16):1568–1575.

132. Rosenbaum M, Goldsmith R, Bloomfield D, et al. Low-dose leptin reverses skeletal muscle, autonomic, and neuroendocrine adaptations to maintenance of reduced weight. J Clin Invest 2005;115(12):3579–3586.

133. Rosenbaum M, Murphy EM, Heymsfield SB, et al. Low dose leptin administration reverses effects of sustained weight-reduction on energy expenditure and circulating concentrations of thyroid hormones. J Clin Endocrinol Metab 2002;87(5):2391–2394.

134. Arsenijevic D, Onuma H, Pecqueur C, et al. Disruption of the uncoupling protein-2 gene in mice reveals a role in immunity and reactive oxygen species production. Nat Genet 2000;26(4):435–439.

135. Gong DW, Monemdjou S, Gavrilova O, et al. Lack of obesity and normal response to fasting and thyroid hormone in mice lacking uncoupling protein-3. J Biol Chem 2000;275(21):16,251–16,257.

136. Vidal-Puig AJ, Grujic D, Zhang CY, et al. Energy metabolism in uncoupling protein 3 gene knockout mice. J Biol Chem 2000;275(21):16,258–16,266.

137. Zhang CY, Baffy G, Perret P, et al. Uncoupling protein-2 negatively regulates insulin secretion and is a major link between obesity, beta cell dysfunction, and type 2 diabetes. Cell 2001;105(6):745–755.

138. Clapham JC, Arch JR, Chapman H, et al. Mice overexpressing human uncoupling protein-3 in skeletal muscle are hyperphagic and lean. Nature 2000;406(6794):415–418.

139. Stuart JA, Harper JA, Brindle KM, et al. Physiological levels of mammalian uncoupling protein 2 do not uncouple yeast mitochondria. J Biol Chem 2001;276(21):18,633–18,639.

140. Hesselink MK, Greenhaff PL, Constantin-Teodosiu D, et al. Increased uncoupling protein 3 content does not affect mitochondrial function in human skeletal muscle in vivo. J Clin Invest 2003;111(4): 479–486.

141. Walder K, Norman RA, Hanson RL, et al. Association between uncoupling protein polymorphisms (UCP2-UCP3) and energy metabolism/obesity in Pima Indians. Hum Mol Genet 1998;7(9):1431–1435.

142. Cases S, Smith SJ, Zheng YW, et al. Identification of a gene encoding an acyl CoA:diacylglycerol acyltransferase, a key enzyme in triacylglycerol synthesis. Proc Natl Acad Sci USA 1998;95(22): 13,018–13,023.

143. Cases S, Stone SJ, Zhou P, et al. Cloning of DGAT2, a second mammalian diacylglycerol acyltransferase, and related family members. J Biol Chem 2001;276(42):38,870–38,876.

144. Chen HC, Smith SJ, Ladha Z, et al. Increased insulin and leptin sensitivity in mice lacking acyl CoA:diacylglycerol acyltransferase 1. J Clin Invest 2002;109(8):1049–1055.

145. Chen HC, Farese RV, Jr. Inhibition of triglyceride synthesis as a treatment strategy for obesity: lessons from DGAT1-deficient mice. Arterioscler Thromb Vasc Biol 2005;25(3):482–486.

146. Chen HC, Ladha Z, Smith SJ, et al. Analysis of energy expenditure at different ambient temperatures in mice lacking DGAT1. Am J Physiol Endocrinol Metab 2003;284(1):E213–E218.

147. Ludwig EH, Mahley RW, Palaoglu E, et al. DGAT1 promoter polymorphism associated with alterations in body mass index, high density lipoprotein levels and blood pressure in Turkish women. Clin Genet 2002;62(1):68–73.

148. Munday MR. Regulation of mammalian acetyl-CoA carboxylase. Biochem Soc Trans 2002;30 (Pt 6):1059–1064.

149. Tong L. Acetyl-coenzyme A carboxylase: crucial metabolic enzyme and attractive target for drug discovery. Cell Mol Life Sci 2005;62(16):1784–1803.

150. Abu-Elheiga L, Oh W, Kordari P, et al. Acetyl-CoA carboxylase 2 mutant mice are protected against obesity and diabetes induced by high-fat/high-carbohydrate diets. Proc Natl Acad Sci USA 2003;100(18):10,207–10,212.

151. Abu-Elheiga L, Matzuk MM, Abo-Hashema KA, et al. Continuous fatty acid oxidation and reduced fat storage in mice lacking acetyl-CoA carboxylase 2. Science 2001;291(5513):2613–2616.

152. Oh W, Abu-Elheiga L, Kordari P, et al. Glucose and fat metabolism in adipose tissue of acetyl-CoA carboxylase 2 knockout mice. Proc Natl Acad Sci USA 2005;102(5):1384–1389.

153. Harwood HJ, Jr., Petras SF, Shelly LD, et al. Isozyme-nonselective N-substituted bipiperidylcarboxamide acetyl-CoA carboxylase inhibitors reduce tissue malonyl-CoA concentrations, inhibit fatty acid synthesis, and increase fatty acid oxidation in cultured cells and in experimental animals. J Biol Chem 2003;278(39):37,099–37,111.

154. Perusse L, Rankinen T, Zuberi A, et al. The human obesity gene map: the 2004 update. Obes Res 2005;13(3):381–490.

155. Neel JV. The "thrifty genotype" in 1998. Nutr Rev 1999;57(5 Pt 2):S2–S9.

156. Weyer C, Pratley RE, Salbe AD, et al. Energy expenditure, fat oxidation, and body weight regulation: a study of metabolic adaptation to long-term weight change. J Clin Endocrinol Metab 2000;85(3): 1087–1094.

157. Chen AS, Marsh DJ, Trumbauer ME, et al. Inactivation of the mouse melanocortin-3 receptor results in increased fat mass and reduced lean body mass. Nat Genet 2000;26(1):97–102.

158. Huszar D, Lynch CA, Fairchild-Huntress V, et al. Targeted disruption of the melanocortin-4 receptor results in obesity in mice. Cell 1997;88(1):131–141.

159. Shimada M, Tritos NA, Lowell BB, et al. Mice lacking melanin-concentrating hormone are hypophagic and lean. Nature 1998;396(6712):670–674.

160. Hahm S, Mizuno TM, Wu TJ, et al. Targeted deletion of the Vgf gene indicates that the encoded secretory peptide precursor plays a novel role in the regulation of energy balance. Neuron 1999;23(3):537–548.

161. Cummings DE, Brandon EP, Planas JV, et al. Genetically lean mice result from targeted disruption of the RII beta subunit of protein kinase A. Nature 1996;382(6592):622–626.

162. Elchebly M, Payette P, Michaliszyn E, et al. Increased insulin sensitivity and obesity resistance in mice lacking the protein tyrosine phosphatase-1B gene. Science 1999;283(5407):1544–1548.
163.   Miller KA, Gunn TM, Carrasquillo MM, et al. Genetic studies of the mouse mutations mahogany and mahoganoid. Genetics 1997;146(4):1407–1415.

II CLINICAL MANAGEMENT

9

Socioeconomics of Obesity

Roland Sturm, PhD, and Yuhua Bao, PhD

CONTENTS

INTRODUCTION
OBESITY EPIDEMIC AND HEALTH AND COST CONSEQUENCES
SOCIOECONOMIC DISPARITIES IN OBESITY AND DIABETES
POSSIBLE MECHANISMS UNDERLYING OBESITY AND DIABETES
    TRENDS AND DISPARITIES
IMPLICATIONS FOR THE TREATMENT OF OBESE AND DIABETIC
    PATIENTS
ACKNOWLEDGMENTS
REFERENCES

Summary

The past two decades have seen a dramatic increase in the prevalence of obesity in the US population. Although increasing obesity was observed in every sociodemographic group, at every point in time groups with lower education, African Americans and Native Americans, and women in lower income households had higher rates of obesity and related chronic conditions such as diabetes. Also noteworthy is the much faster increase of severe obesity compared with moderate obesity, which added further strain to the health care system and proved especially challenging to health care providers. We provide data on the populationwide trends in weight gain, economic consequences of health care cost growth and the socioeconomic disparities in obesity and diabetes. We further discuss the socioeconomic and environmental changes that are likely underlying mechanisms for the obesity epidemic and related disparities. We conclude the chapter by discussing implications of these trends for the prevention and treatment of diabetes and challenges and opportunities faced by the health care system and providers.

Key Words: Body mass index; health disparities; time use; diet; physical activity.

INTRODUCTION

The past two decades have seen an astonishing increase in obesity rates, and it is generally thought that socioeconomic and environmental changes are the primary causes *(1–3)*. When talking about socioeconomic issues, we need to distinguish between two phenomena. The first is trend over time, which is related to societal and economic changes that affect everyone. Indeed, over the past two decades, the average increase in body mass index (BMI) has been surprisingly similar in all sociodemographic groups *(4,5)*. This trend puts an increasing stress on the health care system. The second phenomenon is the disparity in obesity rates between groups at every point in time, which is

From: *Contemporary Endocrinology: Treatment of the Obese Patient*
Edited by: R. F. Kushner and D. H. Bessesen © Humana Press Inc., Totowa, NJ

related to socioeconomic differences across subgroups. As a rule, obesity rates tend to be higher in groups with lower education levels, African Americans and Native Americans, and women in lower-income households *(5,6)*. Disparities in health status across socioeconomic groups mirror disparities in obesity rates.

The time trend is paralleled by the increasing prevalence of diabetes and, to a lesser extent, the prevalence of other chronic conditions. Medical care, especially developments in pharmacological treatments, has weakened the relationship between obesity and major cardiovascular risk factors, such as high cholesterol and hypertension, over time *(7)*. In addition, the cardiovascular health of Americans has improved over time as the strong positive effect of the falling smoking rates have outweighed the adverse effect of increasing obesity rates.

Nevertheless, the obesity epidemic imposes several new burdens on providers, hospitals, and the health care system in general. The proportion of the population that is severely obese, defined by a BMI over 40 or about 100 lb overweight for men and 80 for women, has been growing particularly quickly, and severely obese individuals face different challenges. As yet, many physicians' offices and even hospitals are not equipped to meet the needs of severely obese patients, who may not fit standard imaging equipments, operating tables, or wheelchairs. Even seemingly minor equipment limitations could conceivably affect quality of care and invite lawsuits. And, again, there are differences across populations. For example, among African-American women, one-third of diabetics have a BMI over 35, whereas in other groups a smaller share of diabetics are that heavy.

This chapter provides data on several issues. In the next section, we address trends in weight gain and economic consequences for health care. Typically, cited numbers are based on the definition of obesity as having a BMI over 30. However, as we will show, the time trend for moderate obesity differed from that for severe obesity, which has important economic implications for physician practices. The following section turns to cross-sectional (at a point in time) differences and provides data on socioeconomic disparities in obesity and diabetes, in particular on the interaction among race/ethnicity, income, education, severity of obesity, and diabetes. The next section discusses socioeconomic and environmental factors believed to be related to obesity and diabetes rates. We discuss both the general time trend and possible mechanisms underlying cross-sectional socioeconomic disparities in obesity and diabetes. We then discuss implications of these socioeconomic and environmental trends for the prevention and treatment of diabetes and challenges and opportunities faced by the health care system and providers. Unless indicated otherwise, all the results shown in this chapter are nationally representative for all adults, are based on self-reported height and weight (which means that objectively measured BMIs are likely to be higher), and measure diabetes by an indicator of physician-diagnosed diabetes or borderline diabetes (i.e., undiagnosed diabetes is not included).

OBESITY EPIDEMIC AND HEALTH AND COST CONSEQUENCES

The proportion of the US population that is considered obese has seen a marked increase in the past two decades. Data based on the most recent National Health and Nutrition Examination Survey (NHANES) (1999–2000) *(8),* which uses objectively measured height and weight, indicate that 30.5% had a BMI over 30 *(6)*, more than twice

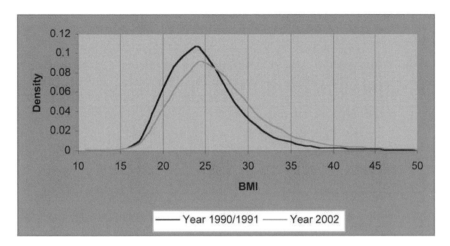

Fig. 1. The population distribution of BMI is shifting. Source: Author's calculation based on the Behavioral Risk Factor Surveillance System (BRFSS).

the rate in early 1980s (14.5% based on the second NHANES, conducted in 1976–1980) *(8,9)*. Moreover, none of the major sociodemographic groups of the population has been immune to the epidemic: rapid weight gain has been found in both genders, all racial/ ethnic groups, and all educational levels *(5,10)*; the entire population weight distribution is moving to the right. Figure 1 is a depiction of the shift of the BMI (based on self-reported weight and height) distribution among the US adult population from the early 1990s to the early 2000s.

There is another, possibly more disturbing, phenomenon. The distribution is becoming flatter—i.e., a smaller proportion of the population is now in the center of the distribution (which is shifting as well), and a larger proportion further out in the right tail, i.e., in the "obese" range. This picture does little to reveal what is going on at the more extreme end of the weight distribution—i.e., in the "severe obesity" range.

Does severe obesity simply parallel the general trend in obesity? Or is there something fundamentally different about clinically severe obesity? Two conflicting opinions exist about the trends in clinically severe obesity. Clinicians tend to consider clinically severe obesity a rare pathological condition that is not affected by behavioral changes in the general population. This view would suggest that severe obesity changes little over time and that the number of patients with these extraordinary health problems and care needs remains roughly constant, even as there are more moderately obese individuals. Epidemiologists tend to lean toward the opposite view, namely that severe obesity is part of the general population distribution and small increases in the population BMI would have proportionally larger effects in the extreme tail *(11)*. Which of those views better describes reality is an empirical question, but the answer has major ramifications for health care systems *(12)*.

Figure 2 shows the time trend in obesity prevalence by severity of obesity, adjusted for sociodemographic changes to isolate the unique trend in obesity rates. In addition to the standard "obese" category, defined as having a BMI greater than 30, the groups of primary interest here are the more extreme categories: BMI greater than 35, BMI greater than 40, BMI greater than 45, and BMI greater than 50.

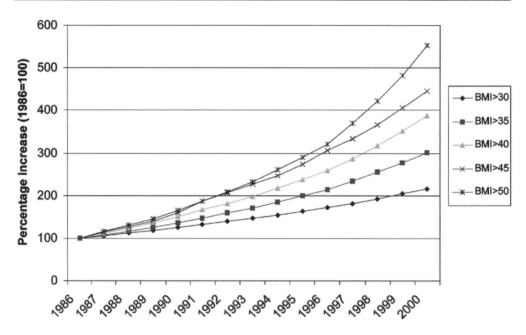

Fig. 2. Prevalence growth by severity of obesity. Source: Ref. *12*.

Between 1986 and 2000, the prevalence of BMI over 40 quadrupled from about 1 in 200 adult Americans to 1 in 50; the prevalence of BMI over 50 increased by a factor of 5, from about 1 in 2000 to 1 in 400 *(12)*. In contrast, obesity defined as a BMI of over 30 roughly doubled during the same time period, from about 1 in 10 to 1 in 5. The rate of increase for the BMI greater than 30 group is significantly lower than for the BMI greater than 40 group, which in turn is significantly lower than that for the BMI greater than 50 group. This trend has continued since those calculations were first published; from 2000 to 2004, we calculate that the prevalence of a BMI over 40 has increased to 2.7%, or more than 1 in 40 compared to 1 in 50 only 4 yr earlier; the prevalence of a BMI over 50 has increased to 1 in 300 (0.33%). These rates are all based on self-reported height and weight, which substantially underestimate higher weight categories.

The immediate consequence is that the economic burden of obesity in the health care system will increase at a much faster rate than the growth rate of moderate obesity. On average, an obese adult incurs health care costs that are about one-third higher than an otherwise similar normal-weight adult *(13)*. Yet when we distinguish weight categories among Americans 54 to 69 years old, a BMI of 35 to 40 is associated with twice the increase in health care expenditures (about a 50% increase) relative to normal weight compared with a BMI of 30 to 35 (about 25% increase); a BMI of over 40 doubled health care costs (approx 100% higher costs) compared with those with normal weight *(14)*.

A key factor behind the large differences in health care costs by weight is the prevalence of major chronic conditions associated with obesity. Figure 3 shows how quickly the prevalence of diabetes increases with BMI. We measure diabetes here by self-reported, doctor-diagnosed diabetes or borderline diabetes, which obviously excludes what is likely to be a sizable number of undiagnosed cases.

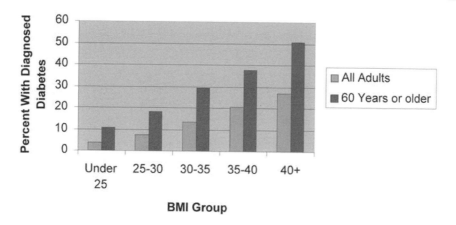

Fig. 3. Prevalence of diabetes among adults by body mass index. Source: Authors' calculation based on BRFSS 2004.

SOCIOECONOMIC DISPARITIES IN OBESITY AND DIABETES

So far, we have discussed overall trends. At every point in time, obesity and diabetes rates are higher in some populations than in others. Populations with higher rates generally include groups with less education, lower household income, blacks, and Native Americans, but there are some noticeable variations and interactions depending on whether we distinguish between moderate and severe obesity. For example, obesity as defined by a BMI of over 30 has been higher among men than women (although that gap has narrowed noticeably). However, severe obesity (BMI > 40) has been much higher among women for some time, and women also make up the vast majority (close to 85%) of bariatric surgery patients *(15)*.

Table 1 shows descriptive prevalence statistics for obesity, severe obesity, and diagnosed diabetes for men and women and by socioeconomic characteristics. Individuals without health insurance are, on average, 10 yr younger than those with health insurance (partly an effect of Medicare), yet have somewhat higher obesity rates and much higher severe obesity rates. Or, put in another way, severely obese patients who have the highest need for treatment are less likely to have health insurance. Largely because of the age difference between the insured and the uninsured populations, diagnosed diabetes is less common among the uninsured. But once age and sociodemographic variables (but not obesity) are adjusted for, the rate of diagnosed diabetes is slightly higher in the uninsured than in the insured population. However, it is less than what would be expected given the differences in obesity rates, suggesting that there is a higher rate of undetected diabetes among the uninsured. There are several reasons for this. People without insurance are far less likely to have a usual source of care—nearly 50% of the nonelderly uninsured, compared with about 10% of the insured, reported no usual source of health care—and a usual source of care and a sustained patient–physician relationship are strongly associated with use of preventive care *(16,17)*. Low-socioeconomic status (SES) patients are less likely to receive regular screening for common health risk factors. Using the third NHANES study (1988–1994) *(8,9)*, Qi Zhang at the University of Chicago estimated that undiagnosed diabetes was twice as common among adults without a high school diploma than among those with higher levels of education (Zhang, personal communication).

Table 1
Socioeconomic Status and Prevalence of Obesity, Severe Obesity, and Diabetes

	BMI > 30		*BMI > 40*		*% Diabetes*	
	Women	*Men*	*Women*	*Men*	*Women*	*Men*
All adults	22.4	23.4	3.4	1.8	7.7	8.4
By insurance						
Uninsured (mean age = 37)	25.6	23.0	4.4	2.6	6.2	5.4
Insured (mean age = 47)	21.9	23.5	3.3	1.8	8.0	9.0
By annual household income						
<$15,000	31.0	24.9	6.4	3.4	14.4	14.3
>$50,000	16.9	22.9	2.2	1.5	3.5	6.0
By education						
Less than high school	30.8	27.0	5.4	2.4	15.5	11.6
Completed college	15.3	18.7	2.1	1.3	4.2	7.0
By race/ethnicity						
Non-Hispanic white	19.9	22.9	2.9	1.8	7.1	8.0
Non-Hispanic black	36.8	28.6	7.5	2.9	11.5	11.1
Asian	6.6	7.7	0.2	0.1	3.6	7.4
Native American	32.2	29.7	5.8	2.5	13.2	12.4
Hispanic	26.0	25.2	3.3	2.2	7.9	8.0

Source: Authors' calculation based on BRFSS 2004

For women, a strong income gradient exists in obesity prevalence: those with annual household income less than $15,000 had an obesity rate that was almost twice as high as that among women with household income above $50,000. There is no such effect for men—obesity rates are fairly similar throughout the income range, a fact that many authors have noted. However, the same is not true for severe obesity, where there is an income gradient for both men and women. As we saw in Fig. 3, diagnosed diabetes is more prevalent among the severely obese than the moderately obese. The prevalence of diabetes therefore displays an income gradient for men as well as for women. This gradient exists even after adjusting for age (retirees have lower incomes) and other sociodemographics.

The causal direction of these associations is unclear. Severe obesity can cause disabilities that prevent people from working, and obesity therefore becomes the cause of lower income. At least for women, obesity also has been implicated as the cause of marrying lower-income spouses, lower educational achievements, and lower wage rates. Alternatively, low income may be a cause of obesity, as hypothesized by several authors and discussed in the next section. It is also possible that other factors cause both low income and obesity. One of the most prominent factors is severe mental illness, especially psychotic disorders. Some of the newer antipsychotics are strongly associated with weight gain and hyperglycemia (18,19) and mental illness obviously limits earning capacity. However, we tried to calculate to what extent this group drives the income gradient and realized that mental illness is not the reason for the association between lower income and severe obesity or diabetes.

Table 2
BMI and Employment Status

BMI	% homemaker, women	% Working for pay, women	% Working for pay, men
<25	13.6	58.5	59.7
25–30	12.1	59.3	63.6
30–35	12.0	55.7	62.8
35–40	11.9	54.9	59.9
40+	10.7	46.7	52.0

Source: BRFSS 2002, work for pay excludes self-employment

For both men and women, education is a socioeconomic factor that is strongly associated with obesity and diabetes. Among women, the rates of both obesity and severe obesity are more than twice as high in the group with less than a high school education than in the group of college graduates. There are noticeable race differences, with Asians having much lower rates of obesity and diabetes, and blacks and Native Americans having the highest rates. These differences remain after adjusting for age, income, and education, except that after this adjustment, Asians are no longer at lower risks for diabetes. Table 1 also shows the high rates of severe obesity among black and Native American women.

For women, several other adverse socioeconomic outcomes are associated with obesity (and although causality runs both ways, it is thought that the main effect is from obesity to adverse social outcomes). The effects appear to be larger for white women than for black or Hispanic women. Obese women are less likely to be married, tend to have lower family income, and are more likely to live in poverty. Table 2 shows additional details for employment status. The heavier a woman is, the less likely she is to work for pay and also less likely to be a homemaker. Women in higher weight categories are increasingly likely to be unemployed or unable to work. For men, there is no similar gradient: the BMI 35–40 group has the same employment rate as the BMI less than 25 group. Only in the severe obesity range—i.e., with a BMI over 40—do we see an adverse employment effect for men. For that group, employment rates are about 10 percentage points lower than that for moderate obese men. The primary reason reported by severely obese men is "unable to work," which is 10 times more common among severely obese men than among moderately obese men.

So far, we have discussed existing disparities in recent years, but there are concerns that current obesity epidemic will increase gaps. Figures 4–6 show that average weight gain has been fairly similar across all sociodemographic groups. Even the more advantaged groups, such as those with higher education and the non-Hispanic white, have seen large increases in BMI.

However, the weight distribution is more skewed to the right among those with less education, African Americans, and women. If we focus on the heaviest individuals, there actually may be an increasing gap by race or education and a decreasing gap by gender. Compare Fig. 7, which shows the 80th percentile, with Fig. 6, which shows the mean. Even though men have a higher mean BMI and this gap has not narrowed much, at the 80th percentile, the story is quite different. Based on self-reported height and weight,

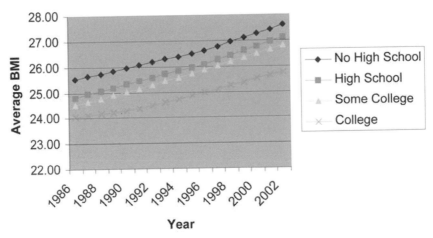

Fig. 4. Average body mass index by education. Source: Authors' calculation based on the BRFSS. Reprinted with permission from ref. *54*.

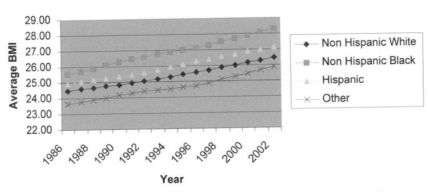

Fig. 5. Average body mass index by race. Source: Authors' calculation based on the BRFSS.

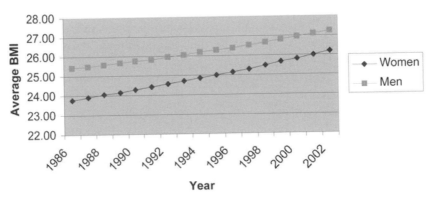

Fig. 6. Average body mass index by gender. Source: Authors' calculation based on the BRFSS.

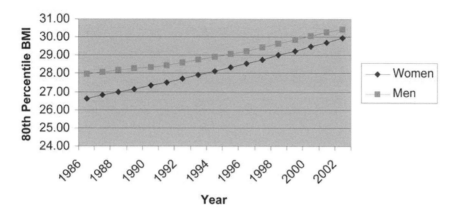

Fig. 7. Eightieth percentile body mass index by gender. Source: Authors' calculation based on the BRFSS.

women have been catching up very rapidly (Fig. 7). In fact, when measuring weight objectively, a BMI of over 30 has already become more common among women than men, a dramatic reversal of the situation 20 yr ago *(6)*. Furthermore, as we saw in Table 1, severe obesity rates are already much higher among women than among men (the lines would cross if we plotted the 90th percentile).

POSSIBLE MECHANISMS UNDERLYING OBESITY AND DIABETES TRENDS AND DISPARITIES

What are the underlying causes for these trends? Among researchers there has been an increasing consensus that changes in dietary and physical activity patterns are driven by changes in the environment and by the changing incentives that people face *(1,2)*. Many factors have been suggested as causes of the "obesity epidemic" and related health disparities—automobiles, television, fast food, computer use, vending machines, suburban housing developments, food portion sizes, and countless others. These are also the same factors that will either simplify or complicate adherence to recommended behavioral changes to maintain weight or manage diabetes. Putting a multitude of isolated data points into a coherent picture is a challenging but necessary task to assess whether proposed solutions are promising or likely to lead us down a blind alley.

Time Use: Do Americans Have Less Time for Exercise?

Over the past four decades, there have been some major changes in the lives of Americans, though some are quite different from common perceptions. Big increases in time use occurred in leisure or free time and time spent in transportation. Leisure time has increased substantially since 1965—by more than 4 h per week *(20,21)*. Occupation and productive activities at home (cooking, cleaning, repairing things, child care) have diminished to make room for increases in leisure time. Thus, increasing weight has been accompanied by increased, not reduced, leisure/free time. Free time between 1965 and 1985 increased by 4.9 h for women (to a total of 39), despite increasing labor force participation, and by 4.7 h (to a total of 40) for men *(20)*. Women spend more time in the

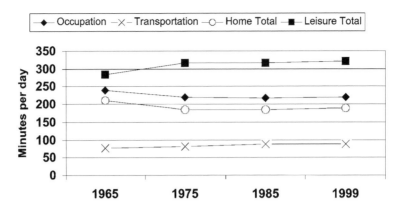

Fig. 8. Changes in time allocation. Source: Reprinted with permission from ref. *21.*

labor force than before, but that increase is more than offset by declines in home production. We plot time trends in Fig. 8 for the several main categories.

What are the possible economic drivers behind this change? A reduction in the relative prices for prepared meals (relative to, for example, the price for women's time in the labor market) has reduced home production (cooking and cleaning up), leaving more time for leisure. Technological changes have also made (largely sedentary) leisure activities (DVDs, cable TV, games, surround-sound) more attractive relative to work or household production.

One persistent myth is that Americans are exercising less. In reality, there has been a consistent increase in active sports or walking/hiking. Between 1985 and 1999, active sports increased by 20 min a week based on two time-use surveys *(21).* Median leisure time physical activity in the Behavioral Risk Factor Surveillance System from 1990 to 2000 increased by 20 min a week, whereas there was a consistent decline in sedentary behavior *(21).* Obviously, a rather small proportion of the increased free time went into active leisure activities, but Americans are exercising more in their leisure time than ever before.

In terms of industry output, the growth of industries associated with leisure time far exceeded gross domestic product (GDP) growth. Between 1987 and 2001, GDP in constant 1996 dollars increased by about 50% (from $6113 billion to $9215 billion), whereas retail of sporting goods and bicycles more than doubled (from $4.7 billion to $11.4 billion). Sports/fitness clubs also more than doubled, and similar growth rates exist in smaller "active" industries, such as dance studios. However, this is dwarfed by the explosive growth of home entertainment retail, an industry that was smaller than sporting goods in 1987 and now is four times as large (Fig. 9). This appears to be a fairly consistent trend: leisure-time industries are growing faster than other industries, paralleling time use. But "sedentary" industries are growing even faster than "active" industries, just as more of the increase in leisure time has gone to sedentary activities than to physical activity *(21).*

In contrast to adults, who now have more free time than ever, children's free time has substantially declined as a consequence of increased time away from home, primarily in school, day care, and after-school programs (a consequence of increased labor force participation among parents), as shown in Fig. 10. Participation in organized activities

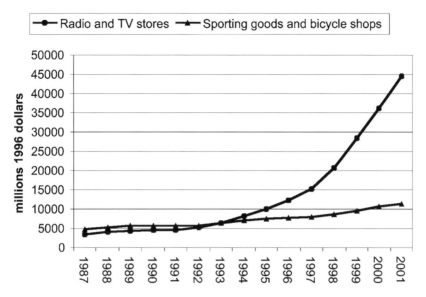

Fig. 9. Retail: sports and television. Source: Sturm, 2004 based on Bureau of Economic Activity, Constant Dollar Gross Output for Double-Deflated Industries; detailed data in constant 1996 dollars.

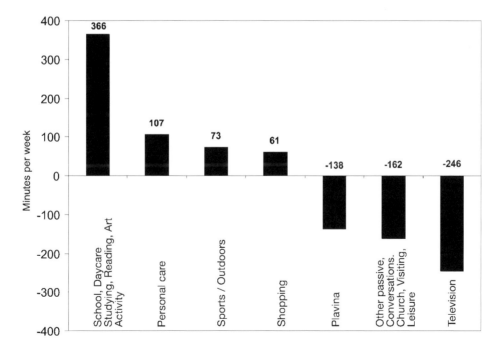

Fig. 10. Changes in weekly minutes spent on activities from 1981 to 1997, ages 3–12.

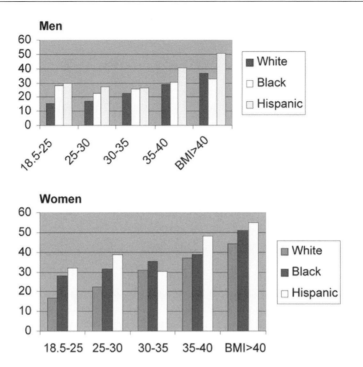

Fig. 11. Americans reporting no leisure-time physical activity for major racial/ethnic groups, by body mass index. Source: Authors' calculation from BRFSS 2004.

(including sports) also increased. To make room for this, play time decreased, but so did time in some sedentary activities such as watching TV, conversations, or other passive leisure, which fell at the same time that obesity became a major public health concern *(22)*. As time away from home in structured settings increases, so does the importance of physical activity in those settings and we know little what is going on there. Certainly, with the decline in discretionary free time, behavioral changes to increase physical activity are harder for youth than for adults. Thus, over the past few decades, time barriers to complying with recommendations to increase leisure time physical activity have been lowered for adults, but increased for youth. Whether there are differential trends for sociodemographic subgroups is not known.

Even though the proportion of adults reporting no leisure-time physical activity at all has been falling across all groups, and three-fourths of the population now reports some activity, there are some groups with inactivity rates over 50%: severely obese Hispanic men and women and severely obese black women. Figure 11 shows that inactivity rates increase quickly with obesity, but also that there are noticeable racial differences even in the normal weight range, which might predict future weight gain as these individuals age. Given the high rates of inactivity in the heavier populations, maybe the counseling message should emphasize any activity, rather than trying to achieve guideline levels of activity.

Leisure-time physical activity is only a component of total physical activity; how total physical activity has changed depends also on labor force and home production as well as transportation patterns. Transportation is part of everyday life, not just for commuting to work, but also for an array of other essential life components such as running errands, dining out, shopping, and visiting family and friends. It could also be a key factor of changes in physical activity because small shifts in travel modes noticeably alter energy expenditures. Some small increases in utilitarian walking may have large health benefits for diabetic and obese patients. Adults in the United States spend well over an hour a day—more than ever before—traveling. Just between 1995 and 2001, time in vehicles increased by 10%, although distance traveled remained about the same *(23)*. Over the past few decades, transportation time, together with leisure time, has increased substantially at the expense of occupation and household activities.

Unfortunately, existing data do not tell us much more about physical activity involved in transportation. The Nationwide Personal Transportation Surveys have shown a consistent proportional shift from walking or biking to driving as the means of trips taken, but the number of trips has also increased. Since 1969, the share of total trips that were for the purpose of commuting to and from work decreased from about one in three to one in six trips. The biggest growth for adults has been in trips for social or recreational purposes. Trips for these purposes increased by about 100 more trips per person per year between 1990 and 2001 *(23)*. The problem, however, is with calculating active travel time, because changes in survey design have made it difficult to calculate trend numbers on physical activity: the 2001 survey prompted for walking trips, but others didn't.

For youth, there has been a substantial decline in walking as a percentage of trips to and from school, falling from 20.2% in 1977 to 12.5% in 2001 *(24)*, indicating a decrease in active travel to school. Although these numbers are often cited as evidence for declining active travel, there has been a substantial increase in the total number of daily trips that could offset declines in the share of walking and biking. However, even the highest estimates based on any of the available surveys indicate that active travel accounts for less than 10 min a day *(24)*. Thus, active transportation is not an important source of physical activity for youth and has not been one for at least 25 yr.

It is not clear how these populationwide trends would exacerbate or narrow socioeconomic disparities in obesity and diabetes. Suburban sprawl has been associated with higher rates of obesity, less walking, and related chronic conditions, after controlling for individual sociodemographic characteristics. But neighborhoods with suburban sprawl characteristics (low density, poorly connected streets, and single land use neighborhoods) tend to have higher income and fewer minorities than more urban (higher density, more connected streets, more land use mix) neighborhoods *(25–28)*.

It is also not known to what extent environmental constraints make it more difficult for obese or diabetic patients to increase utilitarian walking. Urban design plays a crucial role because unless there are locations to walk to (stores, work, schools), there will be little utilitarian walking. Even seemingly minor recommendations, such as increasing stair use, are hard to follow when stairs are hard to find, have alarmed exit doors, and are poorly maintained.

Food Supply and Dietary Changes

Changes in diet have been implied in the rising obesity and diabetes rates. One intriguing theory focuses on the economics of food supply, noting that the price for foods with higher energy density is much lower than that of less energy-dense foods in terms of price per calorie and that maintaining energy balance is more difficult with foods that have

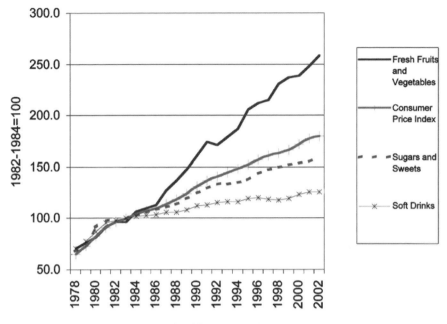

Fig. 12. Price indices.

higher energy density *(29,30)*. An alternative theory to the energy-density argument centers around the glycemic index (a measure of the insulin response to ingested carbohydrate) of food. A diet with a high glycemic index encourages higher total caloric intake *(31–33)*.

Figure 12 shows how prices for different types of foods changed differentially over the past two decades. The price index for fruits and vegetables (foods that have both low energy density and low glycemic loads) has increased much faster than the consumer price index, or general rate of inflation. In contrast, sugars, sweets, and soft drinks, foods either with high energy density or high glycemic index, have become relatively cheaper.

Figure 13 shows how macronutrients changed in the American diet. Whereas fat and protein stayed fairly constant, since the early 1980s there has been a steady increase in the consumption of carbohydrates, and in particular caloric sweeteners (Fig. 14).

If the price per unit of energy for energy-dense products and for sweetened products is much lower than that for food such as fresh produce, lean meats, and fish, a differential dietary pattern would develop between income groups if people of low income are more sensitive to the price of food *(29)*. The evidence is unclear, although low-income families are less likely to purchase fresh produce and they spend less money on it *(34)*. The secular decline of prices for energy-denser foods and sugars relative to produce or fish would suggest widening gaps in obesity and related chronic conditions (such as diabetes) between populations of different socioeconomic status, but there is no strong evidence for such an effect. Nevertheless, these economic effects point to differential challenges in managing diabetes across socioeconomic groups. We do see that children, even at an early age, in communities with higher relative prices for produce gain more weight, and the effect appears to be more pronounced for children in low-income households *(35)*.

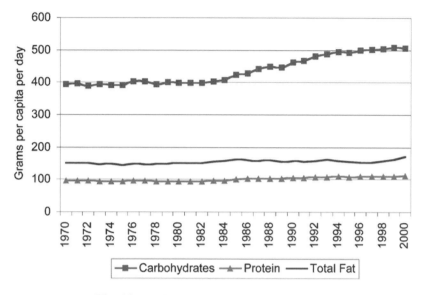

Fig. 13. US food supply for macronutrients.

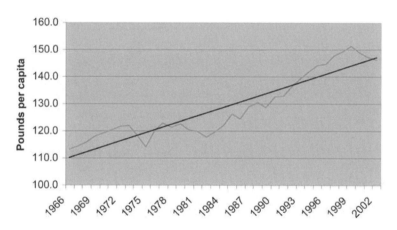

Fig. 14. US production of caloric sweeteners.

IMPLICATIONS FOR THE TREATMENT OF OBESE AND DIABETIC PATIENTS

Socioeconomic and environmental trends are the driving forces behind increasing obesity and diabetes rates. This section focuses on the challenges and opportunities that confront the health care system, especially as they relate to socioeconomic disparities in diabetes and diabetic treatment.

SES Disparities in Access to Health Care

Previous studies have shown that both lifestyle changes and medication (e.g., metformin) were effective in preventing or delaying the onset of diabetes among people at elevated risk for the condition (36–40). However, people of low SES are likely to be

Table 3
Treatment of Diabetes by Patient Education (%)

	Less than high school	High school	Some college	College or higher
Ever seen health professional past 12 mo for diabetes	89.1	92.1	90.7	91.0
Health professional ever checked hemoglobin A1C past 12 mo	72.7	85.5	87.7	87.7
Health professional ever checked feet last 12 mo	63.8	69.6	70.3	68.3
Ever had eye exam past 12 mo	63.8	69.3	71.7	74.3

Estimates based on the 2002 BRFSS. Rates apply to the subpopulation that had diagnosed diabetes.

disadvantaged in both regards because of their lower access to health care and possibly lower quality of health care they receive compared with that received by their high-SES counterparts. In 2002, almost one-third of the nonelderly population living in poverty was without any health insurance coverage, compared with 10.9% among people of the same age but with a household income above 200% of the poverty line (8). A similar pattern is observed by education: in 2001, nonelderly adults without a high school diploma had an uninsurance rate of 40.6%, compared with 21.1% among those with a high school diploma, 10.7% among those with some college education, and 9.5% among those with a college degree (authors' calculation based on the 2001 National Health Interview Survey).

Individuals without insurance, with low educational achievement, or with low household income are less likely to receive proper interventions to prevent the onset of diabetes, and once diagnosed with diabetes, are less likely to receive regular and effective clinical management of the condition. Data from the 2002 Behavioral Risk Factor Surveillance System (BRFSS) indicate that, of all the adults with a diagnosis of diabetes, those who did not have a high school diploma consistently lagged behind adults with higher education in terms of getting essential care for their condition (Table 3), even though these diabetic patients of different education all seemed to have seen their providers for diabetes for at least once in the past year.

Disparities in access to quality health care may develop even among people with similar insurance coverage. One important factor at the systems level is the uneven distribution of medical care resources across communities of different SES. Physicians serving in low-income, minority communities are more likely to be graduates of foreign medical schools and less likely to be board-certified (41–44). There is further evidence that physicians serving disproportionately more low-income patients are not as knowledgeable about national guidelines for preventive care (45) and therefore are less likely to discuss preventive care issues with their patients including primary and secondary prevention of diabetes.

Additionally, even when treated by the same physicians, patients with lower education are likely to receive less physician advice regarding lifestyle and behavior changes and such disparities may exist even after behavior-related conditions develop. Data from the 2001 National Health Interview Survey (NHIS) indicate that among all adults who

Table 4
Rates of Physician Advice on Diet and Physical Activity by Patient Education (%)

	Less than high school	High school	Some college	College or higher
Physician advice on diet				
Unconditional	42.4	42.7	43.1	44.2
Precondition	30.2^b	31.6^b	33.9^a	37.1
Postcondition	52.2	53.9	52.6	52.6
Physician advice on physical activity				
Unconditional	42.2^b	44.1^b	46.9	48.0
Pre-condition	32.2^b	33.6^b	37.3	40.8
Post-condition	47.4^b	50.2^a	52.0	52.7

Rates are based on logistic models that adjust for patient demographics, insurance coverage, and income. The "pre(post)condition" results are derived by conducting the analysis on the subsample of individuals who did not have (already had) chronic conditions related to diet/physical activity. The group with college or higher education is the reference group for comparison by education. Statistically significant difference relative to the reference group is indicated by $^a p < 0.05$ and $^b p < 0.01$.

had at least one visit to their regular health care providers in the past year, low-education patients were less likely to have received advice for diet and physical activity. Even among patients with diagnosed conditions that would benefit from physical activity, low education was associated with a lower rate of advice on physical activity (Table 4).

Disparities in Access to Other Resources

Both lifestyle changes and adherence to diabetic treatment regimens are especially challenging to patients of low SES for both personal/cognitive and environmental reasons. The ability to understand the medical necessity of glycemic control and to internalize the consequences of nonadherence to prescribed regimens is closely related to one's education. The ability to adjust one's diet to include more fresh produce or lean meats and the ability to have regular leisure-time physical activity are partly determined by one's income. On the other hand, communities where low-SES patients reside are associated with special environmental constraints for lifestyle changes. Low-income neighborhoods have fewer supermarkets compared with wealthier communities, although they do have more smaller grocery stores *(35,46)*. Because supermarkets offer a wider variety of food at lower prices, such features of the low-income neighborhoods further constrain the ability of the residents to change the structure of their diets. Low-SES neighborhoods also lack safe environments for outdoor physical activities *(47,48)*. Social supports and personal efficacy and control are likely to be lower and depression and hostility higher among the low-SES population *(49,50)*, which may further impair the ability of low-SES patients to effectively manage serious health problems such as diabetes.

Role of Health Care Providers

Although preventing and managing diabetes is ultimately the responsibility of the patient, health care providers play an important role in patient education and clinical management of diabetes. In addition, providers may also play an active role in assisting patients with effective utilization of community resources for self-management.

Despite the fact that health information is now available through a variety of sources, including the Internet, health care providers remain the most authoritative and dominant source of such information. When asked the main reason that they did not comply with national cancer screening guidelines, for example, individuals were most likely to respond with "I didn't know I need it" and "Dr. did not recommend it" *(51)*. Reliance on health care providers for health information and knowledge is likely to be greater for patients with low education and/or low health literacy, given their limited exposure to other informational and educational sources. Health care providers should therefore take the opportunity of clinical encounters to educate patients about the relationship between health behaviors (such as diet and physical activity) and diabetes and the importance of glycemic control through behavior changes and/or medical management of one's blood glucose level.

Patient knowledge alone, however, will not be enough to lead to desired health outcomes *(52)*. Providers need to make sure that not only do patients understand self-management strategies, but that these strategies can also be carried out in a patient's daily life and, if not, what the barriers are. Increasing utilitarian physical activity is feasible only in walkable neighborhoods and changing diets is possible only when healthful foods are available at reasonable prices. Low-SES patients face special challenges in managing obesity or diabetes. Disease-management programs may need to be tailored to the need of low-SES patients by, for example, administering more intensive clinical management relative to self-management *(53)*, directly providing access to resources (e.g., referral to a diabetic patients' support group), or teaming up with community entities so that patients can more effectively utilize local resources (e.g., discount at local gyms for diabetic patients, coupons for fresh produce at farmers' markets).

ACKNOWLEDGMENTS

We are grateful to Khoa Truong for creating Figs. 4–7 and to Qi Zhang, PhD, for his estimates of undiagnosed diabetes. Funding for preparing this paper was provided by the National Institute of Environmental Health Sciences, grant no. P50ES012383.

REFERENCES

1. Hill JO, Peters JC. Environmental contributions to the obesity epidemic. Science 1998;280(5368): 1371–1374.
2. Hill JO, Wyatt HR, Reed GW, et al. Obesity and the environment: where do we go from here? Science 2003;299(5608):853–855.
3. Popkin BM, Duffey K, Gordon-Larsen P. Environmental influences on food choice, physical activity and energy balance. Physiol Behav 2005;86:603–613.
4. Chang VW, Lauderdale DS. Income disparities in body mass index and obesity in the United States, 1971–2002. Arch Intern Med 2005;165(18):2122–2128.
5. Truong KD, Sturm R. Weight gain trends across sociodemographic groups in the United States. Am J Public Health 2005;95(9):1602–1606.
6. Flegal KM, Carroll MD, Ogden CL, et al. Prevalence and trends in obesity among US adults, 1999–2000. JAMA 2002;288(14):1723–1727.
7. Gregg EW, Cheng YJ, Cadwell BL, et al. Secular trends in cardiovascular disease risk factors according to body mass index in US adults. JAMA 2005;293(15):1868–1874.
8. National Center for Health Statistics. Health, United States. Hyattsville, MD: 2004.
9. Flegal KM, Carroll MD, Kuczmarski RJ, et al. Overweight and obesity in the United States: prevalence and trends, 1960–1994. Int J Obes Relat Metab Disord 1998;22(1):39–47.

10. Mokdad AH, Bowman BA, Ford ES, et al. The continuing epidemics of obesity and diabetes in the United States. JAMA 2001;286(10):1195–1200.
11. Rose G. Sick individuals and sick populations. Int J Epidemiol 1985;14(1):32–38.
12. Sturm R. Increases in clinically severe obesity in the United States, 1986–2000. Arch Intern Med 2003;163(18):2146–2148.
13. Sturm R. The effects of obesity, smoking, and drinking on medical problems and costs. Obesity outranks both smoking and drinking in its deleterious effects on health and health costs. Health Aff (Millwood) 2002;21(2):245–253.
14. Andreyeva T, Sturm R, Ringel JS. Moderate and severe obesity have large differences in health care costs. Obes Res 2004;12(12):1936–1943.
15. Encinosa WE, Bernard DM, Steiner CA, et al. Use and costs of bariatric surgery and prescription weight-loss medications. Health Aff (Millwood) 2005;24(4):1039–1046.
16. Parchman ML, Burge SK. The patient-physician relationship, primary care attributes, and preventive services. Fam Med 2004;36(1):22–27.
17. Xu KT. Usual source of care in preventive service use: a regular doctor versus a regular site. Health Serv Res 2002;37(6):1509–1529.
18. Newcomer JW. Abnormalities of glucose metabolism associated with atypical antipsychotic drugs. J Clin Psychiatry 2004;65 Suppl 18:36–46.
19. Wirshing DA. Schizophrenia and obesity: impact of antipsychotic medications. J Clin Psychiatry 2004;65 Suppl 18:13–26.
20. Robinson JP, Godbey GG. Time for Life: The Surprising Ways Americans Use Their Time. 2nd ed. Pennsylvania State University Press, University Park, PA: 1999.
21. Sturm R. The economics of physical activity: societal trends and rationales for interventions. Am J Prev Med 2004;27(3 Suppl):126–135.
22. Sturm R. Childhood obesity—what we can learn from existing data on societal trends, part 1. Prev Chronic Dis 2005;2(1):A12.
23. National Household Transportation Survey. Summary of Travel Trends: 2001 National Household Travel Survey. Available at http://nhts.ornl.gov/2001/reports.shtml.
24. Sturm R. Childhood obesity—what we can learn from existing data on societal trends, part 2. Prev Chronic Dis 2005;2(2):A20.
25. Ewing R, Schmid T, Killingsworth R, et al. Relationship between urban sprawl and physical activity, obesity, and morbidity. Am J Health Promot 2003;18(1):47–57.
26. Saelens BE, Sallis JF, Black JB, et al. Neighborhood-based differences in physical activity: an environment scale evaluation. Am J Public Health 2003;93(9):1552–1558.
27. Saelens BE, Sallis JF, Frank LD. Environmental correlates of walking and cycling: findings from the transportation, urban design, and planning literatures. Ann Behav Med 2003;25(2):80–91.
28. Sturm R, Cohen DA. Suburban sprawl and physical and mental health. Public Health 2004;118(7): 488–496.
29. Drewnowski A. Obesity and the food environment: dietary energy density and diet costs. Am J Prev Med 2004;27(3 Suppl):154–162.
30. Drewnowski A, Darmon N. The economics of obesity: dietary energy density and energy cost. Am J Clin Nutr 2005;82(1 Suppl):265S–273S.
31. Ludwig DS. Dietary glycemic index and obesity. J Nutr 2000;130(2S Suppl):280S–283S.
32. Ludwig DS. The glycemic index: physiological mechanisms relating to obesity, diabetes, and cardiovascular disease. JAMA 2002;287(18):2414–24123.
33. Ludwig DS. Dietary glycemic index and the regulation of body weight. Lipids 2003;38(2):117–121.
34. Blisard N, Stewart H, Joliffe D. Low-Income Households' Expenditures on Fruits and Vegetables. ERS Research Brief. Available online at http://www.ers.usda.gov/publications/aer833/aer833_researchbrief. pdf. US Department of Agriculture, May 2004.
35. Sturm R, Datar A. Body mass index in elementary school children, metropolitan area food prices and food outlet density. Public Health 2005;119(12):1059–1068.
36. Buchanan TA, Xiang AH, Peters RK, et al. Preservation of pancreatic beta-cell function and prevention of type 2 diabetes by pharmacological treatment of insulin resistance in high-risk hispanic women. Diabetes 2002;51(9):2796–2803.
37. Chiasson JL, Josse RG, Gomis R, et al. Acarbose for prevention of type 2 diabetes mellitus: the STOP-NIDDM randomised trial. Lancet 2002;359(9323):2072–2077.

38. Knowler WC, Barrett-Connor E, Fowler SE, et al. Reduction in the incidence of type 2 diabetes with lifestyle intervention or metformin. N Engl J Med 2002;346(6):393–403.
39. Pan XR, Li GW, Hu YH, et al. Effects of diet and exercise in preventing NIDDM in people with impaired glucose tolerance. The Da Qing IGT and Diabetes Study. Diabetes Care 1997;20(4):537–544.
40. Tuomilehto J, Lindstrom J, Eriksson JG, et al. Prevention of type 2 diabetes mellitus by changes in lifestyle among subjects with impaired glucose tolerance. N Engl J Med 2001;344(18):1343–1350.
41. Bellochs C, Carter AB. Building Primary Health Care in New York City's Low-income Communities. Community Health Service Society of New York, New York: 1990.
42. Fosset JW, Peroff JD, Peterson JA, et al. Medicaid in the inner city: the case of maternity care in Chicago. Milbank Quarterly 1990;68:111–141.
43. Mitchell JB. Physician participation in Medicaid revisited. Med Care 1991;29(7):645–653.
44. Mitchell JB, Cromwell J. Large Medicaid practices and Medicaid mills. JAMA 1980;244(21):2433–2437.
45. Ashford A, Gemson D, Sheinfeld Gorin SN, et al. Cancer screening and prevention practices of inner-city physicians. Am J Prev Med 2000;19(1):59–62.
46. Morland K, Wing S, Diez Roux A, et al. Neighborhood characteristics associated with the location of food stores and food service places. Am J Prev Med 2002;22(1):23–29.
47. Gomez JE, Johnson BA, Selva M, et al. Violent crime and outdoor physical activity among inner-city youth. Prev Med 2004;39(5):876–881.
48. Molnar BE, Gortmaker SL, Bull FC, et al. Unsafe to play? Neighborhood disorder and lack of safety predict reduced physical activity among urban children and adolescents. Am J Health Promot 2004;18(5):378–386.
49. House JS, Lepkowski JM, Kinney AM, et al. The social stratification of aging and health. J Health Soc Behav 1994;35(3):213–234.
50. Marmot MG, Smith GD, Stansfeld S, et al. Health inequalities among British civil servants: the Whitehall II study. Lancet 1991;337(8754):1387–1393.
51. Finney Rutten LJ, Nelson DE, Meissner HI. Examination of population-wide trends in barriers to cancer screening from a diffusion of innovation perspective (1987–2000). Prev Med 2004;38(3):258–268.
52. Kenkel D. Health behavior, health knowledge, and schooling. J Polit Econ 1991;99(2):287–305.
53. Goldman DP, Smith JP. Can patient self-management help explain the SES health gradient? Proc Natl Acad Sci USA 2002;99(16):10,929–10,934.
54. Truong KD, Sturm R. Weight gain trends across sociodemographic groups in the United States. Am J Pub Health 2005;95:1602–1606.

10 Assessment of the Obese Patient

Daniel H. Bessesen, MD

CONTENTS

IMPORTANCE OF EVALUATING OBESITY IN CLINICAL PRACTICE
DEFINING OBESITY
ASSESSING WEIGHT HISTORY
ASSESSING FOR SECONDARY CAUSES OF OBESITY
ASSESSING FOR HEALTH COMPLICATIONS OF OBESITY
ASSESSING ENERGY INTAKE
ASSESSING ENERGY EXPENDITURE
OTHER ASPECTS OF BEHAVIORAL EVALUATION
ROLE OF ALLIED HEALTH PROFESSIONALS IN ASSESSMENT
    OF THE OBESE PATIENT
CONCLUSION
REFERENCES

Summary

There is a growing consensus on the importance of addressing obesity in clinical practice. This consensus is the product of clear evidence that obesity has become an extremely common condition, that it is associated with adverse health consequences, and that treatment modalities are available that can not only reduce weight, but improve some of the associated comorbidities. In this chapter, some of the evidence that obesity, as defined by body mass index and waist circumference, is associated with adverse health consequences will be reviewed. An approach to the assessment of the obese patient that involves a focused weight history, evaluating diet and physical activity habits, and determining the patient's goals and readiness for treatment will be discussed. Assessing for secondary causes of weight gain and risk stratification based on a history, physical exam, and laboratory evaluation are also discussed. The role of other health professionals in a multidisciplinary approach to assessment is proposed. Later chapters in this volume will discuss a variety of treatment approaches that can be used with obese patients.

Key Words: Obesity; assessment; diet, Physical Activity; waist circumference; metabolic syndrome.

IMPORTANCE OF EVALUATING OBESITY IN CLINICAL PRACTICE

Epidemiology of Obesity

The prevalence of obesity has increased dramatically over the past 30 yr. From 1985 to 2004, the Centers for Disease Control and Prevention (CDC) determined the prevalence of obesity by self-report across the country through the Behavioral Risk Factor

From: *Contemporary Endocrinology: Treatment of the Obese Patient*
Edited by: R. F. Kushner and D. H. Bessesen © Humana Press Inc., Totowa, NJ

Surveillance System (BRFSS). Despite the fact that self-reported weights underestimate the true prevalence of obesity, the CDC obesity maps (www.cdc.gov/nccdphp/dnpa/ obesity/trend/maps/) document a dramatic rise in obesity in every state of the country over the past 20 yr. More accurate composite data on the prevalence of obesity in the United States come from a series of studies that directly measured height and weight in carefully selected, nationally representative samples of adults in the National Health and Nutrition Examination Surveys (NHANES). In the most recent NHANES report from 2001 to 2002, the prevalence of overweight or obesity among adults was 65.7%. The prevalence of obesity (body mass index [BMI] > 30 kg/m^2) was 30.6% and the prevalence of severe obesity (BMI > 40) was 5.1% (1). Perhaps even more troubling were the numbers for children and adolescents. Among young people age 6 to 19, 31.5% were at risk for overweight and 16.5% were overweight.

Morbidity and Mortality Associated With Obesity

Obesity is common and is associated with increased rates of mortality and morbidity. The effect of obesity on mortality risk has been addressed by a large number of studies over the past 20 yr. There are unfortunately a number of important methodological issues that have made it difficult to establish a clear relationship between these variables. For example, smokers weigh less than nonsmokers but have increased mortality related to their smoking, not their reduced weight. People with undiagnosed cancer may lose weight and have an increased risk of mortality that, again, is not related to their reduced weight. In an effort to correct for these factors, many modern studies exclude smokers and first 2- to 5-yr mortality (this period begins when BMI/weight is first measured) when looking at the effects of obesity on mortality. When this has been done, there remain some questions about whether mortality rates are increased in overweight individuals (BMI 25–30), but it is clear that obesity(BMI > 30) is associated with increased mortality. In one study, those with a BMI > 30 had a 70% greater risk of dying than lean individuals (2). Another study estimated that a man 20 to 30 yr old with a BMI > 45 would lose 13 yr of life expectancy owing to his excess weight (3). Obesity is felt by many to now rival cigarette smoking as a potentially modifiable contributor to mortality (4).

Many previous analyses, however, used older data sets obtained at a time when the screening and treatment of cardiovascular disease risk factors and diabetes were less aggressive than is currently the case. In a recent controversial analysis, Flegal et al. used NHANES data to make new estimates of excess deaths associated with underweight, overweight, and obesity (5). This analysis did not "correct" for the presence of comorbid conditions such as treated hypertension or treated hyperlipidemia. The results demonstrated that those with a BMI between 25 and 30 had a lower mortality rate than those with either a lower or higher BMI. Those with a BMI greater than 35 clearly had increased mortality. It appeared that the increased risk of mortality associated with obesity was higher in earlier cohorts, suggesting that current treatments for comorbid conditions may be improving the health of obese people. In a related study, Gregg et al. examined longitudinal trends in the management of cardiovascular disease risk factors in the NHANES cohorts (6). The authors looked at the prevalence of hypertension, hyperlipidemia, and diabetes in people of varying BMIs over time. If a person had, for example, a blood pressure that was <140/90 mmHg because of treatment with antihypertensive medications, they were considered to not have hypertension for purposes of this analysis. A similar approach was used for hyperlipidemia. This study found that whereas hypertension and hyperlipidemia were more common in obese than in lean individuals at all time points, because of more aggressive screening and treatment, an obese person in 2000 was less likely to have high blood pressure or hyperlipidemia than a thin person in 1960. The changes were dramatic and represented marked increases in the use of anti-hypertensive and lipid-lowering medications over the past 40 yr. The one exception to this pattern was in the area of diabetes. The prevalence of diagnosed diabetes has increased dramatically over the past 40 yr and is, in fact, more common now among obese individuals than it was in 1960. This is in part because the average obese person in 2000 weighed more than the average obese person did in 1960. The situation appears to be that whereas obesity has increased in prevalence, more aggressive treatment of hyperlipidemia, hypertension, and diabetes have minimized the effect that this rising prevalence has had on mortality. One might ask, though, if this is the public health strategy that we want to pursue for the next 40 yr.

Costs Associated With Obesity

In addition to the impact of obesity on mortality and comorbid health, there are now a great deal of data demonstrating that obesity is responsible for increased medical costs, job absenteeism, and a reduced quality of life for both adults and adolescents *(7,8)*. Obese individuals have more visits to primary care providers and are the recipients of more diagnostic and specialty services *(9)*. In a study of more than 16,000 Medicare recipients, Daviglus et al. found that individuals who were either obese or severely obese in middle age generated $2020 and $6469 more per year in attributable health care charges than their lean counterparts when they entered the Medicare program at age 65 *(10)*. Other studies have also documented an increase in health care costs associated with increasing weight in people covered by indemnity or preferred provider organization (PPO) health insurance plans, as well as those enrolled in health maintenance organizations *(11–13)*. The net effect of health-related economic costs attributable to obesity, including paid sick leave, life insurance, and disability, amount to more than $4 billion *(14)*. Obesity then results in not only health problems but also a substantial economic drain on the health care system and private business.

Consensus That Addressing Obesity Is Important

As a result of the increasingly compelling data on the growing prevalence of obesity, the adverse effects of obesity on health, and the costs of the condition, a broad consensus has emerged that evaluating patients for obesity should be an integral part of usual clinical care. One of the first groups to provide guidance on this topic was the National Heart, Lung, and Blood Institute (NHLBI) Clinical Guidelines on the Identification, Evaluation, and Treatment of Overweight and Obesity in Adults, which was first published in *Obesity Research* in 1998 *(15)*. More recently, a comprehensive evaluation of the evidence for screening for obesity in adults was published by the US Preventive Services Task Force (USPSTF) *(16)* along with recommendations for clinical evaluation *(17)*. This organization, which is relatively conservative and firmly evidence-based, felt that determining BMI in adult patients was justified and that there was fair evidence that high-intensity counseling produces modest, sustained weight loss. More recently, following the publication of the USPSTF report, the American College of Physicians (ACP), the professional organization that represents the field of internal medicine, published meta-analyses of pharmacotherapy *(18)* and surgical therapy *(19)* for obesity and took the position that it was reasonable to discuss these interventions with obese patients who had not reached a weight-loss goal through behavioral means alone *(20)*. A large number of organizations have taken positions advocating more awareness of obesity as a health problem, encouraging screening for associated illnesses and a more aggressive approach to counseling patients about diet and physical activity. These include the American Heart Association *(21)*, the American Academy of Pediatrics *(22)*, the American Gastroenterological Association *(23)*, the American College of Preventive Medicine *(24)*, the American Diabetes Association *(25)*, and the Surgeon General *(26)*, to name just a few. It seems clear that addressing weight as a health issue with patients in primary and specialty care has been recognized as a legitimate even mainstream part of clinical care.

Most Clinicians Currently Do Not Address Obesity

Despite the weight of the evidence and the broad consensus, there remains a great deal of clinical inertia against making a diagnosis of obesity and advising patients to lose weight. One study of more than 55,000 ambulatory care visits from the mid-1990s found that physicians reported obesity in only 38% and counseled only one-quarter of their obese patients *(27)*. In another study of more than 12,000 obese adults, only 42% were advised to lose weight, and yet those who were so advised were more likely to try to do so *(28)*. One might think that things have improved over the past 10 yr, but a recent study found that the number of patients who received advice to lose weight was actually lower in 2000 than it was in 1994 (40%, down from 44%) *(29)*. Physicians feel that there are many barriers to counseling their patients about weight loss. These include insufficient confidence, knowledge, and skills, as well as a perception that there are no effective therapies *(30)*. Physicians seem more likely to discuss weight management with their patients who have comorbid illnesses or are severely obese, or with those who are more educated and have a higher socioeconomic status *(29,31)*. This is despite the fact that helping patients change their lifestyle behaviors, use weight loss medications, or have bariatric surgery results in measurable health benefits *(32,33)*. The health benefits of treating obese patients are discussed in more detail in other parts of this book. Perhaps as physicians gain broader experience in the treatment of obese patients and health care delivery systems invest in the management of this chronic disorder, this unfortunate circumstance will change. Obesity is a diagnosis that is easy to make and one for which proven treatment modalities exist *(34)*.

DEFINING OBESITY

Body Mass Index

There is general agreement that BMI, which is the weight adjusted for height, is the best way to initially evaluate patients for obesity. BMI, generally expressed as kg/m^2, is easily determined using measured height and weight and a table such as the one provided in the NHLBI and North American Association for the Study of Obesity's (NAASO, the Obesity Society) Practical Guide on the Identification, Evaluation, and Treatment of Overweight and Obesity in Adults (Table 1) *(35)*. An individual patient can then be placed in a risk category based on the BMI (Table 2). A healthy weight is defined as a BMI between 18.5 and 24.9, with overweight being defined by a BMI between 25 and 29.9 and obesity being the appropriate diagnosis when the BMI exceeds 30. The BMI is widely advocated for diagnosis and risk stratification because of its documented association with adverse health consequences and ease of determination in usual clinical practice.

Waist Circumference

One might wonder what aspect of body composition is most closely associated with the adverse health risks attributable to excess body weight and whether BMI is the best measure for risk stratification. Is the critical factor total fat mass, the relative amount of subcutaneous versus intra-abdominal fat, or ectopic fat deposition, to name just a few possibilities? A growing body of evidence suggests that adverse consequences of obesity are most closely associated with an accumulation of intra-abdominal fat *(36–38)*. The adverse health effects of increases in intra-abdominal fat are independent of other factors such as total fat, insulin resistance, or serum levels of nonesterified fatty acids. This compartment of adipose tissue can be estimated by measuring waist circumference. Waist circumference is most easily measured with a tape measure parallel to the floor, at the level of the superior iliac crest, while the patient is standing, at the end of a relaxed expiration (Fig. 1). Waist circumference is most useful in risk stratifying patients with a BMI between 25 and 35. When people have a BMI > 35, their health risks are quite high and waist circumference adds little to risk assessment. Table 2 depicts the cut-points advocated by the NHLBI and other consensus organizations for excess risk associated with an increase in waist circumference. These cutoffs are >40 in. for men and >35 in. for women.

Special Considerations for Specific Ethnic Groups

Even though a growing body of data suggests that waist circumference is a better predictor of health risks associated with obesity as compared with BMI *(39)*, it has become increasingly clear that the cut-points generally advocated for risk stratification have limitations. As one might expect, there appears to be a curvilinear relationship between waist circumference and health risks, as opposed to a "threshold effect." This means that health risks rise incrementally as waist circumference increases. Recent evidence suggests that the generally advocated cut-points may be too conservative for Caucasians *(39)*. There appear to be even greater concerns in the use of these cut-points for individuals from different ethnic groups. Zhu and coworkers examined data from NHANES to determine appropriate cutoffs for African Americans and Mexican Americans *(40)*. They found that cutoffs for African American men were 5 to 6 cm lower than the value for Caucasian men. Mexican American men were intermediate. There were few differences in waist-circumference cutoffs for women from different race–ethnicity groups found in this study. They concluded that waist-circumference measurements that correlated with BMIs of 25 and 30 overall for the three race–ethnicity groups examined were 89 and 101 cm for men and 83 and 94 cm for women. These numbers could then be used to classify people as overweight or obese based on waist circumference as opposed to BMI. Asian individuals also appear to have a greater risk of metabolic diseases at lower waist circumferences than Caucasian individuals. Some of this difference may relate to the lower average height in this ethnic group. Ethnic group specific cut points for waist circumference have recently been proposed by the International Diabetes Foundation in the context of its new definition for metabolic syndrome *(41)* (see below).The waist-to-height ratio is another anthropometric measure, which has been

Table 1
Body Mass Index

BMI	19	20	21	22	23	24	25	26	27	28	29	30	31	32	33	34	35
Height (inches)								Body weight (pounds)									
58	91	96	100	105	110	115	119	124	129	134	138	143	148	153	158	162	167
59	94	99	104	109	114	119	124	128	133	138	143	148	153	158	163	168	173
60	97	102	107	112	118	123	128	133	138	143	148	153	158	163	168	174	179
61	100	106	111	116	122	127	132	137	143	148	153	158	164	169	174	180	185
62	104	109	115	120	126	131	136	142	147	153	158	164	169	175	180	186	191
63	107	113	118	124	130	135	141	146	152	158	163	169	175	180	186	191	197
64	110	116	122	128	134	140	145	151	157	163	169	174	180	186	192	197	204
65	114	120	126	132	138	144	150	156	162	168	174	180	186	192	198	204	210
66	118	124	130	136	142	148	155	161	167	173	179	186	192	198	204	210	216
67	121	127	134	140	146	153	159	166	172	178	185	191	198	204	211	217	223
68	125	131	138	144	151	158	164	171	177	184	190	197	203	210	216	223	230
69	128	135	142	149	155	162	169	176	182	189	196	203	209	216	223	230	236
70	132	139	146	153	160	167	174	181	188	195	202	209	216	222	229	236	243
71	136	143	150	157	165	172	179	186	193	200	208	215	222	229	236	243	250
72	140	147	154	162	169	177	184	191	199	206	213	221	228	235	242	250	258
73	144	151	159	166	174	182	189	197	204	212	219	227	235	242	250	257	265
74	148	155	163	171	179	186	194	202	210	218	225	233	241	249	256	264	272
75	152	160	168	176	184	192	200	208	216	224	232	240	248	256	264	272	279
76	156	164	172	180	189	197	205	213	221	230	238	246	254	263	271	279	287

BMI	36	37	38	39	40	41	42	43	44	45	46	47	48	49	50	51	52	53	54
58	172	177	181	186	191	196	201	205	210	215	220	224	228	234	239	244	248	253	258
59	178	183	188	193	198	203	208	212	217	222	227	232	237	242	247	252	257	262	267
60	184	189	194	199	204	209	215	220	225	230	235	240	245	250	255	261	266	271	276

61	190	195	201	206	211	217	222	227	232	238	243	248	254	259	264	269	275	280	285
62	196	202	207	213	218	224	229	235	240	245	251	256	262	267	273	278	284	289	295
63	203	208	214	220	225	231	237	242	248	254	259	265	270	278	282	287	293	299	304
64	209	215	221	227	232	238	244	250	256	262	267	273	279	285	291	296	302	308	314
65	216	222	228	234	240	245	252	258	264	270	276	282	288	294	300	306	312	318	324
66	223	229	235	241	247	253	260	266	272	278	284	291	297	303	309	315	322	328	334
67	230	236	242	248	255	261	268	274	280	287	293	299	306	312	319	325	331	338	344
68	236	243	249	256	262	269	276	282	289	295	302	308	315	322	328	335	341	348	354
69	243	250	257	263	270	277	284	291	297	304	311	318	324	331	338	345	351	358	365
70	251	257	264	271	278	285	292	299	306	313	320	327	334	341	348	355	362	369	376
71	257	265	272	279	286	293	301	308	315	322	329	338	343	351	358	365	372	378	386
72	265	272	279	287	294	302	309	316	327	331	338	346	353	361	368	375	383	390	397
73	272	280	288	295	302	310	318	325	333	340	348	355	363	371	378	386	393	401	408
74	280	287	295	303	311	319	326	334	342	350	358	365	373	381	389	396	404	412	420
75	287	295	303	311	319	3274	335	343	351	359	367	375	383	391	399	407	415	423	432
76	295	304	312	320	328	336	344	353	361	369	377	385	394	402	410	418	426	435	443

Table 2
Increased Disease Risk Associated With Waist Circumference

	BMI (kg/m²)	Obesity class	Disease risk[a] (Relative to normal weight and waist circumference)	
			Men ≤40 in. (≤102 cm) Women ≤35 in. (≤88 cm)	>40 in. (>102 cm) >35 in. (>88 cm)
Underweight	<18.5		—	—
Normal[b]	18.5–24.9		—	—
Overweight	25.0–29.9		Increased	High
Obesity	30.0–34.9	I	High	Very High
	35.0–39.9	II	Very High	Very High
Extreme Obesity	≤40	III	Extrememly High	Extrememly High

[a]Disease risk for type 2 diabetes mellitus, hypertension, and CVD.
[b]Increased waist circumference can also be a marker for increased risk even in persons of normal weight.
Adapted from ref. *15*.

advocated by Hsieh and others to more accurately assess risk in overweight and obese individuals of Asian descent *(42)*. In a study of more than 8000 Japanese adults, a waist-to-height ratio (W/Ht) of ≤0.5 was found to be the factor most closely associated with an adverse metabolic risk profile *(43)*.

Measures of Body Composition

Some have advocated the use of bioelectrical impedance in an effort to provide patients with more specific information on lean body mass as well as body fat content *(44)*. Unfortunately, at this time there are technical limitations with this measure in those with a high BMI that limit its accuracy. As a result, there is not wide support for the use of bioelectrical impedance in the assessment of obese patients in clinical practice *(45)*. Measurements of skinfold thickness, air displacement plethysmography, underwater weighing, and dual-energy X-ray absorptiometry all can provide information on body fat and regional fat distribution. However, in routine practice, BMI and waist circumference provide adequate information for clinical assessment and initial risk stratification.

ASSESSING WEIGHT HISTORY

The pattern of weight change over time in an individual patient often gives important clues as to likely causes of weight gain, past successes and challenges in weight loss, and the reasons that the person is seeking assistance with their weight at this time. Asking questions about the history of weight gain including maximum lifetime weight, factors that were associated with periods of weight gain, and previous periods of weight loss with a focus on events that precipitated previous weight-loss attempts and relevant events associated with the termination of previous attempts at weight loss can be very revealing. One way to get at this information efficiently is to have patients draw a graph of their own weight over time *(46)*. In this manner, triggers for weight gain such as pregnancy, smoking cessation, introduction of a new medication, depression, or a mus-culoskeletal injury can be identified and the clinician can help the patient see the con-

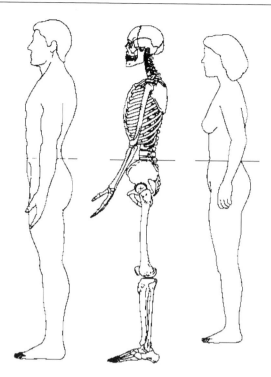

Fig. 1. Measuring tape position for waist (abdominal) circumference.

nection between these events and weight gain. A history of obesity during adolescence with progressive weight gain during adulthood strongly argues against a medical condition such as Cushing's syndrome as the cause of obesity.

Assessing previous weight-loss attempts is also important. Some patients comment with frustration that "diets never work for me." Often, though, when discussed in greater detail, previous efforts are revealed that produced an expected degree of weight loss (3–8%) that was not maintained because of difficulties in sustaining the chosen weight-loss strategy. Acknowledging and exploring these previous weight-loss attempts can provide a useful platform for discussing the amount of weight that is commonly lost with a diet and exercise program and to explore strategies that were or were not successful previously as a prelude to a discussion of potential future approaches to treatment. It is common to hear a person say that he or she tried Weight Watchers or the Atkins diet and had some success, but then encountered difficulties. This kind of discussion allows the clinician to provide empathy and support around what are extremely common, almost expected, periods of relapse. In addition, the patient's own experiences can be leveraged to emphasize the critical need for long-term behavior change strategies if maintenance of weight loss is the goal. It is important to emphasize to patients that it is possible to learn from previous weight-loss attempts and that if they do, future attempts need not be a replay of prior attempts. By learning what did and did not work from those previous attempts at weight loss, an improved, potentially more successful, approach can be crafted. Elements of treatment such as cost, time commitment, social support, types of foods consumed, self-monitoring, exercise, and the impact of special occasions, chronic illnesses, vacations, and work can be explored. Things that did work, as well as barriers to success, can be identified and incorporated into a new plan.

ASSESSING FOR SECONDARY CAUSES OF OBESITY

Endocrine Causes of Obesity

Many patients are concerned that they have a "metabolic" or "glandular" cause for their obesity. This may be a reflection of the frustration that some of these individuals feel over the difficulties that they have had in battling a weight problem over many years. They may be looking for a "medical" explanation of why they have not succeeded in their goal of losing weight. Endocrine causes of serious obesity are not common. The three most commonly cited are hypothyroidism, Cushing's syndrome, and hypothalamic obesity. To evaluate the patient for hypothyroidism, questions can be asked about cold intolerance, constipation, irregular menses, fatigue, or depression. The presence of easy bruisability, proximal muscle weakness (difficulty getting out of a chair, trouble getting things out of a high cupboard), a change in appearance, or osteoporosis may be signs of hypercortisolism. The patient can be examined for signs of hypothyroidism including bradycardia, cool dry skin, a firm palpable thyroid, and delayed reflexes. Cushing's syndrome, though often cited as an endocrine cause of obesity, is rarely found. Central obesity, enlarged supraclavicular fat pads, and a buffalo hump are features of hypercortisolism, but they are not very specific for the condition. More specific physical findings include a recent change in habitus demonstrated from old photographs, objective evidence of proximal muscle weakness, wide (>2 cm) violaceous striae, and visible unexplained bruising. Hypothalamic obesity is exceedingly rare and is associated with headaches, visual field defects, and evidence of hypothalamic/pituitary dysfunction. A serum thyroid-stimulating hormone (TSH) is the best test to rule out the presence of hypothyroidism. A 24-h urinary free cortisol level or an overnight 1-mg dexamethasone suppression test are the most widely used screening tests for hypercortisolism, although these tests have false negative and false positive results in a significant number of cases *(47,48)*. In particular, obese individuals, depressed persons, and chronic alcoholics may have increased cortisol on these screening tests that is not caused by any of the usual causes of Cushing's syndrome (ACTH-secreting tumor, ectopic ACTH secretion, or an adrenal tumor) *(49)*. Some have recently advocated a nighttime salivary cortisol as a good screening test; however this assay is not as widely available as the more traditional measures. The most common cause of hypothalamic obesity is the presence of a retrochiasmatic tumor such as a craniopharyngioma. This condition is predominantly encountered in children and obesity occurs following surgical resection in 25 to 75% of those affected.

Medications That Cause Obesity

Far more common, however, is weight gain associated with the introduction of medications to treat comorbid illnesses *(50)*. These include antidiabetic medications (sulfonylureas, thiazolidinediones, insulin) as well as a wide range of psychotropic medications. The antipsychotic drugs clozapine, olanzepine, risperidone, and quetiapine have all been associated with weight gain, as well as abnormalities in glucose homeostasis *(51)*. A number of antidepressant medications, incuding amitriptyline, mirtazapine, and some serotonin reuptake inhibitors, may promote weight gain in some patients. Other drugs that are used as mood stabilizers—including lithium, valproic acid, and carbamazepine—can cause weight gain. Finally, the antiepileptic drugs valproate, carbamazepine, and gabapentin can promote weight gain. Historically, psychiatrists and neurologists may have paid little attention to the weight-gaining properties of some of the medications that they prescribed. This is fortunately changing, but it is still common for a patient to be placed on a psychotropic medication or an antiepileptic medication and experience substantial weight gain without the knowledge of the provider who initially prescribed the medication.

Fortunately there are alternatives for each of these medications that could be considered if drug-associated weight gain is a serious problem. Metformin and newer GLP-1 analogs offer people with diabetes the benefits of glucose-lowering without weight gain and, in some patients, even mild weight loss. Bupropion is an antidepressant medication that has some weight-loss properties, although it does not have an FDA indication for weight loss (52). Topiramate is a medication that is FDA-approved as an antiepileptic medication and also for use in the treatment of migraines. It has some utility as a mood stabilizer and in the treatment of neuropathic pain. It has moderate weight-loss promoting properties (53,54). Topiramate has a number of side effects that limit its usefulness as a weight-loss drug and it is not FDA-approved for weight loss. However, if a patient has a seizure disorder or migraines, especially if weight gain has resulted from the use of other medications for these conditions, topiramate may be a reasonable alternative.

ASSESSING FOR HEALTH COMPLICATIONS OF OBESITY

Clinical Evaluation for Diseases Associated With Obesity

It is clear that obesity is associated with a wide range of adverse health consequences (55). These include type 2 diabetes, hypertension, hyperlipidemia, coronary artery disease, degenerative joint disease, depression, polycystic ovarian syndrome, some forms of cancer, sleep apnea, urinary stress incontinence, and erectile dysfunction, among others. Therefore, when evaluating an obese patient, it is important to tailor the visit in part around looking for evidence of these associated comorbid conditions. The initial evaluation should involve performing a directed history and physical examination with particular emphasis on signs or symptoms of these disorders. Evidence of the presence of any of these not only warrants further evaluation, but also has implications on the interventions that will be suggested to manage weight. Gallstones are more common in obese patients, and an inquiry should be made for symptoms consistent with episodic biliary obstruction. Symptoms of reflux esophagitis or urinary stress incontinence may be present as a result of increased intra-abdominal pressure, which is a feature of serious obesity. A history of polycystic ovarian disease in women and erectile dysfunction in men may be found, as both have a well-documented association with obesity. Daytime hypersomnolence, morning headaches, and a history of snoring may alert the clinician to the presence of obstructive sleep apnea.

The physical examination should include measurement of blood pressure in the seated position with an appropriately sized cuff. The Joint National Commission has given clear guidelines on the management of hypertension that can then be used to make decisions based on this measured blood pressure (56). Acanthosis nigricans and skin tags are cutaneous manifestations of insulin resistance and hyperinsulinemia that may be seen. Because of the increased risk of cancer in obese patients, it is important to do a breast or prostate exam where appropriate and make sure that appropriate screening for colorectal cancer, including stool hemoccult testing, is done.

Laboratory Evaluation of the Obese Patient

Although one could make a case for obtaining a large number of biochemical tests in the evaluation of an obese patient, a more limited initial screen seems warranted. A fasting sample of blood for glucose; total, LDL, and HDL cholesterol; and triglyceride levels is clearly indicated. These tests, along with an appropriate history, will provide the information necessary for cardiovascular risk stratification and can be used to rule out diabetes or impaired fasting glucose *(25,57)*. Some have advocated obtaining a glycosylated hemoglobin (HbA1C) level to screen for diabetes. Although this test should be useful in the diagnosis of diabetes, the assay method has not been standardized and at this time there is no widely accepted diagnostic criteria for diabetes based on an HbA1C level. In addition, some have advocated obtaining a fasting insulin level to determine whether insulin resistance is present. Unfortunately, here again, methods for assaying insulin have not been standardized and there are no widely accepted diagnostic criteria for diagnosing insulin resistance based on an insulin level. Although metrics such as the homeostasis model assessment (HOMA) calculation, which use the fasting insulin and glucose levels, have a greater ability to estimate insulin action, the same problem with nonstandardized insulin assays apply, so this approach is not yet appropriate for general clinical use. In fact, the waist circumference and fasting triglyceride and glucose levels give almost as much information about insulin action as a HOMA calculation *(58)*. A plasma measure of high high-sensitivity C-reactive protein (hsCRP) appears to also provide useful information in risk-stratifying patients for cardiovascular disease (CVD) risk *(59)*. It is increasingly becoming clear that inflammation plays an important role in CVD risk, and the level of hsCRP provides an indication of the degree of inflammation present in an individual patient *(60)*. Statin therapy has been shown to reduce hsCRP levels, and CVD outcomes correlate with the degree of hsCRP achieved following statin therapy *(61,62)*. However, the exact role of measuring hsCRP levels in overall CVD risk management remains undefined at this time.

Metabolic Syndrome

It is clear that obesity is often associated with a cluster of metabolic disorders that increase the risk of cardiovascular disease and diabetes. These include insulin resistance, glucose intolerance, hypertension, hyperlipidemia, activation of inflammatory pathways, endothelial dysfunction, and nonalcoholic steatohepatitis, to name just a few. This cluster of disorders has been called syndrome X, insulin resistance syndrome, and other names, but most now refer to this condition as metabolic syndrome. Initially proposed by a number of thoughtful clinical investigators including Dr. Gerald Reaven, metabolic syndrome came into broader awareness when formal diagnostic criteria were proposed first by the World Health Organization and then the National Cholesterol Education Program in its Adult Treatment Panel III guidelines (NCEP-ATPIII) *(57)*. There have been a number of other diagnostic criteria proposed by a range of professional organizations since then. The most recent, and perhaps best formulated, diagnostic criteria have come from the American Heart Association in conjunction with the National Heart Lung and Blood institute (AHA/NHLBI) *(63)* and the International Diabetes Federation (IDF) *(41)*. In the paper from the AHA/NHLBI an updated version of the NCEP criteria for defining metabolic syndrome is proposed, and is shown in Table 3. The criteria have changed little with the exception that the criterion for increased fasting glucose has been

Table 3
Criteria for Clinical Diagnosis of Metabolic Syndrome

Measure (any 3 of 5 constitute diagnosis of metabolic syndrome)	Categorical cut-points
Elevated waist circumference[a,b]	≥102 cm (≥40 in.) in men ≥88 cm (≥35 in.) in women
Elevated triglycerides	≥150 mg/dL (1.7 mmol/L) or On drug treatment for elevated triglycerides[c]
Reduced HDL-C	<40 mg/dl (1.03 mmol/L) in men <50 mg/dL (1.3 mmol/L) in women or On drug treatment for reduced HDL-C[c]
Elevated blood pressure	≥130 mmHg systolic blood pressure or ≥85mmHg diastolic blood pressure or On antihypertensive drug treatment in a patient with a history of hypertension
Elevated fasting glucose	≥100 mg/dL or On drug treatment for elevated glucose

[a]To measure waist circumference, locate top of right iliac crest. Place a measuring tape in a horizontal plane around abdomen at level of iliac crest. Before reading tape measure, ensure that tape is snug but does not compress the skin and is parallel to the floor. Measurement is made at the end of a normal expiration.
[b]Some US adults of non-Asian origin (e.g., white, black, Hispanic) with marginally increased waist circumference (e.g., 94–101 cm [37–39 in.] in men and 80–87 cm [31–34 in.] in women) may have strong genetic contribution to insulin resistance and should benefit from changes in lifestyle habits, similar to men with categorical increases in waist circumference. A lower waist circumference cut-point (e.g., ≥ 90 cm [35 in.] in men and ≥80 cm [31 in.] in women) appears to be appropriate for Asian Americans.
[c]Fibrates and nicotinic acid are the most commonly used drugs for elevated TG and reduced HDL-C. Patients taking one of these drugs are presumed to have high TG and low HDL.

reduced from 110 to 100 mg/dL in line with the new definition for impaired fasting glucose from the American Diabetes Association, and lipid and blood pressure criteria now explicitly state that if a person is on a medication to treat one of these conditions, he or she is considered to have that condition. In recognition of the evidence that Asian Americans may experience increased metabolic risk at a smaller waist circumference, alternative cut-points for waist circumference of 35 in. in men and 31 in. in women are proposed for individuals from this ethnic background. The IDF has proposed a definition that requires central obesity, defined by an increased waist circumference, to be present in conjunction with other criteria. The details of this definition are depicted in Table 4. The IDF definition gives a range of ethnic specific waist cut-points (Table 5).

Table 4
IDF Definition of Metabolic Syndrome

Central obesity
Waist circumference[a]—ethnicity-specific (*see* Table 3)
Plus any two:
  Raised triglycerides
    >150 mg/dL (1.7 mmol/L)
    Specific treatment for this lipid abnormaligy
  Reduced HDL-cholesterol
    <40 mg/dL (1.03 mmol/L) in men
    <50 mg/dL (1.29 mmol/L) in women
    Specific treatment for this lipid abnormality
  Raised blood pressure
    Systolic ≥130 mmHg
    Diastolic ≥85 mmHg
    Treatment of previously diagnosed hypertension
  Raised fasting plasma glucose[b]
    Fasting plasma glucose $100 mg/dL (5.6 mmol/L)
    Previously diagnosed type 2 diabetes
    If above 5.6 mmol/L or 100 mg/dL, oral glucose tolerance test is strongly recommended,
    but is not necessary to define presence of syndrome

[a]BMI is over 30 kg/m2, central obesity can be assumed and waist circumference does not need to be measured.
[b]In clinical practice, impaired glucose tolerance is also acceptable, but all reports of prevalence of metabolic syndrome should use only fasting plasma glucose and presence of previously diagnosed diabetes to define hyperglycemia. Prevalences also incorporating 2-h glucose results can be added as supplementary findings.

In a controversial recent paper, the American Diabetes Association (ADA) and the European Association for the Study of Diabetes (EASD) took the provocative position that there is currently inadequate information available to accurately define metabolic syndrome and that this designation should not be used in routine clinical practice (64). This view grew out of a belief that the root cause of this clustering is not known and could include obesity, insulin resistance, or inflammation. The authors of this paper also felt that although the clustering of these conditions increases the risk of cardiovascular disease, it was not clear that the syndrome had any greater risk than the sum of the component parts. This alternative view from a respected organization has caused confusion for many physicians.

The confusion over definitions and the appropriateness of the diagnosis of metabolic syndrome, however, should not take away from what all agree on. It is clear that the presence of abdominal obesity, hyperlipidemia, hypertension, insulin resistance, glucose intolerance, and inflammation are very common (65) and increase a person's risk for both CVD (66,67) and diabetes (68). It is clear that each of these parameters has predictive power for both diabetes and CVD. The term "syndrome" refers simply to a clustering of signs and symptoms; it doesn't necessarily mean that we have a clear etiology, and a lack of consensus on the etiology doesn't necessarily mean that there is no value in identifying the condition. It seems that the designation of "metabolic syn-

Table 5
Waist Circumference Cut-Points for Various Ethnic Groups

Ethnic group	Waist circumference(as measure of central obesity)
Europids[a]	
Men	≥94 cm
Women	≥80 cm
South Asians	
Men	≥90 cm
Women	≥80 cm
Chinese	
Men	≥90 cm
Women	≥80 cm
Japanese	
Men	≥85 cm
Women	≥90 cm
Ethnic south and central Americans	Use south Asian recommendations until more specific data are available
Sub-Saharan Africans	Use European data until more specific data are available
Eastern Mediterranean and middle east (Arab) populations	Use European data until more specific data are available

Data are pragmatic cutoffs and better data are required to link them to risl, Ethnicity should be basis for classifications, not country of residence.

[a]In the United States, Adult Treatment Panel values (102 cm male, 88 cm female) are likely to continue to be used for clinical purposes. In future epidemiological studies of populations of Europid origin (white people of European origin, regardless of where they live in the world), prevalence should be given, with both European and North American cutoffs to allow better comparisons.

drome" by the AHA/NHLBI/NCEP has been useful in raising awareness about the role of obesity and other factors in increasing CVD risk. It also seems that, although there remains no clear consensus on the definition or treatment, continuing to use the NCEP criteria as a screening strategy for this clustering is a reasonable clinical strategy that likely represents the mainstream of clinical care at this time. The designation may especially be useful as a way to convey to patients a sense of their CVD risk and help them come to decisions about modifying diet and physical activity behaviors.

ASSESSING ENERGY INTAKE

Weight change is produced by a long-term imbalance between energy intake (EI) and energy expenditure (EE). Weight gain occurs only when EI > EE, and weight loss will occur only when EE > EI. If weight is stable, then EE = EI. The problem is that it is extremely difficult to accurately measure either EI or EE in a clinical environment. An extensive body of research demonstrates that virtually everyone underestimates EI when asked to self-report food intake. The best measure of EE is a method known as doubly labeled water. This method can accurately determine EE over a period of weeks in free-living individuals. In a number of studies, self-reported food intake underestimated measured EE by an average of almost 30% *(69)*. A number of factors, including BMI, previous weight-loss history, and fear of negative evaluation, have been shown to be associated with underreporting of EI *(70)*.

The reality that people tend to underreport food intake, however, does not undermine the importance of gaining as much information as is reasonably possible on this important parameter. Information on food intake can be easily obtained in an office visit using a 24-h, 3-d, or 7-d dietary recall or a food frequency questionnaire. Information about meal patterns, fast food consumption, calories consumed in beverages, and "trigger foods" that tend to be overeaten can be identified. Even though the information may not be completely accurate, asking for a self-report of food intake such as a 24-h dietary recall on each office visit emphasizes to the patient that the clinician feels that this information is critical in assessing weight health. Diet-record forms can be printed and made available in the office so that patients can collect more extensive information between visits. Handy tools that help patients estimate portion sizes can help improve the quality of information obtained from diet records as well as building a foundation on which dietary interventions can be built. In fact, self-monitoring of the diet appears to be a key feature of both successful short- and long-term weight loss *(71)*. For those patients who use the Internet and computer programs regularly, a number of diet-monitoring tools are available for either PDA- or PC-based use. These are outlined, along with tools for self-monitoring of exercise, in Table 6.

Taking a good diet history can provide useful information about situations and precipitating factors associated with overeating. The patient can be encouraged to look for a "chain of events" that led to a loss of control over food choices. Were meals skipped? Was stress involved? What were the circumstances by which the particular foods overeaten were available? Was food eaten while the person was engaged in other activities, such as television watching? In this manner the patient can begin to identify points along this sequence of events that could be modified through alternative approaches to similar situations that will likely recur in the future. Although a busy clinician may not have time to completely explore these issues in a brief office visit, some attention should be paid to diet at both the initial and subsequent visits where weight is discussed.

ASSESSING ENERGY EXPENDITURE

Energy Expenditure and Obesity

Energy expenditure is made up of three components: basal metabolic rate (BMR), which can be estimated as resting energy expenditure (REE), which has also been called resting metabolic rate (RMR); thermic effect of food, which makes up only a small fraction of total daily energy expenditure; and energy expended in physical activity (EEPA), which is by far the most variable among individuals. Although patients often complain that they have a "low metabolic rate," careful studies have conclusively shown that REE is linearly related to lean body mass *(72)*. This means that heavier people have higher REE than thin individuals, and as a result need to eat more on average each day to maintain their higher weight. It is likely that the rise in the prevalence of obesity is the result not only of increased EI associated within the modern food environment, but also of a reduction in the habitual levels of EEPA associated with a modern environment filled with technologies designed to reduce the need for physical labor *(73)*. There is

Table 6
Popular Internet Diet and Exercise Tracking Tools

Program Name/Website	PDA/PC	Comments	Cost
Balance Log	Both		$29.95 PDA
www.healthetech.com	(software)		$49.94 Both
BeNutriFit	PC		$19.95 PC
www.benutrifit	(software)		
Calorie King	Both		$19.95 PDA
www.calorieking.com	(software)		$29.95 PC
Crosstrainer	Both	In addition to tracking, provides exercise	$49.95 PC
www.crosstrainer.ca	(software)	prescription	$64.95 Both
Diet and Exercise Assistant	Both		$19.95 PDA
www.keyoe.com	(software)		$9.95 PC
DietPro	PC	In addition to tracking, provides	$64.95 PC
www.dietpro.net	(software)	menu plans/diet prescription	
FitDay	PC	Tracks mood in addition	$29.95 PC
www.fitday.com	(Internet and software)	to diet and exercise	
Health Fit Counter	Both		$29.95 PDA
www.heatlthcoutner.com	(software)	$29.95 PC	
Mealformation	PC	No exercise tracking. Focuses on food	$49.00 basic
www.mealformation.com	(software)	menu plans, and shopping lists	$169.00 expanded
My Food Diary	PC	In addition to tracking, provides	$108/year
www.myfooddiary.com	(Internet)	social support for sharing ideas, recipes,	
		and social support	
My Sport Training	Both	In addition to tracking	$24.95 PDA
www.mysporttraining.com	(software)	provides exercise prescription	$24.95 PDA
Nutrawatch	PC		$14.95/year
www.nutrawatch.com	(Internet)		
Nutrigenie	PC	In addition to tracking, provides	$49.00 PC
www.nutrigenie.biz	(software)	menu plans/diet prescripton	
Small Steps	PC	No diet tracking, only	Free
www.smallstep.gov	(Internet)	exercise tracking	
USDA Food Pyramid	PC	In addition to tracking, provides	Free
www.mypyramid.com	(Internet)	basic menu plans and exercise prescription	

increasing evidence that the low levels of physical activity that characterize a sedentary lifestyle are associated with not only obesity *(74)* and type 2 diabetes *(75)*, but also increased mortality *(76,77)*. Conversely, increased levels of physical activity and high levels of cardiorespiratory fitness are associated with reduced levels of morbidity and cardiovascular mortality *(78–80)*.

Physical Activity

Clinicians can and should solicit information about usual levels of physical activity as part of the initial evaluation and at follow-up visits. Questions such as "how often do you engage in planned physical activity?" or "do you ever walk for exercise?" can be helpful. Asking about participation in sports or active pursuits in the past can also provide a useful background on which plans for increases in physical activity to manage weight can be based. Questions about the amount of time spent in sedentary activities such as television watching, using the computer, or reading also provide useful information about habitual activity levels. In addition, time spent in these sedentary activities may be available for active pursuits should the person choose to increase his or her physical activity level. A number of physical activity questionnaires are available to obtain more in-depth information on energy expended in activities of daily living, as well as planned bouts of exercise. As is the case with assessing EI, there are substantial limitations to the measurement of EE in clinical practice. If people tend to underreport food intake, they tend to overreport levels of physical activity. Adults overestimate EEPA by as much as 50% *(81)*. Overreporting EEPA tends to be a greater problem in obese individuals as compared with lean ones, and in some groups tends to get worse following the initiation of a weight-loss program *(82)*.

More objective information about habitual levels of physical activity can be obtained through the use of physical activity monitoring systems. The simplest of these is the pedometer or step counter. These devices are worn at the waist and count the number of steps accumulated over a day or week (83,84). A pedometer can be purchased for $10 to $30 and can be used to characterize an individual as sedentary (2000–5000 steps/d), normal activity (5000–8000 steps/d), meeting guidelines for PA at a level to prevent weight gain (8000–11,000 steps/d), or highly active or active at a level commensurate with that needed to produce and maintain weight loss (11,000–15,000 steps/d). Pedometers have limitations: some cheaper models may be inaccurate, and accuracy may be reduced in obese individuals owing to difficulties in keeping the device in a proper vertical alignment when worn on the belt and reduced sensitivity with slow walking speeds. Like dietary self-monitoring, physical activity self-monitoring using either a pedometer or minutes of moderate physical activity per week is valuable not only in assessing the causes of weight gain, but also for laying a foundation for subsequent interventions *(85)*. A number of newer devices may become more widely available to provide more accurate information on EEPA in free-living individuals. These include the SenseWear armband made by Body Media, the Actiwatch and Actical physical activity monitors made by Mini Mitter, and StayHealthy's RT3 (formerly known as the Tritrack R3D) triaxial accelerometer. These devices and others under development combine measures of movement in space with other physiological measures such as heart rate, skin temperature, and galvanic skin response to estimate EEPA in free-living individuals. These systems tend to be moderately complex and require specialized software for analysis, making them much less user-friendly than the pedometer.

Indirect Calorimetry to Measure Energy Expenditure

Another tool that can be used clinically to measure energy expenditure is indirect calorimetry. The indirect calorimeter measures air flow and the difference in the concentration of oxygen between inspired and expired air to determine oxygen consumption, which is then used to calculate energy expenditure in kcal/h. When measured in the resting state, indirect calorimetry gives an estimate of REE/RMR that can be used to estimate daily energy requirements. For most people, total daily energy expenditure (which equals daily energy intake for weight maintenance) is roughly 1.3 to 1.5 times RMR. A number of indirect calorimetry systems are commercially available to consumers and health care providers for the measurement of RMR. These include the MedGem and BodyGem devices made by Healthetech (www.healthetech.com) and the ReeVue device made by Korr (www.korr.com), to name just a few. These indirect calorimeter devices are designed to directly measure oxygen consumption. However, this is a very technically difficult measurement to make and it is not clear how accurate these devices are in a real clinical environment. Overall it is not clear at this time that these devices add substantially to clinical assessment. However, in the future it seems likely that devices such as these will increasingly be incorporated into the clinical management of overweight and obese patients.

OTHER ASPECTS OF BEHAVIORAL EVALUATION

In addition to gaining information on the weight history and usual diet and physical activity patterns, it is important, if appropriate, to ask patients about their reasons for thinking about weight loss at this time, their weight loss goals, and their readiness for various treatment modalities. These behavioral factors will have a direct bearing on the weight-management advice given. Clinical experience and clinical studies demonstrate that many obese patients seeking treatment have unrealistic expectations of what their weight will be after treatment *(86)*. When patients seeking treatment for obesity were asked what their dream weight loss would be, they reported a 38% weight loss. When asked what level of weight loss would be disappointing—not successful in any way—they reported a 15% weight loss. As most behavioral treatment programs give an average of a 5 to 10% weight loss, patients seeking treatment are likely to be disappointed. However, it seems that despite these high expectations, patients can find satisfaction with more modest degrees of weight loss. It seems that encouraging patients to "lower their expectations" does not improve treatment outcomes *(87)*.

At a minimum, it may be useful to ask patients what their expectations of treatment are. If they articulate a desire for dramatic weight loss, it may be useful to acknowledge this as a common goal in patients embarking on a treatment plan, but that there appear to be clear health benefits to more modest degrees of weight loss. The care provider can place more emphasis on achievable behavioral goals such as changes in food intake, making regular physical activity a priority, or even smaller goals such as self-monitoring of the diet or purchasing a pedometer as a place to start.

Depression and anxiety are common in obese patients seeking treatment. This is true for men *(88,89)* as well as women *(90)*. It is important to ask patients about the presence of symptoms of depression and determine whether there is a history of depression in the past. Feelings about the benefits and shortcomings of previous periods of treatment for depression can be explored. It is often difficult to determine with certainty whether the obesity is causing/exacerbating the depression or whether depression is promoting weight gain. Having said this, it may be difficult for patients to succeed in the difficult task of modifying diet and physical activity behaviors when they are feeling extremely depressed. In situations where patients report a lack of energy, feelings of hopelessness, and a sense of lack of control over their mood, and certainly if there is any suggestion of suicidal ideation, referral to a mental health professional may be the best first step before embarking on any discussion of weight management. As patients may fear abandonment, the care provider can reassure the patient that the goal is only to have the patient succeed in the attempt at losing weight and that the provider will continue to follow the patient on a regular basis while he or she is exploring treatment for an underlying depression.

A formal psychological assessment is particularly important before weight-loss surgery (91). This evaluation ensures that the patient is making an informed and reasoned decision, allows for optimization of the psychological state prior to surgery, and forms a therapeutic foundation should postoperative depression become a problem. Although weight-loss surgery has been shown to produce an improvement in mood over the long run (92), a significant number of patients experience a period of depression in the 6 mo following bariatric surgery. Whereas the presence of a serious or unstable psychological disorder is a contraindication to bariatric surgery, there remains controversy about exactly what degree of pathology justifies this step in an individual who is otherwise a good candidate. In the past it was felt that the patient needed to maintain a high level of dietary compliance following the surgery. More recently, as evidence has accumulated that bariatric surgery may have a biological mechanism of action, some have performed this procedure in patients with stable but serious psychiatric diagnoses or binge-eating disorder and have had acceptable levels of success. Clearly the input of an experienced psychiatrist or psychologist in the evaluation of these patients is extremely important.

ROLE OF ALLIED HEALTH PROFESSIONALS IN ASSESSMENT OF THE OBESE PATIENT

The evaluation proposed here is extensive. It may be unrealistic to expect a busy clinician to obtain, evaluate, and counsel around all the information that could be discussed with an obese patient. An alternative is to identify individuals with unique skills and specialized resources in the clinical environment who can be brought into service during the evaluation and treatment of these patients. Examples include registered dieticians to assist in evaluation of the diet, exercise physiologists who help with assessing exercise capacity and the safety of initiating an exercise program, psychologists or psychiatrists to help evaluate and treat psychological comorbidities such as depression, pharmacists who have an interest in weight loss medications, and surgeons who have experience in bariatric surgery. If a clinician is interested in taking a more active role in managing obesity in his or her practice it will be useful to identify resources in the community to refer patients to. Having written materials available to patients in the office will make these referrals more efficient for both the care provider and the patient.

CONCLUSION

Obesity is common and growing in prevalence. It is associated with an increased risk for a wide range of comorbid conditions, increased health care costs, and disability. Clinicians are in a unique position to have a positive impact on the health of their obese patients. There is a broad consensus now that the BMI should be calculated for all adult patients and that this number should be used in risk stratification. For those with a BMI between 25 and 35, the waist circumference adds clinically useful information and should also be obtained.

Overweight and obese patients should have a complete history and physical to screen for comorbid conditions. Targeted laboratory studies should also be obtained to both look for disorders that can cause obesity as well as to screen for diseases that are associated with obesity. Assessing food intake and physical activity behaviors is the foundation on which treatment recommendations can be built. A number of tools are now available to assist the clinician in assessing these parameters, which are subject to inaccurate self-reports. To successfully manage obesity the clinician should take care to assess the patient's readiness to change, as well as ask questions that will help reveal the presence of any comorbid psychological conditions. Finally, the clinician should develop relationships with other professionals such as dieticians, psychologists, exercise physiologists, and pharmacists to help them in the evaluation and management of their obese patients. Other chapters in this book will provide specific advice on treatment approaches that can be used to help overweight and obese patients lose weight and maintain a reduced state.

REFERENCES

1. Hedley AA, Ogden CL, Johnson CL, et al. Prevalence of overweight and obesity among US children, adolescents, and adults, 1999–2002. JAMA 2004;291(23):2847–2850.
2. Ajani UA, Lotufo PA, Gaziano JM, et al. Body mass index and mortality among US male physicians. Ann Epidemiol 2004;14(10):731–739.
3. Fontaine KR, Redden DT, Wang C, et al. Years of life lost due to obesity. JAMA 2003;289(2):187–193.
4. Peeters A, Barendregt JJ, Willekens F, et al. Obesity in adulthood and its consequences for life expectancy: a life-table analysis. Ann Intern Med 2003;138(1):24–32.
5. Flegal KM, Graubard BI, Williamson DF, et al. Excess deaths associated with underweight, overweight, and obesity. JAMA 2005;293(15):1861–1867.
6. Gregg EW, Cheng YJ, Cadwell BL, et al. Secular trends in cardiovascular disease risk factors according to body mass index in US adults. JAMA 2005;293(15):1868–1874.
7. Bungum T, Satterwhite M, Jackson AW, et al. The relationship of body mass index, medical costs, and job absenteeism. Am J Health Behav 2003;27(4):456–462.
8. Swallen KC, Reither EN, Haas SA, et al. Overweight, obesity, and health-related quality of life among adolescents: the National Longitudinal Study of Adolescent Health. Pediatrics 2005;115(2):340–347.
9. Bertakis KD, Azari R. Obesity and the use of health care services. Obes Res 2005;13(2):372–379.
10. Daviglus ML, Liu K, Yan LL, et al. Relation of body mass index in young adulthood and middle age to Medicare expenditures in older age. JAMA 2004;292(22):2743–2749.
11. Wang F, Schultz AB, Musich S, et al. The relationship between National Heart, Lung, and Blood Institute Weight Guidelines and concurrent medical costs in a manufacturing population. Am J Health Promot 2003;17(3):183–189.
12. Wee CC, Phillips RS, Legedza AT, et al. Health care expenditures associated with overweight and obesity among US adults: importance of age and race. Am J Public Health 2005;95(1):159–165.
13. Quesenberry CP, Jr., Caan B, Jacobson A. Obesity, health services use, and health care costs among members of a health maintenance organization. Arch Intern Med 1998;158(5):466–472.
14. Thompson D, Edelsberg J, Kinsey KL, et al. Estimated economic costs of obesity to U.S. business. Am J Health Promot 1998;13(2):120–127.
15. Clinical Guidelines on the Identification, Evaluation, and Treatment of Overweight and Obesity in Adults—The Evidence Report. National Institutes of Health. Obes Res 1998;6 Suppl 2:51S–209S.
16. McTigue KM, Harris R, Hemphill B, et al. Screening and interventions for obesity in adults: summary of the evidence for the U.S. Preventive Services Task Force. Ann Intern Med 2003;139(11):933–949.

17. US Preventive Services Task Force. Screening for obesity in adults: recommendations and rationale. Ann Intern Med 2003;139(11):930–932.
18. Li Z, Maglione M, Tu W, et al. Meta-analysis: pharmacologic treatment of obesity. Ann Intern Med 2005;142(7):532–546.
19. Maggard MA, Shugarman LR, Suttorp M, et al. Meta-analysis: surgical treatment of obesity. Ann Intern Med 2005;142(7):547–559.
20. Snow V, Barry P, Fitterman N, et al. Pharmacologic and surgical management of obesity in primary care: a clinical practice guideline from the American College of Physicians. Ann Intern Med 2005;142(7):525–531.
21. Klein S, Burke LE, Bray GA, et al. Clinical implications of obesity with specific focus on cardiovascular disease: a statement for professionals from the American Heart Association Council on Nutrition, Physical Activity, and Metabolism: endorsed by the American College of Cardiology Foundation. Circulation 2004;110(18):2952–2967.
22. Krebs NF, Jacobson MS. Prevention of pediatric overweight and obesity. Pediatrics 2003;112(2):424–430.
23. American Gastroenterological Association medical position statement on obesity. Gastroenterology 2002;123(3):879–881.
24. Nawaz H, Katz DL. American College of Preventive Medicine Practice Policy statement. Weight management counseling of overweight adults. Am J Prev Med 2001;21(1):73–78.
25. American Diabetes Association. Standards of medical care in diabetes. Diabetes Care 2005;28 Suppl 1:S4–S36.
26. Jackson Y, Dietz WH, Sanders C, et al. Summary of the 2000 Surgeon General's listening session: toward a national action plan on overweight and obesity. Obes Res 2002;10(12):1299–1305.
27. Stafford RS, Farhat JH, Misra B, et al. National patterns of physician activities related to obesity management. Arch Fam Med 2000;9(7):631–638.
28. Galuska DA, Will JC, Serdula MK, et al. Are health care professionals advising obese patients to lose weight? JAMA 1999;282(16):1576–1578.
29. Jackson JE, Doescher MP, Saver BG, et al. Trends in professional advice to lose weight among obese adults, 1994 to 2000. J Gen Intern Med 2005;20(9):814–818.
30. Huang J, Yu H, Marin E, Brock S, et al. Physicians' weight loss counseling in two public hospital primary care clinics. Acad Med 2004;79(2):156–161.
31. Simkin-Silverman LR, Gleason KA, King WC, et al. Predictors of weight control advice in primary care practices: patient health and psychosocial characteristics. Prev Med 2005;40(1):71–82.
32. Gregg EW, Gerzoff RB, Thompson TJ, et al. Trying to lose weight, losing weight, and 9-year mortality in overweight U.S. adults with diabetes. Diabetes Care 2004;27(3):657–662.
33. Gregg EW, Gerzoff RB, Caspersen CJ, et al. Relationship of walking to mortality among US adults with diabetes. Arch Intern Med 2003;163(12):1440–1447.
34. Kushner RF, Roth JL. Assessment of the obese patient. Endocrinol Metab Clin North Am 2003;32(4):915–933.
35. National Heart, Lung, and Blood Institute (NHLBI) and North American Association for the Study of Obesity (NAASO). Practical Guide on the Identification, Evaluation, and Treatment of Overweight and Obesity in Adults. NIH Publication No. 00-4084. National Institues of Health, Bethesda, MD: 2000.
36. Piche ME, Weisnagel SJ, Corneau L, et al. Contribution of abdominal visceral obesity and insulin resistance to the cardiovascular risk profile of postmenopausal women. Diabetes 2005;54(3):770–777.
37. Goodpaster BH, Krishnaswami S, Harris TB, et al. Obesity, regional body fat distribution, and the metabolic syndrome in older men and women. Arch Intern Med 2005;165(7):777–783.
38. Gastaldelli A, Miyazaki Y, Pettiti M, et al. Separate contribution of diabetes, total fat mass, and fat topography to glucose production, gluconeogenesis, and glycogenolysis. J Clin Endocrinol Metab 2004;89(8):3914–3921.
39. Wang Y, Rimm EB, Stampfer MJ, et al. Comparison of abdominal adiposity and overall obesity in predicting risk of type 2 diabetes among men. Am J Clin Nutr 2005;81(3):555–563.
40. Zhu S, Heymsfield SB, Toyoshima H, et al. Race-ethnicity-specific waist circumference cutoffs for identifying cardiovascular disease risk factors. Am J Clin Nutr 2005;81(2):409–415.
41. Alberti KG, Zimmet P, Shaw J. The metabolic syndrome—a new worldwide definition. Lancet 2005;366(9491):1059–1062.
42. Hsieh SD, Muto T. The superiority of waist-to-height ratio as an anthropometric index to evaluate clustering of coronary risk factors among non-obese men and women. Prev Med 2005;40(2):216–220.

43. Hsieh SD, Yoshinaga H, Muto T. Waist-to-height ratio, a simple and practical index for assessing central fat distribution and metabolic risk in Japanese men and women. Int J Obes Relat Metab Disord 2003;27(5):610–616.

44. Kyle UG, Bosaeus I, De Lorenzo AD, et al. Bioelectrical impedance analysis—part I: review of principles and methods. Clin Nutr 2004;23(5):1226–1243.

45. Kyle UG, Bosaeus I, De Lorenzo AD, et al. Bioelectrical impedance analysis—part II: utilization in clinical practice. Clin Nutr 2004;23(6):1430–1453.

46. Kushner RF, Blatner DJ. Risk assessment of the overweight and obese patient. J Am Diet Assoc 2005;105(5 Suppl 1):S53–S62.

47. Findling JW, Raff H. Screening and diagnosis of Cushing's syndrome. Endocrinol Metab Clin North Am 2005;34(2):385–402.

48. Raff H, Findling JW. A physiologic approach to diagnosis of the Cushing syndrome. Ann Intern Med 2003;138(12):980–991.

49. Lindsay JR, Nieman LK. Differential diagnosis and imaging in Cushing's syndrome. Endocrinol Metab Clin North Am 2005;34(2):403–421.

50. Ness-Abramof R, Apovian CM. Drug-induced weight gain. Drugs Today (Barc) 2005;41(8):547–555.

51. Bergman RN, Ader M. Atypical antipsychotics and glucose homeostasis. J Clin Psychiatry 2005;66(4):504–514.

52. Jain AK, Kaplan RA, Gadde KM, et al. Bupropion SR vs. placebo for weight loss in obese patients with depressive symptoms. Obes Res 2002;10(10):1049–1056.

53. Wilding J, Van GL, Rissanen A, et al. A randomized double-blind placebo-controlled study of the long-term efficacy and safety of topiramate in the treatment of obese subjects. Int J Obes Relat Metab Disord 2004;28(11):1399–1410.

54. Astrup A, Caterson I, Zelissen P, et al. Topiramate: long-term maintenance of weight loss induced by a low-calorie diet in obese subjects. Obes Res 2004;12(10):1658–1669.

55. Bray GA. Medical consequences of obesity. J Clin Endocrinol Metab 2004;89(6):2583–2589.

56. Chobanian AV, Bakris GL, Black HR, et al. The Seventh Report of the Joint National Committee on Prevention, Detection, Evaluation, and Treatment of High Blood Pressure: the JNC 7 report. JAMA 2003;289(19):2560–2572.

57. Executive Summary of The Third Report of The National Cholesterol Education Program (NCEP) Expert Panel on Detection, Evaluation, and Treatment of High Blood Cholesterol In Adults (Adult Treatment Panel III). JAMA 2001;285(19):2486–2497.

58. McLaughlin T, Abbasi F, Cheal K, et al. Use of metabolic markers to identify overweight individuals who are insulin resistant. Ann Intern Med 2003;139(10):802–809.

59. Libby P, Ridker PM. Inflammation and atherosclerosis: role of C-reactive protein in risk assessment. Am J Med 2004;116 Suppl 6A:9S–16S.

60. Willerson JT, Ridker PM. Inflammation as a cardiovascular risk factor. Circulation 2004;109(21 Suppl 1):II2–II10.

61. Nissen SE. Effect of intensive lipid lowering on progression of coronary atherosclerosis: evidence for an early benefit from the Reversal of Atherosclerosis with Aggressive Lipid Lowering (REVERSAL) trial. Am J Cardiol 2005;96(5A):61F–68F.

62. Kinjo K, Sato H, Sakata Y, et al. Relation of C-reactive protein and one-year survival after acute myocardial infarction with versus without statin therapy. Am J Cardiol 2005;96(5):617–621.

63. Grundy SM, Cleeman JI, Daniels SR, et al. Diagnosis and management of the metabolic syndrome: an American Heart Association/National Heart, Lung, and Blood Institute Scientific Statement. Circulation 2005;112(17):2735–2752.

64. Kahn R, Buse J, Ferrannini E, et al. The metabolic syndrome: time for a critical appraisal. Joint statement from the American Diabetes Association and the European Association for the Study of Diabetes. Diabetologia 2005;48(9):1684–1699.

65. Ford ES. Prevalence of the metabolic syndrome defined by the International Diabetes Federation among adults in the U.S. Diabetes Care 2005;28(11):2745–2749.

66. Ford ES. Risks for all-cause mortality, cardiovascular disease, and diabetes associated with the metabolic syndrome: a summary of the evidence. Diabetes Care 2005;28(7):1769–1778.

67. Rutter MK, Meigs JB, Sullivan LM, et al. Insulin resistance, the metabolic syndrome, and incident cardiovascular events in the framingham offspring study. Diabetes 2005;54(11):3252–3257.

68. Wilson PW, D'Agostino RB, Parise H, et al. Metabolic syndrome as a precursor of cardiovascular disease and type 2 diabetes mellitus. Circulation 2005;112(20):3066–3072.
69. Trabulsi J, Schoeller DA. Evaluation of dietary assessment instruments against doubly labeled water, a biomarker of habitual energy intake. Am J Physiol Endocrinol Metab 2001;281(5):E891–E899.
70. Tooze JA, Subar AF, Thompson FE, et al. Psychosocial predictors of energy underreporting in a large doubly labeled water study. Am J Clin Nutr 2004;79(5):795–804.
71. Wadden TA, Berkowitz RI, Womble LG, et al. Randomized trial of lifestyle modification and pharmacotherapy for obesity. N Engl J Med 2005;353(20):2111–2120.
72. Lichtman SW, Pisarska K, Berman ER, et al. Discrepancy between self-reported and actual caloric intake and exercise in obese subjects. N Engl J Med 1992;327(27):1893–1898.
73. Trends in leisure-time physical inactivity by age, sex, and race/ethnicity—United States, 1994–2004. MMWR Morb Mortal Wkly Rep 2005;54(39):991–994.
74. Ekelund U, Brage S, Franks PW, et al. Physical activity energy expenditure predicts changes in body composition in middle-aged healthy whites: effect modification by age. Am J Clin Nutr 2005;81(5):964–969.
75. Hu FB, Stampfer MJ, Solomon C, et al. Physical activity and risk for cardiovascular events in diabetic women. Ann Intern Med 2001;134(2):96–105.
76. Weinstein AR, Sesso HD, Lee IM, et al. Relationship of physical activity vs body mass index with type 2 diabetes in women. JAMA 2004;292(10):1188–1194.
77. Hu FB, Willett WC, Li T, et al. Adiposity as compared with physical activity in predicting mortality among women. N Engl J Med 2004;351(26):2694–2703.
78. Bassuk SS, Manson JE. Epidemiological evidence for the role of physical activity in reducing risk of type 2 diabetes and cardiovascular disease. J Appl Physiol 2005;99(3):1193–1204.
79. Church TS, LaMonte MJ, Barlow CE, et al. Cardiorespiratory fitness and body mass index as predictors of cardiovascular disease mortality among men with diabetes. Arch Intern Med 2005;165(18):2114–2120.
80. LaMonte MJ, Barlow CE, Jurca R, et al. Cardiorespiratory fitness is inversely associated with the incidence of metabolic syndrome: a prospective study of men and women. Circulation 2005;112(4):505–512.
81. Rzewnicki R, Vanden Auweele Y, De Bourdeaudhuij, I. Addressing overreporting on the International Physical Activity Questionnaire (IPAQ) telephone survey with a population sample. Public Health Nutr 2003;6(3):299–305.
82. Walsh MC, Hunter GR, Sirikul B, et al. Comparison of self-reported with objectively assessed energy expenditure in black and white women before and after weight loss. Am J Clin Nutr 2004;79(6):1013–1019.
83. Wyatt HR, Peters JC, Reed GW, et al. A Colorado statewide survey of walking and its relation to excessive weight. Med Sci Sports Exerc 2005;37(5):724–730.
84. Jordan AN, Jurca GM, Locke CT, et al. Pedometer indices for weekly physical activity recommendations in postmenopausal women. Med Sci Sports Exerc 2005;37(9):1627–1632.
85. Stovitz SD, VanWormer JJ, Center BA, et al. Pedometers as a means to increase ambulatory activity for patients seen at a family medicine clinic. J Am Board Fam Pract 2005;18(5):335–343.
86. Foster GD, Wadden TA, Phelan S, et al. Obese patients' perceptions of treatment outcomes and the factors that influence them. Arch Intern Med 2001;161(17):2133–2139.
87. Foster GD, Phelan S, Wadden TA, et al. Promoting more modest weight losses: a pilot study. Obes Res 2004;12(8):1271–1277.
88. Ahlberg AC, Ljung T, Rosmond R, et al. Depression and anxiety symptoms in relation to anthropometry and metabolism in men. Psychiatry Res 2002;112(2):101–110.
89. Rothschild M, Peterson HR, Pfeifer MA. Depression in obese men. Int J Obes 1989;13(4):479–485.
90. Wadden TA, Sarwer DB, Womble LG, et al. Psychosocial aspects of obesity and obesity surgery. Surg Clin North Am 2001;81(5):1001–1024.
91. Greenberg I, Perna F, Kaplan M, et al. Behavioral and psychological factors in the assessment and treatment of obesity surgery patients. Obes Res 2005;13(2):244–249.
92. Dixon JB, Dixon ME, O'Brien PE. Depression in association with severe obesity: changes with weight loss. Arch Intern Med 2003;163(17):2058–2065.

11
Polycystic Ovary Syndrome

Romana Dmitrovic, MD,
and Richard S. Legro, MD

CONTENTS

INTRODUCTION
ETIOLOGY
OLIGOMENORRHEA/AMENORRHEA
HYPERANDROGENEMIA/HYPERANDROGENISM
POLYCYSTIC OVARIES ON ULTRASOUND
LONG-TERM CONSEQUENCES
TREATMENT OF PCOS
CONCLUSION
REFERENCES

Summary

Polycystic ovary syndrome (PCOS) is a common but poorly understood endocrinopathy diagnosed by the combination of oligomenorrhea, hyperandrogenism, and polycystic ovaries. Many of the women with PCOS are also uniquely and variably insulin-resistant. This can manifest as hyperinsulinemia, glucose intolerance, and frank diabetes. Affected women are plagued by infertility, menstrual disorders, dysfunctional uterine bleeding, and peripheral skin disorders including acne and hirsutism. The etiology of the syndrome is poorly understood. Many, if not most, US women with PCOS are also obese, which exacerbates many of the symptoms of the syndrome. This suggests that lifestyle interventions should be the first line treatment for these obese women. Treatment tends to be symptom-based, although some treatments can address multiple presenting complaints. The two most commonly used medications for chronic treatment, oral contraceptives and insulin sensitizing, do appear to improve multiple aspects of the syndrome simultaneously. Unfortunately, clinical trials have focused primarily on surrogate measures rather than clinical outcomes.

Key Words: Polycystic ovary syndrome; insulin resistance; oligomenorrhea; infertility; hyperandrogenism; hirsutism; insulin-sensitizing agents.

INTRODUCTION

Polycystic ovary syndrome (PCOS) is among the most common endocrine disorders, affecting 5% of women in the developed world *(1)*, yet there are still uncertainties about the pathogenesis of the syndrome, and its etiology remains unknown. In their original description of the syndrome, Stein and Leventhal *(2)* reported the condition character-

From: *Contemporary Endocrinology: Treatment of the Obese Patient*
Edited by: R. F. Kushner and D. H. Bessesen © Humana Press Inc., Totowa, NJ

ized by enlarged ovaries with multiple small subcapsular cysts, associated with amen-orrhea and hirsutism. PCOS, as it is understood today, is a disorder characterized by chronic anovulation, menstrual irregularities, and hyperandrogenism; by various clinical stigmata—hirsutism, acne, male pattern balding, and acanthosis nigricans; and by various biochemical findings—elevated serum adrenal and/or ovarian androgen concentration.

ETIOLOGY

A variety of theories have been proposed to explain the development of PCOS.

Central Hypothesis

The primary defect is thought to be the increased luteinizing hormone (LH) pulse amplitude and frequency. Increased LH secretion (evident as an elevated ratio of LH to follicle-stimulating hormone [FSH]), which stimulates ovarian theca cells to produce excess androgens, may be caused by abnormal gonadotropin-releasing hormone (GnRH) pulsatility (3), sensitization of GnRH receptor to GnRH by endogenous opioids (4,5), or reduced dopaminergic inhibition of LH release (5).

Peripheral (Ovarian) Hypothesis

Ovarian theca cell hypertrophy (6), steroidogenic or mitogenic activity of granulosa cells (7), or dysregulated function of the p450 C17-α in the ovaries and adrenal glands (8–11) may cause an intrinsic ovarian or adrenal defect or block FSH activity at the ovarian level, leading to overproduction of androgens and anovulation. The primary defect may also be inhibin B deficiency. Because inhibin B locally enhances follicular development, its deficiency results in anovulation (12).

Insulin Hypothesis

The discovery of hyperinsulinemia (13) and insulin resistance in women with PCOS (14) led to a de-emphasis on the ovary as a diagnostic criterion, and resulted in the insulin hypothesis. In insulin resistance there is a defect of insulin receptor at the postbinding level, leading to abnormality of postreceptor insulin signaling and glucose transport (15). This leads to overproduction of insulin to compensate for the perceived lack of effect, and over time to β-cell exhaustion and ultimately type 2 diabetes. There is now a relatively substantial body of literature confirming β-cell dysfunction in PCOS, although as in diabetes, there is still considerable debate as to the primacy of the defects and their worsening over time (16).

Women with PCOS may have hyperinsulinemia, insulin resistance, impaired glucose tolerance, or diabetes mellitus (13,17,18). The increase in insulin resistance in women with PCOS compared with appropriate controls (~35–40%), is of a similar magnitude to that seen in type 2 diabetes and is independent of obesity, glucose intolerance, increases in waist-to-hip ratio, and differences in muscle mass (14). Basal insulin levels are increased and insulin secretory response to meals has been shown to be reduced in women with PCOS (19), which is also independent of obesity (20).

It has been proposed that, by a variety of mechanisms, hyperinsulinemia increases ovarian androgen production and contributes to the development of anovulation. Four mechanisms of insulin resistance may lead to androgen overproduction in women with

Table 1
Criteria for Diagnosis of PCOS

1990 NIH Criteria (both 1 and 2)

1. Chronic anovulation and
2. Clinical and/or biochemical signs of hyperandrogenism, and exclusion of other etiologies.

Revised Rotterdam 2003 criteria (2 out of 3)

1. Oligo- and/or anovulation
2. Clinical and/or biochemical signs of hyperandrogenism
3. Polycystic ovaries
   Exclusion of other etiologies—congenital adrenal hyperplasia, androgen-secreting tumors, Cushing's syndrome

PCOS, resulting in abnormal ovarian follicular growth and anovulation, which is the hallmark abnormality of the syndrome.

- The ovaries may be directly stimulated by insulin to produce abnormal amounts of androgen *(11)*.
- Synergism of insulin with LH may lead to theca cell stimulation, hyperandrogenism, and large polycystic ovaries *(21,22)*.
- Hyperinsulinemia may lead to inhibition of sex hormone binding globulin (SHBG) secretion *(12)* and increase in free fraction of androgens.
- An increase in free insulin-like growth factors (IGFs) *(23)* may potentiate LH-stimulated androgen synthesis in theca cells *(24)* and suppress IGF binding protein (IGFBP)-I synthesis *(25,26)*.

These theories, however, are reflective of our limited knowledge of both PCOS and insulin resistance. As the pathophysiology and genetics of these disorders are better elucidated, so too will be the putative pathways.

In the United States, PCOS is recognized as an endocrinopathy of undetermined etiology, characterized by hyperandrogenism and/or hyperandrogenemia, oligo-ovulation, and exclusion of other potential causes such as congenital adrenal hyperplasia, Cushing's syndrome, and androgen-secreting tumors (Table 1). This was summarized in a 1990 National Institutes of Health–National Institute of Child and Human Development (NIH–NICHD) consensus conference on PCOS *(27)*, and has been upheld in similar proceedings in recent years.

In Europe, however, PCOS is often diagnosed based on ultrasound criteria with the history of anovulation, without the biochemical evidence. To unify the criteria, in 2004 an international consensus group *(28)* proposed that the syndrome can be diagnosed if at least two of the following are present: oligomenorrhea or amenorrhea, hyperandrogenemia or hyperandrogenism, and polycystic ovaries as defined by ultrasonography (Table 1). Each of these signs and clinical complaints associated with it will be discussed in the following sections.

A suggested laboratory evaluation of women with PCOS is provided in Table 2, but this remains an area where the cost-effectiveness of such an extensive workup should be justified.

Table 2
Tests to Consider in Women With PCOS

Blood tests	Normal range[a]	Purpose
Total testosterone (consider also free or bioavailable measures)	<60 ng/dL[a]	Determine extent of androgen excess
Fasting blood tests		
17-hydroxyprogesterone	<2 ng/mL	Evaluate for NC-CAH; use <4 ng/mL for random sample, ACTH stimulation test if abnormal
Prolactin	<20 ng/mL	Evaluate for prolactin excess
Glucose	<126 mg/dL	Screen for diabetes
Insulin	<20 microU/mL[a]	Screen for insulin resistance
Glucose-to-insulin ratio	>4.5	Screen for insulin resistance
Cholesterol	<200 mg/dL	Identify cardiovascular risk
HDL	>35 mg/dL (and preferably >45 mg/dL)	Identify cardiovascular risk
LDL	<130 mg/dL	Identify cardiovascular risk
Triglycerides	<200 mg/dL	Identify cardiovascular risk
Dynamic blood tests		
Oral glucose tolerance test, give 75 g glucose in AM after overnight fast	2 h glucose > 140 mg/dL —impaired glucose tolerance 2 h glucose > 200 mg/dL—type 2 diabetes mellitus	Identify or diagnose diabetes, repeat if abnormal

OLIGOMENORRHEA/AMENORRHEA

In the broadest definition, PCOS has been identified by the World Health Organization as type 2 ovulatory dysfunction, or normoestrogenic anovulation. Although chronic anovulation (6 to 8 spontaneous episodes of vaginal bleeding per year) may be the *sine qua non* of the syndrome, only a small percentage of women with PCOS are completely amenorrheic. The majority are oligomenorrheic and experience varying intervals of vaginal bleeding. The cause of this vaginal bleeding may be physiologic (postovulatory withdrawal bleed) or pathologic.

The baseline endogenous ovulatory frequency is unknown in an untreated PCOS population but the ovulation rate in the largest randomized controlled trial in women with PCOS to date demonstrated an almost 30% ovulatory frequency in the placebo-treated arm, indicating either a significant placebo effect and/or a high endogenous rate *(29)*.

Infertility

Chronic anovulation is the cause of the most common reason that women with PCOS present to the gynecologist: infertility *(30)*. As a general rule, PCOS patients represent one of the most difficult groups in which to induce ovulation both successfully and safely. Many women with PCOS are unresponsive to clomiphene citrate and human menopausal gonadotropins, and this is exacerbated by underlying obesity. On the other end of the spectrum are PCOS patients who overrespond to both these medications.

Women with PCOS are at especially increased risks of ovarian hyperstimulation syndrome (OHSS), a syndrome of massive enlargement of the ovaries and transudation of ascites into the abdominal cavity that can lead to rapid and symptomatic enlargement of the abdomen, intravascular contraction, hypercoagulability, and systemic organ dysfunction *(31)*. There is also emerging evidence that baseline hyperinsulinemia may contribute to the increased OHSS risk *(32,33)*. Women with PCOS are also at increased risk for multiple pregnancy.

HYPERANDROGENEMIA/HYPERANDROGENISM

Both the adrenal glands and ovaries contribute to the circulating androgen pool in women. In ovarian theca cells, cholesterol is converted to androstenedione. The adrenal preferentially secretes weak androgens such as dehydroepiandrosterone (DHEA) or its sulfated "depot" form, DHEA-S (up to 90% of adrenal origin). These hormones, in addition to androstenedione, may serve as prohormones and may be converted to more potent androgens such as testosterone or dihydrotestosterone.

The ovary is the preferential source of testosterone; it is estimated that 75% of circulating testosterone originates from the ovary (mainly through peripheral conversion of prohormones by liver, fat, and skin, but also through direct ovarian secretion). Androstenedione, of both adrenal (50%) and ovarian (50%) origin, is the only circulating androgen that is higher in premenopausal women than in men, yet its androgenic potency is only 10% that of testosterone. However, it is often elevated in PCOS patients. Dihydrotestosterone (DHT) is the most potent androgen, although it circulates in negligible quantities, and results primarily from the intracellular 5α-reduction of testosterone.

Thus circulating testosterone may be the androgen of choice to measure; indeed, its circulating levels may offer better discrimination between a control population and the affected population with PCOS. A 14% overlap in elevated androgen levels was noted between women with PCOS and a prospectively recruited cohort of cycling control women *(34)*, versus a 20 to 30% overlap of polycystic ovaries in an normal population *(35,36)*. A circulating total testosterone level was found to be the best hormonal correlate of the combined syndrome of hyperandrogenic chronic anovulation and polycystic ovaries *(37)*. Many prefer either a free testosterone or a bioavailable testosterone level, as that better reflects the suppressive effects of hyperinsulinemia on SHBG *(38)*. Assays are reproducible and eliminate any observer bias in identifying women with androgen excess. However given the interassay variability, it is difficult to assign a uniform and specific level of circulating testosterone as the cutoff for diagnosing PCOS *(39)*.

Hyperandrogenism can also be documented based on clinical stigmata of androgen excess, such as by the presence of acne, hirsutism, or androgenic alopecia, instead of relying on biochemical confirmation of circulating hyperandrogenemia, but ethnic, and presumably underlying genetic, differences in population may result in the presence of hyperandrogenemia without clinical signs of hyperandrogenism *(40)*.

Hirsutism

Hirsutism is defined as excess body hair in undesirable locations and, as such, is a subjective phenomenon that makes both diagnosis and treatment difficult. Most commonly hirsutism associated with PCOS tends to be an androgen-dependent, midline-predominant hair growth. It is important to note that other factors than androgen action may contribute to the development of hirsutism. Hyperinsulinemia that accompanies many benign forms of virilization can also stimulate the pilosebaceous unit directly or indirectly by contributing to hyperandrogenemia.

Hirsutism is heterogeneous and a common disorder with features similar to PCOS, but only 50% of women with hirsutism may actually have PCOS *(41)*. Hirsutism is also not invariably present in a woman with PCOS. There are, for instance, ethnic differences in target tissue sensitivity to circulating androgens and intracellular androgens *(42)*, such that marked androgen excess may not manifest as hirsutism (Asians, for example) *(40)*. Methodology of the assessment of hirsutism and response to treatment has been poorly validated *(43)*.

Hirsutism scores are notoriously subjective *(44)*, and even the most frequently utilized standard of subjective hirsutism scores, the modified Ferriman–Gallwey score, relies excessively on nonmidline, nonandrogen-dependent body hair to make the diagnosis *(45)*. In the largest clinical trial to date in PCOS, 50 to 60% of the 400 women prospectively identified to have hyperandrogenemic chronic anovulation had no evidence of hirsutism (Ferriman–Gallwey score < 6) *(29)*. Also, hirsutism is frequently idiopathic and accompanied by normal circulating androgen levels *(42)*, although other studies with more thorough examination have shown idiopathic hirsutism to be rare (<10% of a hirsute population) *(46)*.

POLYCYSTIC OVARIES ON ULTRASOUND

Different authors have defined PCOS on the basis of the morphology of the ovary found on ultrasound, with multiple 2- to 8-mm subcapsular preantral follicles forming a "black pearl necklace" sign *(47)*. Polycystic ovaries are found in a wide variety of unrelated disorders, including in up to 30% of women with normal menses and normal circulating androgens *(35,36,48)*. The differential diagnosis of polycystic ovaries is extensive, with some syndromes having little overlap with hyperandrogenic chronic anovulation.

There have been reports suggesting that polycystic ovaries *per se* may identify a group of women with some further stigmata of reproductive and metabolic abnormalities found in the endocrine syndrome of PCOS *(49,50)*, but the data have not been consistent *(51)*. It is important to note that not all women with the endocrine syndrome of PCOS have polycystic-appearing ovaries *(51)*, and that polycystic ovaries alone should not be viewed as synonymous with PCOS. Polycystic ovaries appear to be an independent risk factor for OHSS after ovulation induction *(52)* and thus it may make clinical sense to document the morphology of the ovary in infertile patients seeking ovulation induction.

LONG-TERM CONSEQUENCES

Type 2 Diabetes Mellitus

Retrospective studies looking at diabetes prevalence over time have generally noted an increased prevalence with age in women with PCOS. Studies from Scandinavia have shown increased rates of type 2 diabetes and hypertension compared with controls *(53)*. This study used a combination of ovarian morphology and clinical criteria to identify women with PCOS and found that 15% had developed diabetes, compared with 2.3% of the controls *(53)*. A case-control study of PCOS in the United States has shown persistent

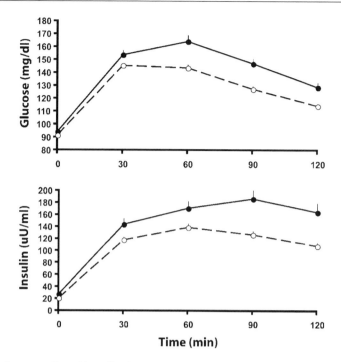

Fig. 1. Glucose (top panel) and insulin (bottom panel) concentrations obtained during a 75-g oral glucose tolerance test (OGTT) in 408 premenopausal women with PCOS (●; positive family history) and without (○; negative family history) a family history of type 2 diabetes. Adapted from ref. *60.*

hyperinsulinemia and dyslipidemia as PCOS patients age, though androgen levels tend to decline in older women with PCOS *(54).* In a population of thin Dutch women, although the overall prevalence of self-reported diabetes by telephone survery was 2.3%, in PCOS patients aged 45 to 54 yr (*n* = 32) the prevalence of diabetes was four times higher (*p* < 0.05) than the prevalence of this condition in the corresponding age group of the Dutch female population as a whole *(55).*

Adult women with PCOS have glucose intolerance rates of 40%, as defined by prevalence of either impaired glucose tolerance (IGT) or type 2 diabetes as diagnosed by a 2-h glucose value after a 75-g oral glucose tolerance test (OGTT) *(56,57).* New data now suggest that adolescents may have soaring rates of glucose intolerance *(58),* comparable with adults, and this appears to be mirrored in the adolescent population with PCOS *(59).* Studies of large cohorts of women with PCOS have demonstrated that the prevalence rates of glucose intolerance are as high as 40% in PCOS patients when the less-stringent WHO criteria are used *(56,57,60).* They have also indicated the importance of family history of diabetes contributing to these high glucose intolerance rates (Fig. 1) *(60).*

These studies are of interest because they have shown nearly identical rates of impaired glucose tolerance and type 2 diabetes among a diverse cohort, both ethnically and geographically, as well as from different investigational groups. It does appear that obesity contributes substantially, as rates of glucose intolerance in a thinner European population with normal weight (BMI 19–25) are lower than in the US population (though still far exceeding control rates) *(61).*

Obesity

Obesity has become epidemic in our society and contributes substantially to reproductive and metabolic abnormalities in PCOS. Obesity is defined by body mass index (BMI; body weight in kilograms divided by height in meters^2) of 30 kg/m^2 or more (62). However, BMI does not take into account patient habitus, so central obesity, which is often present in patients with PCOS, can be diagnosed clinically by measuring the waist circumference (WC) or waist-to-hip circumference ratio (WHR) (62). WC larger than 102 cm for men and 88 cm for women, or WHR greater than 0.95 in men and 0.85 in women in obese individuals with BMI between 25.0 and 34.9 kg/m^2 confer high risk for diabetes, hyperlipidemia, hypertension, atherosclerosis, and insulin resistance (63–67).

Obesity is present in about 50% of patients with PCOS. Both insulin resistance and hyperinsulinemia are magnified in the presence of obesity (68,69). Unfortunately there are no effective treatments that result in permanent weight loss, and it is estimated that 90 to 95% of patients who experience a weight decrease will relapse (70). For obese patients with hirsutism, weight loss is frequently recommended as a potential benefit. Increases in SHBG through improved insulin sensitivity from weight loss may lower bioavailable androgen levels. In one study about 50% of these women who lost weight experienced improvement in their hirsutism (71).

Cardiovascular Risk Factors

Patients with PCOS may have abnormal lipid profiles, including elevated triglyceride, LDL cholesterol, VLDL cholesterol, and decreased HDL. In a study of more than 200 patients with PCOS, Talbott et al. found increased BMI, insulin, triglyceride, cholesterol, LDL, and blood pressure (72). The elevated insulin levels were found to correlate with the increased cardiovascular risk independently in PCOS patients.

The metabolic profile noted in women with PCOS is similar to insulin resistance syndrome, a clustering within an individual of hyperinsulinemia, mild glucose intolerance, dyslipidemia, and hypertension (73). There is a prolific literature identifying obesity, dyslipidemia, glucose intolerance, diabetes, and occasionally hypertension as risk factors for cardiovascular disease in women with PCOS (74–79). However, there is actually little published evidence supporting a link between PCOS and cardiovascular events—i.e., increased mortality from CVD, premature mortality from CVD, or an increased incidence of cardiovascular events (stroke and/or myocardial infarction).

Several surrogate markers for atherosclerotic disease, including carotid wall thickness as determined by B-mode ultrasonography, have been studied in women with PCOS. The University of Pittsburgh performed ultrasonography of the carotid arteries on 125 women with PCOS and 142 control women and found a significantly higher prevalence of abnormal carotid plaque index in women with PCOS (7.2% vs 0.7% in controls) (80). Thus the vast majority of predominantly premenopausal women with PCOS (93%) had no evidence for subclinical carotid atherosclerosis. No difference was noted in the intima–media thickness between PCOS and controls until the age group 45 to 49, after which the difference increased in the oldest age groups (80). Another group recently replicated this finding in a separate group of women with PCOS (81).

In a study from the United Kingdom, 800 women diagnosed with PCOS, primarily by histopathology at the time of an ovarian wedge resection, were followed for an average of 30 yr after the procedure (82). Observed death rates were compared with expected death rates using standardized mortality ratios. There was no increased death from cardiovascular-related causes, although there were an increased number of deaths from complications of diabetes in the PCOS group. In a follow-up study by the same investigative group of 345 of these PCOS patients and 1060 age-matched control women, there was no increased long-term coronary heart disease mortality, although there was evidence of increased stroke related mortality even after adjustment for BMI *(83)*. In a cohort of women with proven coronary artery disease ($N = 143$ and age < 60 yr), polycystic ovaries were noted in 42% of the women, and additionally their presence was associated with more severe coronary artery stenosis (OR 1.7; 95% CI 1.1–2.3 of >50% stenosis with PCO compared with normal ovaries) *(84)*.

Despite the heterogeneous nature of anovulation in a reproductive-age population, some of the best epidemiological studies of menstrual irregularity as a marker for chronic anovulation have showed an increased risk for cardiovascular events. The Dutch breast cancer screening study found a greater incidence of anovulatory cycles during the reproductive years (based on a midluteal urine sample) in women later developing cardiovascular disease *(85)*. Utilizing a prospective cohort design from the Nurses' Health Study *(86),* 2439 female nurses provided information in 1982 on prior menstrual regularity (at ages 20–35 yr) and were followed through 1996 for cardiovascular events. Incident reports of nonfatal myocardial infarction, fatal coronary heart disease (CHD), and nonfatal and fatal stroke were made and confirmed by review of medical records.

Compared with women reporting a history of very regular menstrual cycles, women reporting usually irregular or very irregular cycles had an increased risk for nonfatal or fatal CHD. Increased risks for CHD associated with prior cycle irregularity remained significant after adjustment for BMI and other several potential confounders, including family history of myocardial infarction and personal exercise history. There was a non-significant increase in overall stroke risk as well as in ischemic stroke risk associated with very irregular cycles. The Nurses' Health Study has also identified oligomenorrhea and highly irregular menstrual cycles as risk factors for developing type 2 diabetes, a major risk factor in itself for cardiovascular disease, especially in women *(87)*.

Thus the increased cardiovascular risk ascribed to women with PCOS is still largely inferential, based on risk factors or surrogate markers *(76,79)*, or epidemiologic studies that focus on isolated stigmata of PCOS, such as polycystic ovaries or chronic anovulation, that are even more heterogeneous than PCOS.

Risk for Malignancy

Endometrial cancer is the most commonly diagnosed invasive gynecological cancer in women. Case series have identified women with PCOS at high risk for developing endometrial cancer and often at an early age *(88–91)*, but there is actually little solid epidemiologic evidence to link PCOS and endometrial cancer *(92)*. A stronger association between PCOS and endometrial cancer may be possible if we were able to make the diagnosis of PCOS in menopausal women, but a diagnosis based on hyperandrogenic chronic anovulation becomes difficult to make after ovarian failure and cessation of menses *(93)*.

The mechanism by which women with PCOS may be at increased risk for endometrial hyperplasia and endometrial cancer is thought to be chronic stimulation of the endometrium with weak but bioactive estrogens, combined with the lack of progestin exposure. This condition, known as "unopposed estrogen," is perhaps the clearest hor-monal risk factor for endometrial cancer *(94)*. Women with PCOS have been shown to be normoestrogenic, and perhaps even hypoestrogenic with elevated levels of estrone *(95)*. A Scandanavian study looked at a group of both premenopausal and postmeno-pausal women with endometrial carcinoma and found hirsutism and obesity in both groups of cases compared with controls *(96)*. In the younger group, they additionally noted a recent history of anovulation and infertility, two of the most common presenting complaints of women with PCOS (in addition to hirsutism and obesity) *(30)*. Endome-trial hyperplasia often has been noted in association with anovulation and infertility, common symptoms of PCOS *(90,97,98)*. There are no systematic prospective studies of the prevalence of endometrial hyperplasia/neoplasia in a population with PCOS. Other gynecological cancers have been reported to be more common in women with PCOS, including ovarian cancer *(99)* and breast cancer *(100)*.

Pregnancy Complications

PCOS is associated with increased risk for recurrent miscarriage. When using ovarian morphology as surrogate marker, polycystic ovaries were identified in 82% of women presenting with recurrent miscarriage *(101)*. However, the risk of early first-trimester pregnancy loss in women with PCOS is estimated to be 30%, compared with about 15 to 20 % in the general population *(102,103)*.

Pregnancy complications (gestational diabetes, pre-eclampsia, infants who are small for gestational age, preterm labor, and stillbirth) also appear to be high in patients with PCOS *(104–107)*, although there are reports that did not find such a connection *(108,109)*. Currently, the underlying pathogenesis of early pregnancy loss and pregnancy compli-cations in PCOS is thought to be the result of a combination of several interrelated factors, which include hyperandrogenaemia, insulin resistance, obesity, abnormal folliculogenesis, and infertility therapy itself *(110)*.

TREATMENT OF PCOS

We are currently changing from a symptom-oriented treatment approach to PCOS, which often focused alternatively on either suppression of the ovaries (for hirsutism and menstrual disorders) or stimulation of the ovaries (for infertility), to one that improves insulin sensitivity and treats a variety of stigmata simultaneously *(111)*. Multiple studies have shown that improving insulin sensitivity, be it from lifestyle modifications or from pharmacologic intervention, can result in lowered circulating androgens (primarily mediated through increased SHBG and less bioavailable androgen but also through decreased total testosterone), spontaneous ovulation, and spontaneous pregnancy.

Ovarian-Suppressive Therapies

Women with documented hyperandrogenemia, and stigmata of hirsutism and acne, would theoretically benefit most from this form of therapy. Suppressing the ovary has been achieved with either oral contraceptives, depot progestins, or GnRH analog treat-ment. Oral contraceptives both inhibit ovarian steroid production through lowering of gonadotropins and raise SHBG through their estrogen effect, thus further lowering bioavailable testosterone. They also may inhibit DHT binding to the androgen receptor and 5-α-reductase activity, and increase hepatic steroid clearance. These numerous

Table 3
Treatment of PCOS

Treatment of Hirsutism
- Oral contraceptives
- Spironolactone
- Flutamide
- Finasteride
- Eflornithine hydrochloride (topical)
- Cyproterone acetate
- Insulin-sensitizing agents

Treatment of Obesity
- Sibutramine
- Orlistat

Treatment of Infertility/Anovulation
- Clomiphene citrate
- Gonadotropins
- Laparoscopic ovarian drilling
- Insulin-sensitizing agents

Treatment of Hyperinsulinemia
- Weight reduction
- Exercise/lifestyle modification
- Insulin-sensitizing agents
  - Biguanides (metformin), thiazolidenediones (rosiglitazone, pioglitazone)

---

actions contribute to improving hirsutism *(112)*. There are theoretical reasons for choosing an oral contraceptive using a less androgenic progestin or one with specific androgen-antagonistic properties (such as cyproterone acetate or drospirenone), but few studies have shown a clinical difference between different types of progestins. Although several oral contraceptives (OCPs), including a triphasic OCP containing norgestimate, have been shown to improve acne and have received an FDA indication for this, other pills also appear to offer similar results.

A GnRH agonist may cause greater lowering of circulating androgens, but comparative trials against other agents and combined agent trials have been mixed and have not shown a greater benefit to one or the other or combined treatment *(113–116)*. A GnRH agonist given alone results in unacceptable bone loss *(116)*. Glucocorticoid suppression of the adrenal glands also offers theoretical benefits, but deterioration in glucose tolerance is problematic for women with PCOS, and long-term effects such as osteoporosis are significant concern. It may be useful as adjunctive therapy in inducing ovulation with clomiphene citrate.

Insulin-Sensitizing Agents

Drugs developed initially to treat type 2 diabetes have also been utilized to treat PCOS. None of these agents are currently FDA-approved for the treatment of PCOS or for related symptoms such as anovulation, hirsutism, or acne. These include metformin *(117–119)*, thiazolidinediones, and an experimental insulin sensitizer drug, d-*chiro*-inositol *(120)*.

METFORMIN

Metformin was approved for the treatment of type 2 diabetes by the FDA in 1994, but was used clinically for almost 20 yr before that in other parts of the world. The effects of the drug are therefore well known. Metformin is a biguanide that works primarily by suppressing hepatic gluconeogenesis, and in muscle and fat cells it enhanced glucose uptake and utilization, therefore improving insulin sensitivity in the periphery. This effectively lowers glucose and insulin levels. Its most serious, but rare, side effect is lactic acidosis, which has been reported in individuals with renal deficiency, liver disease, and heart and respiratory failure. The most common side effect is gastrointestinal disturbance, but this rarely is a cause to discontinue the drug. Metformin could also decrease folic acid and vitamin B_{12} absorption.

There have been no reported abnormalities associated with the use of metformin during pregnancy in women with diabetes (121–123) or in women with marked hyperandrogenism during pregnancy (124), or to the small number of women with PCOS who have conceived during treatment (125–127). The combination of metformin and clomiphene markedly improves ovulation in PCOS patients by correcting the underlying metabolic problem.

Metformin, in a meta-analysis of 13 studies in women with PCOS, was shown to significantly reduce fasting insulin levels even in this heterogeneous population (128). Fasting glucose also had a small reduction. Lipid profile was also positively affected by metformin, but in the meta-analysis only LDL cholesterol was significantly reduced after metformin treatment. Furthermore, the meta-analysis has shown that the effects of metformin are independent of BMI changes or of fat distribution as assessed by waist-to-hip ratio (119). There has never been an adequately powered placebo-controlled dose-ranging study.

In a systematic review of seven randomized-controlled trials, it has been shown that women with metformin treatment have a small improvement in ovulation rate—on average, one additional ovulation every 5 mo (129). The Cochrane meta-analysis examined the effectiveness of metformin in spontaneous and clomiphene-induced ovulation (128). Specifically, ovulation was achieved in 46% of the women who received metformin alone (compared with 24% receiving placebo). Pregnancy rates are difficult to interpret, however, owing to the small number of patients, the short follow-up period, and the study design.

Some clinicians advocate the use of metformin during early pregnancy to reduce the miscarriage rate, but the documentation for this claim is poor (130). Studies of longer duration with metformin in PCOS suggest long-term improvement in ovulatory function in about half the patients (131). Unfortunately there have been few well-designed studies that test the effect of metformin on hirsutism.

THIAZOLIDINEDIONES

Thiazolidinediones are peroxisome proliferator activating receptor agonists and are thought to improve insulin sensitivity through a postreceptor mechanism. Insulin resistance is therefore decreased. It is difficult to separate the effects of improving insulin sensitivity from that of lowering serum androgens, as any "pure" improvement in insulin sensitivity can raise SHBG and thus lower bioavailable androgen. Given the long onset of action for improving hirsutism, longer periods of observation are needed. The best data were from a large, randomized, placebo-controlled study, where 305 moderately

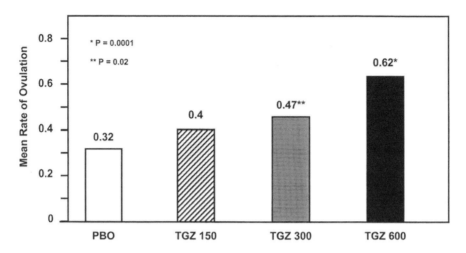

Fig. 2. The mean rate of ovulation in patients with PCOS increased in a dose-related fashion with troglitazone (TGZ) treatment and was significantly different from placebo (PBO) for TGZ 300 mg/d and TGZ 600 mg/d groups, but not for TGZ 150 mg/d patients. Adapted from ref. *132.*

obese women received troglitazone at different doses (150, 300, or 600 mg/d) or placebo. There was a dose-dependent reduction of testosterone, an increase in SHBG levels, an improvement in hirsutism and menstrual cycle, and an increase in ovulation rates in women who received troglitazone *(132)*. Patients treated with 600 mg/d had a 60% ovulation rate compared with a 32% rate among the placebo group (and this placebo rate is greater than that traditionally noted in metformin trials) (Fig. 2). This appeared to be mediated through decreases in hyperinsulinemia and decreases in free testosterone levels.

Troglitazone has been removed from the worldwide market because of hepatotoxicity. The other two thiazolidinediones, rosiglitazone and pioglitazone, have not demonstrated significant hepatotoxicity, and their administration has showed similar results in improving insulin sensitivity, reducing testosterone levels, improving menstrual cycles, and restoring ovulation *(133,134)*. It has been shown that pioglitazone is as effective as metformin in improving insulin sensitivity and hyperandrogenemia, despite an increase in weight, BMI, and waist-to-hip ratio associated with pioglitazone *(135)*.

Anti-Obesity Drugs

Apart from diet, combination with pharmacological treatment with metformin or with weight-reducing agents has been used when required for further weight reduction. It has been reported that the combination of a low-calorie diet with metformin treatment induced greater reduction of body weight and visceral obesity in women with PCOS compared with a low-calorie diet and placebo treatment *(136)*. Weight-reducing agents have been shown to increase the effect of lifestyle modification in reducing the incidence of type 2 diabetes in obese patients *(137)*, and similar effects have been noted in women with PCOS. Sibutramine treatment alone and in combination with ethinyl estradiol and cyproterone acetate in obese women with PCOS has been found to have positive effects on clinical and metabolic risk factors for cardiovascular disease (decrease in waist-to-hip ratio, blood pressure, triglycerides, and insulin levels) *(138)*. Furthermore, orlistat treatment in obese women with PCOS induced a more significant weight reduction than metformin treatment. It also induced a reduction of testosterone levels, which is consistent with the reduction of testosterone levels in overweight women with PCOS after weight loss by dietary changes and exercise *(139)*. However, it is difficult to assess the long-term clinical efficiency of the medications because the literature is rather inconclusive (small number of patients and short-term studies). Common side effects (headache, insomnia) and potentially serious cardiovascular effects (hypertension, arrythmias, etc.) limit the widespread use of sibutramine, and although orlistat generally has a safer side-effect profile, the frequent adverse effects on bowel habits (flatulence, steatorrhea, GI discomfort) are also significant hurdles to its use.

Treatment of Infertility

CLOMIPHENE CITRATE

Clomiphene citrate (CC) has traditionally been the first-line treatment agent for infertility in women with PCOS. It is a nonsteroidal agent and a member of a large family of triphenylethylene derivatives, which includes clorotrianisene and tamoxifen (both of which compare favorably to CC in inducing ovulation). It is a racemic mixture of two isomers, zuclomiphene (longer-acting) and enclomiphene (more potent in inducing ovulation) *(140)*. Clomiphene has a long half-life: only 51% of the oral dose is excreted after 5 d and the zu isomer can be detected in the serum for up to 1 mo after treatment *(141)*. Clomiphene is thought to work as a selective estrogen receptor modulator (SERM) acting as an estrogen antagonist at the hypothalamic–pituitary axis and stimulating GnRH secretion.

A meta-analysis showed CC to be effective in patients with ovulatory dysfunction similar to PCOS *(142)*. Compared with placebo, CC was associated with increased ovulation. CC (all doses) was associated with an increased pregnancy rate per treatment cycle (OR 3.41, 95% CI 4.23–9.48). The odds ratio was better for high doses (50–250 mg/d) (OR 6.82, 95% CI 3.92–11.85) *(142)*.

There are no clear prognostic factors to response, although increasing weight is associated with a larger dose requirement and a greater likelihood for failure *(143)*. Roughly 50% of women with PCOS do not respond to CC. There is no universal definition of resistance to clomiphene citrate, although its simplest rendition would involve failure to ovulate with three progressive dose increases up to 750 mg/cycle. Alternate CC regimens have been developed, including prolonging the period of administration *(144)* and adding dexamethasone *(145)*, both of which, in small studies, have been shown to improve response.

GONADOTROPINS

Gonadotropins are also frequently utilized in both step-up and step-down regimens to induce ovulation in women with PCOS. In one of the largest trial of gonadotropins in women with PCOS to date, women were randomized to a conventional method of ovulation with more aggressive dosing and increases in FSH dosing compared with a low-dose protocol; higher pregnancy rates were achieved with the low-dose protocol (40% vs 20% for the conventional arm) *(146)*. There were fewer cases of multiple pregnancy and ovarian hyperstimulation in the low-dose arm and a higher percentage of monofollicular ovulation (74% vs 27%) *(146)*. Low-dose therapy with gonadotropins offers a high rate on monofollicular development (~50% or greater) with a significantly lower risk of OHSS (20–25%) leading to cycle cancellation or more serious sequelae *(146–150)*. A Cochrane review reports a reduction in the incidence of OHSS with FSH compared with human menopausal gonadotropin (hMG) in stimulation cycles without the concomitant use of a GnRH-a (OR 0.20; 95% CI 0.08–0.46) and a higher overstimulation rate when a GnRH-a is added to gonadotropins (OR 3.15; 95% CI 1.48–6.70) *(151)*. Despite theoretical advantages, urinary-derived FSH preparations did not improve pregnancy rates when compared to traditional and cheaper hMG preparations; their only demonstrable benefit was a reduced risk of OHSS in cycles when administered without the concomitant use of a GnRH-a. A meta-analysis found no studies of adequate power to confirm the benefit of pulsatile GnRH-a to induce ovulation in PCOS *(152)*.

Nonfertility Treatments —Acne and Hirsutism

Oral contraceptive pills will increase SHBG, and insulin-sensitizing agents will lower insulin levels, resulting in less free testosterone. Many of the aforementioned generalized treatments are also applicable to the treatment of hirsutism. Most medical methods, however, although they improve hirsutism, do not produce the dramatic results patients desire. In general, combination therapies appear to produce better results than single-agent approaches, response with medical therapies often take 3 to 6 mo to notice improvement, and adjunctive mechanical removal methods are often necessary. However, the majority of women will experience improvement in their hirsutism. There are unfortunately no universally accepted techniques for assessing hirsutism and response to treatment. Trials have been hampered by the aforementioned methodology concerns as well as by the small number of subjects. For instance, although spironolactone has had a long and extensive use as an antiandrogen and multiple clinical trials have been published showing a benefit, the overall quality of the trials and small numbers enrolled have limited the ability of a meta-analysis to document its benefit in the treatment of hirsutism *(153)*.

Spironolactone *(154)* antagonizes the binding of testosterone and other androgens to the androgen receptor. However, it is teratogenic and poses a risk of feminization of the external genitalia in a male fetus should the patient conceive *(155)*. About 20% of women treated with spironolactone will experience increased menstrual frequency; this is one reason for combining this therapy with the oral contraceptive *(156)*. Cyproterone acetate, which is not available commercially in the United States, is a progestogen with antiandrogen properties. It is frequently combined in an oral contraceptive. Acne has also been successfully treated with spironolactone *(157)*. Ornithine decarboxylase inhibitor eflornithine is used as a facial cream against hirsutism and has been FDA-approved for this indication. Flutamide is another nonsteroidal antiandrogen that has been shown to be effective against hirsutism *(158)*. There is greater risk of teratogenicity with this compound and contraception should be used.

The 5α-reductase inhibitor finasteride has been found to be effective for the treatment of hirsutism in women *(159,160)*. Finasteride is better tolerated than other antiandrogens, but has the highest and clearest risk for teratogenicity in a male fetus and adequate contraception must be used. Randomized trials have found that spironolactone, flutamide, and finasteride all have similar efficacy in improving hirsutism *(161,162)*.

Surgical Treatment

Stein and Leventhal performed ovarian wedge resection more than 80 yr ago and noted regular menses and spontaneous pregnancy in some patients (2). Many studies utilizing ovarian wedge resection or ovarian drilling have been performed over the years, some with impressive results. The beneficial influence of such destructive ovarian interventions has been suggested (163–165), but not proven, and the value of laparoscopic ovarian drilling as a primary treatment for subfertile patients with anovulation and PCOS is undetermined according to a Cochrane review (166).

There is insufficient evidence to determine a difference in ovulation or pregnancy rates when compared with gonadotropin therapy as a secondary treatment for clomiphene-resistant women (166), although a recent study suggested that the pregnancy rates were equivalent (167). None of the various drilling techniques appears to offer obvious advantages (166). The results of the ovarian drilling may in some cases also be temporary (168). Surgery, consisting of total abdominal hysterectomy and bilateral salpingo-oophorectomy, is not a usual initial treatment option for androgen excess, but may be indicated in some cases of refractory ovarian hyperandrogenism.

Exercise /Lifestyle Modification

There is some evidence that lifestyle modification (diet and exercise) may be an effective adjunct to the treatment of PCOS. The use of hypocaloric diets improves the metabolic derangements in those patients, and low-calorie, low-fat diets have been shown to improve clinical parameters and lower insulin and testosterone levels in PCOS patients (169,170). Weight reduction has also been shown to increase noradrenalin sensitivity in PCOS patients, as PCOS patients have a marked reduction in the lipolytic effects of noradrenalin owing to a decreased number of noradrenalin receptors on fat cells (171), resulting in dyslipidemia. Metformin, in addition to a hypocaloric diet, improves hirsutism, menstrual function, visceral adipose tissue, and glucose-stimulated insulin secretion (172,173). Thus, it appears that diet and medication in combination may be helpful in patients with PCOS.

It is reasonable to assume that exercise would have the same beneficial effects in women with PCOS as in women with type 2 diabetes (174). Moreover, exercise by itself, such as regular walking, has been reported to reduce waist-to-hip ratio and homocysteine levels in overweight PCOS patients (175).

Many popular sources advocate a high-protein diet as the diet of choice for women with PCOS. There are few studies to support this, and there are theoretical concerns about the adverse effects of high protein on renal function in a population at high risk for diabetes, as well as the adverse effects of the increased fat composition of these diets on dyslipidemia.

Other Treatments

Minoxidil has mild efficacy in increasing hair growth in women with alopecia. Ketoconazole is an inhibitor of the P450 enzyme system and thus inhibits androgen biosynthesis, but has hepatotoxicity. Others have given aromatase inhibitors to induce ovulation and lower circulating androgens, although hirsutism has not been the primary focus to date (176).

Mechanical hair removal (shaving, plucking, waxing, depilatory creams, electrolysis, and laser vaporization) can control hirsutism, and often is the front-line treatment used by women. Laser vaporization is receiving increasing attention. Hair is damaged using the principle of selective photothermolysis, with wavelengths of light well absorbed by follicular melanin and pulse durations that selectively thermally damage the target without damaging surrounding tissue. Patients with dark hair and light skin are ideal candidates; this process appears to be most effective during anagen.

CONCLUSION

Polycystic ovary syndrome is a common endocrinopathy, but it is poorly understood. It is a disorder clearly heterogeneous in etiology; conditions associated with PCOS may include menstrual abnormalities and infertility due to chronic anovulation, hirsutism and acne caused by hyperandrogenism, glucose intolerance and diabetes mellitus owing to profound peripheral resistance to insulin, and cardiovascular disease.

Considering the long-term consequences, especially the risk for developing type 2 diabetes mellitus and cardiovascular disease, treatment should be directed at preventing such complications. Unfortunately there are few randomized controlled trials of any treatment of PCOS to provide us with clear treatment guidelines. Therefore, treatment tends to be symptom-based, although lifestyle interventions and pharmaceutical treatments directed at improving insulin sensitivity appear to improve multiple stigmata of the syndrome. For obese women with PCOS, lifestyle modification should be a central component of the overall treatment strategy.

REFERENCES

1. Knochenhauer ES, Key TJ, Kahsar-Miller M, et al. Prevalence of the polycystic ovary syndrome in unselected black and white women of the southeastern United States: a prospective study. J Clin Endocrinol Metab 1998;83(9): 3078−3082.
2. Stein IF, Leventhal ML. Amenorrhea associated with bilateral polycystic ovaries. Am J Obstet Gynecol 1935;29:181–191.
3. Yen S,,Vela S, Rankin J. Inappropriate secretion of follicle-stimulating hormone and luteinizing hormone in polycystic ovarian disease. J Clin Endocrinol Metab 1970;30(4):435–442.
4. Marshall JC, Eagleson CA. Neuroendocrine aspects of polycystic ovary syndrome. Endocrinol Metab Clin North Am 1999;28(2):295–324.
5. Barnes RB, Lobo RA. Central opioid activity in polycystic ovary syndrome with and without dopaminergic modulation. J Clin Endocrinol Metab 1985;61(4):779–782.
6. Poretsky L, Cataldo NA, Rosenwaks Z, Giudice LC. The insulin-related ovarian regulatory system in health and disease. Endocr Rev 1999;20(4):535–582.
7. Rosenfield RL. Ovarian and adrenal function in polycystic ovary syndrome. Endocrinol Metab Clin North Am 1999;28(2):265–293.
8. Rosenfield RL, Bames RB, Cara JF, Lucky AW. Dysregulation of cytochrome P450c 17 alpha as the cause of polycystic ovarian syndrome. Fertil Steril 1990;53(5):785–791.
9. Ehrmann DA, Rosenfield RL, Barnes RB, Brigell DF, Sheikh Z. Detection of functional ovarian hyperandrogenism in women with androgen excess. N Engl J Med 1992;327(3):157–162.
10. Zhang LH, Rodriguez H, Ohno S, Miller WL. Serine phosphorylation of human P450c17 increases 17,20-lyase activity: implications for adrenarche and the polycystic ovary syndrome. Proc Natl Acad Sci USA 1995;92(23):10,619–10,623.
11. Nestler JE, Jakubowicz DJ. Decreases in ovarian cytochrome P450c17 alpha activity and serum free testosterone after reduction of insulin secretion in polycystic ovary syndrome. N Engl J Med 1996;335(9):617–623.
12. Welt CK, Taylor AE, Martin KA, Hall JE. Serum inhibin B in polycystic ovary syndrome: regulation by insulin and luteinizing hormone. J Clin Endocrinol Metab 2002;87(12):5559–5565.
13. Chang RJ, Nakamura RM, Judd HL, Kaplan SA. Insulin resistance in nonobese patients with polycystic ovarian disease. J Clin Endocrinol Metab 1983;57(2):356–359.

14. Dunaif A, Segal KR, Futterweit W, Dobrjansky A. Profound peripheral insulin resistance, independent of obesity, in polycystic ovary syndrome. Diabetes 1989;38(9):1165–1174.
15. Ciaraldi TP, el-Roeiy A, Madar Z, et al. Cellular mechanisms of insulin resistance in polycystic ovarian syndrome. J Clin Endocrinol Metab 1992;75(2):577–583.
16. Pimenta W, Korytkowski M, Mitrakou A, et al. Pancreatic beta-cell dysfunction as the primary genetic lesion in NIDDM. Evidence from studies in normal glucose-tolerant individuals with a first-degree NIDDM relative. JAMA 1995;273(23):1855–1861.
17. Dunaif A. Insulin resistance and the polycystic ovary syndrome: mechanism and implications for pathogenesis. Endocr Rev 1997;18(6):774–800.
18. Chang RJ, Geffner ME. Associated non-ovarian problems of polycystic ovarian disease: insulin resistance. Clin Obstet Gynaecol 1985;12(3):675–685.
19. O'Meara NM, Blackman JD, Ehrmann DA, et al. Defects in beta-cell function in functional ovarian hyperandrogenism. J Clin Endocrinol Metab 1993;76(5):1241–1247.
20. Dunaif A, Finegood DT. Beta-cell dysfunction independent of obesity and glucose intolerance in the polycystic ovary syndrome. J Clin Endocrinol Metab 1996;81(3):942–947.
21. Yen SS. The polycystic ovary syndrome. Clin Endocrinol (Oxf) 1980;12(2):177–207.
22. Poretsky L, Clemons J, Bogovich K. Hyperinsulinemia and human chorionic gonadotropin synergistically promote the growth of ovarian follicular cysts in rats. Metabolism 1992;41(8):903–910.
23. Singh A, Hamilton-Fairley D, Koistinen R, et al. Effect of insulin-like growth factor-type I (IGF-I) and insulin on the secretion of sex hormone binding globulin and IGF-I binding protein (IBP-I) by human hepatoma cells. J Endocrinol 1990;124(2):R1–R3.
24. Anttila L, Ding YQ, Ruutiainen K, et al. Clinical features and circulating gonadotropin, insulin, and androgen interactions in women with polycystic ovarian disease. Fertil Steril 1991;55(6):1057–1061.
25. Suikkari AM, Koivisto VA, Rutanen EM, et al. Insulin regulates the serum levels of low molecular weight insulin-like growth factor-binding protein. J Clin Endocrinol Metab 1988;66(2):266–272.
26. Poretsky L, Chandrasekher YA, Bai C, et al. Insulin receptor mediates inhibitory effect of insulin, but not of insulin-like growth factor (IGF)-I, on IGF binding protein 1 (IGFBP-1) production in human granulosa cells. J Clin Endocrinol Metab 1996;81(2):493–496.
27. Zawadski JK, Dunaif A. Diagnostic criteria for polycystic ovary syndrome; towards a rational approach in Polycystic Ovary Syndrome. In: Dunaif A, Haseltine F, Merriam GR, eds. 1992, Blackwell Scientific:Boston; pp.377–384.
28. The Rotterdam ESHRE/ASRM-Sponsored PCOS consensus workshop group. Revised 2003 consensus on diagnostic criteria and long-term health risks related to polycystic ovary syndrome (PCOS). Hum Reprod 2004;19(1):41–47.
29. Azziz R, Ehrmann D, Legro RS, et al. Troglitazone improves ovulation and hirsutism in the polycystic ovary syndrome: a multicenter, double blind, placebo-controlled trial. J Clin Endocrinol Metab 2001;86(4):1626–1632.
30. Goldzieher JW, Axelrod LR. Clinical and biochemical features of polycystic ovarian disease. Fertil Steril 1963;14:631–653.
31. Elchalal U, Schenker JG. The pathophysiology of ovarian hyperstimulation syndrome—views and ideas. Hum Reprod 1997;12(6):1129–1137.
32. Fulghesu AM, Villa P, Pavone V, et al. The impact of insulin secretion on the ovarian response to exogenous gonadotropins in polycystic ovary syndrome. J Clin Endocrinol Metab 1997;82(2):644–648.
33. Dale PO, Tanbo T, Haug E, Abyholm T. The impact of insulin resistance on the outcome of ovulation induction with low-dose follicle stimulating hormone in women with polycystic ovary syndrome. Hum Reprod 1998;13(3):567–570.
34. Legro RS, Driscoll D, Strauss JF, 3rd, Foxx J, Dunaif A. Evidence for a genetic basis for hyperandrogenemia in polycystic ovary syndrome. Proc Natl Acad Sci USA 1998;95(25):14,956–14,960.
35. Farquhar CM, Birdsall M, Manning P, Mitchell JM, France JT. The prevalence of polycystic ovaries on ultrasound scanning in a population of randomly selected women. Aust NZ J Obstet Gynaecol 1994;34(1):67–72.
36. Polson DW, Adams J, Wadsworth J, Franks S. Polycystic ovaries—a common finding in normal women. Lancet 1988;1(8590): 870–872.
37. Robinson S, Rodin DA, Deacon A, Wheeler MJ, Clayton RN. Which hormone tests for the diagnosis of polycystic ovary syndrome? Br J Obstet Gynaecol 1992;99(3):232–238.

38. Nestler JE. Sex hormone-binding globulin: a marker for hyperinsulinemia and/or insulin resistance? J Clin Endocrinol Metab 1993;76(2):273–274.

39. Boots LR, Potter S, Potter D, Azziz R. Measurement of total serum testosterone levels using commercially available kits: high degree of between-kit variability. Fertil Steril 1998;69(2):286–292.

40. Carmina E, Koyama T, Chang L, Stanczyk FZ, Lobo RA. Does ethnicity influence the prevalence of adrenal hyperandrogenism and insulin resistance in polycystic ovary syndrome? Am J Obstet Gynecol 1992;167(6):1807–1812.

41. Moran C, Tapia MC, Hernandez E, et al. Etiological review of hirsutism in 250 patients. Arch Med Res 1994;25(3):311–314.

42. Lobo RA, Goebelsmann U, Horton R. Evidence for the importance of peripheral tissue events in the development of hirsutism in polycystic ovary syndrome. J Clin Endocrinol Metab 1983;57(2):393–397.

43. Barth JH. How robust is the methodology for trials of therapy in hirsute women? Clin Endocrinol (Oxf), 1996;45(4):379–380.

44. Holdaway IM, Fraser A, Sheehan A, et al. Objective assessment of treatment response in hirsutism. Horm Res 1985;22(4): 253–259.

45. Hatch R, Rosenfield RL, Kim MH, Tredway D. Hirsutism: implications, etiology, and management. Am J Obstet Gynecol 1981;140(7):815–830.

46. Azziz R,Waggoner WT, Ochoa T, Knochenhauer ES, Boots LR. Idiopathic hirsutism: an uncommon cause of hirsutism in Alabama. Fertil Steril 1998;70(2):274–278.

47. Franks S. Polycystic ovary syndrome. N Engl J Med 1995;333(13):853–861.

48. Koivunen R, Laatikainen T, Tomas C, et al. The prevalence of polycystic ovaries in healthy women. Acta Obstet Gynecol Scand 1999;78(2):137–141.

49. Chang PL, Lindheim SR, Lowre C, et al. Normal ovulatory women with polycystic ovaries have hyperandrogenic pituitary-ovarian responses to gonadotropin-releasing hormone-agonist testing. J Clin Endocrinol Metab 2000;85(3):995–1000.

50. Carmina E, Wong L, Chang L, et al. Endocrine abnormalities in ovulatory women with polycystic ovaries on ultrasound. Hum Reprod 1997;12(5):905–909.

51. Loucks TL, Talbott EO, McHugh KP, et al. Do polycystic-appearing ovaries affect the risk of cardiovascular disease among women with polycystic ovary syndrome? Fertil Steril 2000;74(3):547–552.

52. Enskog A, Henriksson M, Unander M, Nilsson L, Brannstrom M. Prospective study of the clinical and laboratory parameters of patients in whom ovarian hyperstimulation syndrome developed during controlled ovarian hyperstimulation for in vitro fertilization. Fertil Steril 1999;71(5):808–814.

53. Dahlgren E, Johansson S, Lindstedt G, et al. Women with polycystic ovary syndrome wedge resected in 1956 to 1965: a long-term follow-up focusing on natural history and circulating hormones. Fertil Steril 1992;57(3):505–513.

54. Talbott E, Clerici A, Berga SL, et al. Adverse lipid and coronary heart disease risk profiles in young women with polycystic ovary syndrome: results of a case-control study. J Clin Epidemiol 1998;51(5):415–422.

55. Elting MW, Korsen TJ, Bezemer PD, Schoemaker J. Prevalence of diabetes mellitus, hypertension and cardiac complaints in a follow-up study of a Dutch PCOS population. Hum Reprod 2001; 16(3):556–560.

56. Ehrmann DA, Barnesss RB, Rosenfield RL, Cavaghan MK. Prevalence of impaired glucose tolerance and diabetes in women with polycystic ovary syndrome. Diabetes Care 1999;22(1):141–146.

57. Legro RS, Kunselman AR, Dodson WC, Dunaif A. Prevalence and predictors of risk for type 2 diabetes mellitus and impaired glucose tolerance in polycystic ovary syndrome: a prospective, controlled study in 254 affected women. J Clin Endocrinol Metab 1999;84(1):165–169.

58. Sinha R, Fisch G, Teague B, et al. Prevalence of impaired glucose tolerance among children and adolescents with marked obesity. N Engl J Med 2002;346(11):802–810.

59. Palmert MR, Gordon CM, Kartashov AI, et al. Screening for abnormal glucose tolerance in adolescents with polycystic ovary syndrome. J Clin Endocrinol Metab 2002;87(3):1017–1023.

60. Ehrmann DA, Kasza K, Azziz R, Legro RS, Ghazzi MN. Effects of race and family history of type 2 diabetes on metabolic status of women with polycystic ovary syndrome. J Clin Endocrinol Metab 2005;90(1):66–71.

61. Gambineri A, Pelusi C, Manicardi E, et al. Glucose intolerance in a large cohort of mediterranean women with polycystic ovary syndrome: phenotype and associated factors. Diabetes 2004;53(9):2353–2358.

62. Klein S, Romijin JA, Obesity, in Williams Textbook of Endocrinology, Larsennn, Kronenberg, Melmed, eds. 2002, Saunders: Philadelphia, PA.

63. Janssen I, Katzmarzyk PT, Ross R. Body mass index, waist circumference, and health risk: evidence in support of current National Institutes of Health guidelines. Arch Intern Med 2002;162(18):2074–2079.

64. Kissebah AH, Vydelingum N, Murray R, et al. Relation of body fat distribution to metabolic complications of obesity. J Clin Endocrinol Metab 1982;54(2):254–260.

65. Larsson B, Svardsudd K, Welin L, et al. Abdominal adipose tissue distribution, obesity, and risk of cardiovascular disease and death: 13 year follow up of participants in the study of men born in 1913. Br Med J (Clin Res Ed) 1984;288(6428):1401–1404.

66. Lapidus L, Bengtsson C. Regional obesity as a health hazard in women—a prospective study. Acta Med Scand Suppl 1988;723:53–59.

67. Lapidus L, Bengtsson C, Lissner L. Distribution of adipose tissue in relation to cardiovascular and total mortality as observed during 20 years in a prospective population study of women in Gothenburg, Sweden. Diabetes Res Clin Pract 1990;10 Suppl 1:S185–S189.

68. Rabinowitz D, Zierler KL. Forearm metabolism in obesity and its response to intra-arterial insulin. Characterization of insulin resistance and evidence for adaptive hyperinsulinism. J Clin Invest 1962;41:2173–2181.

69. Peiris AN, Struve MF, Kissebah AH. Relationship of body fat distribution to the metabolic clearance of insulin in premenopausal women. Int J Obes 1987;11(6):581–589.

70. Rosenbaum M, Leibel RL, Hirsch J. Obesity. N Engl J Med 1997;337(6):396–407.

71. Pasquali R, Antenucci D, Casimirri F, et al. Clinical and hormonal characteristics of obese amenorrheic hyperandrogenic women before and after weight loss. J Clin Endocrinol Metab 1989;68(1):173–179.

72. Talbott EO, Zborowski JV, Sutton-Tyrrell K, McHugh-Pemu KP. Cardiovascular risk in women with polycystic ovary syndrome. Obstet Gynecol Clin North Am 2001;28(1):111–133, vii.

73. Reaven GM. Banting Lecture 1988. Role of insulin resistance in human disease. Diabetes 1988;37(12):1595–1607.

74. Legro RS, Kunselman AR, Dunaif A. Prevalence and predictors of dyslipidemia in women with polycystic ovary syndrome. Am J Med 2001;111(8):607–613.

75. Wild RA, Grubb B, Hartz A, et al. Clinical signs of androgen excess as risk factors for coronary artery disease. Fertil Steril 1990;54(2):255–259.

76. Dahlgren E, Janson PO, Johansson S, Lapidus L, Oden A. Polycystic ovary syndrome and risk for myocardial infarction. Evaluated from a risk factor model based on a prospective population study of women. Acta Obstet Gynecol Scand 1992;71(8):599–604.

77. Prelevic GM, Bekjic T, Balint-Peric L, Ginsburg J. Cardiac flow velocity in women with the polycystic ovary syndrome. Clin Endocrinol (Oxf) 1995;43(6):677–681.

78. Temple R. Are surrogate markers adequate to assess cardiovascular disease drugs? JAMA 1999;282(8):790–795.

79. Wild RA. Polycystic ovary syndrome: a risk for coronary artery disease? Am J Obstet Gynecol 2002;186(1):35–43.

80. Talbott EO, Guzick DS, Sutton-Tyrrell K, et al. Evidence for association between polycystic ovary syndrome and premature carotid atherosclerosis in middle-aged women. Arterioscler Thromb Vasc Biol 2000;20(11):2414–2421.

81. Vryonidou A, Papatheodorou A, Tavridou A, et al. Association of hyperandrogenemic and metabolic phenotype with carotid intima-media thickness in young women with polycystic ovary syndrome. J Clin Endocrinol Metab 2005;90(5):2740–2746.

82. Pierpoint T, McKeigue PM, Isaacs AJ, Wild SH, Jacobs HS. Mortality of women with polycystic ovary syndrome at long-term follow-up. J Clin Epidemiol 1998;51(7):581–586.

83. Wild S, Pierpoint T, McKeigue P, Jacobs H. Cardiovascular disease in women with polycystic ovary syndrome at long-term follow-up: a retrospective cohort study. Clin Endocrinol (Oxf) 2000; 52(5):595–600.

84. Birdsall MA, Farquhar CM, White HD. Association between polycystic ovaries and extent of coronary artery disease in women having cardiac catheterization. Ann Intern Med 1997;126(1):32–35.

85. Gorgels WJ, vd Graaf Y, Blankenstein MA, et al. Urinary sex hormone excretions in premenopausal women and coronary heart disease risk: a nested case-referent study in the DOM-cohort. J Clin Epidemiol 1997;50(3):275–281.

86. Solomon CG, Hu FB, Dunaif A, et al. Menstrual cycle irregularity and risk for future cardiovascular disease. J Clin Endocrinol Metab 2002;87(5):2013–2017.

87. Solomon CG, Hu FB, Dunaif A, et al. Long or highly irregular menstrual cycles as a marker for risk of type 2 diabetes mellitus. JAMA 2001;286(19):2421–2426.

88. Coulam CB, Annegers JF, Kranz JS. Chronic anovulation syndrome and associated neoplasia. Obstet Gynecol 1983;61(4):403–407.
89. Smyczek-Gargya B, Geppert M. Endometrial cancer associated with polycystic ovaries in young women. Pathol Res Pract 1992;188(7):946–948; discussion 948–950.
90. Ho SP, Tan KT, Pang MW, Ho TH. Endometrial hyperplasia and the risk of endometrial carcinoma. Singapore Med J 1997;38(1):11–15.
91. Dockerty MB, Jackson RL. The Stein-Leventhal syndrome: analysis of 43 cases with special reference to association with endometrial carcinoma. Am J Obstet Gynecol 1957;73(1):161–173.
92. Hardiman P, Pillay OC, Atiomo W. Polycystic ovary syndrome and endometrial carcinoma. Lancet 2003;361(9371):1810–1812.
93. Legro RS, Spielman R, Urbanek M, et al. Phenotype and genotype in polycystic ovary syndrome. Recent Prog Horm Res 1998;53:217–256.
94. Gambrell RD Jr, Bagnell CA, Greenblatt RB. Role of estrogens and progesterone in the etiology and prevention of endometrial cancer: review. Am J Obstet Gynecol 1983;146(6):696–707.
95. Lobo RA, Granger L, Goebelsmann U, Mishell DR, Jr. Elevations in unbound serum estradiol as a possible mechanism for inappropriate gonadotropin secretion in women with PCO. J Clin Endocrinol Metab 1981;52(1):156–158.
96. Dahlgren E, Friberg LG, Johansson S, et al. Endometrial carcinoma; ovarian dysfunction—a risk factor in young women. Eur J Obstet Gynecol Reprod Biol 1991;41(2):143–150.
97. Aksel S, Wentz AC, Jones GS. Anovulatory infertility associated with adenocarcinoma and adenomatous hyperplasia of the endometrium. Obstet Gynecol 1974;43(3):386–391.
98. Chamlian DL, Taylor HB. Endometrial hyperplasia in young women. Obstet Gynecol 1970;36(5):659–666.
99. Schildkraut JM, Schwingl PJ, Bastos E, Evanoff A, Hughes C. Epithelial ovarian cancer risk among women with polycystic ovary syndrome. Obstet Gynecol 1996;88(4 Pt 1):554–559.
100. Anderson KE, Sellers TA, Chen PL, et al. Association of Stein-Leventhal syndrome with the incidence of postmenopausal breast carcinoma in a large prospective study of women in Iowa. Cancer 1997;79(3):494–499.
101. Sagle M, Bishop K, Ridley N, et al. Recurrent early miscarriage and polycystic ovaries. BMJ 1988;297(6655):1027–1028.
102. Wang JX, Davies MJ, Norman RJ. Polycystic ovarian syndrome and the risk of spontaneous abortion following assisted reproductive technology treatment. Hum Reprod 2001;16(12):2606–2609.
103. Balen AH,Tan SL, MacDougall J, Jacobs HS. Miscarriage rates following in-vitro fertilization are increased in women with polycystic ovaries and reduced by pituitary desensitization with buserelin. Hum Reprod 1993;8(6): 959–964.
104. Sir-Petermann T, Hitchsfeld C, Maliqueo M, et al. Birth weight in offspring of mothers with polycystic ovarian syndrome. Hum Reprod 2005;20(8):2122–2126.
105. Weerakiet S, Srisombut C, Rojanasakul A, et al. Prevalence of gestational diabetes mellitus and pregnancy outcomes in Asian women with polycystic ovary syndrome. Gynecol Endocrinol 2004;19(3):134–140.
106. Bjercke S, Dale PO, Tanbo T, et al. Impact of insulin resistance on pregnancy complications and outcome in women with polycystic ovary syndrome. Gynecol Obstet Invest 2002;54(2):94–98.
107. Kashyap S, Claman P. Obstetric outcome in women with polycystic ovarian syndrome. Hum Reprod 2001;16(7):1537.
108. Haakova L, Cibula D, Rezabek, K, et al. Pregnancy outcome in women with PCOS and in controls matched by age and weight. Hum Reprod 2003;18(7):1438–1441.
109. Mikola M, Hiilesmaa V, Halttunen M, Suhonen L, Tiitinen A. Obstetric outcome in women with polycystic ovarian syndrome. Hum Reprod 2001;16(2):226–229.
110. Balen AH, Tan SL, Jacobs HS. Hypersecretion of luteinising hormone: a significant cause of infertility and miscarriage. Br J Obstet Gynaecol 1993;100(12):1082–1089.
111. Nestler JE. Role of hyperinsulinemia in the pathogenesis of the polycystic ovary syndrome, and its clinical implications. Semin Reprod Endocrinol 1997;15(2):111–122.
112. Givens JR, Andersen RN, Wiser WL, Umstot ES, Fish SA. The effectiveness of two oral contraceptives in suppressing plasma androstenedione, testosterone, LH, and FSH, and in stimulating plasma testosterone-binding capacity in hirsute women. Am J Obstet Gynecol 1976;124(4):333–339.
113. Azziz R, Ochoa TM, Bradley EL, Jr, Potter HD, Boots LR. Leuprolide and estrogen versus oral contraceptive pills for the treatment of hirsutism: a prospective randomized study. J Clin Endocrinol Metab 1995;80(12):3406–3411.

114. Heiner JS, Greendale GA, Kawakami AK, et al. Comparison of a gonadotropin-releasing hormone agonist and a low dose oral contraceptive given alone or together in the treatment of hirsutism. J Clin Endocrinol Metab 1995;80(12):3412–3418.

115. Elkind-Hirsch KE, Anania C, Mack M, Malinak R. Combination gonadotropin-releasing hormone agonist and oral contraceptive therapy improves treatment of hirsute women with ovarian hyperandrogenism. Fertil Steril 1995;63(5):970–978.

116. Carr BR, Breslau NA, Givens C, et al. Oral contraceptive pills, gonadotropin-releasing hormone agonists, or use in combination for treatment of hirsutism: a clinical research center study. J Clin Endocrinol Metab 1995;80(4):1169–1178.

117. Velazquez EM, Mendoza S, Hamer T, Sosa F, Glueck CJ. Metformin therapy in polycystic ovary syndrome reduces hyperinsulinemia, insulin resistance, hyperandrogenemia, and systolic blood pressure, while facilitating normal menses and pregnancy. Metabolism 1994;43(5):647–654.

118. Nestler JE, Jakubowicz DJ. Lean women with polycystic ovary syndrome respond to insulin reduction with decreases in ovarian P450c17 alpha activity and serum androgens. J Clin Endocrinol Metab 1997;82(12):4075–4079.

119. Costello MF, Eden JA. A systematic review of the reproductive system effects of metformin in patients with polycystic ovary syndrome. Fertil Steril 2003;79(1):1–13.

120. Nestler JE, Jakubowicz DJ, Reamer P, Gunn RD, Allan G. Ovulatory and metabolic effects of D-chiro-inositol in the polycystic ovary syndrome. N Engl J Med 1999;340(17):1314–1320.

121. Coetzee EJ, Jackson WP. Metformin in management of pregnant insulin-independent diabetics. Diabetologia 1979;16(4):241–245.

122. Coetzee EJ, Jackson WP. Pregnancy in established non-insulin-dependent diabetics. A five-and-a-half year study at Groote Schuur Hospital. S Afr Med J 1980;58(20):795–802.

123. Callahan TL, Hall JE, Ettner SL, et al. The economic impact of multiple-gestation pregnancies and the contribution of assisted-reproduction techniques to their incidence. N Engl J Med 1994; 331(4): 244–249.

124. Sarlis NJ, Weil SJ, Nelson LM. Administration of metformin to a diabetic woman with extreme hyperandrogenemia of nontumoral origin: management of infertility and prevention of inadvertent masculinization of a female fetus. J Clin Endocrinol Metab 1999;84(5):1510–1512.

125. Diamanti-Kandarakis E, Kouli C, Tssianateli T, Bergiele A. Therapeutic effects of metformin on insulin resistance and hyperandrogenism in polycystic ovary syndrome. Eur J Endocrinol 1998; 138(3):269–274.

126. Vandermolen DT, Ratts VS, Evans WS, et al. Metformin increases the ovulatory rate and pregnancy rate from clomiphene citrate in patients with polycystic ovary syndrome who are resistant to clomiphene citrate alone. Fertil Steril 2001;75(2):310–315.

127. Velazquez E, Acosta A, Mendoza SG. Menstrual cyclicity after metformin therapy in polycystic ovary syndrome. Obstet Gynecol 1997;90(3):392–395.

128. Lord JM, Flight IH, Norman RJ. Insulin-sensitising drugs (metformin, troglitazone, rosiglitazone, pioglitazone, D-chiro-inositol) for polycystic ovary syndrome. Cochrane Database Syst Rev 2003(3):CD003053.

129. Harborne L, Fleming R, Lyall H, Norman J, Sattar N. Descriptive review of the evidence for the use of metformin in polycystic ovary syndrome. Lancet 2003;361(9372):1894–1901.

130. Glueck CJ, Phillips H, Cameron D, Sieve-Smith L, Wang P. Continuing metformin throughout pregnancy in women with polycystic ovary syndrome appears to safely reduce first-trimester spontaneous abortion: a pilot study. Fertil Steril 2001;75(1):46–52.

131. Moghetti P, Casello R, Negri C, et al. Metformin effects on clinical features, endocrine and metabolic profiles, and insulin sensitivity in polycystic ovary syndrome: a randomized, double-blind, placebo-controlled 6-month trial, followed by open, long-term clinical evaluation. J Clin Endocrinol Metab 2000;85(1):139–146.

132. Azziz R, Ehrmann D, Legro RS, et al. Troglitazone improves ovulation and hirsutism in the polycystic ovary syndrome: a multicenter, double blind, placebo-controlled trial. J Clin Endocrinol Metab 2001;86(4):1626–1632.

133. Belli SH, Graffigna MN, Oneto A, et al. Effect of rosiglitazone on insulin resistance, growth factors, and reproductive disturbances in women with polycystic ovary syndrome. Fertil Steril 2004;81(3): 624–629.

134. Brettenthaler N, DeGeyter C, Huber PR, Keller U. Effect of the insulin sensitizer pioglitazone on insulin resistance, hyperandrogenism, and ovulatory dysfunction in women with polycystic ovary syndrome. J Clin Endocrinol Metab 2004;89(8):3835–3840.

135. Ortega-Gonzalez C, Luna S, Hernandez L, et al. Responses of serum androgen and insulin resistance to metformin and pioglitazone in obese, insulin-resistant women with polycystic ovary syndrome. J Clin Endocrinol Metab 2005;90(3):1360–1365.

136. Pasquali R, Gambineri A, Biscotti D, et al. Effect of long-term treatment with metformin added to hypocaloric diet on body composition, fat distribution, and androgen and insulin levels in abdominally obese women with and without the polycystic ovary syndrome. J Clin Endocrinol Metab 2000;85(8):2767–2774.

137. Torgerson JS, Hauptman J, Boldrin MN, Sjostrom L. XENical in the prevention of diabetes in obese subjects (XENDOS) study: a randomized study of orlistat as an adjunct to lifestyle changes for the prevention of type 2 diabetes in obese patients. Diabetes Care 2004;27(1):155–161.

138. Sabuncu T, Harma M, Nazligul Y, Kilic F. Sibutramine has a positive effect on clinical and metabolic parameters in obese patients with polycystic ovary syndrome. Fertil Steril 2003;80(5):1199–1204.

139. Jayagopal V, Kilpatrick ES, Holding S, Jeeennings PE, Atkin SL. Orlistat is as beneficial as metformin in the treatment of polycystic ovarian syndrome. J Clin Endocrinol Metab 2005;90(2):729–733.

140. Glasier AF, Irvine DS, Wickings EJ, Hillier SG, Baird DT. A comparison of the effects on follicular development between clomiphene citrate, its two separate isomers and spontaneous cycles. Hum Reprod 1989;4(3):252–256.

141. Mikkelson TJ, Kroboth PD, Cameron WJ, et al. Single-dose pharmacokinetics of clomiphene citrate in normal volunteers. Fertil Steril 1986;46(3):392–396.

142. Hughes E, Collins J, Vandekerckhove P. Ovulation induction with urinary follicle stimulating hormone versus human menopausal gonadotropin for clomiphene-resistant polycystic ovary syndrome. Cochrane Database Syst Rev 2000(2):CD000087.

143. Shepard MK, Balmaceda JP, Leija CG. Relationship of weight to successful induction of ovulation with clomiphene citrate. Fertil Steril 1979;32(6):641–645.

144. Lobo RA, Granger LR, Davajan V, Mishell DR, Jr. An extended regimen of clomiphene citrate in women unresponsive to standard therapy. Fertil Steril 1982;37(6):762–766.

145. Lobo RA, Paul W, March CM, Granger L, Kletzky OA. Clomiphene and dexamethasone in women unresponsive to clomiphene alone. Obstet Gynecol 1982;60(4):497–501.

146. Homburg R, Levy T, Ben-Rafael Z. A comparative prospective study of conventional regimen with chronic low-dose administration of follicle-stimulating hormone for anovulation associated with polycystic ovary syndrome. Fertil Steril 1995;63(4):729–733.

147. Ergur AR, Yergok YZ, Ertekin A, et al. Clomiphene citrate-resistant polycystic ovary syndrome. Preventing multifollicular development. J Reprod Med 1998;43(3):185–190.

148. Dale O, Tanbo T, Lunde O, Abyholm T. Ovulation induction with low-dose follicle-stimulating hormone in women with the polycystic ovary syndrome. Acta Obstet Gynecol Scand 1993;72(1):43–46.

149. Strowitzki T, Seehaus D, Korell M, Hepp H. Low-dose follicle stimulating hormone for ovulation induction in polycystic ovary syndrome. J Reprod Med 1994;39(7):499–503.

150. Sagle MA, Hamilton-Fairley D, Kiddy DS, Franks S. A comparative, randomized study of low-dose human menopausal gonadotropin and follicle-stimulating hormone in women with polycystic ovarian syndrome. Fertil Steril 1991;55(1): 56–60.

151. Nugent D, Vandekerckhove P, Hughes E, Arnot M. Gonadotrophin therapy for ovulation induction in subfertility associated with polycystic ovary syndrome. Cochrane Database Syst Rev 2000(4): CD000410.

152. Bayram N, van Wely M, Vandekerckhove P, Lilford R, van Der Veen F. Pulsatile luteinising hormone releasing hormone for ovulation induction in subfertility associated with polycystic ovary syndrome. Cochrane Database Syst Rev 2000(2): CD000412.

153. Lee O, Farquhar C, Toomath R, Jepson R. Spironolactone versus placebo or in combination with steroids for hirsutism and/or acne. Cochrane Database Syst Rev 2000(2):CD000194.

154. Eil C, Edelson SK. The use of human skin fibroblasts to obtain potency estimates of drug binding to androgen receptors. J Clin Endocrinol Metab 1984;59(1):51–55.

155. Groves TD, Corenblum B. Spironolactone therapy during human pregnancy. Am J Obstet Gynecol, 1995;172(5):1655–1656.

156. Helfer EL, Miller JL, Rose LI. Side-effects of spironolactone therapy in the hirsute woman. J Clin Endocrinol Metab 1988;66(1):208–211.

157. Muhlemann MF, Carter GD, Cream JJ, Wise P. Oral spironolactone: an effective treatment for acne vulgaris in women. Br J Dermatol 1986;115(2):227–232.

158. Fruzzetti F, De Lorenzo D, Ricci C, Fioretti P. Clinical and endocrine effects of flutamide in hyperandrogenic women. Fertil Steril 1993;60(5):806–813.

159. Moghetti P, Castello R, Magnani CM, et al. Clinical and hormonal effects of the 5 alpha-reductase inhibitor finasteride in idiopathic hirsutism. J Clin Endocrinol Metab 1994;79(4):1115–1121.

160. Fruzzetti F, de Lorenzo D, Parrini D, Ricci C. Effects of finasteride, a 5 alpha-reductase inhibitor, on circulating androgens and gonadotropin secretion in hirsute women. J Clin Endocrinol Metab 1994;79(3):831–835.

161. Moghetti P, Tosi F, Tosti A, et al. Comparison of spironolactone, flutamide, and finasteride efficacy in the treatment of hirsutism: a randomized, double blind, placebo-controlled trial. J Clin Endocrinol Metab 2000;85(1):89–94.

162. Wong IL, Morris RS, Chang L, et al. A prospective randomized trial comparing finasteride to spirono-lactone in the treatment of hirsute women. J Clin Endocrinol Metab 1995;80(1):233–238.

163. Greenblatt E, Casper RF. Endocrine changes after laparoscopic ovarian cautery in polycystic ovarian syndrome. Am J Obstet Gynecol 1987;156(2):279–285.

164. Katz M, Carr PJ, Cohen BM, Millar RP. Hormonal effects of wedge resection of polycystic ovaries. Obstet Gynecol 1978;51(4):437–444.

165. Adashi EY, Rock JA, Guzick D, et al. Fertility following bilateral ovarian wedge resection: a critical analysis of 90 consecutive cases of the polycystic ovary syndrome. Fertil Steril 1981;36(3):320–325.

166. Farquhar C, Vandekerckhove P, Arnot M, Lilford R. Laparoscopic "drilling" by diathermy or laser for ovulation induction in anovulatory polycystic ovary syndrome. Cochrane Database Syst Rev 2000(2):CD001122.

167. Farquhar CM, Williamson K, Gudex G, et al. A randomized controlled trial of laparoscopic ovarian diathermy versus gonadotropin therapy for women with clomiphene citrate-resistant polycystic ovary syndrome. Fertil Steril 2002;78(2):404–411.

168. Donesky BW, Adashi EY. Surgically induced ovulation in the polycystic ovary syndrome: wedge resection revisited in the age of laparoscopy. Fertil Steril 1995;63(3):439–463.

169. Kiddy DS, Hamilton-Fairley D, Bush A, et al. Improvement in endocrine and ovarian function during dietary treatment of obese women with polycystic ovary syndrome. Clin Endocrinol (Oxf) 1992;36(1):105–111.

170. Jakubowicz DJ, Beer NA, Beer RM, Nestler JE. Disparate effects of weight reduction by diet on serum dehydroepiandrosterone-sulfate levels in obese men and women. J Clin Endocrinol Metab 1995;80(11):3373–3376.

171. Faulds G, Ryden M, Ek I, Wahrenberg H, Arner P. Mechanisms behind lipolytic catecholamine resistance of subcutaneous fat cells in the polycystic ovarian syndrome. J Clin Endocrinol Metab 2003;88(5):2269–2273.

172. Haas DA, Carr BR, Attia GR. Effects of metformin on body mass index, menstrual cyclicity, and ovulation induction in women with polycystic ovary syndrome. Fertil Steril 2003;79(3):469–481.

173. Pasquali R, Gambineri A, Biscotti D, et al. Effect of long-term treatment with metformin added to hypocaloric diet on body composition, fat distribution, and androgen and insulin levels in abdominally obese women with and without the polycystic ovary syndrome. J Clin Endocrinol Metab 2000;85(8):2767–2774.

174. Braun B, Zimmermann MB, Kretchmer N. Effects of exercise intensity on insulin sensitivity in women with non-insulin-dependent diabetes mellitus. J Appl Physiol 1995;78(1):300–306.

175. Randeva HS, Lewandowski KC, Drzewoski, J, et al. Exercise decreases plasma total homocysteine in overweight young women with polycystic ovary syndrome. J Clin Endocrinol Metab 2002;87(10):4496–4501.

176. Mitwally MF, Casper RF. Use of an aromatase inhibitor for induction of ovulation in patients with an inadequate response to clomiphene citrate. Fertil Steril 2001;75(2):305–309.

12 Weight Management in Diabetes Prevention

Translating the Diabetes Prevention Program Into Clinical Practice

F. Xavier Pi-Sunyer, MD, MPH

CONTENTS

INTRODUCTION
THE DIABETES PREVENTION PROGRAM
CONCLUSION
REFERENCES

Summary

Obesity and impaired glucose tolerance (IGT) are associated with a greater health risk for a number of conditions, including insulin resistance, diabetes mellitus, hypertension, dyslipidemia, coagulation abnormalities, inflammatory markers, and coronary heart disease. Lifestyle changes can delay or prevent the development of type 2 diabetes in patients with obesity and IGT. The risks improve with weight loss and increased physical activity. A decrease of 7 to 10% or more from baseline weight can have a significant effect. This has now been documented in a number of randomized controlled studies. This essay is directed on how the Diabetes Prevention Program approach to lifestyle change can be translated in a meaningful way to routine clinical care practice settings.

Key Words: Diabetes; prevention; physical activity; weight loss; diet; impaired glucose tolerance.

INTRODUCTION

Impaired glucose tolerance (IGT) is a pathophysiological state that exists between normal glucose homeostasis and frank diabetes mellitus. It is defined by the level of plasma glucose 2 h after an oral glucose load. The conversion rate to diabetes has varied in differing population groups, but is about 5 to 6% per year *(1)*. IGT is a risk factor not only for diabetes, but also for macrovascular disease *(2,3)* and for cardiovascular mortality. Because diabetes is increasing rapidly around the globe *(4)* and is predicted to continue to do so *(5)*, it is important to attempt to prevent it, and persons with IGT are obvious targets. The most important predictors of conversion are a higher 2-h blood glucose and greater weight. Another predictor is a low level of physical activity *(6)*.

From: *Contemporary Endocrinology: Treatment of the Obese Patient*
Edited by: R. F. Kushner and D. H. Bessesen © Humana Press Inc., Totowa, NJ

Increase in Prevalence of Obesity

The National Health and Nutrition Examination Survey (NHANES) III, which was conducted from 1988 to 1994, showed that 59.4% of men and 50.7% of women in the United States are overweight or obese. In the period between the second NHANES survey and the third, the prevalence of obesity rose from 14.5% to 22.5% *(7)*. More recent data has put the figure at 30.5% for obesity and 64.5% for overweight *(8)*. Obesity is also increasing rapidly in other parts of the world *(8)*. Global obesity increased from an estimated 200 million adults in 1995 to more than 300 million in 2000 *(9)*. Childhood obesity has also increased. During the past 30 yr, childhood obesity in the United States has more than doubled *(10)*. As obesity increases, it leads to an increased disease burden *(11,12)*, increased mortality *(13)*, and a shortened life span *(14)*. It brings with it not only an increased incidence of type 2 diabetes, but also of dyslipidemia, hypertension, and cardiovascular disease.

Abnormal Glucose Metabolism and Type 2 Diabetes

Excess weight is the most important modifiable risk factor for the development of type 2 diabetes. The incidence of diabetes rises as obesity prevalence increases *(15)*. The prevalence of reported diabetes is 2.9 times higher in overweight than in nonoverweight persons in the NHANES data *(16)*. Obesity is associated with type 2 diabetes mellitus in both women *(17)* and men *(18)*. Also, the longer that people are obese, the higher becomes their risk of developing diabetes *(19)*. From 1990 to 1998, the prevalence of type 2 diabetes increased by 33%. More than 85% of type 2 diabetic patients are overweight or obese *(20)*. Type 2 diabetes accounts for 90 to 95% of the 20.8 million cases of diabetes mellitus in the United States today *(21)*.

Fat distribution is also very important in diabetes risk *(22–25)*. Central or upper body fat deposition is independently associated with insulin resistance *(23)*, diabetes *(24,25)*, and cardiovascular disease *(26)*. Intra-abdominal or visceral obesity is strongly associated with insulin resistance, as well as with dyslipidemia, hypertension, and glucose intolerance *(27–30)*. In Japanese American men intra-abdominal fat deposition was closely correlated with type 2 diabetes, whereas subcutaneous fat deposits in the abdomen, thorax, or thigh were not statistically significant predictors *(31)*.

A lack of adequate physical activity is another important risk factor for the development of type 2 diabetes. Men who habitually engage in moderate levels of physical activity have a substantially reduced risk of diabetes compared with physically inactive men, even after adjustment for age, body mass index (BMI), and other risk factors *(32)*. Physical training can reduce insulin resistance *(33)* and high physical activity can lower insulin levels *(34–37)*. Adopting a regular exercise style also improves lipids, due to both an independent effect of the exercise and to a loss of fat, particularly visceral fat *(38)*.

Weight Loss in IGT

Weight loss can prevent or delay the progression to diabetes in obese patients. In the Nurses' Health Study, Colditz et al. found that women who lost more than 5 kg over a 10-yr period reduced their risk of diabetes by 50% or more—a remarkable benefit for a relatively modest loss *(39)*. Will et al. *(40)* examined retrospectively the 13-yr incidence of diabetes in a large cohort of subjects from the first Cancer Prevention Study. The authors also found that intentional weight loss was associated with a significant reduction in the rate of developing diabetes. In the Swedish Obese Subjects (SOS) study, there was a weight loss averaging 28 ± 15 kg (mean ± SD) at 2 yr, and this was associated with an improvement of cardiovascular risk factors including glucose and insulin levels *(41,42)*. Thus, weight loss improves insulin sensitivity, leading to lower risk factors for diabetes and cardiovascular disease *(43–45)*. There have been a number of trials that have tested the effect of lifestyle change on the development of diabetes in persons with IGT. These have included generally both diet and exercise to effect weight loss and improve fitness *(46–49)*.

THE DIABETES PREVENTION PROGRAM

The Diabetes Prevention Program (DPP) asked whether lifestyle intervention or treatment with metformin can prevent or delay the progression from IGT to diabetes, and whether their effectiveness differs according to age, sex, race, or ethnic group *(50)*. This randomized trial engaged 27 centers in the United States and included 3234 individuals *(50)*. Subjects were selected who had impaired fasting glucose of 95 to 125 and/or postprandial glucose of 140 to 200. The mean BMI of this group was 34 kg/m^2. These persons were therefore at high risk of developing diabetes. Individuals were randomized to an intensive lifestyle arm, a metformin arm (850 mg bid), a troglitazone arm, and a placebo "usual care" arm. The troglitazone arm was stopped after about a year because of hepatic toxicity.

The lifestyle intervention goals were as follows *(50)*: the weight loss goal was 7% from baseline and the physical activity goal was at least 150 min/week. The study was terminated early by the Data Safety Monitoring Board because of the superior effectiveness of the lifestyle intervention in preventing diabetes. Patients had been followed for up to 4 yr and the average length of follow-up was 2.8 yr. The weight loss effects are shown in Fig. 1 and the physical activity results in Fig. 2 *(50a)*. The goal of 7% weight loss from baseline was reached at 6 mo. Thereafter there was a gradual return toward baseline weight. With this amount of weight loss in the lifestyle arm, there was a 58% reduction in the development of diabetes in the lifestyle intervention group as compared with the usual care placebo group. The metformin group had a reduction of diabetes of 31%. The progression to diabetes in the three arms is shown in Fig. 3. The incidence of diabetes was 11.0 cases per 100 person-years in the placebo group, 7.8 in the metformin group, and 4.8 in the lifestyle group. The results were highly significant for both metformin and lifestyle ($p < 0.001$). These results did not differ by sex, race, or ethnic group. The lifestyle intervention was highly effective in all subgroups *(50a)*. Nearly half the participants were from minority groups, who have an increased risk for developing type 2 diabetes. Also, it is interesting to note that preliminary data from the DPP suggest that weight loss rather than physical activity was most responsible for the reduction of the incidence of type 2 diabetes with the intensive lifestyle intervention.

The DPP showed that it is possible to significantly reduce the development of diabetes in persons with IGT with a program of a hypocaloric diet and exercise that will drop weight by about 7% and is at least partially sustained for up to 4 yr. This has prompted the American Diabetes Association and the National Institute of Diabetes and Digestive and Kidney Disease to put forth lifestyle intervention as the first line of treatment in attempting to prevent diabetes *(51)*.

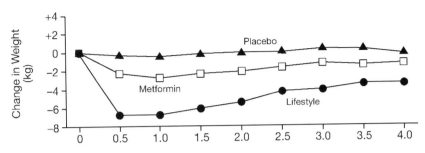

Fig. 1. Changes in body weight according to study group. Each data point represents the mean value for all participants examined at that time. The number of participants decreased over time because of the variable length of time that persons were in the study. For example, data on weight were available for 3085 persons at 0.5 yr, 3064 at 1 yr, 2887 at 2 yr, and 1510 at 3 yr. Changes in weight over time differed significantly among the treatment groups ($p < 0.001$). Reprinted from ref. *50a* with permission.

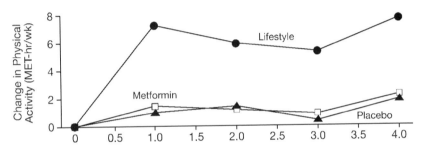

Fig. 2. Changes in leisure physical activity according to study. Each data point represents the mean value for all participants examined at that time. The number of participants decreased over time because of the variable length of time that persons were in the study. Changes in physical activity over time differed significantly among the treatment groups ($p < 0.001$). Reprinted from ref. *50a* with permission.

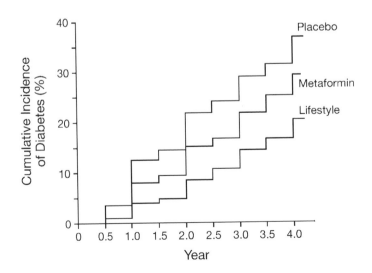

Fig. 3. Cumulative incidence of diabetes according to study group. Reprinted from ref. *50a* with permission.

Intervention in Clinical Practice

The National Institutes of Health (NIH) Roadmap *(52)* has placed great emphasis on the translation of clinical research to clinical care in a timely and effective manner. The DPP was developed to compare two strategies to prevent or delay type 2 diabetes in individuals with IGT. The primary research goal was a comparison of the efficacy and safety of each of three interventions (an intensive lifestyle [ILS] intervention or standard lifestyle recommendations combined with either metformin or placebo) in preventing or delaying the development of diabetes. We discuss below the nature of the ILS intervention and how it might be translated to general clinical practice.

What have we learned from the DPP and how we can apply it to routine clinical practice?

For adequate translation, translators are needed. These will be informed physicians and other health professionals who feel comfortable in approaching the issue of weight loss with their patients. This requires education programs that will provide physicians with the tools they need for the task. Many physicians feel, and are, inadequately trained for such a task and will therefore not embark on it. For translating DPP, the first issue is to put physicians at ease about dealing with the issue of weight loss. Modern schools of medicine do almost nothing to train practitioners who are conversant and comfortable with treating people for obesity. As a result, these practitioners are very poorly equipped to give advice to patients *(53)*. Much stronger nutritional knowledge and more training in counseling skills are necessary to allow them to be effective in facilitating lifestyle changes in their patients. This will require better understanding of nutrition, exercise physiology, behavior modification, and pharmacotherapy *(53)*.

It is not only the physician who can be an agent of change. Nurses are also well positioned in clinical practice to become the persons who take on much of the task of patient behavior change. In some clinical practices, dietitians are also present; if they are, they can also play a large role in providing support, training, and follow-up that is needed *(54)*.

There has been criticism that the ILS intervention is much too expensive and complicated for translation to routine clinical practice settings. As the success of the ILS arm of the trial is undoubted, it seems reasonable to try to dissect what might be possible and not possible in the translation of this program to clinical care settings. Much of the cost of the DPP was due to the fact that essentially all of the core curriculum and much of the post-core were done individually by case managers. The study was designed in this way to try to ensure that the weight loss occurred. The DPP was an effectiveness study, not an efficacy study. The goal was thus to see if the weight loss was effective in changing outcome, not whether we could produce weight loss.

A criticism is that although we showed that we could reduce the progression to diabetes, we did not show how a physician can be successful in promoting weight loss and preventing diabetes in a routine clinical practice. We had an "unreal" budget, an "unreal" staff, a coordinating center, trained and knowledgeable investigators, coordinators, case managers, and so on. How can all this be translatable to the average clinician's office? The way to do this is to try to dissect what was done, simplify it as much as possible without emasculating it, and try it in physicians' offices. One obvious step is to change the patient–staff contacts from individual ones to groups. This has been done in the Look AHEAD *(55)* trial that is currently under way. This is a trial trying to reduce cardiovascular outcomes in diabetic patients through weight loss and physical activity. There is good evidence that the same degree of motivation and efficacy in weight loss can be achieved in groups as in individual counseling *(56,57)*. In fact, there is substantial evidence suggesting that groups may actually be better. Physicians can organize patients in groups and either meet them themselves or designate someone else in the office (nurse, dietitian) to do it. This reduces costs greatly without reducing efficacy. Exercise testing can be done so that submaximal, three-step tests, or some other form of less expensive and sophisticated testing, can be done to ensure safety in the exercise program. The diaries, self-monitoring, and questionnaires can be done more quickly, cheaply, and efficiently on Palm Pilots or other electronic programs that are becoming rapidly available.

The ILS intervention was based on previous literature suggesting that obesity and a sedentary lifestyle may both independently increase the risk of developing type 2 diabetes *(58)*. The DPP focused on two of the modifiable risk factors for diabetes, sedentary lifestyle and overweight. The DPP participants had a mean BMI of 34.5 kg/m^2 and a mean age of 51 yr, with age ranging from 25 to 85 yr. Two-thirds of the DPP participants were women, and 45% were from high-risk minority groups (20% African American, 16% Hispanic, 5% American Indian, and 4% Asian American) *(59)*. They were therefore quite representative of the American population. The retention rate was more than 90% over 4 yr.

Goals

It is important in a behavior modification program to set goals. It is common for patients beginning a weight-loss program to have faulty and unrealistic beliefs about how rapidly they can lose weight *(60)*. There is a need to instruct them in this regard to prevent disappointment and attrition. The goals for the ILS intervention were to achieve and maintain a weight reduction of at least 7% of initial body weight through healthy eating and physical activity, and to achieve and maintain a level of physical activity of at least 150 min/wk (equivalent to about 700 kcal/wk) through moderate-intensity activity (such as walking or bicycling).

Were these goals reasonable? And why were they selected?

Attempting to lose 7% of body weight seemed a reasonable goal to set even though it meant that most of the participants would not reach their ideal body weight. The goal was set on the basis that a number of clinical trials had been carried out that were successful in reaching that level *(61)*. It was felt that trying to set the goal more aggressively would be counterproductive in that most of the participants would not be able to achieve this, become disappointed, and drop out of the study. Retention was considered extremely important for a landmark trial such as this.

The physical activity goal of 150 min/wk was in agreement with the national physical activity recommendations of the Centers for Disease Control and Prevention and the American College of Sports Medicine at the time *(62)*. The feasibility of using behavior modification for the prevention of type 2 diabetes had been shown in two smaller previous trials *(46,63)*.

A number of interactive interventions were used: training in diet, exercise, and behavior modification skills; frequent (no less than monthly) support for behavior change; diet and exercise interventions that are flexible, sensitive to cultural differences, and acceptable in the specific communities in which they are implemented; a combination of individual and group intervention; a combination of a structured protocol (in which all participants receive certain common information) and the flexibility to tailor strategies individually to help a specific participant achieve and attain the study goals; and emphasis on self-esteem, empowerment, and social support. A Lifestyle Resource Core developed intervention materials and provided ongoing training and support for intervention staff *(50,64,65)*.

The intervention was conducted by case managers with training in nutrition, exercise, or behavior modification who met with an individual patient for at least 16 sessions in the first 24 wk and contacted the participant at least bimonthly thereafter (with in-person contacts at least every 2 mo throughout the remainder of the program). The initial 16 sessions represent a core curriculum, with general information about diet and exercise and behavior strategies such as self-monitoring, goal setting, stimulus control, problem solving, and relapse prevention training. Individualization was facilitated by use of several different approaches to self-monitoring and flexibility in deciding how to achieve the changes in diet and exercise. All participants were encouraged to achieve the weight loss and exercise goals within the first 24 wk.

The focus of the exercise intervention was a gradual increase in brisk walking or other activities of similar intensity. Two supervised group exercise sessions per week were provided to help participants achieve their exercise goal, but participants could also achieve the exercise goal on their own and were given the flexibility in choosing the type of exercise to perform. Exercise tolerance tests (performed in individuals with preexisting coronary heart disease, and in men aged greater than 40 yr and post-menopausal women not using hormone replacement therapy who had at least two coronary heart disease risk factors) were used to modify the individual's exercise program.

For individuals having difficulty achieving or maintaining the weight loss or exercise goal, a "tool-box" approach was used to add new strategies for the participant. Strategies included incentives such as items of nominal value. Additional tool-box approaches could include lending of aerobic exercise tapes or other home exercise equipment, enrolling the participant in a class at an exercise facility, additional telephone reminders, a buddy system, structured menus, and use of more structured eating plans, liquid formula diets, or home visits. Also, individuals could be seen more often. Group courses were also offered quarterly during maintenance, with each course lasting 4 to 6 wk and focusing on topics related to exercise, weight loss, or behavioral issues. These courses were designed to help participants achieve and maintain the weight-loss and exercise goals.

Lifestyle participants were to complete the 16-module core curriculum during the first 24 wk of participation. It introduced basic skills related to nutrition, exercise, and behavior change. Subsequently, participants were expected to be seen in person at least once every 2 mo, either individually or in group sessions. This 16-module course is available on an NIH website. It is self-explanatory and can be used by any physician or nurse in a clinical care facility. After the curriculum was completed, the participant moved on to post-core intervention activities. These consisted of bimonthly visits with a lifestyle coach to discuss issues arising from the need to reach the goal or maintain it. After 6 mo, participants were expected to be seen in person. Active case management involved scheduling quarterly outcome assessment visits for participants within appropriate time windows, reporting and documenting any adverse events, reviewing each participant's progress with lifestyle goals at weekly team meetings, and referring participants when appropriate to the exercise specialist or psychologist on the team.

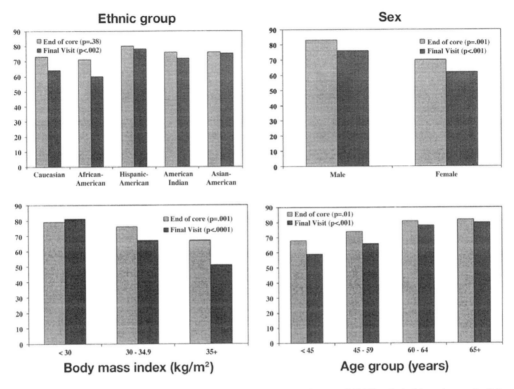

Fig. 4. Percentage of participants who achieved the exercise goal (150 min/wk) at the end of the core curriculum and at the final intervention visit by ethnic group, sex, baseline BMI, and baseline age. Reprinted from ref. *65* with permission.

In the DPP, 49% of the participants met the weight loss goals and 74% met the activity goals initially (37% and 67%, respectively, met these goals long-term). At the first intervention session, participants weighed, on average, 94.5 ± 21.0 kg with weights ranging from 49.1 kg to 200.9 kg. The average BMI was 33.9 ± 6.8. Weight loss over the core curriculum averaged 6.5 ± 4.7 kg, or 6.9 ± 4.5% of initial body weight. At the final intervention visit, participants had maintained an average weight loss of 4.5 ± 7.6 kg or 4.9 ± 7.4% of initial body weight *(65)*. The 7% weight loss goal was achieved by 49% of participants at the end of the core curriculum, and these persons were three times more likely to achieve the goal at study end. Figure 4 shows the percentage of participants who achieved the weight loss goal at both the end of the core curriculum and the final intervention visit in univariate analyses by BMI, age, gender, and ethnicity.

Behavioral Therapy

The DPP cohort was not that different from the usual patient in a physician's office who needs to lose weight. Almost 90% had previously tried to lose weight—45% on at least five occasions—and almost two-thirds had lost and regained more than 20 lb at least once in the past *(66)*. Approximately one-half had never tried a formal weight loss program *(66)*.

The goal of behavioral therapy is twofold: to decrease food intake and to increase physical activity. The behavior of a patient is changed in ways that are possible and in reasonable steps, in concert with a physician or group therapy leader, who helps one patient or, preferably, a group of patients.

The first step in such therapy is to describe the behavior to be controlled. This means helping the patients in self-monitoring so that they become aware of the amount, time, and circumstances of their eating and their activity (or inactivity) patterns. This increases their awareness, which is required before corrective measures can be instituted. The second step is to practice control over stimuli that negatively affect eating behavior. Typical stimuli would be persons or situations that increase stress, anxiety, or hostility. The particular stimuli need to be identified and the patient needs to make an effort to distance himself or herself from them. The third step is to develop techniques to control the act of eating. These include the places where the person eats, the speed of eating, the size of mouthfuls, the number of times eating occurs, and the attention paid to eating. It also includes learning the differences in the caloric value and nutrient content of foods, which is of great importance. Some therapists have suggested that prompt reinforcement of behaviors that delay or control eating is quite helpful. This would mean setting up some reward system (e.g., money, entertainment) as positive reinforcement for improved behavior.

The program is adapted to a patient's goals and skills rather than to a physician's idea of how a patient should behave. This individualization of treatment enhances the chances for success in a motivated person. The advantage of a behavioral approach is that both the patient and the therapist (which may include the group) focus on the specific environmental variables that seem to govern a particular person's behavior. Central to a behavioral analysis is the search by patient and therapist for solutions to problems that are both relatively modest and potentially soluble. This simplifies and focuses therapy. It has been our experience in our weight-control program that conducting behavioral therapy in a group setting is highly efficacious. The group setting leads to inquiry and mutual support and encouragement that are conducive to success. Another advantage of a behavioral approach is that when patients are given the major responsibility for the weight-loss strategy, they can attribute increased power to themselves. This tends to reinforce the treatment, inasmuch as when patients believe that the positive results are attributable to their own efforts, they gain confidence and a desire to continue. The final and most important advantage of a behavioral approach is that it allows patients to learn to eat and exercise under the natural social and environmental conditions with which they live day to day. Thus, the habits learned during weight loss can be continued during the difficult period of weight maintenance. It must be remembered that a behavioral program often produces the slowest initial weight loss because caloric reduction is not radical and patients are encouraged to eat a hypocaloric but balanced and sensible diet. Patients must be advised to develop a long-term view. A goal weight should be set and perseverance encouraged. It is of importance that the goal weight that is set is usually higher than the normal weight for each patient. This needs to be negotiated with the patient with an explanation of the general futility of reaching ideal weight in a person who is significantly obese (67). It is imperative that the patient remain in the treatment program not only until the goal is achieved, but also well into the weight-maintenance period.

One should not underestimate the physician as an agent of change. There have been a number of studies that have shown the powerful effect a physician can have on a patient with regard to motivation and success in carrying through a difficult weight-loss program *(68,69)*. Taking even 5 or 6 min to discuss weight, nutrition, and activity issues with patients can be very empowering. Frequent visits or contacts of some kind are most effective *(70)*. Of course, the more engaged and interested the physician is in the patient, the more effective the contact.

Diet

A crucial component of the DPP program was the diet. The weight-loss goal was attempted initially through a reduction in dietary fat intake to less than 25% of calories. If weight loss did not occur with fat restriction alone, then a calorie goal was added. Energy requirements vary according to weight and activity *(71)*. To lose weight, energy intake must be less than energy expenditure. Energy intake was aimed at in the DPP. Participants weighing 120 to 174 lb (54 to 78 kg) at baseline were instructed to follow a 1200 kcal/d diet (33 g of fat); participants weighing 175 to 219 lb (79 to 99 kg) were instructed to follow a 1500 kcal/d diet (42 g fat); those 220 to 249 lb (100 to 113 kg) were instructed to follow an 1800-kcal/d diet (50 g fat); and those over 250 lb (114 kg) were instructed to follow a 2000 kcal/d diet (55 g fat) *(65)*.

To lose weight successfully, obese persons must lower their caloric intake and sustain such a reduced intake for a prolonged period. It is important to develop a diet program within the framework of a patient's current food habits and preferences. This is sometimes impossible when dietary habits are so poor that a radical restructuring must take place. However, better compliance occurs in patients for whom it can be done, because such patients are familiar and comfortable with the foods that they are already eating. Factors such as available cooking facilities, ethnic background, and economic background cannot be ignored. Documentation of food intake (e.g., diet records) is a good method of tracking dietary pitfalls, patterns, and progress, but physicians must beware of perfect records unaccompanied by weight loss. These should serve as a signal that a patient may not be ready to accept the weight problem or be willing to work seriously on improving it.

Patients were given a food frequency questionnaire to determine their food intake at baseline and to track it over time. The DPP food frequency questionnaire was semiquantitative, designed to collect information via in-person interviews regarding usual intake of food and dietary supplements over the previous year. Implementation and management of the dietary assessment was centralized at the DPP Nutrition Coding Center (NCC). The main body of the questionnaire contained 117 line items, plus an open-ended query for food not included within the line items. Foods added to enhance sensitivity to regional or ethnic food choices were identified through queries to each of the clinical centers *(72)*. Baseline median estimated energy intake was 7676 kj/d (1828 kcal/d) and 8585 kj/d (2044 kcal/d) for women and men respectively. The median percent of energy from fat ranged from 30.6% for Asian American men to 37.5% for American Indian men and women. After 1 yr among the Lifestyle group, the median change in total energy and percent energy from fat was –1897 kj/d (–452 kcal/d) and –6.6%, respectively. Figure 5 shows the change in total kjoules from baseline to 1-year post randomization by treatment group *(72)*.

Decisions about dietary change should be made jointly by the patient and the physician to help promote long-term compliance. A diet must be adequate nutritionally, and this is possible without supplements only in diets of 1100 to 1200 kcal per day or more. To achieve this, patients must be taught to eat certain micronutrient-rich foods that they

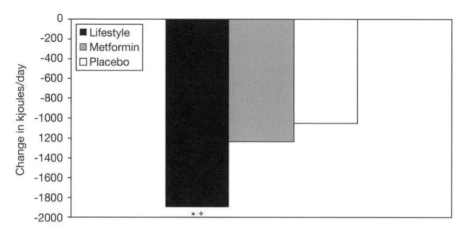

Fig. 5. Change in total kjoules, baseline to 1 yr postrandomization, by treatment group. Statistical significance for pairwise comparisons ($p < 0.003$) is shown only when overall treatment effect was demonstrated ($p < 0.01$). *indicates statistically significant difference between lifestyle and metformin; + indicates statistically significant difference between lifestyle and placebo. There were no statistically significant differences between metformin and placebo. Reprinted from ref. *72* with permission.

may not be used to eating. With very hypocaloric diets, the nutrients most likely to be in deficit are iron, folic acid, vitamin B_6, and zinc. If kilocalorie values fall below 1100, vitamin and mineral supplements become necessary and should be prescribed by the physician; a multivitamin–multimineral tablet once a day is enough. In the DPP, we opted to give everyone in the ILS a multivitamin tablet daily. This was done to ensure that no patient would be deficient in micronutrient ingestion. This seems a good practice with no known downsides. Extra macrominerals (sodium, potassium, calcium) are usually not necessary, unless patients go on very-low-calorie diets (300–600 kcal), which we did not recommend for long-term use.

During weight loss, the emphasis should be on reduction of adipose rather than lean tissue. Although there is some obligate loss of lean body mass, it should be kept to a minimum. Lean body mass can generally be spared during weight loss with a protein intake of 1.0 to 1.5 g/kg of ideal body weight. The dietary sources of protein should be of high biologic value (e.g., egg whites, fish, poultry, lean beef, and low-fat dairy products). A vegetarian diet is perfectly acceptable, but the concept of protein complementing must be explained, encouraged, and monitored. The remainder of calories should come from carbohydrates (preferably high-fiber foods) and fat. Although the macronutrient ratio can vary according the patient's preferences, it is important to obtain some of the antiketogenic and digestive high-fiber benefits of carbohydrates and to get adequate amounts of fat-soluble vitamins and essential fatty acids from the dietary fat.

In all cases of weight reduction, the emphasis should be on micronutrient-dense food choices and away from empty calorie selections. A brief discussion of basic nutrition should help alert the patient to the most appropriate food choices to maximize caloric restriction. A patient must be taught that alcohol and sweets are not sources of any essential micronutrients. These should therefore be avoided, especially in the early stages of weight reduction, because they provide little more than excess calories. It should be made clear that although some fats are less atherogenic than others, all fats are

high-energy, low-micronutrient foods. As mentioned, in the DPP, they were restricted
to less than 25% of total daily calories. Gram for gram, pure fat has more than double the
caloric concentration of carbohydrate or protein (9 cal/g vs 4 cal/g). Because carbohydrate often absorbs water on cooking, the actual caloric density of hydrated carbohydrate
on the plate may be as low as 1 to 2 cal/g. Thus, eliminating or decreasing high-fat foods
from the diet should provide a substantial caloric decrease, even if pure-carbohydrate
foods are substituted. In general, high-fat spreads, condiments, sauces, and gravies are
far more detrimental in a weight-reduction program than are bread, potatoes, pasta, and
rice, if the latter are eaten in moderate portion sizes and in conjunction with other foods.

Many of the more popular media-touted diets have little scientific basis and simply
play on vulnerable people's desperation to lose weight. They often completely ignore the
concept of balanced nutrition by totally eliminating or providing insufficient amounts of
a particular macronutrient (e.g., protein, carbohydrate, or fat) (73). In time, this can result
in a concurrent micronutrient imbalance. Such diets are clearly unsound, and if they are
followed for any significant length of time, serious health consequences such as electrolyte imbalances, deficiency syndromes, or protein malnutrition may ensue (73).

Very-low-calorie diets (300–500 kcal/d) are counterproductive and potentially dan-
gerous. Although weight loss can be large on such diets, the results are generally short-
lived (74). A return to pre-diet weight after solid foods are resumed is the rule. Unless
such diets are undertaken in the context of a complete medically supervised, stepwise
program in which the very-low-calorie diet is replaced after a few weeks by a high-
calorie balanced diet and intensive behavior modification program, they accomplish
little except for an initial loss of water and electrolytes. However, the use of formula diets
or bars to substitute for regular food for one or two meals a day for a period of time,
particularly initially, can be quite helpful. This was done in the DPP with good results.

Instruction in the use of low-energy-density diets is also helpful. This consists of
relatively large volumes of low-energy foods. Preferred foods are those that are high in
volume and require more time for ingestion, with the calories generally diluted by fiber
and water. Vegetables, fruit, and starches are emphasized, whereas sweets and fats and
oils are not. This has been shown to be a good strategy for losing weight and maintaining
weight loss.

To help the patient adhere to a diet balanced in micronutrients and vitamins, it is wise
to introduce the concept of the basic food groups and the food pyramid. These consist
of the following: (1) grains: bread, cereal, rice and pasta; (2) fruits; (3) vegetables; (4)
milk and milk products: milk, yogurt, cheese; (5) meat, poultry, fish, dry beans, eggs,
nuts and seeds; (6) legumes; (7) fats, oils, and sweets (use sparingly). By selecting
judiciously from these groups, patients can obtain adequate nutrients. Patients should be
encouraged to select a wide variety of food choices within these basic food groups to help
alleviate a lack of compliance caused by boredom or monotony. The number of servings
per day from each food group will vary according to the individual's caloric restriction
and macronutrient breakdown. Because portion sizes are crucial, they should be explained in terms of common household measures (e.g., cups, ounces) and with the aid of
food models.

The macronutrient composition of the diet in the DPP was much like the Step 1 diet
of the AHA or the National Heart, Lung, and Blood Institute (NHLBI) Guidelines (75).
In order to be successful in reaching the goal, a great deal of emphasis was placed on self-
monitoring. This has been shown to enhance weight loss (76). But this can be improved

if, as self-monitoring diaries are reviewed, education on estimating portion size, reading food labels, nutrient density of foods, and recording of food intake shortly after a meal are stressed. The more that meal plans are structured for individuals, the more likely they will be successful. Prescribed individualized menus can also be helpful *(77)*.

Formula diets can also be very helpful *(77,78)*. One can prescribe 1200 to 1500 kcal/d and the patient may find this much more convenient. This is particularly helpful at the start of a weight-loss program. Individuals can then gradually move from three times per day to two times per day to once per day over time but continue to use these effective dietary aids indefinitely.

Exercise

Physical activity seems to be very helpful for weight maintenance but not so much for weight loss *(79–82)*. But increased physical activity in very sedentary individuals is helpful in a number of ways. It helps in inducing a deficit in calories, preserves lean body mass, enhances fat loss, and improves cardiovascular fitness.

It is important to discuss two types of physical activity: programmed and lifestyle. Lifestyle activity occurs in the course of a regular day as one goes about normal activities. If one is conscious of it, one can increase energy expenditure by changing activities such as using stairs rather than elevators, choosing distant parking spaces, and so on. Programmed activity is actually planning exercise bouts (such as biking, walking, swimming, etc.). Both types of activity are helpful *(7)*. The more activity a person engages in, the greater the weight loss he or she is able to achieve *(83)*. This is shown in Fig. 6. This can easily be initiated by a physician and monitored closely.

Because exercise expends calories, it is a logical part of any weight-loss program. Overweight persons are generally inactive, spending much of their day sitting or lying down *(84,85)*. Many of them, particularly the heavier ones, have a real problem walking even short distances and climbing steps and tend to avoid situations that require such activities. By remaining as sedentary as they do, they are essentially almost at their resting metabolic rate for most of the day. These persons must be taught first to walk, then to walk faster, and then to run or bicycle or do aerobic dance. An exercise program must start slowly. If an obese person is pushed too rapidly, discomfort and avoidance occur. Careful observation for and treatment of skin intertrigo, dependent edema, and foot or joint injuries is mandatory.

The ILS intervention stressed brisk walking as the means to achieving the activity goal, although other activities of similar intensity (aerobics, dance, bicycle riding, skating, swimming) could also be applied to the goal. (No more than 75 min/wk of strength training could be applied to the goal.) Participants were encouraged to increase their activity slowly and to exercise at least three times per day 5 d/wk for at least 10 min per session. Although most participants completed their activity on their own, two supervised exercise classes were offered at all clinics each week. Participants at high risk for adverse events related to underlying coronary artery disease were given an exercise tolerance test before starting the activity intervention.

Participants were instructed to self-monitor minutes of physical activity and fat grams consumed every day during the core curriculum and then 1 wk per month over the remainder of the trial. These self-monitoring records and measures of body weight taken at each intervention visit were used to assess success at achieving the intervention goals. Participants were sometimes missing values for weight, fat grams, and physical activity

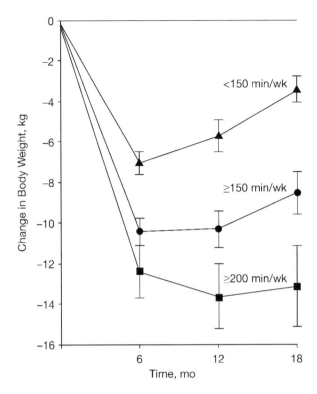

Fig. 6. Dose response of exercise on weight loss across 18 mo of treatment (mean [SEM]). For time, group, and group×time, all $p < 0.001$. Error bars indicate standard error of the mean. Printed from ref. *83* with permission.

for a variety of reasons, including a lack of a scale for occasional visits conducted outside the usual clinic or lack of self-monitoring information. These participants were excluded from analyses where these values were required.

ILS participants reported completing an average of 224 min/wk of physical activity at the end of the core curriculum and 227 min/wk at the final intervention visit. The goal of >150 min/wk of activity was achieved by 74% of participants at the end of the core curriculum and 67% at the final intervention visit *(65)*. Figure 4 shows the percentage of participants who achieved the activity goal at the end of the core curriculum and at the final intervention visit according to baseline demographic characteristics *(65)*.

It is helpful to educate the patient about how many calories are spent in an individual exercise activity. Most tables of caloric expenditure with given levels of activity have been compiled to reflect total caloric expenditure, not the amount over the resting metabolic rate. As a result, the caloric contribution of exercise must be calculated as the difference between the calories expended per minute during the exercise and the calories that a person would have expended just sitting. It is instructive and often disappointing to patients to discover just how much exercise they must do to expend a significant number of calories. For instance, if an overweight woman's basal metabolic rate is 1400 kcal/d, lying down awake she expends 1.1 kcal/min; sitting, about 1.2 kcal/min; walking slowly, about 1.9 kcal/min; and walking a treadmill at 4.0 miles per hour, 7.2 kcal/min. Thus, the difference in caloric expenditure between sitting quietly and walking fast on a treadmill (at 4.0 miles per hour) is 6.0 kcal/min. In an hour, therefore, the energy expended by walking 4 miles is only 360 kcal higher than the subject would have expended just sitting quietly. It is important to emphasize that a significant and persistent commitment to exercise must be present for exercise to have any substantial effect on caloric balance and weight loss.

Drugs

The DPP allowed the use of drugs in the ILS arm. The drug orlistat was used as a rescue operation in individuals who were unable to achieve their goal or to maintain it over time. At the time (and also at present) the only two drugs that were approved in the United States for long-term weight loss were orlistat and sibutramine. Sibutramine is a norepinephrine and serotonin reuptake inhibitor. As a result of its effect on norepinephrine, it has cardiovascular side effects. These include a potential for an increase in blood pressure and heart rate *(86,87)*. For this reason, the DPP investigators did not consider the drug to be safe to give to overweight prediabetic individuals who have a high incidence of metabolic syndrome and of cardiovascular disease. As a result, only orlistat was provided.

Orlistat, a gastrointestinal lipase inhibitor, reduces dietary fat absorption by approximately 30% *(88)*. Four 2-yr trials demonstrated the efficacy and safety of orlistat. Two multicenter, double-blind, 2-yr studies, an 18-center US study *(25)* and a 15-center European study *(89)*, randomized patients to receive orlistat (120 mg tid) in conjunction with a hypocaloric diet for 1 yr and orlistat in conjunction with a eucaloric weight-maintenance diet for the second year. Both studies showed that orlistat-treated patients lost more weight than placebo-treated patients during the first year (9% to 10%, respectively, vs 6% of initial body weight) *(88,89)*. In the US trial, patients who switched from placebo to orlistat lost weight during the second year of treatment *(88)*. The European Multicentre Orlistat Study compared two dosage regimens of orlistat (60 vs 120 mg) in the weight-maintenance phase of the trial. Patients treated with 120 mg orlistat throughout the 2-yr study period regained less weight during the second year (3.2 kg; 35.2% regain) than did those treated with 60 mg orlistat (4.26 kg; 51.3% regain) or placebo (5.3 kg; 63.4% regain). Two other multicenter randomized controlled trials, the Orlistat Primary Care Study *(90)* and the European Orlistat Obesity Study *(91)*, compared orlistat in 120 mg tid and 60 mg tid regimens versus placebo over a 2-yr period. At the end of the first year in the US and European trials, the percentage of body weight lost from initial body weight was greatest among patients treated with the higher orlistat dose: 9.7 and 7.9%, respectively. During the second-year maintenance period, orlistat, particularly the 120 mg dose, was associated with less weight gain in both trials. In the second year of the US study, only 6.6% of patients in the placebo group compared with 18.6% of those in the 120 mg orlistat group ($p = 0.001$) and 14.6% in the 60 mg orlistat group ($p = 0.008$) sustained a weight loss of >10% of initial body weight *(90)*. Thus, four multicenter trials showed that orlistat in conjunction with diet promoted sustained weight loss over a 2-yr period. The only side effect of orlistat observed in clinical trials was a small decline in fat-soluble vitamins (within the normal range). Gastrointestinal side effects, such as steatorrhea, or soft and frequent stools, have also been reported in all the trials.

Using medication can be helpful in weight loss and also in weight maintenance. Randomized controlled trials with both sibutramine and orlistat reported that patients on the drug maintained weight loss almost twice as high as those on placebo. Also, the Storm trial showed a similar ability to maintain an impressive weight loss with medication *(87)*.

Weight Maintenance

Maintaining reduced weight once a loss has been achieved is very difficult. There is a persistent tendency to regain the weight , and there is experimental evidence that the metabolic rate is abnormally depressed after weight loss *(92)* and that lipogenic pathways enhancing the reaccretion of fat may be particularly efficient. Although the diet may be liberalized after the goal weight has been reached, it must be done gradually, with daily weight monitoring. A limitation of caloric intake will be required indefinitely *(93)*. All the lifestyle changes learned during the weight-loss period need to be continued, including the exercise program. More long-term experience with the efficacy and safety of drugs for longer than 2 yr of use is necessary. Perri et al. *(70,94,95)* have reported the positive influence of frequent contact on weight maintenance.

Depressive symptoms were unrelated to success at achieving the activity or weight-loss goals in DPP. This may result, in part, from the low levels of depressive symptoms in our participants and the paucity of individuals with clinical depression. Prior behavioral weight loss studies, however, have also failed to show a relationship between baseline depressive symptoms and weight loss, although depression has, in some cases, been related to the risk of dropping out of the program. As a result, depressive symptoms should not deter a physician from initiating a weight loss attempt with a patient.

The DPP study suggests that getting patients off to a good start is important for long-term success. Both for weight loss and physical activity, success at achieving the goal at the end of the core curriculum was strongly related to the probability of success at study end. This evidence supports the behavioral approach of incorporating frequent contacts and more aggressive approaches at the start of the treatment program *(68,96,97)*.

One of the key issues is for the physician to stay involved after weight loss, so that weight maintenance is successful. The DPP recognized the need for continued and frequent contact with the patient, and this needs to be done by the physician. The contacts can be quite short, but they are crucial to the maintenance.

Costs

What about costs? A careful cost analysis was done in the DPP *(98)*. The direct medical cost of laboratory tests to identify one subject with impaired glucose tolerance was $139. Over three years, the direct medical costs of the interventions were $79 per participant in the placebo group and $2780 in the ILS. The direct medical costs of care outside the DPP were $432 less per participant in the ILS compared with the placebo. Indirect costs were $174 less in the ILS than placebo. From the perspective of a health care system, the cost of lifestyle intervention was $2269 per participant over 3 yr. From the perspective of society, the cost of ILS intervention relative to the placebo intervention was $3540 per participant over 3 yr. Thus, the ILS was associated with modest incremental costs. The costs of such prevention strategies must be balanced against the savings related to averted disease. Utilizing a group approach, the cost of the ILS could be considerably reduced.

Metabolic Syndrome and Lifestyle Change

Metabolic syndrome (MS) has been defined by the National Cholesterol Education Program (NCEP). It has been reported that the MS increases the risk of cardiovascular disease and the risk of cardiovascular disease mortality. In the DPP, 53% of the subjects had MS. Of the components, an elevated waist circumference was the most common (73%) and high fasting glucose was the least common (33%). The prevalence of MS between baseline and follow-up increased from 55 to 61% in the placebo group, remained unchanged in the metformin group (54 to 55%), and was reduced in the lifestyle group from 51 to 43%. The study showed that an ILS intervention with weight loss and increased physical activity is more effective in reducing the onset of diabetes, but is also more effective in reducing the other components of MS. This may mean that, over the long run, it is more effective in reducing the incidence of cardiovascular disease.

CONCLUSION

Type 2 diabetes affects more than 150 million adults worldwide; this figure is expected to double over the next 25 yr. Lifestyle changes reduced the incidence of diabetes in persons at high risk, and the lifestyle intervention was more effective than metformin. Because the lifestyle changes worked equally well in all racial/ethnic groups in the DPP, they should be applicable to high-risk populations worldwide and may be able to reduce the projected progressive rise in the incidence of diabetes.

REFERENCES

1. Edelstein SL, Knowler WC, Bain RP, et al. Predictors of progression from impaired glucose tolerance to NIDDM: an analysis of six prospective studies. Diabetes 1997;46:701–710.
2. De Courten M, Bennet PH, Tuomilehto J, et al. Epidemiology of NIDDM in non-europids. In: Alberti KG, DeFronzo RA, Keen H, et al., eds. International Textbook of Diabetes Mellitus. John Wiley & Sons, Chichester: 1997; pp.1687–1707.
3. Donahue RP, Orchard TJ. Diabetes mellitus and macrovascular complications. An epidemiological perspective. Diabetes Care 1992;15:1141–1155.
4. Zimmet P, Alberti KG, Shaw J. Global and societal implications of the diabetes epidemic. Nature 2001;414(6865):782–787.
5. King H, Aubert RE, Herman WH. Global burden of diabetes, 1995–2025: prevalence, numerical estimates, and projections. Diabetes Care 1998;21:1414–1431.
6. Kriska AM, Blair SN, Pereira MA. The potential role of physical activity in the prevention of non-insulin-dependent diabetes mellitus: the epidemiological evidence. Exerc Sport Sci Rev 1994;22:121–143.
7. Flegal KM, Carroll MD, Kuczmarski RJ, et al. Overweight and obesity in the United States: prevalence and trends, 1960–1994. Int J Obes 1998;22:39–47.
8. Flegal KM, Carroll MD, Ogden CL, et al. Prevalence and trends in obesity among US adults, 1999–2000. JAMA 2002;288(14):1723–1727.
9. World Health Organization. Obesity: preventing and managing the global epidemic. Report on a WHO Consultation Technical Report Series No. 894. Geneva, 1997.
10. Rocchini AP. Childhood obesity and a diabetes epidemic. N Engl J Med 2002;346(11):854–855.
11. Must A, Spadano J, Coakley EH, et al. The disease burden associated with overweight and obesity. JAMA 1999;282(16):1523–1529.
12. Pi-Sunyer FX. Medical hazards of obesity. Ann Intern Med 1993;119:655–660.
13. Allison DB, Fontaine KR, Manson JE, et al. Annual deaths attributable to obesity in the United States. JAMA 1999;282:1530–1538.
14. Fontaine KR, Redden DT, Wang C, et al. Years of life lost due to obesity. JAMA 2003;289(2):187–193.
15. Mokdad AH, Bowman BA, Ford ES, et al. The continuing epidemics of obesity and diabetes in the United States. JAMA 2001;286(10):1195–1200.
16. Harris M, Flegal K, Cowie C, et al. Prevalence of diabetes: impaired fasting glucose and impaired glucose tolerance in U.S. adults. Diabetes Care 1998;21:518–524.
17. Colditz GA, Willett WC, Stampfer MJ, et al. Weight as a risk factor for clinical diabetes in women. Am J Epidemiol 1990;132:501–513.

18. Chan JM, Rimm EB, Colditz GA, et al. Obesity, fat distribution, and weight gain as risk factors for clinical diabetes in men. Diabetes Care 1994;17:961–969.

19. Modan M, Karasik A, Halkin H, et al. Effect of past and concurrent body mass index on prevalence of glucose intolerance and type 2 non-insulin-dependent diabetes and on insulin response. The Israel study of glucose intolerance, obesity and hypertension. Diabetologia 1986;29:82–89.

20. Maggio CA, Pi-Sunyer FX. The prevention and treatment of obesity: application to type 2 diabetes. Diabetes Care 1997;20:1744–1766.

21. American Diabetes Association. All about diabetes. American Diabetes Association, 2006. 3–1–2006. http://www.diabetes.org/about-diabetes.jsp. Accessed November 7, 2006.

22. Sparrow D, Borkan GA, Gerzof SG, et al. Relationship of fat distribution to glucose tolerance. Results of computed tomography in male participants of the Normative Aging Study. Diabetes 1986;35:411–415.

23. Olefsky JM. Insulin resistance and insulin action: an in vivo and in vitro perspective. Diabetes 1981;38:148–162.

24. Lundgren H, Bengtsson C, Blohme G, et al. Adiposity and adipose tissue distribution in relation to incidence of diabetes in women: results from a prospective population study in Gothenburg, Sweden. Int J Obes 1989;13:413–423.

25. Ohlson LO, Larsson B, Svärdsudd K, et al. The influence of body fat distribution on the incidence of diabetes mellitus: 13.5 years of follow-up of the participants in the study of men born in 1913. Diabetes 1985;34:1055–1058.

26. Lapidus L, Bengtsson C, Larsson B, et al. Distribution of adipose tissue and risk of cardiovascular disease and death: a 12 year follow up of participants in the population study of women in Gothenburg, Sweden. Br Med J (Clin Res Ed) 1984;289(6454):1257–1261.

27. Despres JP. The insulin resistance-dyslipidemic syndrome of visceral obesity: effect on patients' risk. Obes Res 1998;6 Suppl 1:8S–17S.

28. Carey DG, Jenkins AB, Campbell LV, et al. Abdominal fat and insulin resistance in normal and overweight women: Direct measurements reveal a strong relationship in subjects at both low and high risk of NIDDM. Diabetes 1996;45:633–638.

29. Colberg SR, Simoneau JA, Thaete FL, et al. Skeletal muscle utilization of free fatty acids in women with visceral obesity. J Clin Invest 1995;95:1846–1853.

30. Jensen MD, Haymond MW, Rizza RA, et al. Influence of body fat distribution on free fatty acid metabolism in obesity. J Clin Invest 1989;83:1168–1173.

31. Boyko EJ, Leonetti DL, Bergstrom RW, et al. Visceral adiposity, fasting plasma insulin, and lipid and lipoprotein levels in Japanese Americans. Int J Obes Relat Metab Disord 1996;20:801–808.

32. Perry IJ, Wannamethee SG, Walker MK, et al. Prospective study of risk factors for development of non-insulin dependent diabetes in middle aged British men. Br Med J 1995;310:560–564.

33. Segal KR, Edano A, Abalos A, et al. Effect of exercise training on insulin sensitivity and glucose metabolism in lean, obese, and diabetic men. J Appl Physiol 1991;71:2402–2411.

34. Regensteiner JG, Mayer EJ, Shetterly SM, et al. Relationship between habitual physical activity and insulin levels among nondiabetic men and women. San Luis Valley Diabetes Study. Diabetes Care 1991;14:1066–1074.

35. Wing RR, Matthews KA, Kuller LH, et al. Environmental and familial contributions to insulin levels and change in insulin levels in middle-aged women. JAMA 1992;268(14):1890–1895.

36. Manolio TA, Savage PJ, Burke GL, et al. Correlates of fasting insulin levels in young adults: the CARDIA study. J Clin Epidemiol 1991;44:571–578.

37. Lamarche B, Despres JP, Pouliot MC, et al. Is body fat loss a determinant factor in the improvement of carbohydrate and lipid metabolism following aerobic exercise training in obese women? Metabolism 1992;41:1249–1256.

38. Lemieux S, Despres JP. Metabolic complications of visceral obesity: contribution to the aetiology of type 2 diabetes and implications for prevention and treatment. Diabetes Metab 1994;20:375–393.

39. Colditz GA, Willett WC, Rotnitzky A, et al. Weight gain as a risk factor for clinical diabetes mellitus in women. Ann Intern Med 1995;122:481–486.

40. Will JC, Williamson DF, Ford ES, et al. Intentional weight loss and 13-year diabetes incidence in overweight adults. Am J Public Health 2002;92:1245–1248.

41. Sjöström CD, Lissner L, Sjöström L. Relationships between weight change, body composition and incidence of cardiovascular risk factors. Int J Obes 1996;20:95.

42. Sjöström CD, Lissner L, Wedel H, et al. Reduction in incidence of diabetes, hypertension and lipid disturbances after intentional weight loss induced by bariatric surgery: the SOS Intervention Study. Obes Res 1999;7:477–484.

43. Goldstein DJ. Beneficial health effects of modest weight loss. Int J Obes 1992;16:397–415.

44. Pi-Sunyer FX. Short-term medical benefits and adverse effects of weight loss. Ann Intern Med 1993;119:722–726.

45. Pi-Sunyer FX. A review of long-term studies evaluating the efficacy of weight loss in ameliorating disorders associated with obesity. Clin Therap 1996;18:1006–1035.

46. Eriksson KF, Lindgarde F. Prevention of type 2 non-insulin-dependent diabetes mellitus by diet and physical exercise. The 6-year Malmo feasibility study. Diabetologia 1991;34:891–898.

47. Pan XR, Li GW, Hu YH, et al. Effects of diet and exercise in preventing NIDDM in people with impaired glucose tolerance. The Da Qing IGT and Diabetes Study. Diabetes Care 1997;20:537–544.

48. Tuomilehto J, Lindstrom J, Eriksson JG, et al. Prevention of type 2 diabetes mellitus by changes in lifestyle among subjects with impaired glucose tolerance. N Engl J Med 2001;344:1343–1350.

49. Erikkson J, Franssila-Kallunki A, Ekstrand A, et al. Early metabolic defects in persons at increased risk for non-insulin-dependent mellitus. N Engl J Med 1989;321:337–344.

50. The Diabetes Prevention Program Research Group. Design and methods for a clinical trial in the prevention of type 2 diabetes. Diabetes Care 1999;22:623–634.

50a. Diabetes Prevention Program Research Group. Reduction in the incidence of type 2 diabetes with lifestyle intervention or metformin. N Engl J Med 2002;346:393–403.

51. American Diabetes Association. Standards of medical care for patients with diabetes. Diabetes Care 2003;26:S62–S69.

52. National Institutes of Health. NIH roadmap for clinical research. National Institutes of Health, 2006. 3-1-2006. http://nihhroadmap.nih.gov/. Accessed November 7, 2006.

53. Pi-Sunyer X. A clinical view of the obesity problem. Science 2003;299(5608):859–860.

54. Wylie-Rosett J, Delahanty L. An integral role of the dietitian: implications of the Diabetes Prevention Program. J Am Diet Assoc 2002;102:1065–1068.

55. Ryan DH, Espeland MA, Foster GD, et al. Look AHEAD (Action for Health in Diabetes): design and methods for a clinical trial of weight loss for the prevention of cardiovascular disease in type 2 diabetes. Control Clin Trials 2003;24:610–628.

56. Wing RR. Behavioral strategies for weight reduction in obese type II diabetic patients. Diabetes Care 1989;12:139–144.

57. Wadden TA. The treatment of obesity: an overview. In: Stunkard AJ, Wadden T, eds. Obesity Theory and Therapy. Raven Press, New York: 1993; pp. 197–218.

58. Tuomilehto J, Knowler WC, Zimmet P. Primary prevention of non-insulin-dependent diabetes mellitus. Diabetes Metab Rev 1992;8:339–353.

59. The Diabetes Prevention Program: baseline characteristics of the randomized cohort. The Diabetes Prevention Program Research Group. Diabetes Care 2000;23(11):1619–1629.

60. Foster G, Wadden T, Vogt R, et al. What is a reasonable weight loss? Patients' expectations and evaluations of obesity treatment outcomes. J Consul Clin Psych 1997;65:79–85.

61. National Heart Lung and Blood Institute. Clinical Guidelines on the Identification, Evaluation, and Treatment of Overweight and Obesity in Adults—The Evidence Report. Obes Res 1998;6,suppl 2:51S–210S.

62. Pate RR, Pratt M, Blair SN, et al. Physical activity and public health. A recommendation from the Centers for Disease Control and Prevention and the American College of Sports Medicine. JAMA 1995;273(5):402–407.

63. Pan X, Li G, Hu Y, et al. Effects of diet and exercise in preventing NIDDM in people with impaired glucose tolerance. Diabetes Care 1997;20:537–544.

64. The Diabetes Prevention Program (DPP) Research Group. The Diabetes Prevention Program (DPP): description of lifestyle intervention. Diabetes Care 2002;25(12):2165–2171.

65. Wing RR, Hamman RF, Bray GA, et al. Achieving weight and activity goals among diabetes prevention program lifestyle participants. Obes Res 2004;12:1426–1434.

66. Delahanty LM, Meigs JB, Hayden D, et al. Psychological and behavioral correlates of baseline BMI in the Diabetes Prevention Program (DPP). Diabetes Care 2002;25(11):1992–1998.

67. USDA/DHHS. Dietary Guidelines for Americans, 4th ed. Home and Garden Bulletin 232: 1995.

68. Wadden TA, Berkowitz RI, Vogt RA, et al. Lifestyle modification in the pharmacologic treatment of obesity: a pilot investigation of a potential primary care approach. Obes Res 1997;5:218–226.

69. Wadden TA, Berkowitz RI, Womble LG, et al. Randomized trial of lifestyle modification and pharmacotherapy for obesity. N Engl J Med 2005;353(20):2111–2120.

70. Perri MG, McAdoo WG, McAllister DA, et al. Effects of peer support and therapist contact on long-term weight loss. J Consult Clin Psychol 1987;55:615–617.

71. Melanson K, Dwyer J. Popular diets for treatment of overweight and obesity. In: Wadden TA, Stunkard AJ, eds. Handbook of Obesity Treatment. Guilford Press, New York: 2002; pp.249–275.

72. Mayer-Davis EJ, Sparks KC, Hirst K, et al. Dietary intake in the diabetes prevention program cohort: baseline and 1-year post randomization. Ann Epidemiol 2004;14(10):763–772.

73. Freedman MR, King J, Kennedy E. Popular diets: a scientific review. Obes Res 2001;9 Suppl 1:1S–40S.

74. Larsson B, Svärdsudd K, Welin L, et al. Obesity, adipose tissue distribution and health: the study of men born in 1913. In: Björntorp P, Rossner S, eds. Obesity in Europe 88. John Libbey, London: 1989; pp. 49–54.

75. Després JP, Tremblay A, Talbot J, et al. Regional adipose tissue distribution and plasma lipoproteins. In: Bouchard C, Johnson FE, eds. Fat Distribution During Growth and Later Health Outcomes. Alan R. Liss, New York: 1988: pp. 221–242.

76. Baker RC, Kirschenbaum DS. Self-monitoring may be necessary for successful weight control. Behav Ther 1993;24:377–394.

77. Ditschuneit HH, Flechtner-Mors M, Johnson TD, et al. Metabolic and weight-loss effects of a long-term dietary intervention in obese patients. Am J Clin Nutr 1999;69:198–204.

78. Ashley JM, St Jeor ST, Schrage JP, et al. Weight control in the physician's office. Arch Intern Med 2001;161(13):1599–1604.

79. Kayman S, Bruvold W, Stern JS. Maintenance and relapse after weight loss in women: behavioral aspects. Am J Clin Nutr 1990;52:800–807.

80. Klem ML, Wing RR, McGuire MT, et al. A descriptive study of individuals successful at long-term maintenance of substantial weight loss. Am J Clin Nutr 1997;66:239–246.

81. Wing RR. Physical activity in the treatment of the adulthood overweight and obesity: current evidence and research issues. Med Sci Sports Exerc 1999;31:S547–S552.

82. Pronk N, Wing RR. Physical activity and long-term maintenance of weight loss. Obes Res 1994;2:587–599.

83. Jakicic JM, Winters C, Lang W, et al. Effects of intermittent exercise and use of home exercise equipment on adherence, weight loss, and fitness in overweight women: a randomized trial. JAMA 1999;282(16):1554–1560.

84. Levine JA, Lanningham-Foster LM, McCrady SK, et al. Interindividual variation in posture allocation: possible role in human obesity. Science 2005;307(5709):584–586.

85. Levine JA, Eberhardt NL, Jensen MD. Role of nonexercise activity thermogenesis in resistance to fat gain in humans. Science 1999;283(5399):212–214.

86. Smith IG, Goulder MA. Randomized placebo-controlled trial of long-term treatment with sibutramine in mild to moderate obesity. J Fam Pract 2001;50(6):505–512.

87. James WPT, Astrup A, Finer N, et al. Effect of sibutramine on weight maintenance after weight loss: a randomised trial. STORM study group. Sibutramine Trial of Obesity Reduction and Maintenance. Lancet 2000;356:2119–2125.

88. Davidson MH, Hauptman J, DiGirolamo M, et al. Weight control and risk factor reduction in obese subjects treated for 2 years with orlistat: a randomized controlled trial. JAMA 1999;281(3):235–242.

89. Sjöström L, Rissanen A, Andersen T, et al. Randomised placebo-controlled trial of orlistat for weight loss and prevention of weight regain in obese patients. European Multicentre Orlistat Study Group. Lancet 1998;352:167–172.

90. Hauptman J, Lucas C, Boldrin MN, et al. Orlistat in the long-term treatment of obesity in primary care settings. Arch Fam Med 2000;9:160–167.

91. Rossner S, Sjostrom L, Noack R, et al. Weight loss, weight maintenance, and improved cardiovascular risk factors after 2 years treatment with orlistat for obesity. European Orlistat Obesity Study Group. Obes Res 2000;8(1):49–61.

92. Rosenbaum M, Goldsmith R, Bloomfield D, et al. Low-dose leptin reverses skeletal muscle, autonomic, and neuroendocrine adaptations to maintenance of reduced weight. J Clin Invest 2005;115(12): 3579–3586.

93. Build and Blood Pressure study Chicago, Society of Actuaries and Association of Life Insurance Directors of America: 1979, 1980.

94. Perri MG, Shapiro RM, Ludwig WW, et al. Maintenance strategies for the treatment of obesity: an evaluation of relapse prevention training and posttreatment contact by mail and telephone. J Consult Clin Psychol 1984;52(3):404–413.

95. Perri MG, McAdoo WG, Spevak PA, et al. Effect of a multicomponent maintenance program on long-term weight loss. J Consult Clin Psychol 1984;52(3):480–481.

96. Jeffery RW, Wing RR, Mayer RR. Are smaller weight losses or more achievable weight loss goals better in the long term for obese patients? J Consult Clin Psychol 1998;66(4):641–645.

97. Wing R, Venditti F, Jakicic J, et al. Lifestyle intervention in overweight individuals with a family history of diabetes. Diabetes Care 1998;21:350–360.

98. Herman WH, Hoerger TJ, Brandle M, et al. The cost-effectiveness of lifestyle modification or metformin in preventing type 2 diabetes in adults with impaired glucose tolerance. Ann Intern Med 2005;142(5):323–332.

13 Reductions in Dietary Energy Density as a Weight Management Strategy

Jenny H. Ledikwe, PhD, Heidi M. Blanck, PhD, Laura Kettel Khan, PhD, Mary K. Serdula, MD, Jennifer D. Seymour, PhD, Beth C. Tohill, PhD, and Barbara J. Rolls, PhD

CONTENTS

INTRODUCTION
WHAT IS ENERGY DENSITY?
POPULATION-BASED STUDIES
EXPERIMENTAL STUDIES
CLINICAL INTERVENTIONS
PRACTICAL STRATEGIES TO REDUCE ENERGY DENSITY
CONCLUSIONS
ACKNOWLEDGMENTS
REFERENCES

Summary

Reducing caloric intake is the cornerstone of dietary therapy for long-term healthy weight management. Strategies individuals have typically used include limiting portion sizes, food groups, or certain macronutrients. Although such restrictive approaches can lead to weight loss in the short term, they can result in feelings of hunger or dissatisfaction, which can limit their acceptability, sustainability, and long-term effectiveness. An alternative positive strategy to manage energy intake is for individuals to eat more foods that are low in calories for a given measure of food—that is, they are low in energy density (kcal/g). Data have shown that people eat a fairly consistent amount of food on a day-to-day basis; therefore, the energy density of the foods an individual consumes influences energy intake. Encouraging patients to eat more foods low in energy density and to substitute these foods for those higher in energy density allows them to decrease their energy intake while eating satisfying portions, thereby controlling hunger and lowering energy intake. This type of diet fits with the current *Dietary Guidelines for Americans* in that it incorporates high quantities of fruits, vegetables, and fiber, which are often suboptimal in typical low-calorie diets, and it provides ample intakes of numerous micronutrients. Moreover, studies have found that individuals who consume lower-energy-dense diets consume more food by weight and have lower body weights compared

From: *Contemporary Endocrinology: Treatment of the Obese Patient*
Edited by: R. F. Kushner and D. H. Bessesen © Humana Press Inc., Totowa, NJ

with individuals who consume higher-energy-dense diets. This chapter reviews the evidence supporting the use of diets rich in low-energy-dense foods for weight management and provides practical approaches to lowering the energy density of the diet.

   Key Words: Energy density; energy intake; satiety; body weight; obesity.

INTRODUCTION

   To prevent gradual weight gain over time, the *2005 Dietary Guidelines for Americans*
recommend small decreases in energy from foods and beverages and increases in physical activity *(1)*. For individuals who need to lose weight, the guidelines encourage a slow,
steady weight loss by decreasing energy intake while maintaining an adequate nutrient
intake and increasing physical activity. Strategies individuals have typically used to
reduce energy intake include limiting portion sizes, food groups, or certain macronutrients. Clinical trials have found that restrictive approaches such as low-fat or low-carbohydrate regimens, because of decreased caloric intake, have led to weight loss in the short
term (6 mo or less) *(2,3)*. Restrictive approaches may, however, result in feelings of
hunger or dissatisfaction, which can limit their acceptability, sustainability, and long-
term effectiveness *(4–6)*. An alternative positive strategy to manage energy intake is for
individuals to eat more foods that are low in calories for a given measure of food—that
is, they are low in energy density (kcal/g). Encouraging individuals to eat these types of
foods is one of the dietary strategies recommended in the *Dietary Guidelines for Americans* to manage energy intake. In the following sections, energy density as a dietary
strategy for management of weight is discussed.

WHAT IS ENERGY DENSITY?

   Energy density is the amount of energy in a particular weight of food. It is generally
presented as the number of calories in a gram (kcal/g). Foods with a low energy density
provide less energy relative to their weight than foods with a high energy density.
Therefore, for the same amount of energy, a larger, more satisfying portion size of food
can be consumed of a food low in energy density, compared with a food high in energy
density.

   Energy density values, which are influenced by the moisture content and macronutrient composition of foods, range from 0 kcal/g to 9 kcal/g (Fig. 1). The component of food
with the greatest impact on energy density is water *(7)*. Water has an energy density of
0 kcal/g, as it contributes weight but not energy to foods. Fiber also has a relatively low
energy density, providing 1.5 to 2.5 kcal/g, and can lower the energy density of foods.
On the opposite end of the energy density spectrum, fat is the most energy-dense component of food. Fat provides 9 kcal/g, more than twice as much energy as carbohydrates
or protein, which provide 4 kcal/g. Although most high-fat foods have a high energy
density, increasing the water content lowers the energy density of all foods, even those
high in fat.

   The energy density of a food can be calculated easily by using information that is
readily available on the Nutrition Facts Panel of food labels. In order to better understand
which foods are low or high in energy density, Table 1 classifies foods into four categories. Water-rich foods, such as nonstarchy fruits and vegetables and broth-based soups,
are very low in energy density (<0.6 kcal/g) *(8,9)* and should constitute a large proportion
of each meal, be eaten as snacks, and be chosen as appetizers. In addition to foods with
a very low energy density, low-energy-dense foods (0.6 to 1.5 kcal/g) such as starchy

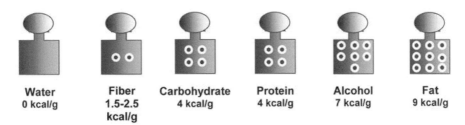

Fig. 1. Energy density values, which vary from 0 to 9 kcal/g, are influenced by the water content and macronutrient composition of foods. This is illustrated using 1-g scale weights in which each dot on the scales represents 1 kcal.

Table 1
Typical Energy Density Values for Different Types of Foods

Food examples	Typical energy density	Description
Nonstarchy fruits and vegetables, and broth-based soups	0 to 0.6	Very low energy density
Starchy fruits and vegetables, cooked grains, beans and legumes, lean meats, low-fat diary foods, and low-fat mixed dishes such as chili and spaghetti	0.6 to 1.5	Low energy density
Eggs, dried fruits, bread and bagels, jelly, fried vegetables, and part-skim mozzarella cheese	1.5 to 4.0	Medium energy density
Low-moisture foods such as crackers, cookies, chips, and high-fat foods such as croissants, peanut butter, margarine, and bacon	4.0 to 9.0	High energy density

Adapted from refs. *8* and *9.*

fruits and vegetables, cooked grains, legumes, lean meat and fish, and low-fat mixed dishes should accompany and/or be incorporated with very-low-energy-dense foods as the primary focus of meals. Foods with a medium (1.5 to 4.0 kcal/g) and high (4.0 to 9.0 kcal/g) energy density should be consumed less frequently and attention should be given to limiting their portion size.

By consuming a diet low in energy density, caloric intake can be reduced without strictly limiting food portions. Figure 2 depicts the total amount of food that can be consumed on a 1600-kcal diet depending on the overall energy density of the diet. The energy density values in this figure correspond to a low- (1.4 kcal/g), medium- (1.9 kcal/ g), or high-energy-dense (2.2 kcal/g) diet, as defined by the average dietary energy density of a representative group of US adults *(10,11)*. When consuming a diet with an energy density of 1.4 kcal/g, which would be rich in low-energy-dense foods, more than 1100 g of foods can be consumed for 1600 kcal. However, only 725 g can be consumed on the high-energy-dense, 2.2 kcal/g diet. At any energy level, the lower the energy density of the diet, the greater the amount of food that can be consumed.

This review will focus on several types of scientific evidence, including population-based studies, laboratory-based studies, and clinical trials, showing the influence of

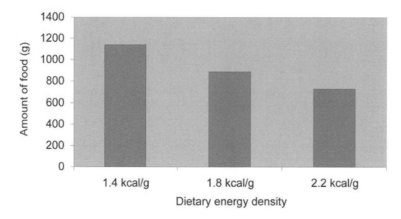

Fig. 2. The amount of food a person consumes on a 1600 kcal/d diet varies depending on the energy density of the diet. At a given calorie level, a greater amount of food is consumed on a low-energy-dense diet. The energy density values in this figure were based on values corresponding to a low-, medium-, and high-energy-dense diet, as defined using food intake data from a representative group of US adults *(10,11)*.

Table 2
Information Important for Understanding Why Diets Low in Energy Density Are Effective at Reducing Energy Intake and Managing Body Weight

- Energy density (kcal/g) (also called calorie density) is the amount of energy (calories) in a specific amount of food.
- A food that is high in energy density provides a large amount of calories in a small weight, whereas a food of low energy density has fewer calories for the same weight.
- For the same number of calories, one can consume a larger portion of a food lower in energy density than a food higher in energy density.
- On a day-to-day basis, people generally eat a similar amount of food, by weight.
- Choosing foods with a lower energy density allows people to consume their usual amount of food while they reduce their energy intake.

energy density on energy intake, satiety, and body weight. Concepts important in understanding why diets low in energy density are effective at reducing energy intake and managing body weight are highlighted in Table 2.

POPULATION-BASED STUDIES

Population-based studies suggest that energy density is associated with energy intake, the amount of food consumed, diet quality, and weight status. Data from studies examining the foods people habitually consume in the course of their everyday lives provide a first level of evidence that energy density is associated with energy intake and the amounts of food individuals consume. A nationally representative study of US adults found that men and women who reported eating a lower-energy-dense diet consumed more food, by weight, yet had lower energy intakes than persons with a higher-energy-dense diet *(11)*. Studies among free-living Mediterranean *(12)*, Chinese *(13)*, and French

(14) adults have also found that people with a diet low in energy density consume less energy.

Epidemiological studies also provide information about the foods selected by individuals consuming a diet low in energy density. Components common to a diet low in energy density include grains, dairy foods, and meat/meat alternatives with a low fat content, a high micronutrient content, or a high water content. Increased consumption of fruits and vegetables is a critical component of a lower-energy-dense diet. Although lower-energy-dense diets tend to be relatively low in fat, this is not always the case. Even the energy density of diets that are moderately high in fat can be reduced by the addition of fruits and vegetables. Among a nationally representative group of adults, consumption of nine or more servings of fruits and vegetables was associated with relatively low dietary energy density values, even for diets moderately high in fat *(11)*.

Additionally, several epidemiological studies indicate that the energy density of an individual's typical diet is related to weight status *(11,13,15–17)*. Normal-weight adults have been shown to consume diets with a lower energy density than obese individuals *(11)*. Data have also shown that the prevalence of obesity was lowest among those individuals with a high intake of fruits and vegetables; this was found even among individuals with a diet relatively high in fat (>30% of kcal). This highlights the importance of fruits and vegetables in weight management and their potential to lower the energy density even in diets relatively high in fat.

Many weight-management diets focus on reductions in certain macronutrients or food groups, which may lead to inadequate nutrient intakes *(18)*. Diets low in energy density, however, encourage consumption of a variety of foods from all groups. Data from a nationally representative survey of US adults indicate that people consuming a lower-energy-dense diet do eat a balanced diet by making specific choices within each food group in the Food Guide Pyramid *(19)*, generally choosing foods that were low-fat, micronutrient-dense, or with high water content *(10)*. These food choices led to higher intakes of fiber, vitamin A, vitamin C, and folate, compared with foods consumed in a higher-energy-dense diet. These data indicate that choosing lower-energy-dense foods can lead to food patterns consistent with a healthy diet based on the *Dietary Guidelines for Americans (1)*.

These epidemiological data suggest that a diet low in energy density allows people to reduce their energy intake without necessarily decreasing the amount of food they consume and is associated with a more favorable nutrition profile and weight status.

EXPERIMENTAL STUDIES

Further information regarding the influence of energy density on food intake is provided by experimental studies indicating that energy density affects energy intake, hunger, and satiety. In a study conducted in 1983, Duncan and colleagues *(20)* showed that providing people with a diet rich in lower-energy-dense foods was associated with a spontaneous decrease in energy intake without a significant increase in reported hunger. Obese and nonobese participants ate all meals over 5 d in a hospital on two separate occasions in which the diets varied in both fat and energy density. On one occasion a lower-fat, lower-energy-dense diet was provided, which included substantial amounts of fresh fruits, vegetables, whole grains, and beans; the other diet included large amounts of high-fat meats and desserts. Participants reported that each diet satisfied hunger similarly, and they consumed comparable weights of food during each 5-d session, which resulted in a 50% lower energy intake on the lower-fat, lower-energy-dense diet.

In a longer-term study, Shintani and colleagues *(21,22)* provided participants with a traditional Hawaiian diet, rich in fruits and vegetables, for 3 wk. This diet was considerably lower in energy density and in fat than the participants' habitual diet. They consumed a similar amount of food, by weight, with both diets, which led to a reduction in daily energy intake on the low-energy-dense traditional diet. Despite the reduction in energy intake, the subjects reported the diet to be moderately to highly satiating. These findings are supported by studies lasting up to 11 wk in which the energy density of the diet was lowered by reducing the fat content of the available foods *(23–25)*. Again the participants consumed a similar weight of food so that the diet that was reduced in energy density was associated with lower energy intake.

It is not clear from these studies whether it was the reduction in the fat content of the diet or the reduction in energy density that affected energy intake. Although fat intake and energy density are closely linked, energy density can be reduced independent of changes in fat by adding water-rich fruits and vegetables to the diet. Bell and colleagues *(26)* provided normal-weight women with all their meals for 2 d on three occasions. On each occasion, the women were served mixed dishes with varying amounts of vegetables, which changed the energy density of the meals but not the fat content. Although they could eat as much or as little as they liked, the women ate similar amounts of food, by weight, over the 2-d sessions (Fig. 3). Consequently, reducing the energy density of the diet by 30% through the addition of extra vegetables led to a 30% reduction in energy intake. Despite the substantial reduction in energy intake, subjects rated themselves equally full and satisfied. This indicates that when individuals continue to consume their normal amount of food, reducing the energy density of the diet by adding water-rich vegetables is an effective way to decrease energy intake.

Conversely, lowering the fat content of the diet without reducing the energy density has not been shown to affect energy intake *(27,28)*. For example, when men were provided with diets varying in fat (20, 40, or 60% of energy) that did not differ in energy density for 2-wk periods, energy intakes were comparable in each diet condition *(29)*.

Studies suggest that a practical approach to help moderate energy intake is to consume a satisfying portion of low-energy-dense food, such as salad or soup, at the start of a meal. Whereas large portions of energy-dense foods have been shown to increase energy intake *(30–36)*, recent laboratory-based studies indicate that having a large portion of a low-energy-dense food at the beginning of a meal decreases energy intake *(30,37)*. In one study, subjects consumed a first-course salad, which was varied in energy density and portion size on different days; this was followed by a main course of pasta consumed *ad libitum*. Compared to having no first course, consuming a low-energy-dense salad as a first course led to a decrease in total energy intake at the meal (Fig. 4). This reduction in energy intake was greater when the subjects were served the larger rather than the smaller low-energy-dense salad. It is, however, important to note that the energy content of the low-energy-dense salads was fairly low, less than 150 kcal. Consumption of a low-energy-dense soup at the start of a meal has also been shown to reduce overall meal intake *(39)*. This indicates that when choosing a first course, patients can enhance satiety and reduce overall energy intake by selecting large portions of foods low in energy density.

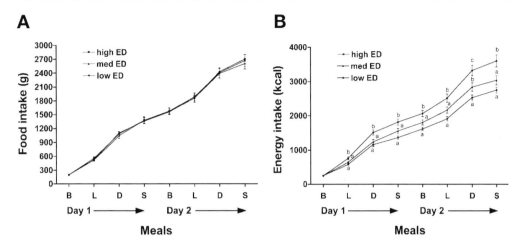

Fig. 3. When provided with meals varying in energy density over 2 d on three separate occasions, participants ate similar amounts of food, by weight, over each 2-d session. As mean cumulative food consumption was similar in each condition, mean cumulative energy intake was lowest when participants were provided with low-energy-dense meals. (Means with different letters are significantly different at each time point [$p < 0.05$]. B, breakfast; L, lunch; D, dinner; S, evening snack.) Reproduced with permission from ref. *26*.

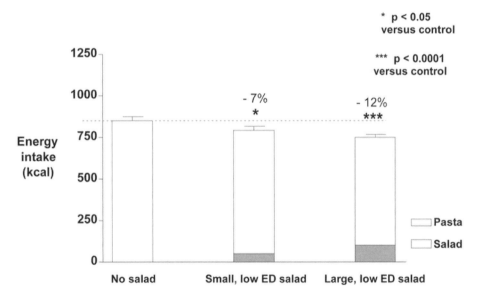

Fig. 4. As part of a laboratory-based study, participants consumed a low-energy-dense salad as a first course that varied in portion size on different days, followed by a main course of pasta consumed *ad libitum*. Compared to having no first course, consuming either a small or large low-energy-dense salad as a first course lead to a decrease in total energy intake at the meal. This reduction in energy intake was greater when participants were served the large salad rather than the smaller low-energy-dense salad. Reproduced with permission from ref. *30*.

CLINICAL INTERVENTIONS

Clinical interventions indicate that counseling patients to consume a lower-energy-dense diet is an effective strategy for weight management. Multiple studies indicate that individuals consistently consume less energy when presented with a lower-energy-dense diet than with a diet consisting of similar foods having a higher energy density. An important question is whether reductions in energy density can be successfully employed to manage body weight *(38)*. The effectiveness of consuming a diet rich in low-energy-dense foods for weight loss and maintenance was first demonstrated by Fitzwater and colleagues *(39)*. A group of more than 200 obese people were counseled to consume a reduced-energy diet emphasizing foods that were low in energy density such as fresh fruits, vegetables, whole grains, and beans. Over 7 mo, the participants lost an average of 6.3 kg. At a follow-up approx 2 yr after the intervention, 77% of the participants were below their pretreatment weight, and 53% were below the weight they had achieved immediately after completion of the intervention. Even though detailed food intake information was not collected as part of the study, these findings suggest that advice to consume a diet rich in lower-energy-dense foods is an effective strategy for weight loss and maintenance.

Stronger evidence regarding long-term effects of energy density on body weight has been provided by controlled clinical trials that collected detailed food intake data. Rolls and colleagues *(40)* examined the effectiveness of incorporating a single low-energy-dense food into a reduced-energy diet. In a year-long clinical trial, 200 overweight or obese men and women were randomly assigned to one of four intervention groups and provided with one of the following items, which provided 100 kcal/serving, to incorporate into their daily diet: one serving of a low-energy-dense soup, two servings of a low-energy-dense soup, two servings of a high-energy-dense snack food, or no special food. Over the course of the year, incorporating soup into the diet led to the greatest decrease in energy density (1.23 vs 1.73 kcal/g at 1 yr). The percentage of weight lost during the first month of the study was correlated with the participants' decrease in the energy density of their diet (Fig. 5). Furthermore, when all dietary and subject characteristics were considered, dietary energy density was the main predictor of weight loss during the first 2 mo of the study, which was when the majority of the weight loss occurred and when adherence was likely to be highest. After 1 yr, weight loss among those consuming two servings of low-energy-dense soup a day was 50% greater than among those consuming two servings of high-energy-dense dry snacks (7.2 vs 4.8 kg). Thus, incorporating a single low-energy-dense food into a reduced-energy diet increased the magnitude of the weight loss and helped participants to maintain this loss.

In the studies mentioned thus far, participants were counseled to consume a reduced-energy diet. Ello-Martin and colleagues *(41)* recently tested the effects of two strategies to reduce the energy density of the diet on weight loss with 71 obese women. Participants were not given specific limits for energy intake. One group was counseled to decrease the energy density of their diet by increasing consumption of water-rich foods, such as fruits and vegetables, and choosing reduced-fat foods. A comparison group was counseled to eat less fat. Both groups lowered the energy density of their diets, and both groups lost weight. However, after 12 mo, the group counseled to eat more fruits and vegetables while also reducing fat intake had a greater reduction in the energy density of their diet and lost 23% more weight (7.9 vs 6.4 kg) than the group told just to eat less fat. Even though they lost more weight, participants eating the lower-energy-dense diet

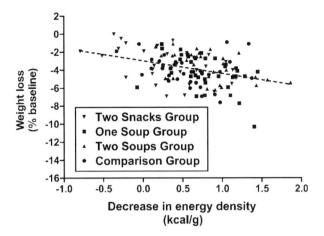

Fig. 5. In a year-long clinical trial, the decrease in food energy density (from baseline value) was significantly correlated ($r = 0.36$) with the percentage weight loss and was the best dietary predictor of weight loss at 1 mo. Subjects followed an energy-restricted diet plan and either incorporated low-energy-dense soup or high-energy-dense snacks (one or two servings daily) or did not incorporate any special foods (comparison group). Reproduced with permission from ref. *40.*

reported consuming an average of 25% more food by weight. Furthermore, they reported less hunger than participants who reduced the energy density of their diet by simply reducing fat intake. Thus, dietary advice to reduce the energy density of the diet was shown to be an effective strategy for long-term weight management. Furthermore, achieving reductions in energy density by combining fat reduction with increased consumption of fruits and vegetables was more effective for weight management than simply reducing fat intake.

PRACTICAL STRATEGIES TO REDUCE ENERGY DENSITY

The overall goal of any dietary strategy for weight loss is to reduce energy intake below expenditure in a manner that is both nutritious and sustainable. Consuming a diet low in energy density is not only associated with a healthy balance of foods, but it also allows individuals to eat satisfying food portions while reducing their energy intake. This section examines practical strategies to reduce the energy density of the diet, which, along with physical activity, can be an important part of a healthy, lifelong weight management plan.

Choose Foods Low in Energy Density

Palatability and preferences play a critical role in food selection *(42)*; therefore, modifying the energy density of a patient's existing diet pattern increases the likelihood of achieving lasting dietary changes. When providing patients with guidance for decreasing the energy density of their diet, the main goals should be to increase fruit and vegetable intake and decrease fat intake. These strategies can be used to lower the energy density of many food items with a high energy content. For instance, instead of having a cup of ice cream for dessert, which has an energy density of 2.4 kcal/g and provides approx 235 kcal, consuming half a cup of reduced-fat ice cream with half a cup of fruit will decrease the energy density of this snack to 0.96 kcal/g and lower the calorie content to 130 kcal.

The energy density of mixed dishes can also be reduced by adding water-rich ingredients such as fruits and vegetables or by reducing the amount of added fat. For example, the energy density of lasagna can be lowered by increasing the amount of vegetables in the dish (add chopped spinach, shredded carrots, or broccoli) and reducing the fat content (choose lower-fat meat and cheese, or simply use less). When consuming mixed dishes such as this, studies indicate that people will likely consume their usual portion, but will ingest less energy (26,37,43–45). This can help patients meet prescribed reductions in energy intake while feeling full and satisfied with their diet.

Two sample menus are listed in Table 3 to demonstrate how food choices can influence the energy density, energy content, and the amount of food that a person consumes. The first menu is a typical moderate-fat diet (35% fat) providing 2000 kcal. It provides approx 955 g of food. The second menu is lower in fat (25% fat) and energy (1500 kcal), but provides more food—almost 2000 g of food. This lower-energy-dense menu contains foods that are both lower in fat and have a higher water content. The main lunch entrée included in the sample menus is an example of how food selections can influence the energy content and the amount of food an individual is able to consume. Compared with the fried chicken sandwich, the grilled chicken salad with a low-fat dressing contains less fat and more water-rich vegetables. It contains more than 50% fewer calories (240 vs 510 kcal), yet provides approx 100 more grams of food. Although reductions in energy density can be accomplished by decreasing the fat content of the diet or increasing the consumption of water-rich foods, the most substantial reductions in energy density are achieved when both these strategies are used simultaneously (41–46).

Encourage Consumption of First-Course Foods Low in Energy Density

A practical approach to help moderate energy intake is to consume a satisfying portion of low-energy-dense food at the start of a meal. Evidence indicates that when choosing a first course, patients can achieve the greatest enhancement of satiety and reduction in overall energy intake by selecting large portions of foods low in energy density, such as broth-based soups and low-energy-dense salads, which provide 100 to 150 kcal (30).

Avoid Large Portions of Foods High in Energy Density

In addition to modifying high-energy-dense foods to decrease their energy density, patients should be counseled to consume smaller portions of energy-dense foods. Along with energy density, food portion size has been shown to influence energy intake.

Specifically, studies have found that people consume more energy when presented with large portions of food (30–36). This has been shown for a variety of foods, including foods served in units such as sandwiches (35) or prepackaged potato chips, or foods with an amorphous shape such as macaroni and cheese (33). The effect of portion size on intake persisted when all foods in a 2-d period were increased in size (36). Given the pervasiveness of large portions of energy-dense foods in today's society, recent studies have examined the combined influence of energy density and portion size on food intake (30–32). In one such study (32), participants were provided with a variety of popular commercially available foods over two consecutive days on four occasions. The foods were varied in energy density and presented in either reduced or standard portion sizes.

Table 3
Sample Menus for 2000-kcal and 1500-kcal Diets of Varying Energy Density

Typical, moderate-fat, 2000-kcal diet

	Energy (kcal)	Weight (g)	Energy Density (kcal/g)
Breakfast			
Waffles (2) with syrup (1/4 c) and butter (1 t)	305	115	2.65
Cottage cheese (1/2 c)	100	115	0.87
Snack			
Snack crackers with peanut butter (3)	105	20	5.25
Lunch			
Fried chicken sandwich	510	220	2.32
Yogurt and fruit parfait	160	150	1.07
Dinner			
Meatloaf (3 oz)	180	85	2.12
Macaroni and cheese (3/4 c)	270	165	1.64
Green beans (1/2 c)	20	60	0.33
Garlic bread (1)	95	25	3.80
Ice cream (3/4 c) with strawberry topping (1.5 T)	255	110	2.32
Total	2000 kcal	1065 g	1.88 kcal/g
	35% fat		
	49% carbohydrate		
	16% protein		

Reduced-energy-density, reduced-fat 1500-kcal diet

	Energy (kcal)	Weight (g)	Energy Density (kcal/g)
Breakfast			
Oatmeal (1 c) with strawberries (3/4 c) and walnuts (1.5 T)	255	355	0.72
Cottage cheese (1/2 c) with blueberries (1/2 c)	140	185	0.76
Snack			
Melon (1 c)	50	165	0.30
Lunch			
Grilled chicken salad with vinaigrette dressing	240	325	0.74
Yogurt and fruit parfait	160	150	1.07
Minestrone soup (1 c)	80	240	0.33
Dinner			
Lean beef (3 oz) stir-fried with vegetables (1.5 c), soy sauce (1 T), and oil (1 t)	290	280	1.04
Brown rice (1/2 c)	110	100	1.1
Fortune cookie (1)	30	10	3.0
Lite ice cream (1/5 c) with peaches (1)	145	160	0.91
	1500 kcal	1970 g	0.76 kcal/g
	25% fat		
	49% carbohydrate		
	26% protein		

The effects of energy density and portion size were combined so the participants consumed the least amount of energy when provided with the reduced portions of the lower-energy-dense foods, and the greatest amount of energy when provided with the standard portions of the higher-energy-dense foods. Over the 2 d, they consumed 1625 kcal less when both portion size and energy density were decreased. Although longer-term studies are needed, these data suggest that habitual exposure to large portions of energy-dense foods is likely to be problematic for weight management. Energy-dense foods do not need to be completely eliminated from the diet, but rather should be consumed in moderate portions along with foods that are predominantly low in energy density.

CONCLUSIONS

Dietary strategies that help individuals maintain a healthy body weight and prevent weight gain are important to reverse current trends in overweight and obesity. In addition, for those who are already overweight, sound and practical strategies are needed to reduce daily energy intake by the recommended 500 or more kcal/d *(1,47)*. However, weight management plans should not only reduce energy intake; they should also satisfy hunger, meet nutritional requirements, take food preferences into account, and include physical activity. Practical approaches for incorporating energy density principles with other dietary recommendations to achieve a balanced diet are summarized in Table 4. Two important points for lowering the energy density of the diet are highlighted below:

- Individuals should ensure that meals include a large proportion of very-low-energy-dense fruits and vegetables and are accompanied by low-energy-dense foods such as starchy fruits and vegetables, cooked grains, legumes, lean meats, low-fat dairy foods, and low-fat mixed dishes.
- High-energy-dense foods, such as low-moisture foods and high-fat foods, should not be completely eliminated from the diet; however, they should be consumed in small or moderate portions.

Achieving and maintaining a healthy body weight is a challenge for a large percentage of the population. Diet, along with physical activity, continues to be a cornerstone of weight management *(47,48)*. Data support the suggestion that choosing a diet rich in low-energy-dense foods is a nutritionally sound eating strategy that can help individuals manage their energy intake while being able to enjoy satisfying portions of food. Because the energy density of a variety of eating patterns can be lowered, this type of diet encourages the adoption of lifelong healthy eating habits, which is integral to weight management.

ACKNOWLEDGMENTS

Preparation of this chapter was supported in part by an appointment to the Research Participation Program at the Centers for Disease Control and Prevention (CDC), National Center for Chronic Disease Prevention and Health Promotion, Division of Nutrition and Physical Activity, which was administered by the Oak Ridge Institute for Science and Education through an interagency agreement between the US Department of Energy and CDC (JHL). Additional support was provided by National Institutes of Health grant R37DK039177 (BJR). The conclusions in this report are those of the authors and do not necessarily represent the views of the funding agency.

Table 4
Practical Approaches for Incorporating Energy Density Principles With Key Recommendations
From the Dietary Guidelines for Americans (DGA) 2005

DGA focus area	DGA 2005 key recommendation	Strategies for incorporating energy density principles with the DGA (8,9)
Adequate nutrients within calorie needs	Consume a variety of nutrient-dense foods and beverages within and among the basic food groups while choosing foods that limit the intake of saturated and *trans* fats, cholesterol, added sugars, salt, and alcohol.	Choose plenty of foods with a very low or low energy density and moderate portions of higher-energy-dense foods.
Weight management		
Prevention of gradual weight gain	To prevent gradual weight gain over time, make small decreases in food and beverage calories and increase physical activity.	A reduction of 50 to 100 calories per day may prevent gradual weight gain.
Weight loss	Those who need to lose weight should aim for a slow, steady weight loss by decreasing calorie intake and increasing physical activity.	For patients who are overweight or obese, a reduction of usual intake by 500 calories per day can lead to a loss of a pound per week.
Food groups to encourage		
Fruits and vegetables	Consume a sufficient amount of fruits and vegetables while staying within energy needs. Two cups of fruit and 2.5 cups of vegetables per day are recommended for a 2,000-calorie intake, with higher or lower amounts depending on the calorie level. Choose a variety of fruits and vegetables each day. In particular, select from all five vegetable subgroups (dark green, orange, legumes, starchy vegetables, and other vegetables) several times a week.	Nonstarchy fruits and vegetables are very low in energy density (<0.6 kcal/g); make these items a large proportion of each meal and consume them as snacks and appetizers. Have starchy fruits and vegetables as an accompaniment with lower-energy-dense fruits and vegetables at meals.

(continued)

277

Table 4 (Continued)

DGA focus area	DGA 2005 key recommendation	Strategies for incorporating energy density (8,9)
Whole grains	Consume 3 or more ounce-equivalents of whole-grain products per day, with the rest of the recommended grains coming from enriched or whole-grain products. In general, at least half the grains should come from whole grains.	Select nutrient-rich whole grains such as fiber-rich breakfast cereals and whole-wheat pasta.
Dairy products	Consume 3 cups per day of fat-free or low-fat milk or equivalent milk products.	Choose reduced-fat, low-fat, or fat-free dairy foods.
Fats	Limit intake of fats and oils high in saturated and/or *trans* fatty acids, and choose products low in such fats and oils.	Choose low-fat or reduced-fat foods with a low energy density.
	Consume less than 10% of calories from saturated fatty acids and less than 300 mg/d of cholesterol, and keep *trans* fatty acid consumption as low as possible. When selecting and preparing meat, poultry, dry beans, and milk or milk products, make choices that are lean, low-fat, or fat-free.	Have beans, low-fat fish, lean meats, and low-fat dairy foods as an accompaniment to lower-energy-dense fruits and vegetables at meals.
Carbohydrates	Choose fiber-rich fruits, vegetables and whole grains often.	Emphasize carbohydrates from whole grains, vegetables, and fruits.
	Choose and prepare foods and beverages with little added sugars or caloric sweeteners	
Sodium and Potassium	Choose and prepare foods with little salt. At the same time, consume potassium-rich foods, such as fruits and vegetables. Emphasize carbohydrates from whole grains, vegetables, and fruits.	
Alcohol	Those who choose to drink alcoholic beverages should do so sensibly and in moderation — defined as the consumption of up to one drink per day for women and up to two drinks per day for men.	Alcohol is high in energy density with 7 calories per gram, and it is often mixed with sugar-laden liquids. Those who choose to drink alcoholic beverages should budget those calories into their overall dietary plan.

Adapted from ref. *1.*

278

REFERENCES

1. US Department of Health and Human Services, US Department of Agriculture. Dietary Guidelines for Americans 2005. 6th ed. Washington, DC: 2005.
2. Dansinger ML, Gleason JA, Griffith JL, et al. Comparison of the Atkins, Ornish, Weight Watchers, and Zone diets for weight loss and heart disease risk reduction: a randomized trial. JAMA 2005; 293(1):43–53.
3. Foster GD, Wadden TA, Peterson FJ, et al. A controlled comparison of three very-low-calorie diets: effects on weight, body composition, and symptoms. Am J Clin Nutr 1992;55(4):811–817.
4. Cuntz U, Leibbrand R, Ehrig C, et al. Predictors of post-treatment weight reduction after in-patient behavioral therapy. Int J Obes Relat Metab Disord 2001;25 Suppl 1:S99–S101.
5. Pasman WJ, Saris WH, Westerterp-Plantenga MS. Predictors of weight maintenance. Obes Res 1999; 7(1):43–50.
6. Elfhag K, Rossner S. Who succeeds in maintaining weight loss? A conceptual review of factors associated with weight loss maintenance and weight regain. Obes Rev 2005;6(1):67–85.
7. Rolls BJ, Bell EA. Dietary approaches to the treatment of obesity. In: Jensen MD, ed. Medical Clinics of North America. W.B. Saunders, Philadelphia: 2000; pp. 401–418.
8. Rolls B, Barnett RA. The Volumetrics Weight-Control Plan. Quill, New York: 2000.
9. Rolls B. The Volumetrics Eating Plan. HarperCollins Publishers, New York: 2005.
10. Ledikwe JH, Blanck HM, Kettel-Khan L, et al. Food patterns and diet quality of US adults with a low-energy-dense diet. J Am Dietetic Assn 2006;106(8):1172–1180.
11. Ledikwe JH, Blanck HM, Khan LK, et al. Dietary energy density is associated with energy intake and weight status in US adults. Am J Clin Nutr 2006;83(6):1362–1368.
12. Cuco G, Arija V, Marti-Henneberg C, et al. Food and nutritional profile of high energy density consumers in an adult Mediterranean population. Eur J Clin Nutr 2001;55(3):192–199.
13. Stookey JD. Energy density, energy intake and weight status in a large free-living sample of Chinese adults: exploring the underlying roles of fat, protein, carbohydrate, fiber and water intakes. Eur J Clin Nutr 2001;55:349–359.
14. Drewnowski A, Almiron-Roig E, Marmonier C, et al. Dietary energy density and body weight: is there a relationship? Nutr Rev 2004;62:403–413.
15. Marti-Henneberg C, Capdevila F, Arija V, et al. Energy density of the diet, food volume and energy intake by age and sex in a healthy population. Eur J Clin Nutr 1999;53(6):421–428.
16. Cox DN, Mela DJ. Determination of energy density of freely selected diets: methodological issues and implications. Int J Obes Rel Metab Disord 2000;24(1):49–54.
17. Kant AK, Graubard BI. Energy density of diets reported by American adults: association with food group intake, nutrient intake, and body weight. Int J Obes (Lond) 2005;29(8):950–956
18. Foote JA, Murphy SP, Wilkens LR, et al. Dietary variety increases the probability of nutrient adequacy among adults. J Nutr 2004;134(7):1779–1785.
19. MyPyramid. 2005. Accessed April 2005, at www.mypyramid.gov.
20. Duncan KH, Bacon JA, Weinsier RL. The effects of high and low energy density diets on satiety, energy intake, and eating time of obese and nonobese subjects. American J Clin Nutr 1983;37:763–767.
21. Shintani TT, Beckham S, Brown AC, et al. The Hawaii Diet: ad libitum high carbohydrate, low fat multi-cultural diet for the reduction of chronic disease risk factors: obesity, hypertension, hypercholesterolemia, and hyperglycemia. Hawaii Med J 2001;60:69–73.
22. Shintani TT, Hughes CK, Beckham S, et al. Obesity and cardiovascular risk intervention through the ad libitum feeding of traditional Hawaiian diet. Am J Clin Nutr 1991;53:1647S–1651S.
23. Lissner L, Levitsky DA, Strupp BJ, et al. Dietary fat and the regulation of energy intake in human subjects. Am J Clin Nutr 1987;46:886–892.
24. Kendall A, Levitsky DA, Strupp BJ, et al. Weight loss on a low-fat diet: consequence of the imprecision of the control of food intake in humans. Am J Clin Nutr 1991;53:1124–1129.
25. Rolls BJ, Shide DJ. Dietary fat and the control of food intake. In: Fernstrom JD, Miller GD, eds. Appetite and Body Weight Regulation: Sugar, Fat, and Macronutrient Substitutes. CRC Press, Boca Raton, FL: 1994; pp. 167–177.
26. Bell EA, Castellanos VH, Pelkman CL, et al. Energy density of foods affects energy intake in normal-weight women. Am J Clin Nutr 1998;67:412–420.
27. Saltzman E, Dallal GE, Roberts SB. Effect of high-fat and low-fat diets on voluntary energy intake and substrate oxidation: studies in identical twins consuming diets matched for energy density, fiber and palatability. Am J Clin Nutr 1997;66:1332-9.

28. van Stratum P, Lussenburg RN, van Wezel LA, et al. The effect of dietary carbohydrate:fat ratio on energy intake by adult women. Am J Clin Nutr 1978;31:206–212.

29. Stubbs RJ, Harbron CG, Prentice AM. Covert manipulation of the dietary fat to carbohydrate ratio of isoenergetically dense diets: effect on food intake in feeding men ad libitum. Int J Obes 1996;20:651–660.

30. Rolls BJ, Roe LS, Meengs JS. Salad and satiety: energy density and portion size of a first course salad affect energy intake at lunch. J Am Dietetic Assn 2004;104:1570–1576.

31. Kral TVE, Roe LS, Rolls BJ. Combined effects of energy density and portion size on energy intake in women. Am J Clin Nutr 2004;79:962–968.

32. Rolls BJ, Roe LS, Meengs JS. Reducing the energy density and portion size of foods decreases energy intake over two days. Obes Res 2004;12:A5.

33. Rolls BJ, Morris EL, Roe LS. Portion size of food affects energy intake in normal-weight and over-weight men and women. Am J Clin Nutr 2002;76:1207–1213.

34. Diliberti N, Bordi P, Conklin MT, et al. Increased portion size leads to increased energy intake in a restaurant meal. Obes Res 2004;12:562–568.

35. Rolls BJ, Roe LS, Meengs JS, et al. Increasing the portion size of a sandwich increases energy intake. J Am Dietetic Assn 2004;104:367–372.

36. Rolls BJ, Roe LS, Meengs JS. Larger portion sizes lead to sustained increase in energy intake over two days. J Am Dietetic Assn 2006;106(4):543–549.

37. Rolls BJ, Bell EA, Thorwart ML. Water incorporated into a food but not served with a food decreases energy intake in lean women. Am J Clin Nutr 1999;70:448–455.

38. Hedley AA, Ogden CL, Johnson CL, et al. Prevalence of overweight and obesity among US children, adolescents, and adults, 1999–2002. JAMA 2004;291(23):2847–2850.

39. Fitzwater SL, Weinsier RL, Wooldridge NH, et al. Evaluation of long-term weight changes after a multidisciplinary weight control program. J Am Dietetic Assn 1991;91:421–426, 429.

40. Rolls BJ, Roe LS, Beach AM, et al. Provision of foods differing in energy density affects long-term weight loss. Obes Res 2005;13:1052–1060.

41. Ello-Martin JA, Roe LS, Rolls BJ. A diet reduced in energy density results in greater weight loss than a diet reduced in fat. Obes Res 2004;12:A23.

42. Drewnowski A. Energy density, palatability, and satiety: implications for weight control. Nutr Rev 1998;56:347–353.

43. Bell EA, Rolls BJ. Energy density of foods affects energy intake across multiple levels of fat content in lean and obese women. Am J Clin Nutr 2001;73:1010–1018.

44. Kral TV, Rolls BJ. Energy density and portion size: their independent and combined effects on energy intake. Physiol Behav 2004;82(1):131–138.

45. Rolls BJ, Bell EA, Castellanos VH, et al. Energy density but not fat content of foods affected energy intake in lean and obese women. Am J Clin Nutr 1999;69:863–871.

46. Rolls BJ, Drewnowski A, Ledikwe JH. Changing the energy density of the diet as a strategy for weight management. J Am Dietetic Assn 2005;105:98–103.

47. National Institutes of Health. Clinical Guidelines on the Identification, Evaluation, and Treatment of Overweight and Obesity in Adults. NIH Publication No. 98-4083. Department of Health and Human Services, National Institutes of Health, National Heart, Lung, and Blood Institute, Bethesda, MD: 1998.

48. National Institutes of Health. The Practical Guide. Identification, Evaluation, and Treatment of Over-weight and Obesity in Adults. NIH Publication No. 02-4084. Department of Health and Human Services, National Institutes of Health, National Heart, Lung, and Blood Institute, Bethesda, MD: 2002.

14   Glycemic Index, Obesity, and Diabetes

Cara B. Ebbeling, PhD,
and David S. Ludwig, MD, PhD

CONTENTS

INTRODUCTION
CLASSIFYING CARBOHYDRATE-CONTAINING FOODS
PROPOSED PHYSIOLOGICAL MECHANISMS
EXPERIMENTAL EVIDENCE FOR CLINICAL UTILITY
    OF GLYCEMIC INDEX
PRACTICAL APPLICATION
CONCLUSION
REFERENCES

Summary

Prescribing diets to treat obese patients and to prevent type 2 diabetes poses a challenge to clinicians. Overemphasis on carbohydrate-to-fat ratio, with insufficient attention directed toward diet quality, may partially explain disappointing outcomes with available approaches. The glycemic index (GI) is an alternative system for classifying carbohydrate-containing foods according to postprandial blood glucose responses to portions containing a standard amount of available carbohydrate, thereby providing a measure of carbohydrate quality. Because GI is based on standardized portions, glycemic load (GL; product of GI and carbohydrate amount) values are used to describe how portions differing in both quality and quantity of carbohydrate affect postprandial glycemia. Plausible physiologic mechanisms link high-GI or -GL meals with disease processes. Selecting carbohydrate sources to reduce dietary GI—either without altering the contribution of carbohydrate to total energy intake or in combination with a moderate decrease in carbohydrate consumption—is a promising weight management strategy that can be implemented using a pragmatic approach.

Key Words: Glycemic index; glycemic load; dietary carbohydrate; body weight; obesity; hyperglycemia; type 2 diabetes.

INTRODUCTION

Diet therapy is the cornerstone of obesity treatment, with the spectrum of available approaches ranging from very-low-carbohydrate to very-low-fat prescriptions. Although short-term weight loss can be achieved with diets varying widely in carbohydrate-to-fat ratio, few individuals are successful in maintaining weight at a reduced level over the long term *(1–4)*. Weight loss in response to energy-restricted low-fat diet prescriptions

From: *Contemporary Endocrinology: Treatment of the Obese Patient*
Edited by: R. F. Kushner and D. H. Bessesen © Humana Press Inc., Totowa, NJ

rarely exceeds 5% at 12 to 18 mo of follow-up *(1–10)*. Although very-low-carbohydrate diets seem to be more efficacious than low-fat diets during the initial 6 mo of treatment *(2,4,11,12)*, several studies have indicated no differences in body weight at 12 mo *(2,4,10)*. In a recent clinical trial, Dansinger et al. *(10)* compared four popular diets that traversed the spectrum of available approaches. Consistent with previous studies, weight losses approximated only 2 to 3% of initial body weight at 12 mo and did not differ between the very-low-fat Ornish diet (70–75% of energy from carbohydrate, ≤10% from fat) and the very-low-carbohydrate Atkins diet (≤10% of energy from carbohydrate, 60% from fat). Moreover, outcomes of these two extreme diets did not differ from more moderate approaches, including the Weight Watchers diet (variable carbohydrate-to-fat ratio) and Zone diet (40% of energy from carbohydrate, 30% from fat).

Disappointing results may be due, in part, to insufficient attention directed toward diet quality. Emerging data suggest that the quality (i.e., source) of carbohydrate and fat may be as important as, or possibly even more important than, quantity (i.e., carbohydrate-to-fat ratio) when considering optimal diet therapy for long-term weight management and disease prevention *(9,13–15)*. This chapter focuses on carbohydrate; the reader is directed elsewhere for a discussion on dietary fat *(13,16)*. First, we explore the glycemic index (GI) as a method for classifying carbohydrate-containing foods. Because debate concerning the GI has caused confusion among clinicians and patients, we briefly address methodological issues, arguing that much of the controversy arises from improperly controlled or underpowered studies. Second, we present proposed physiologic mechanisms linking dietary glycemic index with disease processes. Third, we summarize experimental evidence for the clinical utility of the GI for promoting weight loss and preventing comorbidities, including type 2 diabetes mellitus (T2DM) and cardiovascular disease (CVD), in obese patients. (Treatment strategies for T2DM and CVD have been addressed previously *[13,16]* and are beyond the scope of this chapter.) Finally, we provide a pragmatic approach to diet prescription for treating obesity, informed by the GI.

CLASSIFYING CARBOHYDRATE-CONTAINING FOODS

Chemical Structure vs Glycemic Index

All dietary carbohydrates, regardless of chemical structure, can be digested or metabolically converted to glucose. Classification as "simple sugar" or "complex carbohydrate" is based on the premise that rates of digestion and absorption are dependent on saccharide chain length. Based on this classification system, recommendations to consume complex carbohydrate, often in the form of starchy foods, and to restrict sugary products are inherent to most conventional low-fat diets *(17,18)*. However, the overlapping postprandial responses to foods containing carbohydrates that vary in saccharide chain length suggest that this system is overly simplistic and has limited physiological relevance *(19,20)*. For example, Wahlqvist et al. *(19)* observed similar blood glucose and insulin responses in research subjects who consumed glucose as a monosaccharide, disaccharide, oligosaccharide, or polysaccharide. Bantle et al. *(20)* found that meals containing sucrose did not cause greater increases in blood glucose than those containing potato or wheat starch. Nevertheless, these findings do not negate the importance of carbohydrate source to health in general or body weight regulation in particular. There are marked differences in responses to ingestion of carbohydrate-controlled portions of foods such as white bread vs pasta *(21)*, rolled oats vs steel-cut oats *(22,23)*, and potatoes vs dried peas *(24)*. Recognizing the potential influence of carbohydrate source on post-prandial metabolism, Jenkins et al. *(25)* proposed the GI as an alternative classification system.

The GI describes the 2-h postprandial blood glucose response following consumption of a food portion containing a standard amount of available carbohydrate (i.e., total carbohydrate minus dietary fiber) *(25)*. To calculate GI, the incremental area under the blood glucose response curve after consuming 50 g of available carbohydrate from a test food is divided by the area under the curve after consuming the same amount of carbo-hydrate from a reference food (i.e., either glucose or white bread) *(26)*. High-GI foods are rapidly digested and absorbed or metabolically converted to glucose, whereas low-GI foods elicit a less dramatic response. The GI of any given food is influenced by variables such as degree of food processing, type of starch, soluble fiber content, and acidity, as previously reviewed *(27)*.

Glycemic Index vs Glycemic Load

Given that the GI of foods is based on portions containing a standard 50-g amount of carbohydrate, the glycemic load (GL) concept was proposed to describe how portions differing in both quality and quantity of carbohydrate affect postprandial blood glucose responses *(28)*. GL is calculated as the product of GI and carbohydrate amount, as shown in Table 1. In an experimental study designed to systematically validate this arithmetic concept, Brand-Miller et al. *(29)* noted that calculated GL accurately predicted observed postprandial glycemia to foods varying widely in GI and carbohydrate amount. More-over, Wolever and Bolognesi *(30)* reported that the GI of a food and the amount of carbohydrate in a given portion account for approximately equal variability in glycemic responses (i.e., 46–64% vs 47–57%, respectively).

Among those who agree that dietary GL has a significant effect on postprandial metabolism and disease processes, discussion concerning optimal diet prescriptions has focused on determining the best strategies for decreasing GL *(31)*. These include (1) decreasing carbohydrate amount, without altering carbohydrate sources and GI, (2) selecting carbohydrate sources to reduce GI, without altering carbohydrate amount; or (3) moderately decreasing carbohydrate amount while also carefully selecting carbohy-drate sources to reduce GI. Regarding the first strategy, similar glycemic responses were observed following consumption of food portions differing in available carbohydrate by more than twofold in the study by Brand-Miller et al. *(29)*. Moreover, simply decreasing carbohydrate amount, compared with altering carbohydrate source to reduce GI, may have detrimental effects on β-cell function *(32)*, circulating free fatty acid and triglyc-eride concentrations *(33)*, and satiety *(34)*. The relevance of carbohydrate source is underscored by several, although not all *(35–39)*, epidemiologic studies showing an inverse relationship between GI and risk for obesity *(14)*, diabetes and insulin resistance syndrome *(28,40–44)*, or cardiovascular disease *(45–48)*; by comparison, several of these studies showed no associations between total dietary carbohydrate and risk. These findings call into question conventional "carbohydrate counting" regimens and attention directed toward "net carbs" (i.e., a lay term for available carbohydrate) on food labels. Therefore, the primary focus of this chapter is on the latter two strategies listed above for decreasing dietary GL, with consideration for carbohydrate source as informed by the GI.

Before proceeding, it is important to summarize terminology *(49)*. *Glycemic response* is the change in blood glucose concentration following a meal or snack. *Glycemic index*

Table 1
Glycemic Index and Glycemic Load Values for Selected Items from Carbohydrate-Containing Food Groups[a]

Item	Portion Household measure	(g)	Available carbohydrate[b](g)	Glycemic index[c]	Glycemic load[d]
Nonstarchy vegetables					
Broccoli, raw[e]	1 cup	88	3.6	—	—
Carrots, raw[e]	1 cup	155	10.4	47	4.9
Starchy vegetables[f]					
Yam, baked	1 medium	114	19.9	37	7.4
Potato, baked	1 medium	173	32.8	85	27.9
Legumes					
Chickpeas	0.5 cup	82	16.3	28	4.6
Lentils	0.5 cup	99	14.1	28	3.9
Fruit[g]					
Apple	1 medium	138	15.8	38	6.0
Apple juice	1 cup	248	28.7	40	11.5
Dairy					
Milk	1 cup	244	11.0	27	3.0
Grains[f]					
Spaghetti, cooked	0.5 cup	70	18.4	44	8.1
Corn flakes	1 cup	28	23.1	92	21.3
White bread	2 slices	50	24.1	73	17.6
Nuts					
Peanuts	2 tablespoons	18	2.5	14	0.3
Sweets[f]					
Angel food cake	1 slice	75	47.1	67	31.6

[a]The food groups correspond to those delineated in the low-glycemic load food pyramid (Fig. 2) and the food choice lists (Table 2).

[b]Available carbohydrate (total carbohydrate – dietary fiber) was determined using the Nutrition Data System for Research software (NDS-R 2005, Nutrition Coordinating Center, University of Minnesota, Minneapolis).

[c]Values for GI (glucose standard) were derived from the International Table of Glycemic Index and Glycemic Load Values (56).

[d]Values for GL were calculated based on amounts of available carbohydrate in the specified portions, GL = (GI × available carbohydrate) / 100%.

[e]The GI of broccoli is not measurable due to the very large portions that would be required to ingest 50 g of available carbohydrate. The GI of carrots is measurable; however, the amount of carbohydrate, and thus the GL, is minimal.

[f]Starchy vegetables, highly processed grains, and sweets are on Level 4 of the low-glycemic load pyramid (Fig. 2) due to relatively high GI values and dramatic impacts on GL when consumed in large portions. Whole-grain products, high-fiber cereal, and pasta have a lower GI and are on Level 2. Controlled portions of these foods (Table 2) are included in a low-GL diet prescription.

[g]A whole piece of fruit, such as an apple, may have a similar GI as the corresponding juice form. However, patients tend to drink large volumes of juice, thereby increasing GL. Also, a whole piece of fruit offers more nutrition (e.g., more dietary fiber).

provides a system for categorizing carbohydrate-containing foods according to their effects on glycemic response, while controlling for carbohydrate amount. As such, the GI is a measure of carbohydrate quality. *Glycemic load* describes the combined effects of carbohydrate amount and GI on the glycemic response. In this chapter, we do not use these terms interchangeably.

Debate

Much debate surrounds the practical utility of the GI. Critics contend that classification of carbohydrate-containing foods based on the GI does not apply to mixed meals *(50–53)*. Their arguments often are based on studies that lack statistical power because of small sample sizes or are not properly controlled owing to an inappropriate reliance on published GI values instead of rigorous validation *(50,51,54,55)*. Although the International Table of Glycemic Index and Glycemic Load Values *(56)* is a useful reference tool, it has recognized limitations. Tabulated values were derived from studies conducted in laboratories located in several different countries. Variability in GI values for the "same" food (e.g., a starchy vegetable or bread product) may be due to deviation from standard methodology for quantifying GI—such as sampling venous rather than capillary blood for analysis of glucose, using inaccurate glucose analyzers, and calculating absolute rather than incremental area under the glucose-response curve *(57–59)*. Moreover, differences in food production, processing, preparation, and storage may contribute to variability. The latter concerns are not unique to studies of the GI; for example, a published value for the vitamin content of a Macintosh apple does not necessarily apply to any given piece of fruit, at any time of year, from any location, regardless of time in storage.

We argue that the GI differs across major food groups with excellent consistency, ranging from nonstarchy vegetables, legumes, and nontropical fruits at the low end to highly processed grain products at the high end. The cited limitations, therefore, do not detract from the potential importance of carbohydrate source in modulating postprandial metabolism through a variety of physiologic mechanisms. Moreover, most well-controlled experimental studies provide evidence for the efficacy of choosing low-GI carbohydrate sources to decrease dietary GL, and efficacious interventions can be translated to clinical practice using a pragmatic approach.

PROPOSED PHYSIOLOGICAL MECHANISMS

Elegant homeostatic regulatory mechanisms exert tight control over blood glucose concentrations during the postprandial period to ensure a smooth transition from the fed to the postabsorptive state. In the normal fed state, nutrients stimulate release of incretins, including glucagon-like peptide-1 (GLP1) and glucose-dependent insulinotropic polypeptide (GIP), into the circulation from endocrine cells located in the gut. The incretins augment the effects of rising blood glucose in stimulating insulin release from the β-cells. Insulin promotes an anabolic response characterized by glucose uptake in liver and muscle, and fat uptake in adipose tissue. In the postabsorptive state, counter-regulatory hormones (i.e., glucagon, epinephrine, cortisol, growth hormone) antagonize insulin action, stimulating release of stored metabolic fuels to maintain euglycemia. Metabolic fuels are directed away from storage via increased hepatic glycogenolysis, lipolysis, and gluconeogenesis.

Meals that are high in GI challenge these regulatory mechanisms, as presented in Fig. 1. To illustrate the dynamic changes that occur following a meal, the postprandial period can be divided into early, middle, and late phases *(60)*. During the early phase (0–2 h after a meal), hyperglycemia can be more than twofold greater following consumption of a high-GI food (e.g., potatoes) compared with a macronutrient-controlled portion of a low-GI food (e.g., legumes) *(24,61)*. Exaggerated hyperglycemia accentuates release of gut hormones and promotes primary hyperinsulinemia, along with hypoglucagonemia. This hormonal milieu enhances the normal anabolic response to feeding described above. The middle postprandial phase (2–4 h after a meal) is marked by a decline in nutrient absorption from the gastrointestinal tract. However, persistent elevation of circulating insulin relative to glucagon stimulates continued glucose uptake by insulin-sensitive tissues, often causing a rapid drop in blood glucose to concentrations below premeal levels. Suppressed circulating free fatty acid concentrations also indicate continued partitioning of nutrients toward storage and away from oxidation. As the body attempts to restore homeostasis, hunger increases due to limited availability of metabolic fuels. During the late postprandial phase (4–6 h after a meal), an exaggerated counterregulatory response elicits increased glycogenolysis, gluconeogenesis, and hepatic glucose output to restore euglycemia. In addition, there is an increase in lipolysis and elevated circulating free fatty acid concentrations. This metabolic state typically would be expected only after fasting for several hours beyond the postprandial period *(62)*.

The adverse effects of a high-GI meal or snack seem to persist beyond the postprandial period, thereby compromising glucose uptake following a subsequent meal. This phenomenon is known as the "second-meal effect" *(63)*. The underlying mechanism likely involves decreased insulin sensitivity with increased concentrations of circulating free fatty acids during the late postprandial phase *(64)*. The second-meal effect has been observed during the postprandial period following breakfast in response to a high-GI dinner or evening snack on the previous day *(63,65,66)*. Likewise, the GI of breakfast can affect glucose disposal at lunch on the same day *(67–70)*.

Body Weight Regulation

The effect of endocrine-regulated partitioning of metabolic fuels on hunger is a critical aspect of the proposed mechanism linking obesity with high dietary GL, whether modulated by carbohydrate quality or quantity *(60,71)*. With regard to carbohydrate quality, the vast majority of studies on the topic suggest that GI is important in regulating hunger, voluntary energy intake, and satiety *(27)*. Moreover, the drop in blood glucose that occurs during the middle postprandial phase may increase preference for high-GI foods *(72,73)*, leading to repeated cycles of excess hunger followed by hyperphagia that may last for several hours following restoration of euglycemia *(73)*. These vicious cycles, exacerbated by the second-meal effect, may contribute to disappointing long-term weight control with conventional low-fat diet prescriptions that emphasize the importance of consuming starchy foods.

In a study of hormone responses and voluntary food intake to meals varying in GL, obese adolescent boys were fed three different breakfast meals *(23)*. Two of the meals had identical macronutrient composition (64% of total energy from carbohydrate, 20% from fat, 16% from protein) but varied in carbohydrate source to achieve a GI differential (i.e., high-GI instant oatmeal vs moderate-GI steel-cut oats). The third meal, a vegetable

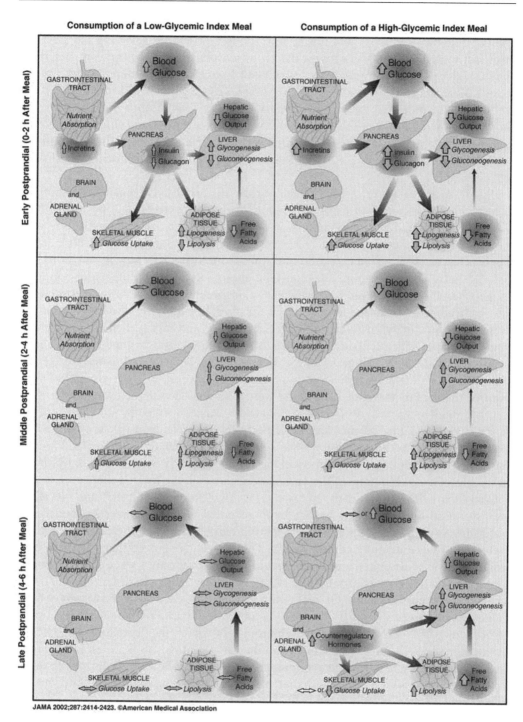

Fig. 1. Dynamic physiological changes occurring during the early, middle, and late phases of the postprandial period, after ingesting a high-glycemic index meal compared with a low-glycemic index meal. Vertical outlined arrows indicate direction and magnitude of change from the preprandial state indicated by horizontal outlined arrows. Reproduced with permission from ref. *60*.

omelet, had a low GL owing to reductions in carbohydrate amount (40% of total energy) and GI. The blood glucose and hormone responses observed following the high-GL breakfast meal were consistent with the proposed physiologic mechanism described above, with responses progressively attenuated following the moderate- and low-GL meals. When adolescents were given the same meals for lunch, the interval between completing the meal and initiating voluntary intake of foods from a buffet platter was shortest following the high-GL meal. Moreover, hunger ratings and cumulative voluntary energy intake over the 5-h postprandial period were highest following the high-GL meal, intermediate following the moderate-GL meal, and lowest following the low-GL meal.

Data from animal research provide support for the proposed mechanism relating GI to nutrient partitioning and energy metabolism. In two experiments by Kabir et al. *(74,75)*, rats were fed diets varying only in carbohydrate source (i.e, high-GI vs low-GI starch) for 3 wk. Based on ^{14}C-glucose tracer studies, insulin-stimulated glucose oxidation was lower, whereas incorporation of glucose into lipid was higher, in rats fed the high-GI diet *(74)*. Furthermore, the high-GI diet provoked changes in insulin-regulated lipogenic and gluconeogenic enzymes as demonstrated by higher fatty acid synthase activity in adipose tissue and lower mRNA for phosphoenolpyruvate carboxykinase in liver *(75)*, respectively. In a study of body composition and energy metabolism, Pawlak et al. *(76)* fed rats identical diets that, like those in the previously cited studies, varied only in the GI of the carbohydrate source. The rats on the high-GI diet seemed to become more energy-efficient, as indicated by a progressive decrease in the amount of food required to maintain the same mean body weight compared with the rats on the low-GI diet. Although mean body weight between groups was controlled by study design, rats on the high-GI vs low-GI diet had more body fat, and less lean tissue, after 18 wk. Interestingly, the insulin concentration at 30 min following an oral glucose load prior to the dietary intervention predicted most of the variance in body weight at week 18 for rats on the high-GI diet but none of the variance for those on the low-GI diet.

Consistent with animal work, emerging data suggest that dietary GI and GL affect energy expenditure in humans. In two feeding studies, GL was reduced by moderately decreasing carbohydrate amount and selecting carbohydrate sources to reduce GI in overweight or obese young adults *(77,78)*. The first study showed that a low-GL diet, providing 50% of estimated total energy requirements over only 1 wk, elicited a smaller decrease in resting energy expenditure (REE) compared with a high-GL diet *(77)*. The second study compared a low-GL diet with a low-fat diet, each designed to reduce body weight by 10% over approx 10 wk *(78)*. As anticipated based on the previous work of Leibel et al. *(79)*, REE decreased in both groups; however, the decrease was 80 kcal/d less with the low-GL diet. The subjects on the low-GL diet also reported less hunger. These findings may be attributed to improved access to metabolic fuels during the active phase of weight loss with the low-GL diet, providing additional support for the proposed physiologic mechanism presented above.

Weight-Independent Mechanisms for Disease Risk

Metabolic events occurring in response to diet-induced hyperglycemia may play an important role in the etiology of T2DM by weight-independent mechanisms that exacerbate the well-documented adverse effects of excess adiposity *(28,40,42,44)*. Hyperglycemia (early postprandial phase) and elevated circulating free fatty acid concentrations (late postprandial phase) in response to high-GL meals may foster progression toward T2DM by promoting insulin resistance and compensatory hyperinsulinemia, β-cell decompensation and relative insulin deficiency, and ultimately β-cell failure *(60,80)*. Moreover, exaggerated postprandial blood glucose and insulin responses to a high-GI meal are thought to increase risk for CVD associated with the insulin resistance syndrome, independent of body weight *(43,45–48)*. Experimental evidence suggests that even small increases in blood glucose levels, less than the difference in postprandial glycemia following high-GL vs low-GL meals, can cause insulin resistance *(81)*. The adverse effects of a high-GL diet on the β-cell (i.e., impaired insulin gene expression, β-cell apoptosis) and CVD risk (e.g., endothelial dysfunction) are likely mediated, in part, by glucose-induced oxidative stress *(82,83)*.

EXPERIMENTAL EVIDENCE FOR CLINICAL UTILITY OF GLYCEMIC INDEX

Short-Term Weight Loss

Selecting carbohydrate sources to reduce GI—either without altering the contribution of carbohydrate to total energy intake or in combination with a moderate decrease in carbohydrate consumption—is a promising weight-management strategy based on several short-term intervention studies of free-living subjects. Bouche et al. *(84)* treated 11 overweight men with low- vs high-GI diets, using a crossover design and controlling for energy and macronutrient composition (39–42% of energy from carbohydrate, 37–38% from fat). After 5 wk of intervention, trunk fat was 500 g less following the low-GI diet. Slabber et al. *(85)* assessed the effects of low- vs high-GI diets (50% of energy from carbohydrate, 30% from fat) in 16 obese hyperinsulinemic women in another crossover study. After 12 wk on the respective diets, body weight decreased more with the low-GI diet (–7.4 vs –4.5 kg). Fasting insulin decreased with the low-GI diet and increased with the high-GI diet (–61 vs +17 pmol/L). Spieth et al. *(86)* conducted a retrospective outcomes assessment of 107 obese children who attended a pediatric obesity clinic. Patients had received an *ad libitum* low-GL diet (45–50% carbohydrate, 30–35% fat), emphasizing low-GI carbohydrate sources, or an energy-restricted low-fat diet (55–60% of energy from carbohydrate, 25–30% from fat). Over a mean follow-up period of 4 mo, those on the low-GL diet lost more weight, such that the group difference was –1.5 kg/m^2 for change in body mass index (BMI). Clapp *(87)* treated 12 pregnant women who were randomly assigned to macronutrient-controlled low- vs high-GI diets (55–60% of energy from carbohydrate, 20–25% from fat) at 8 wk gestation. The mothers on the low-GI diet gained less weight during pregnancy (11.8 vs 19.7 kg) and had smaller babies (3.27 vs 4.25 kg).

Decreasing dietary GL may be especially beneficial for obese patients who have exaggerated insulin responses to an oral glucose load or insulin resistance *(88,89)*. Two controlled feeding studies of low-GL (40% of energy from carbohydrate, 40% from fat) vs high-GL (60% of energy from carbohydrate, 20% from fat) diets have addressed this issue. Cornier et al. *(89)* stratified 44 obese nondiabetic women by insulin sensitivity and randomly assigned them to low-GL vs low-fat diets for 16 wk, modulating GL by altering carbohydrate amount without consideration for GI. The low-GL diet caused more weight loss among women who were insulin-resistant; conversely, the low-fat diet caused greater weight loss among those who were insulin-sensitive. Pittas et al. *(88)* randomly assigned 34 normoglycemic adults to respective dietary interventions for 24 wk, modulating GL by altering carbohydrate source as well as carbohydrate amount. For *post hoc* analyses, subjects were dichotomized based on the 30-min insulin response to a 75-g oral glucose load. Among those who had insulin responses below the median, weight loss did not differ between interventions. However, among those who had higher insulin responses, weight loss was greater for those on the low-GL diet. Findings from the latter study are consistent with the aforementioned animal data, indicating a particularly adverse effect of a high-GI diet among rats with an exaggerated insulin response to an oral glucose load *(76)*. Taken together, these studies suggest that low-GL diets may be especially beneficial for obese patients with higher insulin secretion or lower insulin sensitivity. More research is needed to fully explore this topic.

In two studies, investigators were unable to document an effect of dietary GL on body weight *(54,55)*. Sloth et al. *(54)* prescribed *ad libitum* high-carbohydrate diets (55–60% of energy from carbohydrate, ≤30% from fat) to 45 overweight adults, varying GL between intervention groups by providing comparable low-GI (e.g., *al dente* pasta) or high-GI (e.g., mashed potato) foods. Weight loss did not vary between intervention groups at 10 wk (–1.9 vs –1.3 kg), although this study may have been statistically underpowered in that a progressive divergence in rates of weight loss over time seemed to favor the low-GI treatment. Raatz et al. *(55)* compared two high-carbohydrate diets (60% of energy from carbohydrate, 25% from fat), one low-GI and the other high-GI, with a high-fat diet (45% of energy from carbohydrate, 40% from fat) in 42 obese men and women. No group differences in weight loss were observed among the 22 subjects who completed the 36-wk intervention (i.e., 12-wk controlled feeding phase followed by 24-wk dietary counseling phase). However, analysis of food records obtained during the dietary counseling phase suggested that both groups were consuming relatively low-GL diets, making interpretation of results problematic. In the context of the ongoing debate regarding GI, these studies do not provide sufficient evidence for dismissing the importance of carbohydrate source in dietary treatments for obesity. More large-scale and long-term trials are needed in diverse patient populations.

Long-Term Efficacy

We examined relatively long-term efficacy in a small-scale randomized controlled trial of 16 obese adolescents *(9)*. The *ad libitum* low-GL diet prescription was based on 45 to 50% of energy from carbohydrate, with emphasis on low-GI sources, and 30 to 35% from fat. The low-fat diet (55–60% of energy from carbohydrate, 25–30% from fat) was prescribed using an exchange system to externally impose energy restriction, with emphasis on low-fat sources of complex carbohydrate. Over 12 mo, BMI decreased in adolescents on the low-GL diet and increased in those on the low-fat diet (–1.3 vs +0.7 kg/m²). Insulin resistance, by homeostasis model assessment (HOMA), increased less with the low-GL diet. Moreover, comparing the same diets in 23 obese adults, we observed greater declines in circulating triglyceride and plasminogen activator inhibitor (PAI)-1 concentrations with the low-GL diet prescription, despite similar changes in body weight (–7.8 vs –6.1%) *(90)*. The latter findings extend data from numerous short-term intervention trials showing beneficial changes in CVD risk factors with low-GI diets *(91–94)*.

PRACTICAL APPLICATION

The dietary interventions employed in studies of free-living subjects can be translated to clinical settings, taking a pragmatic approach. Although we use the International Table of Glycemic Index and Glycemic Load Values (56) to inform how foods are categorized in patient education materials, we do not present these values to patients in light of the aforementioned limitations. Rather, we rely on the consistency with which GI differs across major food groups. We counsel patients to reduce GL by replacing high-GI foods with low-GI alternatives or sources of healthful fat. Thus, attention is directed toward quality of dietary carbohydrate and fat, as opposed to quantity (e.g., carbohydrate-to-fat ratio). Although dietary fat is not the focus of this chapter, it is important to note that certain unsaturated fats decrease risk for T2DM and CVD, whereas trans (partially hydrogenated) fat increases risk (15,95).

The diet is operationalized using a low-GL food pyramid (Fig. 2) and corresponding food choice lists (Table 2). The pyramid provides a broad overview of the diet, and the food choice lists offer additional guidance in making appropriate selections within each food group. With regard to carbohydrate sources, we encourage *ad libitum* consumption of low-GL foods located on Level 1 of the pyramid (nonstarchy vegetables, nontropical fruits, legumes), and restricted intake of high-GL foods on Level 4. Moderate-GL grains (e.g., whole-grain products, high-fiber cereal, pasta) are on Level 2. Because we counsel patients to eat an abundance of low-GL foods, we do not present portion sizes for these options in the food choice lists. In contrast, we list recommended portion sizes for moderate- and high-GL foods so that patients have adequate information for monitoring intake, with upper limits of approx 1 to 3 servings per day of moderate-GL and 0 to 2 servings per day of high-GL foods. We encourage patients to complement low-GL foods (Level 1) with reasonable portions of healthful oils (Level 2), nuts (Level 3), and other sources of protein (including low-GL dairy products, Level 3). Foods high in *trans* fat—such as commercial bakery products and packaged snacks—often have a high GL and are on Level 4.

An *ad libitum* approach to diet therapy relies on intrinsic control of energy intake based on the physiologic mechanisms and satiety hypotheses presented above. Thus, we counsel patients to recognize what it means to be hungry using a variety of verbal descriptors for physical sensations. We encourage them to eat when "hungry," rather than waiting until they become "famished," and to stop eating when they are "satisfied," before becoming "stuffed."

CONCLUSION

Much effort has been devoted to treating obese patients using diet therapy, with limited success in achieving significant weight reduction over the long term. We and others contend that available diets, ranging from very-low-carbohydrate to very-low-fat, are not optimal because these approaches do not adequately consider carbohydrate (e.g., low- vs high-GI) or fat (e.g., unsaturated vs saturated) quality (16,60,90). A low-GL diet may represent an ideal compromise between such extremes. Emerging data lend support to proposed physiologic mechanisms linking GI and GL to body weight and obesity-related comorbidites. Although critics argue that the GI is too complex and does not apply to mixed meals (50–53), key concepts can be presented using a pragmatic approach given the consistency of GI values within food groups. Meaningful effects have

Table 2
Food Choice Lists for Low-Glycemic-Load Diet, Informed by Glycemic Index

Carbohydrate	Vegetables	Legumes	Fruit	Dairy	Grains
Low Glycemic Load					
Nonstarchy					
	Alfalfa sprouts	Beans	Apples	Milk	*Bread (1 slice, 1 oz)*
	Artichoke	Black-eyed peas	Apricots		Flourless
	Asparagus	Chickpeas	Berries	Yogurt	Pumpernickel
	Bamboo shoots	Hummus	Cantaloupe	plain,	Stone ground
	Beans (green, wax)	Lentils	Cherries	sugar-free	Whole grain
	Bean sprouts	Split peas	Clementines		*Cereal (1/2 cup)*
	Bok choy		Grapefruit		High-fiber
	Broccoli		Grapes		Steel-cut oats
	Brussels sprouts		Honeydew		*Pasta (1/2 cup)*
	Cabbage		Kiwi		Al dente
	Carrots		Lemon		*Grains (1/2 cup)*
	Cauliflower		Lime		Barley
	Celery		Nectarines		Basmati rice
	Cucumber		Oranges		Brown rice
	Eggplant		Peaches		Bulgur
	Greens		Pears		Kasha
	Kohlrabi		Plums		Parboiled rice
	Leeks		Tangelos		Quinoa
	Lettuce		Tangerines		Wheat berries
	Mushrooms				Wild rice
	Okra				
	Onions				
	Peppers				
	Radishes				
	Salsa				
	Scallions				
	Snow peas				
	Sauerkraut				
	Spinach				
	Summer squash				
	Swiss chard				
	Tomatoes				
	Turnip				
	Water chestnuts				
	Zucchini				
Moderate Glycemic Load					
Starchy (1/2 cup)					
	Acorn squash		Apple sauce (1/2 cup)		
	Beets		Banana (1/2)		
	Butternut squash		Canned fruit (1/2 cup)		
	Green peas		Dried fruit (2 tablespoons)		
	Parsnips		Mango (1/2 cup)		
	Plantain		Papaya (1/2 cup)		
	Pumpkin		Pineapple (1/2 cup)		
	Yam		Watermelon (1 cup cubes)		
High Glycemic Load					
Starchy					
Corn (1/2 cup)		Baked Beans	Fruit juices (1/2 cup)	Yogurt,	*Cereal (1/2 cup)*
French fries		(1/3 cup)	Juice drinks (1/2 cup)	sugar-sweetened	Most varieties
(1/2 small order)				(4 oz)	*Pasta (1/2 cup)*
Potato, boiled					Canned
(1/2 cup)					*Snacks*
Potato, baked					Crackers (6)
(1 small)					*Pizza*
Sweet potato					(1/8 of 12")
(1/2 cup, 1 small)					Popcorn
					(3 cups)
					Pretzels
					Breads
					Bagel (1/4)
					Bread (1 slice, 1 oz)
					Bread stick (1 oz)
					Bun (1 small, 1 oz)
					Cornbread (2")
					Muffin (1 small, 1 oz)
					Pancake (4")
					Pita (1/2 of 6")
					Roll (1 small, 1 oz)
					Stuffing (1/3 cup)

(3/4 oz)
Snack chips (10, 3/4 oz)
Taco shell (6")
Tortilla (6")
Waffle (4")
Grains (1/2 cup)
Couscous
Millet
Rice
Rice cakes (2 large, 7 mini)

Healthful Fat

Nuts	*Seeds*	*Oils*	*Other*
Almonds	Flaxseed	Canola oil	Avocado
Almond butter (natural)	Pumpkin seeds	Mayonnaise	Olives
Brazil nuts	Sesame seeds	Olive oil	
Cashews	Sunflower seeds	Peanut oil	
Hazelnuts		Salad dressing	
Macadamia nuts		(Italian style)	
Peanuts		Soybean oil	
Peanut butter (natural)			
Pecans			
Pine nuts			
Pistachios			
Soy nuts			
Walnuts			

Protein

Cheese	*Eggs*	*Fish and Shellfish not breaded*		*Poultry not breaded*	*Soy products*	*Deli meat*
Cheddar	Egg substitutes	Bass	Mackerel	Chicken	Seitan	Chicken breast
Cottage	Egg whites	Catfish	Mahi mahi	Cornish hen	Tempeh	Turkey breast
Feta	Whole eggs	Cod	Salmon	Duck	Textured vegetable protein	Turkey ham
Monterey Jack		Flounder	Sardines	Turkey	Tofu	
Mozzarella		Grouper	Snapper			
Parmesan		Haddock	Sole			
Ricotta		Halibut	Swordfish			
Swiss		Herring	Trout			
		Tuna	Clams			
		Crab	Lobster			
		Oysters	Scallops			
		Shrimp				

Sweets (100 calories per serving)

High Glycemic Load

Angel food cake (1 slice, 1 oz)	Doughnut, glazed (1/2 Dunkin Donut®)	Ice cream (1/2 cup)	Sweet roll (1 small, 1 oz)
Brownie (2" square)	Energy, sport or breakfast bar (1/2)	Jam, Jelly (1 tablespoon)	Syrup, chocolate (1/2 tablespoons)
Cake, unfrosted (2" square)	Gelatin (1/2 cup)	Pie ("sliver", 1/16 of 9" pie)	Syrup, pancake (1.5 tablespoons)
Cookies (2 small)	Gingersnaps (3)	Pudding (1/4 cup)	Vanilla wafers (5)
Cranberry sauce (1/8 cup)	Granola bar (1)	Sports drinks (8 fl oz)	Whipped topping (1/2 cup)
Danish (1 small, 1 oz)	Honey (1 tablespoon)	Sugar (2 tablespoons)	

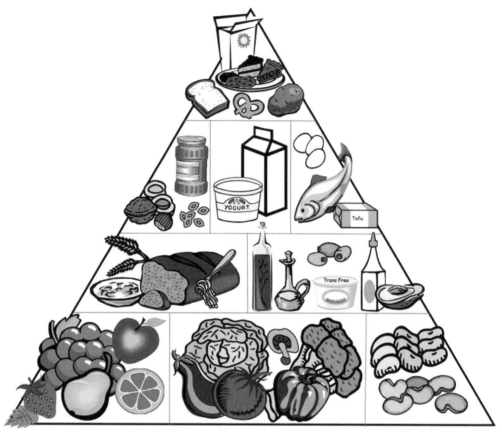

Ebbeling and Ludwig, © 2006

Fig. 2. Low-glycemic load food pyramid (Ebbeling and Ludwig, © 2006). Classification of foods is based on GL values, informed by the GI, as exemplified in Table 1. We supplement the pyramid with the food choice lists presented in Table 2.

been observed in pilot studies of patients consuming self-selected diets based on low-GL prescriptions, with an emphasis on selecting low-GI sources of carbohydrate (9,90). Pending definitive randomized controlled trials, a low-GL diet, focused on carbohydrate and fat quality, would seem to be a promising approach to the treatment of obesity and prevention of type 2 diabetes and associated CVD risk.

REFERENCES

1. Baron JA, Schori A, Crow B, et al. A randomized controlled trial of low carbohydrate and low fat/high fiber diets for weight loss. Am J Public Health 1986;76:1293–1296.
2. Foster GD, Wyatt HR, Hill JO, et al. A randomized trial of a low-carbohydrate diet for obesity. N Engl J Med 2003;348:2082–2090.
3. McManus K, Antinoro L, Sacks F. A randomized controlled trial of a moderate-fat, low-energy diet compared with a low fat, low-energy diet for weight loss in overweight adults. Int J Obes 2001;25:1503–1511.
4. Stern L, Iqbal N, Seshadri P, et al. The effects of low-carbohydrate versus conventional weight loss diets in severely obese adults: one-year follow-up of a randomized trial. Ann Intern Med 2004;140:778–785.

5. Shah M, Baxter JE, McGovern PG, et al. Nutrient and food intake in obese women on a low-fat or low-calorie diet. Am J Health Promot 1996;10:179–182.

6. Jeffery RW, Hellerstedt WL, French SA, et al. A randomized trial of counseling for fat restriction versus calorie restriction in the treatment of obesity. Int J Obes 1995;19:132–137.

7. Pascale RW, Wing RR, Butler BA, et al. Effects of behavioral weight loss program stressing calorie restriction versus calorie plus fat restriction in obese individuals with NIDDM or a family history of diabetes. Diabetes Care 1995;18:1241–1248.

8. Harvey-Berino J. Calorie restriction is more effective for obesity treatment than dietary fat restriction. Ann Behav Med 1999;21:35–39.

9. Ebbeling CB, Leidig MM, Sinclair KB, et al. A reduced-glycemic load diet in the treatment of adolescent obesity. Arch Pediatr Adolesc Med 2003;157:773–779.

10. Dansinger ML, Gleason JA, Griffith JL, et al. Comparison of the Atkins, Ornish, Weight Watchers, and Zone diets for weight loss and heart disease risk reduction: a randomized trial. JAMA 2005;293:43–53.

11. Brehm BJ, Seeley RJ, Daniels SR, et al. A randomized trial comparing a very low carbohydrate diet and a calorie-restricted low fat diet on body weight and cardiovascular risk factors in healthy women. J Clin Endocrinol Metab 2003;88:1617–1623.

12. Yancy WS, Olsen MK, Guyton JR, et al. A low-carbohydrate, ketogenic diet versus a low-fat diet to treat obesity and hyperlipidemia. Ann Intern Med 2004;140:769–777.

13. Hu FB, Willett WC. Optimal diets for prevention of coronary heart disease. JAMA 2002;288:2569–2578.

14. Ma Y, Olendzki B, Chiriboga D, et al. Association between dietary carbohydrates and body weight. Am J Epidemiol 2005;161:359–367.

15. Salmeron J, Hu FB, Manson JE, et al. Dietary fat intake and risk of type 2 diabetes in women. Am J Clin Nutr 2001;73:1019–1026.

16. Hu FB, vanDam RM, Liu S. Diet and risk of type II diabetes: the role of types of fat and carbohydrate. Diabetologia 2001;44:805–817.

17. http://www.health.gov/dietaryguidelines/dga2005/document/pdf/dga2005.pdf (accessed December 15, 2005).

18. Klein S, Sheard NF, Pi-Sunyer X, et al. Weight management through lifestyle modification for the prevention and management of type 2 diabetes: rationale and strategies. Diabetes Care 2004;27:2067–2073.

19. Wahlqvist ML, Wilmshurst EG, Richardson EN. The effect of chain length on glucose absorption and the related metabolic response. Am J Clin Nutr 1978;31:1998–2001.

20. Bantle JP, Laine DC, Castle GW, et al. Postprandial glucose and insulin responses to meals containing different carbohydrates in normal and diabetic subjects. N Engl J Med 1983;309:7–12.

21. Granfeldt Y, Bjorck I, Hagander B. On the importance of processing conditions, product thickness and egg addition for the glycaemic and hormonal responses to pasta: a comparison with bread made from 'pasta ingredients'. Eur J Clin Nutr 1991;45:489–499.

22. Granfeldt Y, Hagander B, Bjorck I. Metabolic responses to starch in oat and wheat products. On the importance of food structure, incomplete gelatinization or presence of viscous dietary fibre. Eur J Clin Nutr 1995;49:189–199.

23. Ludwig DS, Majzoub JA, Al-Zahrani A, et al. High glycemic index foods, overeating, and obesity. Pediatrics 1999;103:e26.

24. Schafer G, Schenk U, Ritzel U, et al. Comparison of the effects of dried peas with those of potatoes in mixed meals on postprandial glucose and insulin concentrations in patients with type 2 diabetes. Am J Clin Nutr 2003;78:99–103.

25. Jenkins DJA, Wolever TMS, Taylor RH, et al. Glycemic index of foods: a physiological basis for carbohydrate exchange. Am J Clin Nutr 1981;34:362–366.

26. Wolever TMS, Jenkins DJA, Jenkins AL, Josse RG. The glycemic index: methodology and clinical implications. Am J Clin Nutr 1991;54:846–854.

27. Ebbeling CB, Ludwig LS. Treating obesity in youth: should dietary glycemic load be a consideration? Adv Pediatr 2001;48:179–212.

28. Salmeron J, Manson JE, Stampfer MJ, et al. Dietary fiber, glycemic load, and risk of non-insulin-dependent diabetes mellitus in women. JAMA 1997;277:472–477.

29. Brand-Miller JC, Thomas M, Swan V, et al. Physiological validation of the concept of glycemic load in lean young adults. J Nutr 2003;133:2728–2732.

30. Wolever TM, Bolognesi C. Source and amount of carbohydrate affect postprandial glucose and insulin in normal subjects. J Nutr 1996;126:2798–2806.

31. Sheard NF, Clark NG, Brand-Miller JC, et al. Dietary carbohydrate (amount and type) in the prevention and management of diabetes: a statement by the American Diabetes Association. Diabetes Care 2004;27:2266–2271.
32. Wolever TM, Mehling C. High-carbohydrate-low-glycaemic index dietary advice improves glucose disposition index in subjects with impaired glucose tolerance. Br J Nutr 2002;87:477–487.
33. Wolever TM, Mehling C. Long-term effect of varying the source or amount of dietary carbohydrate on postprandial plasma glucose, insulin, triacylglycerol, and free fatty acid concentrations in subjects with impaired glucose tolerance. Am J Clin Nutr 2003;77:612–621.
34. Ball SD, Keller KR, Moyer-Mileur LJ, et al. Prolongation of satiety after low versus moderately high glycemic index meals in obese adolescents. Pediatrics 2003;111:488–494.
35. vanDam RM, Visscher AWJ, Feskens EJM, et al. Dietary glycemic index in relation to metabolic risk factors and incidence of coronary heart disease: the Zutphen Elderly Study. Eur J Clin Nutr 2000;54:726–731.
36. Meyer KA, Kushi LH, Jacobs DR, et al. Carbohydrates, dietary fiber, and incident type 2 diabetes in older women. Am J Clin Nutr 2000;71:921–930.
37. Stevens J, Ahn K, Juhaeri, et al. Dietary fiber intake and glycemic index and incidence of diabetes in African-American and white adults: the ARIC study. Diabetes Care 2002;25:1715–1721.
38. Lau C, Faerch K, Glumer C, et al. Dietary glycemic index, glycemic load, fiber, simple sugars, and insulin resistance: the Inter99 study. Diabetes Care 2005;28:1397–1403.
39. Liese AD, Schulz M, Fang F, et al. Dietary glycemic index and glycemic load, carbohydrate and fiber intake, and measures of insulin sensitivity, secretion, and adiposity in the insulin resistance atherosclerosis study. Diabetes Care 2005;28:2832–2838.
40. Salmeron J, Ascherio A, Rimm EB, et al. Dietary fiber, glycemic load, and risk of NIDDM in men. Diabetes Care 1997;20:545–550.
41. Hodge AM, English DR, O'Dea K, Giles GG. Glycemic index and dietary fiber and the risk of type 2 diabetes. Diabetes Care 2004;27:2701–2706.
42. Schulze MB, Liu S, Rimm EB, et al. Glycemic index, glycemic load, and dietary fiber intake and incidence of type 2 diabetes in younger and middle-aged women. Am J Clin Nutr 2004;80:348–356.
43. McKeown NM, Meigs JB, Liu S, et al. Carbohydrate nutrition, insulin resistance, and the prevalence of the metabolic syndrome in the Framingham Offspring Cohort. Diabetes Care 2004;27:538–546.
44. Sahyoun NR, Anderson AL, Kanaya AM, et al. Dietary glycemic index and load, measures of glucose metabolism, and body fat distribution in older adults. Am J Clin Nutr 2005;82:547–552.
45. Frost G, Leeds AA, Dore CJ, Madeiros S, Brading S, Dornhorst A. Glycemic index as a determinant of serum HDL-cholesterol concentration. Lancet 1999;353:1045–1048.
46. Liu S, Willett WC, Stampfer MJ, et al. A prospective study of dietary glycemic load, carbohydrate intake, and risk of coronary heart disease in women. Am J Clin Nutr 2000;71:1455–1461.
47. Liu S, Manson JE, Stampfer MJ, et al. Dietary glycemic load assessed by food-frequency questionnaire in relation to plasma high-density-lipoprotein cholesterol and fasting plasma triacylglycerols in postmenopausal women. Am J Clin Nutr 2001;73:560–566.
48. Ford ES, Liu S. Glycemic index and serum high-density lipoprotein cholesterol concentration among US adults. Arch Intern Med 2001;161:572–576.
49. Barclay AW, Brand-Miller JC, Wolever TM. Glycemic index, glycemic load, and glycemic response are not the same. Diabetes Care 2005;28:1839–1840.
50. Alfenas RC, Mattes RD. Influence of glycemic index/load on glycemic response, appetite, and food intake in healthy humans. Diabetes Care 2005;28:2123–2129.
51. Flint A, Moller BK, Raben A, et al. The use of glycaemic index tables to predict glycaemic index of composite breakfast meals. Br J Nutr 2004;91:979–989.
52. Hollenbeck CB, Coulston AM, Reaven GM. Comparison of plasma glucose and insulin responses to mixed meals of high-, intermediate-, and low-glycemic potential. Diabetes Care 1988;11:323–329.
53. Laine DC, Thomas W, Levitt MD, et al. Comparison of predictive capabilities of diabetic exchange lists and glycemic index of foods. Diabetes Care 1987;10:387–394.
54. Sloth B, Krog-Mikkelsen I, Flint A, et al. No difference in body weight decrease between a low-glycemic-index and a high-glycemic-index diet but reduced LDL cholesterol after 10-wk ad libitum intake of the low-glycemic-index diet. Am J Clin Nutr 2004;80:337–347.
55. Raatz SK, Torkelson CJ, Redmon JB, et al. Reduced glycemic index and glycemic load diets do not increase the effects of energy restriction on weight loss and insulin sensitivity in obese men and women. J Nutr 2005;135:2387–2391.

56. Foster-Powell K, Holt SHA, Brand-Miller JC. International table of glycemic index and glycemic load values: 2002. Am J Clin Nutr 2002;76:5–56.
57. Wolever TM, Vorster HH, Bjorck I, et al. Determination of the glycaemic index of foods: interlaboratory study. Eur J Clin Nutr 2003;57:475–482.
58. Velangi A, Fernandes G, Wolever TM. Evaluation of a glucose meter for determining the glycemic responses of foods. Clin Chim Acta 2005;356:191–198.
59. Wolever TM. Effect of blood sampling schedule and method of calculating the area under the curve on validity and precision of glycaemic index values. Br J Nutr 2004;91:295–301.
60. Ludwig DS. The glycemic index: physiological mechanisms relating to obesity, diabetes, and cardiovascular disease. JAMA 2002;287:2414–2423.
61. Wursch P, Acheson K, Koellreutter B, et al. Metabolic effects of instant bean and potato over 6 hours. Am J Clin Nutr 1988;48:1418–1423.
62. Cahill GF Jr. Starvation in man. Clin Endocrinol Metab 1976;5:397–415.
63. Wolever TM, Jenkins DJ, Ocana AM, et al. Second-meal effect: low-glycemic-index foods eaten at dinner improve subsequent breakfast glycemic response. Am J Clin Nutr 1988;48:1041–1047.
64. Homko CJ, Cheung P, Boden G. Effects of free fatty acids on glucose uptake and utilization in healthy women. Diabetes 2003;52:487–491.
65. Axelsen M, Arvidsson Lenner R, et al. Breakfast glycaemic response in patients with type 2 diabetes: effects of bedtime dietary carbohydrates. Eur J Clin Nutr 1999;53:706–710.
66. Stevenson E, Williams C, Nute M, et al. The effect of the glycemic index of an evening meal on the metabolic responses to a standard high glycemic index breakfast and subsequent exercise in men. Int J Sport Nutr Exerc Metab 2005;15:308–322.
67. Jenkins DJ, Wolever TM, Taylor RH, et al. Slow release dietary carbohydrate improves second meal tolerance. Am J Clin Nutr 1982;35:1339–1346.
68. Wolever TMS, Bentum-Williams A, Jenkins DJA. Physiological modulation of plasma free fatty acid concentrations by diet. Diabetes Care 1995;18:962–970.
69. Liljeberg HG, Akerberg AK, Bjorck IM. Effect of the glycemic index and content of indigestible carbohydrates of cereal-based breakfast meals on glucose tolerance at lunch in healthy subjects. Am J Clin Nutr 1999;69:647–655.
70. Liljeberg H, Bjorck I. Effects of a low-glycaemic index spaghetti meal on glucose tolerance and lipaemia at a subsequent meal in healthy subjects. Eur J Clin Nutr 2000;54:24–28.
71. Willett WC. Reduced-carbohydrate diets: no roll in weight management? Ann Intern Med 2004;140:836–837.
72. Thompson DA, Campbell RG. Hunger in humans induced by 2-deoxy-D-glucose: glucoprivic control of taste preference and food intake. Science 1977;198:1065–1068.
73. Friedman MI, Granneman J. Food intake and peripheral factors after recovery from insulin-induced hypoglycemia. Am J Physiol 1983;244:R374–R382.
74. Kabir M, Rizkalla SW, Champ M, et al. Dietary amylose-amylopectin starch content affects glucose and lipid metabolism in adipocytes of normal and diabetic rats. J Nutr 1998;128:35–43.
75. Kabir M, Rizkalla SW, Quignard-Boulange A, et al. A high glycemic index starch diet affects lipid storage-related enzymes in normal and to a lesser extent in diabetic rats. J Nutr 1998;128:1878–1883.
76. Pawlak DB, Kushner JA, Ludwig DS. Effects of dietary glycaemic index on adiposity, glucose homoeostasis, and plasma lipids in animals. Lancet 2004;364:778–785.
77. Agus MSD, Swain JF, Larson CL, Eckert EA, Ludwig DS. Dietary composition and physiologic adaptations to energy restriction. Am J Clin Nutr 2000;71:901–907.
78. Pereira MA, Swain J, Goldfine AB, et al. Effects of a low-glycemic load diet on resting energy expenditure and heart disease risk factors during weight loss. JAMA 2004;292:2482–2490.
79. Leibel RL, Rosenbaum M, Hirsch J. Changes in energy expenditure resulting from altered body weight. N Engl J Med 1995;332:621–628.
80. Ludwig DS, Ebbeling CB. Type 2 diabetes mellitus in children: primary care and public health considerations. JAMA 2001;286:1427–1430.
81. Rossetti L, Giaccari A, DeFronzo RA. Glucose toxicity. Diabetes Care 1990;13:610–630.
82. Poitout V, Robertson RP. Minireview: Secondary beta-cell failure in type 2 diabetes—a convergence of glucotoxicity and lipotoxicity. Endocrinology 2002;143:339–342.
83. Ceriello A, Motz E. Is oxidative stress the pathogenic mechanism underlying insulin resistance, diabetes, and cardiovascular disease? The common soil hypothesis revisited. Arterioscler Thromb Vasc Biol 2004;24:816–823.

84. Bouche C, Rizkalla SW, Luo J, et al. Five-week, low-glycemic index diet decreases total fat mass and improves plasma lipid profile in moderately overweight nondiabetic men. Diabetes Care 2002;25:822–828.
85. Slabber M, Barnard HC, Kuyl JM, et al. Effects of a low-insulin-response, energy-restricted diet on weight loss and plasma insulin concentrations in hyperinsulinemic obese females. Am J Clin Nutr 1994;60:48–53.
86. Spieth LE, Harnish JD, Lenders CM, et al. A low glycemic index diet in the treatment of pediatric obesity. Arch Pediatr Adol Med 2000;154:947–951.
87. Clapp JF. Diet, exercise, and feto-placental growth. Arch Gynecol Obstet 1997;261:101–108.
88. Pittas AG, Das SK, Hajduk CL, et al. A low-glycemic load diet facilitates greater weight loss in overweight adults with high insulin secretion but not in overweight adults with low insulin secretion in the CALERIE trial. Diabetes Care 2005;28:2939–2941.
89. Cornier MA, Donahoo WT, Pereira R, et al. Insulin sensitivity determines the effectiveness of dietary macronutrient composition on weight loss in obese women. Obes Res 2005;13:703–709.
90. Ebbeling CB, Leidig MM, Sinclair KB, et al. Effects of an ad libitum reduced glycemic load diet on cardiovascular disease risk factors in obese young adults. Am J Clin Nutr 2005;81:976–982.
91. Fontvieille AM, Rizkalla SW, Penfornis A, et al. The use of low glycaemic index foods improves metabolic control of diabetic patients over five weeks. Diabetic Med 1992;9:444–450.
92. Frost G, Wilding J, Beecham J. Dietary advice based on the glycaemic index improves dietary profile and metabolic control in type 2 diabetic patients. Diabet Med 1994;11:397–401.
93. Jenkins DJA, Wolever TMS, Kalmusky J, et al. Low-glycemic index diet in hyperlipidemia: use of traditional starchy foods. Am J Clin Nutr 1987;46:66–71.
94. Wolever TMS, Jenkins DJA, Vuksan V, et al. Beneficial effect of a low glycaemic index diet in type 2 diabetes. Diabetic Med 1992;9:451–458.
95. Hu FB, Stampfer MJ, Manson JE, et al. Dietary fat intake and the risk of coronary heart disease in women. N Engl J Med 1997;337:1491–1499.

15

Low-Carbohydrate Diets

Angela P. Makris, PhD, RD,
and Gary D. Foster, PhD

CONTENTS

    INTRODUCTION
    BACKGROUND
    EFFICACY OF LOW-CARBOHYDRATE DIETS ON WEIGHT LOSS
    EFFICACY OF LOW-CARBOHYDRATE DIETS ON FASTING LIPIDS
    EFFICACY OF LOW-CARBOHYRATE DIETS ON IMFLAMMATORY
        BIOMARKERS
    EFFICACY OF LOW-CARBOHYDRATE DIETS ON LIPOPROTEIN
        SUBFRACTIONS
    EFFICACY OF LOW-CARBOHYDRATE DIETS ON BLOOD PRESSURE
    EFFICACY OF LOW-CARBOHYDRATE DIETS ON INSULIN SENSITIVITY
        AND GLYCEMIC CONTROL
    CONCLUSION
    REFERENCES

Summary

    Traditionally, the gold standard for obesity treatment has been the combination of a low-fat, low-calorie diet with regular physical activity and behavior therapy. This combination has been shown to be safe and effective; however, the best dietary approach to weight loss continues to be a matter of debate among professionals and the public alike. Preliminary short-term findings suggesting that low-carbohydrate diets are effective in reducing body weight and do not appear to increase the risk of cardiovascular disease have generated interest in the low-carbohydrate approach and have spawned further research. This chapter reviews the most recent findings from short- and long-term studies evaluating the effects of low-carbohydrate diets on weight, lipids, lipoprotein subfractions, inflammatory biomarkers, blood pressure, and insulin sensitivity.

    Key Words: Diet; low-carbohydrate; high-protein; weight loss.

INTRODUCTION

Various forms of low-carbohydrate, ketogenic diets have existed for centuries. William Banting's "A Letter on Corpulence Addressed to the Public," published in 1863, has been coined as the first publicized low-carbohydrate diet *(1)*. Ebstein's diet is another

From: *Contemporary Endocrinology: Treatment of the Obese Patient*
Edited by: R. F. Kushner and D. H. Bessesen © Humana Press Inc., Totowa, NJ

example of a low-carbohydrate weight-loss diet that emerged in the early 20th century *(2)*. In addition to the management of obesity, low-carbohydrate diets were also used for the treatment of seizures in the early 20th century *(3)*. Different versions of low-carbohydrate diets, varying in their degree of carbohydrate and calorie restriction, have emerged since that time. In 1972 Dr. Robert Atkins proposed the use of a low-carbohydrate diet for the treatment of obesity. Although it gained some recognition in the 1970s *(4)* and again in the 1990s *(5)*, the popularity of the diet remained dormant until 2002 *(6)*, when it re-emerged as an alternative to conventional low-fat diets. Heightened public interest in the low-carbohydrate approach and the failure of conventional dietary approaches to effectively manage obesity in the long term prompted researchers to study this dietary approach and its effects on a variety of outcomes.

Despite its long history, relatively little is known about the short-term efficacy of low-carbohydrate diets in the treatment of obesity and its effects on body composition, lipids, or insulin insensitivity. Even less is known about its long-term effects. This chapter reviews the most recent findings from short- and long-term studies evaluating the effects of low-carbohydrate diets on weight, lipids, and insulin sensitivity.

BACKGROUND

Unlike low-fat diets, the FDA has not established a clear definition for "low-carbohydrate" diets; however, diets prescribing less than 100 g of carbohydrate or approx 10 to 20%, 25 to 35%, and 55 to 65% of total energy from carbohydrate, protein, and fat, respectively, are generally considered low-carbohydrate *(7)*. The focus of existing low-carbohydrate diets is replacement of foods containing refined carbohydrates (i.e., white bread, rice, pasta, desserts, chips, and sweetened soft drinks) with controlled amounts of nutrient-dense carbohydrate-containing foods (i.e., nonstarchy vegetables, fruits, and whole-grain products). The hypothesis underlying this approach is that high intake of refined carbohydrates results in hyperinsulinemia and insulin resistance, which ultimately leads to weight gain; therefore, lower intakes of carbohydrate and a shift toward consumption of foods that contain nutrients that do not cause a dramatic spike in insulin levels is metabolically advantageous. Although consumption of foods that do not contain carbohydrate (i.e., meats, poultry, fish, as well as butter and oil) is not restricted, the emphasis is on moderation and quality rather than quantity.

The following section will present findings from studies comparing the effects of low-carbohydrate and low-fat diets in the treatment of obesity. The remainder of this chapter will focus on the effects of low-carbohydrate diets on mechanisms of weight loss, effects on lipids, inflammatory biomarkers, lipoprotein subfractions and postprandial lipemic response, blood pressure, and insulin sensitivity.

EFFICACY OF LOW-CARBOHYDRATE DIETS ON WEIGHT LOSS

Five randomized studies conducted over 6 to 12 mo have compared the effects of a low-carbohydrate diet and a calorie-controlled, low-fat diet on weight and body composition in obese adults *(8–13)*. (Note that the Samaha and Stern papers refer to the same study but report 6-mo and 12-mo data, respectively.) With the exception of one study that prescribed nutritional supplements including vitamins, minerals, essential oils, and chromium picolinate to the low-carbohydrate group but not the low-fat group *(12)*, diet prescriptions in these studies were comparable (e.g., a low-carbohydrate diet containing

20–60 g of carbohydrate). Body mass index (BMI) and ages ranged from 33 to 43 kg/m^2 and 43 to 54 yr, respectively, in all five studies. Although there were many similarities in diet prescriptions and participant characteristics, a few differences emerged. The majority of the studies consisted of female participants (8,9,12,13) except for one (10,11). Comorbidities and amount of clinician contact also differed slightly between these studies. Two of the investigations evaluated effects in obese but otherwise healthy adults (8,9); three examined effects in adults with significant comorbidities such as diabetes, metabolic syndrome (MetS) (10,11), hyperlipidemia (12), and other cardiovascular risk factors (13). Treatment occurred primarily in a self-help setting in one study (8) and in individual and/or group treatment in the others (9–13). Only three studies evaluated effects at 1 yr (8,11,13). Findings of these studies are summarized in Table 1.

Participants who consumed a low-carbohydrate diet lost significantly more weight than those who consumed a low-fat diet during the first 6 mo of treatment in four of the five studies (8–12). Despite differences at 6 mo, there were no differences in weight loss at 1 yr (8,11,13) (Table 1). Two studies (8,13) observed weight regain in both groups after 6 mo, with a greater regain in the low-carbohydrate group. Although participants in the low-carbohydrate group did not regain weight in the third 1-yr study, those in the low-fat group continued to lose weight after 6 mo, resulting in similar weight losses at 1 yr (11).

Calories or Carbohydrates?

The focus of the low-carbohydrate approach is on carbohydrate rather than the number of calories consumed. Given that individuals following this approach track the grams of carbohydrate from only a limited number of foods, it is appealing to many dieters because it reduces the burden of accounting for all foods consumed; however, it may also reduce awareness of total calories consumed because the emphasis is placed on altering one's metabolic state rather than altering one's energy balance.

Rather than attribute differences in weight loss between low- and high- carbohydrate diets to differences in energy intake, some suggest that low-carbohydrate diets confer a "metabolic advantage" (i.e., differences in the metabolism of nutrients, increased energy expenditure, etc.) that results in greater weight loss (6,14). Comparing the effects of isocaloric low-carbohydrate and low-fat diets on body weight would test the hypothesis that metabolic factors rather than calories account for the differences in weight loss. If low-carbohydrate diets posses a metabolic advantage over low-fat diets, low-carbohydrate diets should result in greater reductions in body weight despite similar energy intake. One study randomly assigned 43 obese individuals isocaloric diets (1000 kcal/d) composed of either 15% carbohydrate (37 g/d) and or 45% carbohydrate (115 g/d) (15). These diets contained similar amounts of protein, but the low-carbohydrate diet was higher in fat (53% fat) than the high-carbohydrate diet (26% fat). Participants consumed these diets in an inpatient clinic, where food intake was closely monitored for 6 wk. Weight loss between the 15% carbohydrate (8.9 ± 0.6 kg) and 45% carbohydrate (7.5 ± 0.5 kg) diets was not significantly different. These findings are supported by a number of metabolic ward studies that compare isocaloric diets varying in macronutrient composition (16–18). These studies are summarized in a review by Freedman et al (7).

These findings suggest that when calories are held constant, weight loss is similar between low-carbohydrate and low-fat diets, suggesting that a reduction in calories, rather than "metabolic factors," contributes to a decrease in body weight. Differences in

Table 1
Summary of Findings From 6- and 12-Mo Studies

	Brehm (6-mo data)	Yancy (6-mo data)	Stern (12-mo data)	Foster (12-mo data)	Dansinger (12-mo data)
Sample size (n)	53	119	132	63	80
LC	26	59	64	33	40
C	27	60	68	30	40
Sex					
Male	N/A	28 (15 LC/13 C)	109 (51 LC/58 C)	20 (12 LC/8 C)	36 (19 LC/17 C)
Female	53 (26 LC/27 C)	91 (44 LC/47 C)	23 (13 LC/10 C)	43 (21 LC/22 C)	44 (21 LC/23 C)
Age (years)					
LC	44.2	44.2	53.0	44.0	47
C	43.1	45.6	54.0	44.2	49
Baseline BMI (kg/m^2)					
LC	33.2	34.6	42.9	33.9	35.0
C	34.0	34.0	42.9	34.4	35.0
Weight loss (% change)					
LC	-9.3	-12.9	-3.9	-7.3	-3.9
C	-4.2	-6.7	-2.3	-4.5	-4.8
Percent Change					
Triglycerides					
LC	-23.4	-47.2	-28.6	-28.1	N/A
C	1.6	-14.4	2.7	1.4	
Total cholesterol					
LC	-0.4	-3.3	3.4	0.2	-3.8
C	-0.9	-5.6	-4.2	-5.5	-5.7
LDL					
LC	-0.7	1.0	6.2	0.5	-9.9
C	-5.3	-5.0	-3.2	-5.8	-10.0
HDL					
LC	13.4	9.8	-2.8	18.2	13.3
C	8.4	-2.9	-12.3	3.1	11.1

LC = low-carbohydrate diet; C = conventional low-fat diet

weight loss do not appear to be due to differences in physical activity, the thermic effect of food (TEF), or resting energy expenditure (19,20). There is some evidence to suggest that gender (20), menopausal state (21), and degree of insulin sensitivity (22) result in differences in weight-loss outcomes. For example, one study reported that insulin-resistant obese women lost more weight following a hypocaloric, low-carbohydrate diet compared with a hypocaloric, high-carbohydrate diet after 16 wk, whereas insulin-sensitive women lost more weight on a high-carbohydrate diet compared with a low-carbohydrate diet (22). Clearly more research needs to be conducted to understand the mechanisms in which low-carbohydrate diets produce their effects.

It is interesting to note that in four of five studies at 6 mo, participants who were instructed to count carbohydrate consumed fewer calories (i.e., lost more weight) than those who were instructed to count calories (8–10,12). The reasons for this are unknown but may include greater satiety on a higher-protein, low glycemic index (GI) diet and increased structure (i.e., clear boundaries about what foods are allowed). Structured approaches, including meal replacements and food provision, have been shown to increase the magnitude of weight loss (23–30).

EFFICACY OF LOW-CARBOHYDRATE DIETS ON FASTING LIPIDS

A principal concern about low-carbohydrate approaches is that the high-fat content of the diet may adversely affect serum lipids and increase the risk for cardiovascular disease. As discussed in a review by Volek et al. (31), preliminary findings challenge this argument. In studies that compared low-carbohydrate and low-fat diets over the course of 6 to 12 mo, there were no differences in total cholesterol or low-density lipoprotein (LDL) cholesterol concentrations between groups (8–12,21). One study reported that the low-carbohydrate diet was less effective than the low-fat diet in reducing total cholesterol and LDL cholesterol at 1 yr (13). Only one study reported a small, transient increase in total cholesterol and LDL cholesterol during the third month of a 1-yr treatment (8). Furthermore, compared with the conventional group, those in the low-carbohydrate group experienced greater improvements in high-density lipoprotein (HDL) cholesterol (8,12) and triglycerides (8–10,12). Only one study reported decreases in HDL cholesterol in participants following a low-carbohydrate diet, but the decrease was less than the decrease in the low-fat group (11). Findings of these studies are summarized in Table 1. A meta-analysis of these data suggests that whereas the low-carbohydrate diet produced more favorable changes in triglycerides and HDL cholesterol concentrations, the low-fat diet produced more favorable changes in total cholesterol and LDL cholesterol concentrations (32). As such, further research is needed to understand whether the improvements in triglycerides and HDL concentrations outweigh the relatively smaller effects low-carbohydrate diets have on total and LDL cholesterol as compared with low-fat diets.

EFFICACY OF LOW-CARBOHYDRATE DIETS ON INFLAMMATORY BIOMARKERS

Evaluating fasting lipid profiles is one strategy for determining the effects of diets on cardiovascular risk; however, this measurement alone does not provide a complete picture. Other factors, such as inflammatory processes, also significantly contribute to the pathogenesis and progression of cardiovascular risk. Inflammation markers (e.g., interleukin [IL]-6, tumor necrosis factor [TNF]-α, intracellular cell-adhesion molecule-1 [CAMs], and P-selectin) have been associated with increased risk for cardiovascular disease *(33–35)*.

Sharman and Volek compared the effects of short-term (6-wk) consumption of hypocaloric low-carbohydrate and low-fat diets on C-reactive protein (CRP), CAMs, and proinflammatory cytokines (i.e., IL-6, TNF-α, and P-selectin) in 15 overweight but otherwise healthy men *(36)*. Consumption of both low-carbohydrate and low-fat diets resulted in weight loss (–6.5 ± 3.0 kg and –3.7 ± 3.3 kg, respectively). Improvements in inflammatory biomarkers were also observed following both diets (i.e., reductions in IL-6, TNF-α, CRP, and sICAM-1). These data were analyzed further to represent the delta change in inflammatory biomarkers per 1 kg reduction in body weight. There were no significant differences between the diets for IL-6, TNF-α, CRP, and sICAM-1; however, there was a significantly lower response for P-selectin in the low-fat group. Compared with individuals consuming a low-fat diet, greater reductions in CRP have been reported in individuals consuming a low-carbohydrate diet after adjusting for differences in weight loss *(37)*; however, these outcomes were observed only in participants who had high baseline CRP levels (>3 mg/dL) and high mean BMIs (46 kg/m^2). These data support previous findings that weight loss decreases markers of inflammation, but also suggest that improvements in inflammatory markers can also be achieved by diets that vary in macronutrient composition.

EFFICACY OF LOW-CARBOHYDRATE DIETS ON LIPOPROTEIN SUBFRACTIONS

In addition to elevated fasting cholesterol, LDL cholesterol concentrations and inflammatory markers, increased large very-low-density lipoprotein (VLDL) particle concentration, increased chylomicron concentration, small particle size diameter, and elevated postprandial lipemia are associated with increased risk for cardiovascular disease. Lipids and lipoprotein subfractions (i.e., chylomicrons and VLDL, LDL, and HDL subfractions) were evaluated in one study in which 78 obese individuals were randomly assigned to a low-carbohydrate (≤30g/d) or low-fat (≤30% energy from fat) diet for 6 mo *(37)*. Forty percent of these participants had diabetes and 77% of those who did not have diabetes had metabolic syndrome. After 6 mo, participants in the low-carbohydrate group lost more weight than those in the low-fat group (–8.5 ± 9.3 kg vs –3.5 ± 4.9 kg). At 6 mo more participants in the low-carbohydrate group had detectable chylomicron concentrations. In addition, greater decreases in large VLDL concentrations, particularly in men, were observed in the low-carbohydrate group. Decreases in LDL particle number, increases in LDL particle size, and small increases in large HDL concentration were also observed in both groups.

Sharman et al. compared the effect of hypocaloric low-carbohydrate (10% carbohydrate, 60% fat) and low-fat (55% carbohydrate, 25% fat) diets on postprandial lipemic response in 15 overweight men *(38)*. Participants consumed each diet for 6 wk and at the end of the experimental period completed an oral fat tolerance test. Participants were provided a low-carbohydrate, high-fat (11% carbohydrate, 86% fat) test meal and blood samples were taken immediately after the meal and hourly for a total of 8 h. Serum lipids, oxidized LDL, and lipoprotein particle size were measured.

The low-carbohydrate diet produced greater weight loss than the low-fat diet ($-6.1 \pm$ 2.9 kg vs -3.9 ± 3.4 kg). Differences in lipoprotein fractions and particle size were also observed between diets. Significant increases in the larger lipoprotein fractions (LDL-1), decreases in the smaller lipoprotein fractions (LDL-3 and LDL-4), and increases in the mean and peak LDL particle diameters were observed after consumption of the low-carbohydrate diet. Both diets reduced postprandial lipemia compared with baseline, but the magnitude of the reduction was greater under low-carbohydrate conditions. Given that elevated postprandial lipemia and small particle size diameter are associated with conditions that promote atherogenesis *(39,40)*, these findings suggest that weight-reducing low-carbohydrate diets may reduce cardiovascular disease risk; however, given the limited measures of cardiovascular risk biomarkers, small sample size, and short duration of the study, it is unclear whether these findings generalize to the larger population or persist over time. Similar findings have been observed in another study measuring lipid particle size in overweight individuals *(41)*; however, the low-carbohydrate diet provided in this study was supplemented with fish borage and flaxseed oil, which may have affected lipid outcomes.

Volek et al. *(20)* also compared the effect of hypocaloric low-carbohydrate (10% carbohydrate, 60% fat) and low-fat (55% carbohydrate, 25% fat) diets on postprandial lipemic response in 13 normolipidemic, overweight women. Consumption of these diets for 4 wk resulted in modest weight loss, with the low-carbohydrate diet producing larger reductions in weight (-3.0 ± 1.5 kg vs -1.1 ± 2.1 kg). With the exception of lowered VLDL cholesterol following the low-carbohydrate diet, no differences in lipoprotein fractions, LDL size, or the magnitude of postprandial triglyceride concentrations were observed between diets in this study. Based on their prior work in men, Volek et al. suggest that differences in findings in men and women may be caused by differences in baseline lipids and severity of dyslipidemia *(20)*. Whereas 12 of 15 men were characterized as having pattern B dyslipidemia (i.e., having small, dense LDL particles) at baseline, only one woman was classified as having pattern B dyslipidemia.

Taken together, findings from these studies suggest that low-carbohydrate diets are effective in reducing inflammatory biomarkers and are either more or equally effective in improving lipoprotein subfraction profile and postprandial lipemic response. Although these data are clinically useful, they are confounded by weight loss and therefore do not reveal whether effects are due to weight loss or specific characteristics of low-carbohydrate diets. In order to distinguish between the effects of macronutrient composition and weight loss, the effects of low-carbohydrate diets on inflammatory biomarkers and postprandial lipemic response should be studied under conditions of weight maintenance and compared with effects produced by low-fat diets. Short-term studies (4–8 wk) conducted in normal-weight men and women suggest that beneficial effects on postprandial lipemic response (i.e., reduced lipemic response and increased LDL particle size) following low-carbohydrate diets persist when weight is held constant *(42–45)*.

The effects of low-carbohydrate diets on inflammatory biomarkers are less clear. A study measuring CRP and inflammatory cytokines in normal-weight women found no significant changes following low- and high-carbohydrate diets *(46)*. Given that improvements in inflammatory biomarkers were observed in overweight individuals who experienced weight loss following both low- and high-carbohydrate diets and no effects were observed in women who experienced minimal weight loss following low- ($-1.2 \pm$

0.8 kg) and high- (–0.8 ± 1.0 kg) carbohydrate diets, preliminary findings suggest that weight loss rather than the macronutrient composition of the diet may be responsible for improvements in inflammatory biomarkers.

EFFICACY OF LOW-CARBOHYDRATE DIETS ON BLOOD PRESSURE

Weight-reducing low-carbohydrate and low-fat diets both appear to be effective in reducing blood pressure. No significant differences in blood pressure have been observed between groups in any of the long-term studies *(8–12,32)* or short-term studies *(21,47)* that measured blood pressure.

EFFICACY OF LOW-CARBOHYDRATE DIETS ON INSULIN SENSITIVITY AND GLYCEMIC CONTROL

A limited number of studies have compared the effects of low- and high-carbohydrate diets on insulin sensitivity. Differences in methodology preclude a pooled analysis of measures of glucose and insulin *(32)*; however, there is some evidence to suggest that low-carbohydrate diets are effective in improving insulin sensitivity and glycemic control *(10,11,48)*.

Samaha et al. *(10)* measured fasting glucose and mean glycosylated hemoglobin levels in nondiabetic and diabetic participants and insulin sensitivity (measured by the quantitative insulin sensitivity check [QUICK]) in nondiabetic participants. Compared with the low-fat group, greater decreases in fasting glucose were observed in the low-carbohydrate group and a trend toward greater decreases in mean glycosylated hemoglobin levels was observed in diabetic participants consuming a low-carbohydrate diet after 6 mo. After adjustment for the amount of weight lost at 6 mo, the low-carbohydrate diet was no longer a significant predictor of decreased glucose concentrations *(10)*; however, significantly greater decreases in mean glycosylated hemoglobin levels were observed at 1 yr even after adjustment for weight loss, suggesting that the diet had a direct effect on glycemic control *(11)*. In addition, greater increases in insulin sensitivity (6 ± 9% vs –3 ± 8%) were observed at 6 mo in individuals consuming low-carbohydrate diets compared with those consuming a low-fat diet *(10)*; however, these effects did not persist at 1 yr *(11)*. It is important to note that participants in the low-carbohydrate group experienced greater weight loss compared with the low-fat group at 6 mo, but no differences in weight were observed between groups at 1 yr. Another study reported no difference in the area under the glucose curve (as assessed by an oral glucose tolerance test) even with weight loss at 6 mo and 1 yr in individuals consuming low-carbohydrate and low-fat diets *(8)*. Although the area under the insulin curve improved at 1 yr in both groups, there were no differences in the area under the insulin curve or insulin sensitivity between groups at 1 yr when there were no differences in weight loss between groups. Unlike individuals participating in the Samaha study, participants in this study were relatively healthy and did not have any clinically significant illnesses such as type 2 diabetes or metabolic syndrome.

Boden et al. *(48)* examined the effects of a low-carbohydrate diet (approx 20 g of carbohydrate) on blood glucose concentration and insulin sensitivity (measured by euglycemic hyperinsulinemic clamps) in 10 obese individuals with type 2 diabetes admitted to the general clinical research center. The experimental diet was administered for 14 d. An energy deficit of approx 1030 kcal/d resulted in a weight loss of 1.65 kg, which was caused primarily by a reduction of adipose tissue rather than a loss of body water. In addition, 24-h plasma glucose concentrations normalized, hemoglobin A_{1C} decreased (from 7.3% to 6.8%), and insulin sensitivity improved.

In another short-term study, Corneir et al. (22) investigated whether insulin sensitivity was differentially affected in insulin-sensitive and insulin-resistant women consuming hypocaloric (–400 kcal/d) diets varying in macronutrient composition. The effects of low-carbohydrate and low-fat diets on insulin sensitivity (measured by fasting insulin, homeostasis model assessment, and QUICK) were compared in 12 insulin-sensitive and 9 insulin-insensitive obese women. After 16 wk on either a hypocaloric low-carbohydrate or hypocaloric low-fat diet, weight loss was observed in both insulin-sensitive women consuming low-carbohydrate (–6.2 kg) and low-fat (–11.3 kg) diets and insulin-resistant women consuming low-carbohydrate (–11.1 kg) and low-fat diets (–7.42 kg). Fasting insulinemia improved in both groups and insulin sensitivity improved in insulin-resistant women but did not change in insulin-sensitive women. The change in insulin sensitivity was correlated with the degree of weight loss, suggesting that weight loss, rather than macronutrient composition, improved insulin resistance in this study; however, this study also showed that hypocaloric low-carbohydrate diets were as effective as hypocaloric low-fat diets in increasing insulin sensitivity.

One study suggests that low-carbohydrate diets do not confer any advantage over low-fat diets on glucose metabolism and insulin sensitivity when studied under conditions of weight maintenance. Sunehag et al. (49) compared the effects of isocaloric low-carbohydrate (30% carbohydrate, 55% fat) and low-fat (60% carbohydrate, 25% fat) diets on glucose metabolism and insulin sensitivity and secretion in 13 obese but otherwise healthy, nondiabetic but insulin-resistant adolescents. In this crossover design study, participants were instructed to consume a low- or high-carbohydrate diet 7 d prior to metabolic testing. Glucose metabolism, insulin sensitivity, and insulin secretory indices were measured by isotopically labeled tracers and a stable-label iv glucose tolerance test (SLIVGTT). No differences in insulin sensitivity were observed between dietary conditions and neither diet provided beneficial effects on glucose metabolism; therefore, these researchers suggest that treatment of insulin resistance should focus on management of weight rather than the macronutrient composition of the diet.

Taken together, these studies suggest that fasting glucose, glycosylated hemoglobin, and insulin sensitivity improve during weight loss. Greater improvements in insulin sensitivity and glycemic response at 6 mo in individuals consuming a low-carbohydrate diet are associated with greater losses of weight. Improvements in glycemic response and insulin sensitivity may be more prevalent in those with chronic disease.

CONCLUSION

Studies that compare low-carbohydrate and low-fat diets suggest that low-carbohydrate diets are effective in reducing body weight and do not appear to increase risk of cardiovascular disease in the short term (50). In fact, the low-carbohydrate diet produces favorable effects on triglycerides and HDL concentrations, traditional measures of cardiovascular disease risk. Furthermore, low-carbohydrate diets for weight reduction do not appear to confer additional costs compared to low-fat, low-calorie diets (51). These results are preliminary and do not signal a call for revised dietary guidelines. Improvements in lipid profiles associated with low-carbohydrate diets (increased HDL cholesterol and reduced triglycerides) are suggestive of an overall beneficial effect, but the clinical implications of these findings clearly require additional study *(52)*. As suggested by the meta-analysis *(32)*, potential unfavorable changes in total and LDL cholesterol should be weighed against the favorable changes in HDL and triglycerides before low-carbohydrate diets can be recommended for the long-term treatment of obesity. Furthermore, these preliminary data need to be replicated in larger and longer trials that include more comprehensive assessment of safety, including measures of bone health and kidney function. Additional studies comparing the effects of low-carbohydrate and low-fat diets on fasting lipids, inflammatory biomarkers, postprandial lipemic response, and insulin sensitivity under conditions of weight maintenance (i.e., without the confounding factor of weight loss) are also needed to better understand mechanisms and effects.

REFERENCES

1. Banting W. A Letter on Corpulence Addressed to the Public. Harrison and Sons, London: 1863.
2. Carter HS, Howe PE, Mason HH. Nutrition and Clinical Dietetics. Lea & Febiger, Philadelphia: 1917.
3. Sinha SR, Kossoff EH. The ketogenic diet. Neurologist 2005; 11:161–170.
4. Atkins RC. Dr. Atkins' Diet Revolution. David McKay, New York: 1972.
5. Atkins RC. Dr. Atkins' New Diet Revolution. Avon Books, New York: 1992.
6. Atkins RC. Dr. Atkins' New Diet Revolution. Avon Books, New York: 2002.
7. Freedman MR, King J, Kennedy E. Popular diets: a scientific review. Obes Res 2001;9 Suppl 1:1S–40S.
8. Foster GD, Wyatt HR, Hill JO, et al. A randomized trial of a low-carbohydrate diet for obesity. N Engl J Med 2003;348:2082–2090.
9. Brehm BJ, Seeley RJ, Daniels SR, et al. A randomized trial comparing a very low-carbohydrate diet and a calorie-restricted low-fat diet on body weight and cardiovascular risk factors in healthy women. J Clin Endocrin Metab 2003;88:1617–1623.
10. Samaha FF, Iqbal N, Seshadri P, et al. A low-carbohydrate as compared with a low-fat diet in severe obesity. N Engl J Med 2003;348: 2074–2081.
11. Stern L, Iqbal N, Seshadri P, et al. The effects of low-carbohydrate versus conventional weight loss diets in severely obese adults: one-year follow-up of a randomized trial. Ann Intern Med 2004;140:778–785.
12. Yancy WS, Olsen MK, Guyton JR, et al. A low-carbohydrate, ketogenic diet versus a low-fat diet to treat obesity and hyperlipidemia. Ann Intern Med, 2004; 140:769-777.
13. Dansinger ML, Gleason JA, Griffith JL, et al. Comparison of the Atkins, Ornish, Weight Watchers, and Zone diets for weight loss and heart disease risk reduction: a randomized trial. JAMA 2005;293:43–53.
14. Fine EJ, Feinman RD. Thermodynamics of weight loss diets. Nutr Metab 2004;1:15.
15. Golay A, Allaz AF, Morel Y, et al. Similar weight loss with low- or high-carbohydrate diets. Am J Clin Nutr 1996;63:174–178.
16. Werner SC. Comparison between weight reduction on a high-calorie, high fat diet and on an isocaloric regimen high in carbohydrate. N Engl J Med 1985;252:661–664.
17. Pilkington TRE, Gainsborough HJ, Rosenoer VM, et al. Diet and weight reduction in the obese. Lancet 1960; i:856–858.
18. Oleson ES, Quaade F. Fatty food and obesity. Lancet 1960:1048–1051.
19. Brehm BJ, Spang SE, Lattin BL, et al. The role of energy expenditure in the differential weight loss in obese women on low-fat and low-carbohydrate diets. J Clin Endocrinol Metab 2005;90:1475–1482.
20. Volek JS, Sharman MJ, Gomez AL, et al. Comparison of a very low-carbohydrate and low-fat diet on fasting lipids, LDL subclasses, insulin resistance, and postprandial lipemic responses in overweight women. J Am Coll Nutr 2004;23:177–184.
21. Lean ME, Han TS, Prvan T, et al. Weight loss with high and low carbohydrate 1200 kcal diets in free living women. Eur J Clin Nutr 1997;51:243–248.
22. Cornier MA, Donahoo WT, Pereira R, et al. Insulin sensitivity determines the effectiveness of dietary macronutrient composition on weight loss in obese women. Obes Res 2005;13:703–709.

23. Jeffery RW, Wing RR, Thorson C, et al. Strengthening behavioral interventions for weight loss: a randomized trial of food provision and monetary incentives. J Consult Clin Psychol 1993;6:1038–1045.
24. Wing RR, Jeffery RW, Burton LR, et al. Food provision vs structured meal plans in the behavioral treatment of obesity. Int J Obes Relat Metab Disord 1996;20:56–62.
25. Ditschuneit HH, Flechtner-Mors M, Johnson TD, et al. Metabolic and weight loss effects of a long-term dietary intervention in obese patients. Am J Clin Nutr 1999;69:198–204.
26. Ditschuneit HH, Flechtner-Mors M. Value of structured meals for weight management: risk factors and long-term weight maintenance. Obes Res 2001;9:284S–289S.
27. Rothacker DQ, Staniszewski BA, Ellis PK. Liquid meal replacement vs traditional food: a potential model for women who cannot maintain eating habit change. J Am Diet Assoc 2001;101:345–347.
28. Ashley JM, St Jeor ST, Perumean-Chaney S, et al. Meal replacements in weight intervention. Obes Res 2001;9:312S–320S.
29. Hannum SM, Carson L, Evans EM, et al. Use of portion-controlled entrees enhances weight loss in women. Obes Res 2004;12:538–546.
30. Metz JA, Stern JS, Kris-Etherton P, et al. A randomized trial of improved weight loss with a prepared meal plan in overweight and obese patients. Arch Intern Med 2000;160:2150–2158.
31. Volek JS, Sharman MJ, Forsythe CE. Modification of lipoproteins by very low-carbohydrate diets. J Nutr 2005;135:1339–1342.
32. Nordmann AJ, Nordmann A, Briel M, et al. Effects of low-carbohydrate vs low-fat diets on weight loss and cardiovascular risk factors: a meta-analysis of randomized controlled trials. Arch Intern Med 2006;166:285–293.
33. Libby P, Ridker PM, Maseri A. Inflammation and atherosclerosis. Circulation 2002;105:1135–1143.
34. Blake G J, Ridker PM. Inflammatory bio-markers and cardiovascular risk prediction. J Intern Med 2002;252:283–294.
35. Blake GJ, Ridker PM. Novel clinical markers of vascular wall inflammation. Circ Res 2001;89:763–771.
36. Sharman MJ, Volek JS. Weight loss leads to reductions in inflammatory biomarkers after a very-low-carbohydrate diet and a low-fat diet in overweight men. Clin Sci (Lond) 2004;107:365–369.
37. Seshadri P, Iqbal N, Stern L, et al. A randomized study comparing the effects of a low-carbohydrate diet and a conventional diet on lipoprotein subfractions and C-reactive protein levels in patients with severe obesity. Am J Med 2004;117:398–405.
38. Sharman MJ, Gomez AL, Kraemer WJ, et al. Very low-carbohydrate and low-fat diets affect fasting lipids and postprandial lipemia differently in overweight men. J Nutr 2004; 134:880–885.
39. Cohn JS. Postprandial lipemia: emerging evidence for atherogenicity of remnant lipoproteins. Can J Cardiol 1998;14:18B–27B.
40. Roche HM, Gibney MJ. The impact of postprandial lipemia in accelerating atherothrombosis. J Cardiovasc Risk 2000;7:317–324.
41. Westman EC, Yancy WS Jr, Olsen MK, et al. Effect of a low-carbohydrate, ketogenic diet program compared to a low-fat diet on fasting lipoprotein subclasses. Int J Cardiol 2006;110:212–216.
42. Volek JS, Gûmez AL, Kraemer WJ. Fasting lipoprotein and postprandial triacylglycerol responses to a low-carbohydrate diet supplemented with n-3 fatty acids. J Am Coll Nutr 2000;19:383–391.
43. Sharman MJ, Kraemer WJ, Love DM, et al. A ketogenic diet favorably affects serum biomarkers for cardiovascular disease in normal-weight men. J Nutr 2002;132:1879–1885.
44. Volek JS, Sharman MJ, Gûmez AL, et al. An isoenergetic very low-carbohydrate diet is associated with improved serum high-density lipoprotein cholesterol (HDL-C), total cholesterol to HDL-C ratio, triacylglycerols, and postprandial lipemic responses compared to a low-fat diet in normal weight, normolipidemic women. J Nutr 2003;133:2756–2761.
45. Volek JS, Westman EC. Low-carbohydrate weight-loss diets revisited. Clev Clin J Med 2002;69:849–862.
46. Volek JS, Sharman MJ, Gomez AL, et al. An isoenergetic very low-carbohydrate diet improves serum HDL cholesterol and triacylglycerol concentrations, the total cholesterol to HDL cholesterol ratio and postprandial pipemic responses compared with a low-fat diet in normal weight, normolipidemic women. J Nutr 2003;133:2756–2761.
47. Meckling KA, O'Sullivan C, Saari D. Comparison of a low-fat diet to a low-carbohydrate diet on weight loss, body composition, and risk factors for diabetes and cardiovascular disease in free-living, overweight men and women. J Clin Endocrinol Metab 2004;89(6):2717–2723.
48. Boden G, Sargrad K, Homko C, et al. Effect of a low-carbohydrate diet on appetite, blood glucose levels, and insulin resistance in obese patients with type 2 diabetes. Ann Intern Med 2005;142:403–411.

49. Sunehag AL, Toffolo G, Campioni M, et al. Effects of dietary macronutrient intake on insulin sensitivity and secretion and glucose and lipid metabolism in healthy, obese adolescents. J Clin Endocrinol Metab 2005;90:4496–4502.
50. Noble CA, Kushner RF. An update on low-carbohydrate, high-protein diets. Curr Opin Gastroenterol 2006;2:153–159.
51. Tsai AG, Glick HA, Shera D, et al. Cost-effectiveness of a low-carbohydrate diet and a standard diet in severe obesity. Obes Res 2005; 13:1834–1840.
52. Bonow RO, Eckel RH. Diet, obesity, and cardiovascular risk. N Engl J Med 2003;348:2057–2058.

16 Physical Activity and Obesity

John M. Jakicic, PhD, Amy D. Otto, PhD, RD, LDN,
Kristen Polzien, PhD, and Kelli K. Davis, MS

CONTENTS

INTRODUCTION
CONTRIBUTION OF PHYSICAL ACTIVITY TO TOTAL
  ENERGY EXPENDITURE
CAN PHYSICAL ACTIVITY PREVENT WEIGHT GAIN?
PHYSICAL ACTIVITY FOR WEIGHT LOSS AND PREVENTION
  OF WEIGHT REGAIN
DEVELOPMENT OF EXERCISE PRESCRIPTION FOR WEIGHT CONTROL
CONCLUSION
ACKNOWLEDGMENTS
REFERENCES

Summary

There is an increasing prevalence of overweight and obesity in the United States and other developed countries. This can have significant public health implications because of the association of excess body weight with increased risk of chronic diseases. It has been suggested that the increasing prevalence of excess body weight (overweight and obesity) and related diseases also has a significant impact on health care costs. Physical activity can significantly affect weight control and can also have an independent effect on associated chronic disease risk factors. However, physical activity participation is less than optimal. Thus, it is important for health care professionals to understand the role of physical activity in weight loss, the prevention of weight gain, and the prevention of weight regain, and to understand how to provide accurate and meaningful information to their patients.

Key Words: Exercise; overweight; fitness; weight control.

INTRODUCTION

Obesity, physical activity, and poor dietary behaviors have been linked to increased health risk, which may contribute to 300,000 to 400,000 additional deaths per year in the United States (1). This may in part be a result of the increasing prevalence of overweight (body mass index [BMI] ≥ 25.0 kg/m^2) and obesity (BMI ≥ 30.0 kg/m^2), with these rates estimated to be approx 65% and 30% in adults, respectively (2,3). Moreover, it is estimated that 16% of children and adolescents ages 6 to 19 yr are obese (4). The increasing prevalence of overweight and obesity results in associated health risks from an increase

From: *Contemporary Endocrinology: Treatment of the Obese Patient*
Edited by: R. F. Kushner and D. H. Bessesen © Humana Press Inc., Totowa, NJ

in numerous chronic diseases that include heart disease, diabetes, and various forms of cancer *(1)*. These increased obesity-related health risks may contribute to more than $100 billion in annual health care costs. Thus, the development and implementation of interventions that result in weight loss, prevention of weight gain, and prevention of weight regain can significantly reduce the health burden and have an impact on public health.

It has been demonstrated that a reduction in body weight and an increase in physical activity may facilitate the management of body weight and reduce the risk and onset of obesity-related diseases *(1)*. However, it is estimated that only 20% of adults in the United States participate in adequate levels of physical activity to improve their health *(5)*, and it is clear that most children do not participate in adequate amounts of physical activity *(5)*. Thus, it is important for health care professionals to understand the role of physical activity in the prevention of weight gain, weight loss, and the prevention of weight regain, and to understand how to provide accurate and meaningful information to their patients.

CONTRIBUTION OF PHYSICAL ACTIVITY TO TOTAL ENERGY EXPENDITURE

Whether body weight remains stable, increases, or decreases is ultimately dependent on the balance or imbalance between energy intake (calories consumed) and energy expenditure. To reduce body weight, energy expenditure must exceed energy intake, whereas to prevent weight gain or to maintain weight loss, energy expenditure must equal energy intake. Thus, the effect of an increase in energy expenditure on body weight is also dependent on the relative contribution of energy intake to energy balance. This section will focus on the contribution of the components of energy expenditure on energy balance.

There are three basic component of energy expenditure: resting energy expenditure (REE), thermic effect of food (TEF), and voluntary physical activity (Fig. 1). Although it is recognized that REE can vary among individuals, and there are physiological, metabolic, and genetic influences on REE, the REE within a given individual remains relatively stable, provided that weight and health status remain stable. Moreover, despite the large contribution of REE to total energy expenditure, limited studies have shown the ability of lifestyle interventions to increase REE; this is especially true during weight loss when REE tends to decrease *(6,7)*. Thus, it appears that interventions targeting an increase in REE will have a small and limited impact on total energy expenditure for most individuals, which will result in a limited impact on body weight.

TEF is the increase in energy expenditure resulting from the food that is consumed to allow for the necessary components of digestion. Ravussin et al. *(8)* have suggested that TEF is approx 10% of total daily energy expenditure. Moreover, TEF is influenced by the macronutrient content of the food that is consumed. Despite the potential increase in TEF based on dietary composition, this increase in energy expenditure is relatively small compared with the total daily energy expenditure. Moreover, this would require a significant increase in a specific macronutrient content sustained over a relatively long period of time to significantly and independently affect body weight. Thus, attempting to affect body weight solely through an increase in TEF is not practical and will likely result in minimal impact. A more detailed discussion of this issue is not within the scope or focus of this chapter.

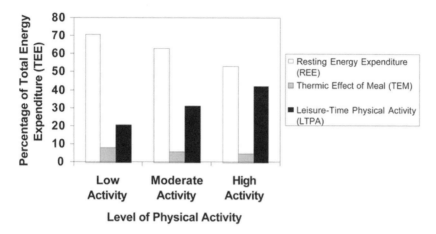

Fig. 1. Contribution of varying levels of leisure-time physical activity (LTPA) to total energy expenditure (TEE) for a fix resting energy expenditure (REE - 1800 kcal/d) and thermic effect of a metal (TEM = 180 kcal/d).

Leisure-time physical activity (LTPA) is the most variable component of energy expenditure. LTPA can occur in the form of structured exercise, lifestyle activity, or other forms of activity that contribute to an increase in energy expenditure. The amount of the increase in energy expenditure varies based on the amount of LPTA that is performed. For example, an individual who is relatively inactive will expend approx 30% more calories above what is expended in REE, with this increasing to approx 50% or 80% for individuals participating in moderate or higher amounts of LTPA, respectively (*see* Fig, 1). Thus, it is important to understand the contribution of an increase in total daily energy expenditure resulting from LTPA on energy balance, which can affect the prevention of weight gain, weight loss, the prevention of weight regain following weight loss.

CAN PHYSICAL ACTIVITY PREVENT WEIGHT GAIN?

Close examination of prevalence data indicates the need to focus intervention efforts on the prevention of weight gain. If effective, this will decrease the likelihood of a transition from normal weight to overweight or obesity, and decrease the transition from overweight to obesity. There is some evidence that LTPA can play a significant role in the prevention of weight gain; this is mostly likely a result of the increase in energy expenditure resulting from an increase in LTPA. For example, there are data from prospective observation studies that appear to support this hypothesis. Lee and Paffenbarger *(9)* concluded that participants in the Harvard Alumni Study who reported levels of physical activity consistent with approx 30 min of moderate-intensity physical activity had a lower body weight when compared with individuals reporting lower levels of physical activity. When change in cardiorespiratory fitness is used as a surrogate for change in LTPA, the data reported by DiPietro et al. *(10)* demonstrate the inverse association between change in fitness and change in body weight, which also supports the importance of physical activity in the prevention of weight gain in adults.

The application of these prospective, observational findings need to be apply to interventions to have a meaningful impact on weight gain prevention. In fact, Sherwood et al. *(11)* reported that an increase in physical activity was predictive of prevention of weight gain. Moreover, preliminary data are available from an ongoing clinical trial that is being conducted in our research center. Results indicated that an increase in physical activity (150 to 300 min/wk) resulted in prevention of weight gain or modest weight loss (1–2 kg) in approx 60% of overweight adults (BMI = 25.0–29.9), with change in fitness predictive of prevention of weight gain (unpublished data).

These findings are important when considered in context of the recommendations for physical activity in the prevention of weight gain that appeared in the 2005 US Dietary Guidelines, which stated that to prevent weight gain there is a need for individuals to "engage in approximately 60 minutes of moderate- to vigorous-intensity activity on most days of the week while not exceeding caloric intake requirements." Clinicians should consider individually tailoring these recommendations based on the response of the participant. For example, it has been established that approx 30 min of moderate-intensity physical activity per day on most days of the week can result in a significant reduction in the risk of chronic diseases. Thus, individuals should increase to this level of activity and determine whether this level of physical activity is sufficient to prevent weight gain. If it is not, the recommended level of physical activity can gradually be increased (e.g, 30 to 35 min/wk, 35 to 40 min/wk, etc.) until weight gain ceases. This is illustrated in the flow chart provided in Fig. 2.

PHYSICAL ACTIVITY FOR WEIGHT LOSS AND PREVENTION OF WEIGHT REGAIN

Short-Term Weight Loss

It has been clearly established that effective behavioral weight-loss interventions result in approximately a 10% weight loss compared to initial body weight within 6 mo of initiating an intervention *(12)*. These results appear to be achievable with the combination of a reduction in energy intake and an increase in energy expenditure *(1)*. However, the contributions of each of these components (reduction in energy intake and increase in energy expenditure) are not equal, with the majority of weight loss resulting from a reduction in energy intake. In response to a 12-wk intervention, Hagan et al. *(13)* reported a reduction in body weight of 8.4% in males and 5.5% in females, with Wing et al. *(14)* reporting 9.1% in response to a 24-wk intervention, with energy intake ranging from 1000 to 1500 kcal/d. The addition of exercise to a reduction in energy intake resulted in weight loss of 11.4% and 7.5%, respectively in males and females *(13)*, with Wing et al. *(14)* reporting weight loss of 10.4%. In these studies, exercise alone resulted in weight loss of 0.3, 0.6, and 2.1%, respectively *(13,14)*. These findings support the conclusions of the clinical guidelines developed by the National Institutes of Health that recommend the combination of a reduction in energy intake and an increase in energy expenditure to maximize weight loss in response to a behavioral intervention *(1)*.

Long-Term Weight Loss and Weight-Loss Maintenance

Despite the minimal effect of exercise on short-term weight loss, exercise appears to be an important component of long-term interventions. This is supported by the 2005 US Dietary Guidelines *(15)*, the Institute of Medicine *(16)*, and extensive reviews of the

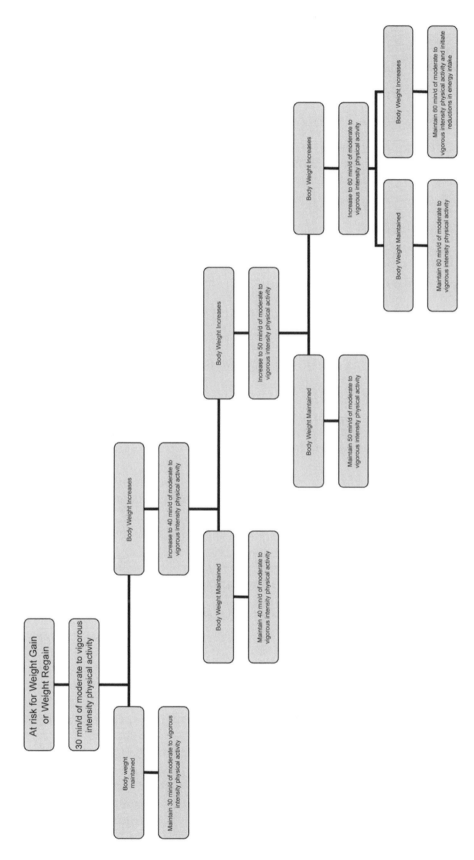

Fig. 2. Example of exercise progression to prevent weight gain or weight regain.

literature *(17,18)*. However, a common conclusion that appears to be supported by cross-sectional data, prospective observational data, and data from clinical trials is that physical activity equivalent to ≥2000 kcal/wk or approx 250 to 300 min/wk is associated with improved long-term weight loss at 12 to 24 mo *(19–24)*. These results appear to support the recommendation of the US Dietary Guidelines that 60 to 90 min/d is required to prevention weight regain following significant weight loss *(15)*.

It appears that adequate levels of physical activity do not act alone to control body weight long-term, but rather work in synergy with appropriate levels of energy intake. For example, Jakicic et al. *(25)* reported that the combination of increased levels of physical activity combined with reduced levels of energy intake were predictive of long-term weight-loss outcomes following an 18-mo intervention. Similar findings were reported by McGuire et al. *(26)* based on data from the National Weight Control Registry. Thus, these data appear to support the importance of maintaining adequate levels of energy balance (energy intake and energy expenditure) to enhance long-term weight loss and prevent weight regain following weight loss. Thus, it is important for clinicians to address these components of energy balance equally when providing interventions for overweight and obese adults.

DEVELOPMENT OF EXERCISE PRESCRIPTION FOR WEIGHT CONTROL

Exercise Mode

The majority of clinical trials have incorporated aerobic forms of physical activity (i.e., brisk walking) into the weight loss interventions; overweight/obese individuals report that walking is the self-selected mode of physical activity for 80 to 90% of activity sessions *(20)*. This may be a result of ease of participation for most individuals, the low cost of participation, and lack of need for special skills to participate in this form of physical activity.

Despite these findings, additional forms of physical activity have been examined for weight control with mixed results. For example, a review of the scientific literature revealed no apparent improvement in weight loss with the addition of resistance exercise *(27)*, and preliminary data from our laboratory appear to support this conclusion *(35)*. Moreover, Jannsen et al. *(28)* reported no significant improvement in risk factors with the addition of resistance exercise when compared with weight loss resulting from diet alone. However, there is initial evidence, that despite these findings, that resistance exercise has been associated with a reduction in all-cause mortality *(29)*. Moreover, resistance exercise will improve muscular strength *(30,31)*, which may affect physical function of overweight and obese adults *(32)*. Despite these potential benefits, resistance exercise has not been shown to be more effective for weight loss or the maintenance of weight loss compared with other forms of physical activity. Thus, although more research is needed to understand the role of resistance exercise for weight control, this form of exercise may be appropriate when used as a complement to other forms of physical activity such as walking.

Because of the potential functional limitations of overweight and obese adults, alternative forms of physical activity may need to be considered. Yoga has been shown to improve range of motion and physical function, while reducing pain *(33,34)*. However, there are limited data to support the addition of yoga to interventions to improve weight loss. Results from a 12-mo weight-loss intervention that included yoga as a complement to aerobic forms of physical activity and a reduction in energy intake demonstrate no improvement in weight loss when compared with interventions not including yoga *(35)*. Another popular recommendation is to include aquatic forms of physical activity for overweight adults, as this may overcome functional limitations in overweight and obese individuals. Again, the limited data in this area of research do not indicate that weight loss is improved with the addition of aquatic exercise compared with other forms of physical activity *(36)*. These factors should be considered by clinicians when recommending physical activity to overweight and obese adults when weight loss is the primary outcome, and used to enhance LTPA and energy expenditure for individuals who find these activities enjoyable.

Physical Activity Intensity vs Volume

Current recommendations for physical activity to control body weight appear to indicate that approx 60 to 90 min/d may be required to prevent weight gain or improve long-term weight loss *(15)*. Moreover, although the accumulation of at least 10,000 steps per day, measured using a pedometer, may be associated with improvements in health-related parameters *(37)*, it has been suggested that it may be necessary to progressively increase daily steps to levels above 10,000 steps per day to improve weight loss *(38)*. Thus, clinicians should focus on progressively increasing the total volume of physical activity to maximize energy expenditure in overweight and obese adults. This could involve increasing duration by 10 min/d or by 1000 steps/d at approximately 4-wk intervals until the desired level of physical activity is attained.

The total volume of physical activity, expressed as energy expenditure, may be more important for weight control than the intensity of the physical activity that is performed. For example, Duncan et al. *(39)* have demonstrated that when total volume of physical activity is held constant, there is no difference in the effect on body weight across different intensities of physical activity. Similar results have been reported by Jakicic et al. *(20)*, who demonstrated that the magnitude of weight loss was affected by volume of physical activity rather than the intensity of physical activity within a 12-mo clinical trial.

Even though total volume of physical activity may be more important than the intensity of physical activity for promoting weight control, this does not suggest that an adequate intensity of physical activity to improve cardiorespiratory fitness is not important. In fact, there is a growing body of literature to support the need for sufficient improvements in cardiorespiratory fitness independent of body weight, with higher levels of fitness reducing health-related risk even in overweight and obese adults *(40–43)*. Moreover, this may also result in a reduction in all-cause mortality independent of body weight *(44)*. However, these data appear to only apply to individuals with a BMI <35, as there are limited data to support the independent effects of physical activity on health-related outcomes and mortality for individuals above this level of BMI.

An additional factor when considering the volume of physical activity is whether this needs to be done in a continuous manner to have an effect on the desired outcomes. In fact, there are numerous studies to support that intermittent exercise performed in multiple bouts of at least 10 min in duration can significantly improve desired outcomes. These outcomes can include cardiorespiratory fitness *(45–47)* and selected risk factors *(46)*. Moreover, intermittent physical activity may provide an effective strategy for improving initial adoption of physical activity in overweight and obese adults *(21,47)*. This may provide a strategy for clinicians when addressing physical activity for individuals who are resistant to traditional forms of physical activity that require continuous exercise for periods ranging from 20 to 60 min per session.

CONCLUSION

Excessive body weight that results in overweight or obesity has been linked to significant health risks for numerous chronic conditions *(1)*. A continuing challenge for clinicians is to address the increasing prevalence of weight gain in patients to prevent overweight or obesity, and to prevent weight regain following initial weight loss. However, it appears that physical activity can contribute to a significant increase in energy expenditure, which will facilitate long-term weight control provided that a sufficient dose of physical activity is performed. It appears that the level of physical activity necessary for prevention of weight gain and to enhance long-term weight loss maintenance ranges from approx 30 to 60 min/d *(15,17–20)*. Therefore, clinicians should encourage patients to progressively increase physical activity to this range (*see* Fig. 2) in addition to maintaining a complementary level of energy intake. This may require clinicians to individually tailor these recommendations to the needs of the patient in a progressive and systematic manner to enhance both weight control and health-related outcomes in overweight and obese adults.

ACKNOWLEDGMENTS

The efforts of Dr. Jakicic, Dr. Otto, Dr. Polzien, and Ms. Davis are supported by research funding from the National Institutes of Health (HL70257, HL67826, DK066150).
Dr. Jakicic is on the scientific advisory boards for the Coca-Cola Beverage Institute for Health and Wellness, the Calorie Control Council, and BodyMedia, Inc.

REFERENCES

1. National Institutes of Health, National Heart, Lung and Blood Institute. Clinical Guidelines on the Identification, Evaluation, and Treatment of Overweight and Obesity in Adults—The Evidence Report. Obes Res 1998;6(suppl.2).
2. Flegal KM, Carroll MD, Ogden CL, et al. Prevalence and trends in obesity among US adults, 1999–2000. JAMA 2002;288(14):1723–1727.
3. Hedley AA, Ogden CL, Johnson CL, et al. Prevalence of overweight and obesity among US children, adolescents, and adults, 1999–2002. JAMA 2004;291:2847–2850.
4. Ogden CL, Flegal KM, Carroll MD, et al. Prevalence and trends in overweight among US children and adolescents, 1999-2000. JAMA 2002;288(14):1728–1732.
5. US Department of Health and Human Services. Physical Activity and Health: A Report of the Surgeon General. US Department of Health and Human Services, Centers for Disease Control and Prevention, National Center for Chronic Disease Prevention and Health Promotion, Atlanta, GA: 1996.
6. Donnelly JE, Pronk NP, Jacobsen DJ, et al. Effects of a very-low-calorie diet and physical-training regimenson body composition and resting metabolic rate in obese females. Am J Clin Nutr 1991;54: 56–61.
7. Geliebter A, Maher MM, Gerace L, et al. Effects of strength or aerobic training on body composition, resting metabolic rate, and peak oxygen consumption in obese dieting subjects. Am J Clin Nutr 1997;66:557–563.

8. Ravussin E, Bogardus C. Relationship of genetics, age, and physical fitness to daily energy expenditure and fuel utilization. Am J Clin Nutr 1989;49:968–975.

9. Lee I-M, Paffenbarger R. Associations of light, moderate, and vigorous intensity physical activity with longevity: the Harvard Alumni Health Study. Am J Epidemiol 2000;151(3):293–299.

10. DiPietro L, Kohl HW, Barlow CE, Blair SN. Improvements in cardiorespiratory fitness attenuate age-related weight gain in healthy men and women: the Aerobics Center Longitudinal Study. Int J Obes 1998;22:55–62.

11. Sherwood NE, Jeffery RW, French SA, et al. Predictors of weight gain in the Pound of Prevention study. Int J Obes 2000;24:395–403.

12. Wing RR. Behavioral weight control. In: Wadden TA, Stunkard AJ, eds. Handbook of Obesity Treatment. Guilford Press, New York: 2002; pp. 301–316.

13. Hagan RD, Upton SJ, Wong L, et al. The effects of aerobic conditioning and/or calorie restriction in overweight men and women. Med Sci Sports Exerc 1986;18(1):87–94.

14. Wing RR, Venditti EM, Jakicic JM, et al. Lifestyle intervention in overweight individuals with a family history of diabetes. Diabetes Care 1998;21(3):350–359.

15. Department of Health and Human Services and Department of Agriculture. Dietary Guidelines for Americans: www.healthierus.gov/dietaryguidelines; 2005.

16. Institute of Medicine. Dietary Reference Intakes for Energy, Carbohydrates, Fiber, Fat, Protein and Amino Acids (Macronutrients): A Report of the Panel on Macronutrients, Subcommittees on Upper Reference Levels of Nutrients and Interpretation and Uses of Dietary Reference Intakes, and the Standing Committee on the Scientific Evaluation of Dietary Reference Intakes. National Academies Press, Washington, DC: 2002.

17. Jakicic JM, Clark K, Coleman E, et al. American College of Sports Medicine position stand: appropriate intervention strategies for weight loss and prevention of weight regain for adults. Med Sci Sports Exerc 2001;33(12):2145–2156.

18. Saris WHM, Blair SN, van Baak MA, et al. How much physical activity is enough to prevent unhealthy weight gain? Outcome of the IASO 1st Stock Conference and consensus statement. Obes Rev 2003;4:101–114.

19. Jakicic JM, Marcus B, Lang W. Effect of varying doses of exercise on 24-month weight loss in overweight adults. Obes Res 2005;13(suppl):A24.

20. Jakicic JM, Marcus BH, Gallagher KI, et al. Effect of exercise duration and intensity on weight loss in overweight, sedentary women. A randomized trial. JAMA 2003;290:1323–1330.

21. Jakicic JM, Winters C, Lang W, et al. Effects of intermittent exercise and use of home exercise equipment on adherence, weight loss, and fitness in overweight women: a randomized trial. JAMA 1999;282(16):1554–1560.

22. Jeffery RW, Wing RR, Sherwood NE, et al. Physical activity and weight loss: Does prescribing higher physical activity goals improve outcome? Am J Clin Nutr 2003;78(4):684–689.

23. Klem ML, Wing RR, McGuire MT, et al. A descriptive study of individuals successful at long-term maintenance of substantial weight loss. Am J Clin Nutr 1997;66:239–246.

24. Schoeller DA, Shay K, Kushner RF. How much physical activity is needed to minimize weight gain in previously obese women. Am J Clin Nutr 1997;66:551–556.

25. Jakicic JM, Wing RR, Winters-Hart C. Relationship of physical activity to eating behaviors and weight loss in women. Med Sci Sports Exerc 2002;34(10):1653–1659.

26. McGuire MT, Wing RR, Klem ML, et al. What predicts weight regain in a group of successful weight losers? J Consult Clin Psychol 1999;67(2):177–185.

27. Donnelly JE, Jakicic JM, Pronk NP, et al. Is resistance exercise effective for weight management? Evidence Based Prev Med 2004;1(1):21–29.

28. Jannsen I, Fortier A, Hudson R, et al. Effects of an energy-restrictive diet with or without exercise on abdominal fat, intermuscular fat, and metabolic risk factors in obese women. Diabetes Care 2002;25(3):431–438.

29. Jurca R, LaMonte MJ, Church TS, et al. Association of muscle strength and aerobic fitness with metabolic syndrome in men. Med Sci Sports Exerc 2004;36(8):1301–1307.

30. Kraemer WJ, Volek JS, Clark KL, et al. Physiological adaptations to a weight-loss dietary regimen and exercise programs in women. J Appl Physiol 1997;83(1):270–279.

31. Kraemer WJ, Volek JS, Clark KL, et al. Influence of exercise training on physiological and performance changes with weight loss in men. Med Sci Sports Exerc 1999;31:1320–1329.

32. Jakicic JM. Physical activity considerations for the treatment and prevention of obesity. Am J Clin Nutr 2005;82(1 Suppl):226S–229S.

33. Oken BS, Zajdel D, Kishiyama S, et al. Randomized, controlled, six-month trial of yoga in healthy seniors: effects on cognition and quality of life. Altern Ther Health Med 2006;12(1):40–47.

34. Williams KA, Petronis J, Smith D, et al. Effect of iyengar yoga therapy for chronic low back pain. Pain 2005;115:107–117.

35. Gallagher KI, Jakicic JM, Otto AD, et al. Examination of twelve month changes in body weight and body composition following alternative forms of exercise. Med Sci Sports Exerc 2005;37(5(suppl): S339.

36. Nagle EF, Otto AD, Jakicic JM, et al. Effects of aquatic plus walking exercise on weight loss and function in sedentary obese females. Med Sci Sports Exerc 2003;35(5 (suppl):S136.

37. Tudor-Locke C, Bassett DR. How many steps/day are enought? Preliminary pedometer indices for public health. Sports Med 2004;34(1):1–8.

38. Yamanouchi K, Takashi T, Chikada K, et al. Daily walking combined with diet therapy is a useful means for obese NIDDM patients not only to reduce body weight but also to improve insulin sensitivity. Diabetes Care 1995;18(6):775–778.

39. Duncan JJ, Gordon NF, Scott CB. Women walking for health and fitness: how much is enough? JAMA 1991;266(23):3295–3299.

40. Barlow CE, Kohl HW, Gibbons LW, et al. Physical activity, mortality, and obesity. Int J Obes 1995;19: S41–S44.

41. Farrell SW, Braun L, Barlow CE, et al. The relation of body mass index, cardiorespiratory fitness, and all-cause mortality in women. Obes Res 2002;10(6):417–423.

42. Lee CD, Blair SN, Jackson AS. Cardiorespiratory fitness, body composition, and all-cause and cardiovascular disease mortality in men. Am J Clin Nutr 1999;69(3):373–380.

43. Wei M, Kampert J, Barlow CE, et al. Relationship between low cardiorespiratory fitness and mortality in normal-weight, overweight, and obese men. JAMA 1999;282(16):1547–1553.

44. Church TS, LaMonte MJ, Barlow CE, et al. Cardiorespiratory fitness and body mass index as predictors of cardiovascular disease mortality among men with diabetes. Arch Intern Med 2005;165:2114–2120.

45. DeBusk R, Stenestrand U, Sheehan M, et al. Training effects of long versus short bouts of exercise in healthy subjects. Am J Cardiol 1990;65:1010–1013.

46. Ebisu T. Splitting the distances of endurance training: on cardiovascular endurance and blood lipids. Jap J Phys Edu. 1985;30:37–43.

47. Jakicic JM, Wing RR, Butler BA, et al. Prescribing exercise in multiple short bouts versus one continuous bout: effects on adherence, cardiorespiratory fitness, and weight loss in overweight women. Int J Obes 1995;19:893–901.

17

Motivational Interviewing in Medical Settings

Application to Obesity Conceptual Issues and Evidence Review

Ken R. Resnicow, PhD, MHS
and Abdul Shaikh, PhD

CONTENTS

INTRODUCTION
OVERVIEW OF MI
IDENTIFICATION OF PRIOR STUDIES
RESEARCH PRIORITIES
CONCLUSION
REFERENCES

Summary

Counseling by health care professionals represents a potentially important component of the public health response to rising rates of obesity in the United States. One promising approach to weight control counseling is motivational interviewing (MI). This manuscript explores conceptual issues related to the application of MI for the prevention and treatment of obesity in medical practice. Given the paucity of studies on MI and obesity, we examine what is known about the application of MI to adult diet and physical activity behaviors, as well as the use of MI to modify weight, diet, and activity in children and adolescents. We begin with a brief overview of MI and describe some nuances of applying this approach to obesity counseling. Recommendations for future research and clinical practice are also presented.

Key Words: Obesity; motivational interviewing; counseling; client-centered.

INTRODUCTION

Obesity and its medical and economic sequelae have risen dramatically in the United States over the past 30 yr *(1–4)*. Although slowing or reversing this trend will require concerted effort at multiple levels of intervention, counseling by health care professionals represents an important component of the public health response. However, there are significant barriers to counseling for health care practitioners, and as a result, both the efficacy and reach of clinical interventions have been substantially limited *(5–8)*.

From: *Contemporary Endocrinology: Treatment of the Obese Patient*
Edited by: R. F. Kushner and D. H. Bessesen © Humana Press Inc., Totowa, NJ

Patients who receive advice on how to control their weight are significantly more likely to try to lose weight, but fewer than half of obese adults report that their health care professional advised them to lose weight *(9–13)*. One study found that although 65% of patients received information on the health benefits of weight loss, only 37% were given specific advice on how to control their weight *(10)*. Obese individuals with obesity-related comorbidities are more likely to receive weight management counseling *(10,11)*, which suggests that counseling is used more for secondary than primary prevention. Key system-level barriers to nutrition and activity counseling include time constraints, lack of organizational support, lack of referral mechanisms, and poor financial incentives *(8,9,12,14)*.

Perhaps more important, health care practitioners report low confidence in their ability to counsel their patients, and they also question the efficacy of behavioral counseling *(6,15–19)*. In one study, for example, 67% of primary care physicians agreed that lack of training in counseling skills was a barrier to nutrition counseling, whereas 50% felt that confidence in their ability to counsel patients about diet was a barrier to nutrition counseling *(6)*. Similar factors appear operative among pediatric practitioners. Kolagotla and Adams *(15)* found that only 30% of pediatricians felt that their efficacy for obesity counseling was good to excellent and only 10% felt obesity counseling was effective. In another study, only 26% of pediatricians felt "quite" to "extremely" competent to counsel overweight youth and only 37% felt "quite" to "extremely" comfortable providing such treatment *(20)*. Almost 80% of pediatricians report feeling "very frustrated" treating pediatric obesity *(20)*.

Low practitioner confidence in the skills and perceptions of treatment futility appear in part to stem from frustration over what practitioners perceive as low patient motivation and poor behavioral adherence *(15,16)*. Perceived patient indifference likely decreases practitioner efficacy as well as perceived treatment utility, which act synergistically to discourage practitioners from attempting to intervene. Importantly, these factors appear to be even more cogent inhibitors than lack of time or reimbursement, and they may be more amenable to intervention. Yet, despite low confidence in their counseling skills, practitioners are interested in improving their behavioral skills *(6,16,17,21)*.

One promising approach to weight control counseling that may address both clinician efficacy and treatment efficacy is motivational interviewing (MI). As originally described by Miller *(22)* and more fully discussed in a seminal text by Miller and Rollnick *(23)*, MI has been used extensively in the addiction field *(22,24–26)*. Numerous randomized trials have demonstrated its clinical efficacy for addictive behaviors *(27,28)*. Over the past 10 yr, there has been considerable interest from health care practitioners in adapting MI to address various nonaddictive, health-related and chronic disease behaviors *(28–38)*.

This chapter will explore conceptual issues related to the application of MI for the prevention and treatment of obesity in adults and youth. Given the paucity of studies on MI and obesity, we will examine what is known about the application of MI to adult diet and physical activity behaviors, as well as investigate the use of MI to modify other behaviors in children and adolescents. We begin with a brief overview of MI and describe some nuances of applying this approach to weight control.

OVERVIEW OF MI

MI is an egalitarian, empathetic "way of being" that manifests through specific techniques and strategies such as reflective listening and agenda setting. One of the goals of

MI is assisting individuals to work through their ambivalence about behavior change. As a result, MI appears to be particularly effective for individuals who are initially less ready to change *(23,25,37,39,40)*. The tone of MI is nonjudgmental, empathetic, and encouraging. Counselors establish a nonconfrontational and supportive climate in which clients feel comfortable expressing both the positive and negative aspects of their current behavior. Ambivalence is fully explored and at least partially resolved prior to moving toward change. Many counseling models rely heavily on therapist insight or traditional patient and nutrition education methods that emphasize information exchange. In contrast, a client engaged in MI is expected to do much of the psychological work. There is generally no direct attempt to dismantle denial, to confront irrational or maladaptive beliefs, or to convince or persuade. Instead, the goal is to help clients think about and verbally express their own reasons for and against change and how their current behavior or health status affects their ability to achieve their life goals or live out their core values. A primary goal of MI is to encourage clients to make fully informed and deeply contemplated life choices, even if the decision is not to change.

To achieve these ends, MI counselors rely heavily on reflective listening and positive affirmations. The assumption is that behavior change is affected more by motivation than information. Whereas the essence of MI lies in its spirit, there are specific techniques and strategies that, when used effectively, help ensure that such a spirit is evoked. In addition to reflective listening, core MI techniques include allowing the client to interpret information, agenda setting, rolling with resistance, building discrepancy, and eliciting self-motivational statements or "change talk." As recently noted by Rollnick et al. *(41)*, MI can be considered a form of guiding, as opposed to more directive methods that rely on advice and persuasion.

Reflective listening can be conceptualized as a form of hypothesis testing. The hypothesis can be stated in generic terms as "If I heard you correctly, this is what I think you are saying ..." or "Where you are going with this..." Reflections, particularly by counselors who are new to the technique, often begin with the phrase "It sounds like..." More skilled counselors often phrase their reflections as more direct statements such as "You are having trouble with ...", leaving off the assumed "It sounds like..." The goals of reflecting include demonstrating that the counselor has heard and is trying to understand the client, affirming the client's thoughts and feelings, and helping the client continue the process of self-discovery. One of the most important elements of mastering MI is suppressing the instinct to respond with questions or advice. Questions can be biased by what the counselor may be interested in hearing about rather than what the client wants or needs to explore. Reflecting helps ensure that the direction of the encounter remains client-driven. Reflections involve several levels of complexity or depth *(42)*.

The simplest level tests whether the counselor understood the content of the client's statement. Deeper levels of reflection explore the meaning or feeling behind what was said. Effective deeper-level reflections can be thought of as the next sentence or next paragraph in the story—i.e., "where the client is going with it." A high level of reflective listening involves selectively reinforcing positive change talk that may be embedded in a litany of barriers. Similarly, skilled MI counselors selectively reflect statements that build efficacy by focusing on prior successful efforts or reframing past unsuccessful attempts as practice rather than failure.

In standard medical practice, practitioners often provide information about the risks of continuing a behavior or the benefits of change with the intent of persuasion. With regard to obesity counseling, a traditional counseling statement might be, "It is very important that get control of your weight. It can cause problems with diabetes and blood pressure and the risks are significant." In this style of communication the practitioner often attempts to push motivation by increasing perceived risk. In contrast, information is presented through MI by first eliciting the person's understanding and information needs, then providing this in a more neutral manner, followed by eliciting what this means for them, with a question such as, "How do you make sense of all this?" MI practitioners avoid persuasion with "predigested" health messages and instead allow clients to process information and find their own personal relevance. To this end, the guideline "elicit-provide-elicit" has been proposed as a framework for exchanging information in the spirit of MI.

Confronting clients can lead to defensiveness, rapport breakage, and, ultimately, poor outcomes (22). Therefore, MI counselors avoid argumentation and instead "roll with resistance." An MI encounter resembles a dance more than a wrestling match (43). For example, if a patient raises doubts that his or her weight poses any problem, MI practitioners are trained to reflect the patient's doubt and then provide opportunities for the patient to voice any concerns he or she may have about remaining overweight or gaining weight rather than stating facts to counter such beliefs. In cases where resistance is severe, practitioners may use an amplified negative reflection. For example, a counselor may comment, "It appears that you see no real problem with your weight." This potentially risky strategy is designed to "unstick" the entrenched client by short-circuiting the "yes-but" cycle.

A core principle of MI is that individuals are more likely to accept and act upon opinions that they voice themselves (44). The more a person argues for a position, the greater his or her commitment to it often becomes. Therefore, clients are encouraged to express their own reasons and plans for change (or lack thereof). This is referred to as eliciting change talk. A technique to elicit change talk is the use of importance/confidence rulers (39,43,45). This strategy begins with two questions: (1) "On a scale from zero to 10, with 10 being the highest, how important is it to you to change your [insert target behavior]?" and (2) "On a scale from zero to 10, with 10 being the highest, assuming you wanted to change this behavior, how confident are you that you could change [insert target behavior]?" These two questions assess the client's importance and confidence for change, respectively (24,45). Clinicians follow these questions with two probes: (1) "Why did you not choose a lower number, like a 1 or a 2?" and (2) "What would it take to get you to a 9 or a 10?" These probes elicit positive change talk and ideas for potential solutions from the client. To help patients establish the discrepancy between their current behavior and their personal core values or life goals, our group has developed a values list tailored for adult patients as well as parents seeking to improve their children's weight (see Table 1). Patients identify what is important to them and practitioners then probe to see if they can find any connections between the values they selected and the health issue at hand.

Three Communication Styles: Route to Integration

A challenge for practitioners is understanding how to fit MI into their everyday practice. Some view it as a highly specialized skill developed and best delivered by psychologists, which is difficult for the typical physician to integrate effectively. Yet, it is also striking how brief consultations by skilled physicians can approach the spirit and even the letter of MI. One resolution to this "intimidation factor," proposed by

Table 1
MI Values List for Counseling Parents of Overweight Children

Values for your child	Values for you	Values for your family
Be healthy	Good parent	Cohesive
Be strong	Responsible	Healthy
Have many friends	Disciplined	Peaceful meals
Be fit	Good spouse	Getting along
Have high self-esteem	Respected at home	Spending time together
Not being teased	On top of things	Be able to communicate feelings
Not feeling left out	Spiritual	Fulfill our potential

Rollnick et al. *(42)*, is to place MI within a model of communication that comprises three naturally occurring communication styles: directing, guiding, and following. When practitioners use a directing style, they primarily inform patients about what the practitioner thinks they should do and why they should do it. This is similar what is often referred to as anticipatory guidance. Conversely, when practitioners use a more guiding style, they rely less on persuasion and instead encourage patients to explore their motivations and aspirations. Following involves understanding and tracking the patient's story, and is typically used in the early phrase of a consultation and under special circumstances like when responding to a bereaved individual. Skillfulness is defined as the ability to move flexibly between these styles according to patient needs; the guiding style is seen as particularly suited to consultations involving health behavior change, and MI is defined as a refined form of this naturally occurring guiding style. Seen in this light, the task for practitioners in obesity counseling is to get better at guiding while also suppressing the instinct to direct.

Applying MI to Obesity: Conceptual and Pragmatic Issues

There are several aspects of obesity counseling that pose unique challenges for the MI counselor. First, for pediatric obesity, depending on the age of the patient, the intervention may occur directly with the parent(s), directly with the child, or both. There is some evidence that older obese children do not benefit from the involvement of their parents, whereas parent involvement may be beneficial for younger children *(46)*. However, it is not known at what ages youth and parents should be seen alone versus together. For both youth and adults, the practitioner needs to understand that obesity is not a behavior *per se*. Therefore, a key task for clinicians is to work with patients to identify what behaviors contribute to their own or their child's weight status and use agenda setting strategies to determine which behaviors they feel are most amenable to intervention (Table 1).

Although MI has been established as a useful method for helping individuals overcome resistance and clarify motivation, it is important to note that additional strategies, such as behavior therapy or cognitive behavioral therapy, may be needed once an individual decides to attempt behavior change. There is an MI-consistent means for delivering treatment and at this stage of care, MI should perhaps be conceived as a platform for treatment delivery rather than the primary treatment modality; as background rather than foreground.

IDENTIFICATION OF PRIOR STUDIES

Studies were identified by electronic search of the Medline database using various combinations of key search terms, including motivational interviewing, motivational enhancement, obesity, nutrition, diet, and physical activity. Additional studies were identified though bibliographies of published studies and informal communication with peers. Given the lack of published randomized trials of MI for treatment or prevention of obesity, we decided to include in our review obesity pilot studies as well as studies of MI to modify diet or physical activity behavior. Both youth and adult studies are reviewed.

Review of Studies

We first review studies in which MI was employed directly to modify weight in children or adolescents. We then examine studies in youth where MI was used to address dyslipidemia *(34)* or diabetes *(47,48)*. Next, we examine adult studies in which MI was used to modify dietary and/or physical activity behaviors *(37,49–54)* (Table 2).

MI Studies Targeting Pediatric Obesity

We identified two studies in which MI was used to intervene in pediatric obesity. The first of these studies, the Healthy Lifestyles Pilot Study, focused on prevention of overweight among children 3 to 7 yr old. The second study, Go Girls, was a multicomponent intervention for overweight African American adolescents aged 12 to 16 that included MI as a key intervention element.

HEALTHY LIFESTYLES PILOT STUDY

The Healthy Lifestyles Study (HLS) (unpublished data) and Go Girls was conducted in 2004–2005 as a partnership of the Centers for Disease Control and Prevention, the American Academy of Pediatrics (AAP), and the American Dietetic Association. The primary aim of the HLS pilot was to examine the feasibility and potential efficacy of pediatrician and dietitian MI counseling for preventing childhood obesity in primary care pediatrics. Study sites were members of the AAP Pediatric Research in Office Settings (PROS) network, which is a practice-based research network established by the AAP in 1986 *(55)*. Fifteen PROS practices were randomly assigned to one of three conditions: control; minimal intervention; or intensive intervention. Five practices were allocated to each arm. The intervention phase lasted 6 mo. Each of the 15 PROS practices was asked to recruit 10 patients. Subject eligibility included children ages 3 to 7 yr with either a BMI-for-age-and-sex between the 85th and 95th percentiles or a combination of at least one parent with a BMI greater than 30 and a BMI-for-age-and-sex between the 50th and 85th percentiles. Parents in all groups were administered questionnaires at baseline and again 6 mo later. The only intervention provided to participants in the control group consisted of two safety education tip sheets. Parents of children in the minimal intervention group received a single, brief MI counseling session from their pediatrician 1 mo after baseline. Pediatricians in the minimal intervention group were trained to provide counseling in a 2-d MI workshop. In contrast, participants in the intensive intervention group engaged in four MI counseling sessions. Two sessions were led by the patient's pediatrician, and two sessions were guided by a dietitian. These counseling sessions were delivered at 1 mo and 3 mo post-enrollment. The physicians

Table 2

MI Pediatric Weight, Diet, and Activity Trials: Study Design

Study	Starting n	Age	Outcome/Design	Intervention	Interventionist
Healthy Lifestyles Dietz, Schwartz Wasserman, Slora Resnicow, Myers Hamre (unpublished)	93	3–7	BMI Pilot	Standard Care Mod = 1 MI (MD) High = 2 MI (MD) + 2 MI (RD)	Pediatricians Dietitians
Go Girls Resnicow et al. 2005	147	12–16	BMI RCT	Multicomponent Group session & 4–6 phone MI	Health Educators Psychologists
DISC Berg-Smith et al. 1999	127	13–17	Diet Lipids No Control	1 in-person MI 1 phone MI	Health Educators Dietitians
DIABETES Channon et al. 2003	40	14–18	HBA1c Nonparticipants as controls	Variable 1–9 mean 4.7	Investigator
Knight et al. 2003	20	13–16	Perceptions about DM	6 1-h sessions Qualitative response	RN Senior registrar

and dietitians were trained at a joint, 2-d MI workshop. The dietitian-led sessions were longer than the sessions with the pediatricians, generally in the range of 30 to 45 min. Sick visits continued as usual for children in both groups. Recruitment occurred from April through November 2004. One minimal intervention practice dropped out, leaving a total of 93 enrolled patients from 14 practices.

To assess competence in MI skill, clinicians participating in the HLS pilot completed a measure of MI fidelity developed by the HLS investigators called the 1-PASS. The 1-PASS consists of self-evaluation rating forms for one or two patient encounters on which performance on several MI dimensions is scored on a scale of 1 to 7. Scores of 4.0 and higher are considered as indicators of adequate to proficient MI skill. Using audiotapes of the HLS intervention encounters, a trained psychologist rated each MI session using One-Pass MI Fidelity Rating Systemm (1-PASS) and then discussed her score with each clinician. Overall scores for the first patient encounters ranged from 3.2 for moderate-intensity pediatricians to 4.4 for high-intensity dietitians. Overall scores were slightly higher in the second encounters, ranging from 3.7 to 5.8 for pediatricians and dietitians combined. For the six clinicians who participated in two supervisor feedback sessions, mean MI skills scores increased 1.1 points between the first and second encounters.

A subset of 16 parents, consisting of eight parents from the minimal intervention group and eight parents from the high-intensity intervention group, was asked to rate their reactions to their counseling sessions. Overall, 88% of parents reported being very satisfied with their pediatrician visit and 100% reported being very satisfied with their dietitian visit. Parents' ratings of the "client-centeredness" (e.g., "listened to me," "asked my opinion") of their encounters with the pediatricians and dietitians were highly positive. In addition, 100% of parents indicated that they talked about the same amount of time as their pediatrician or dietitian during the visit, which is the target proportion of client participation for MI counseling encounters. Results of the trial on BMI will be available in 2007.

Go Girls

Go Girls was a church-based nutrition and physical activity program designed for overweight African American adolescent females (56). Ten predominantly middle-socioeconomic-status churches were randomized to either a high-intensity (20–26 sessions) or moderate-intensity (6 sessions) culturally tailored behavioral group intervention delivered over 6 mo. Each session included an experiential behavioral activity, approx 30 min of physical activity, and preparation and tasting of healthy foods. In the high-intensity group, girls also received 4 to 6 MI telephone counseling calls. Counselors were either health educators with master's degrees or doctorally trained psychologists. All counselors received 2 d of experiential MI training by the first author of this chapter, plus ongoing clinical supervision by doctoral-level psychologists. The telephone calls were synchronized with the group sessions to ensure that the MI calls focused on participants' plans and progress regarding the same topics covered during each weekly group session. The calls lasted approx 20 to 30 min each and were generally conducted in the afternoon or evening.

From the 10 churches, 123 girls completed the baseline and 6-mo follow-up assessments. The primary outcome was BMI. The 6-mo assessments indicated a net difference of 0.5 BMI units between the high and moderate intensity. This difference was not statistically significant ($p = 0.20$). Additionally, there was no association between change in BMI and the number of MI calls completed in the high-intensity group. An additional follow-up assessment was conducted at 1 yr post-baseline, and findings mirrored those found at 6 mo.

MI Studies Addressing Dyslipidemia and Diabetes

DIETARY INTERVENTION STUDY IN CHILDREN

The Dietary Intervention Study in Children (DISC) was a multicenter, randomized controlled trial sponsored by the National Heart, Lung, and Blood Institute to assess the efficacy of dietary counseling to decrease elevated serum lipids (LDL-C). Children with elevated LDL-C entered the initial clinical trial when they were 8 to 10 yr of age *(34)*. As the intervention cohort moved into adolescence, the investigators elected to add an MI-based intervention to "renew" adherence to the prescribed diet among the original intervention group (there was no control group for this phase). The counselors were primarily masters-level health educators and dietitians who received 18 h of MI training. Each study participant received one in-person MI session and one follow-up session that was conducted either in person or by telephone. Twenty-four-hour recall data from the first 127 youths to complete the two-session protocol indicated that the proportion of calories from fat and dietary cholesterol was significantly reduced at the 3-mo follow-up assessment. The mean proportion of calories from fat also decreased from 27.7 to 25.6% ($p < 0.001$), and overall dietary adherence scores improved. When asked about their reaction to the counseling, 74% of the youths reported being satisfied or very satisfied.

OTHER STUDIES TARGETING DIABETES

In a pilot study, Channon et al. tested the impact of MI on 22 adolescents, aged 14 to 18 yr, with diabetes *(47)*. Participating youth received between one and nine MI sessions each, with an average of 4.7 sessions over 6 mo. The focus of the MI sessions consisted of awareness building (analyzing pros and cons), finding alternatives, problem solving, goal setting, and minimizing confrontation. Between 8 wk and 6 mo after the end of the intervention phase, patients who had received MI showed a significant reduction in HbA1c, from an average baseline measure of 10.8% to approx 10.0%.

Knight and et al. *(48)* administered an MI-based group intervention in six weekly, 1-h sessions to six youths, ages 13 to 16, with poorly controlled Type 1 diabetes. The intervention included externalizing conversations as well as MI. Participation in the MI-based group was compared with a "usual care" control group ($n = 14$). At the 6-mo follow-up assessment, adolescents who had received the group MI were more likely than those youtsh in the control group to display positive shifts in their perception of diabetes such as increased feelings of control and acceptance. Changes in behavior or physiologic outcomes were not assessed.

Studies on Diet and Physical Activity Among Adults

We identified eight controlled outcome studies and one pilot study in adults where MI was used to modify diet and physical activity behaviors (*see* Tables 3 and 4) *(35,37,49–54,57–59)*. In none of these studies was weight the primary target.

For adult diet and activity trials in which data were available, outcomes are reported as standardized effect sizes and presented as the mean group differences divided by standard deviations according to the method of Hedges and Olkin *(60)*. Effect sizes were

Table 3
MI Adult Diet and Activity Trials: Study Design

Author	Starting n	Outcome	Design	Interventionist
Resnicow 2001[a] Eat for Life	1011	F & V	Control Self-help Self-help + MI × 2	RD
Resnicow 2004[a] Body & Soul	1022	F & V	Control Churchwide + peer counseling × 2	Peer Counselors
Resnicow 2005[a] Healthy Body/Spirit	1056	F & V Exercise	Control Self-help Self-help + MI × 4	Master or higher Psychologists
Bowen 2002[a]	175	Fat intake	Standard care 3 MI (phone or in person)	Dietitian
Harland, 1999[a]	523	Exercise	No MI 1 MI × 40min 6 MI × 40min	Health educator
Mhurchu, 1998[a]	121	Diet & exercise Weight loss	Standard care Standard integrated with MI	Dietitian
Smith, 1997[a]	22	Diabetes Glycemic control	Standard care Standard care + 3 MI	Psychologists
Woollard, 1995[a]	166	Blood pressure Weight loss	Standard care 5 MI by phone (low) 6 MI face to face (high)	Nurses
Wollard, 2003[a]	212	Blood pressure Weight loss	Standard care Monthly by phone, 10–15 min (low) Monthly face to face, 1 h (high)	Nurses

[a]Randomized trial

either computed directly from data available in published studies, obtained from prior meta-analyses (27,61), or calculated from raw data provided by the study investigators.

Smith et al. (35) conducted a pilot study involving 22 overweight women (41% African American) with non-insulin-dependent diabetes mellitus. Subjects were randomized to receive either a 16-wk behavioral weight control group intervention or the same intervention with the addition of three individual MI sessions delivered by experienced psychologists. One MI session was delivered before the group treatment began, and two were delivered mid-treatment. The MI encounters included individualized feedback on glycemic control to help develop the discrepancy between participants' current status and desired goals. At the 4-mo post-test, the 16 women who received the MI showed significantly better glycemic control, they better monitored their blood glucose, and they attended more sessions than those in comparison group. No group effects on weight loss were observed.

Table 4
MI Adult Diet and Activity Trials: Results

Author	Time to FU (wk)	Outcome	Results/effect size
Resnicow 2001 Eat for Life	52	**F & V** MI vs control MI vs Self-help	$.58^a$ $.51^a$
Resnicow 2004 Body & Soul	24	F & V 2-item F & V 36-item	$.39^a$ $.18^a$
Resnicow 2005 Healthy Body/Healthy Spirit	52	**F & V** MI vs control MI vs self-help **PA** MI vs control MI vs self-help	$.30^a$ $.20^a$ $.24^a$ 0.0
Bowen 2002	52	Fat intake	$.39^a$
Harland 1999	12 12 52 52	PA 1 session PA 6 sessions PA 1 session PA 6 sessions	$.49^a$ $.46^a$ 0 .17
Mhurchu 1998	13	Serum cholesterol BMI	.03 .25
Smith 1997	18	Glycemic control Weight loss	$.36^a$ .34
Woollard 1995	18	SBP DBP Weight	$1.24^{a,b}$ $1.94^{a,b}$ $1.75kg^{a,b}$
Woollard 2003	18	SBP DBP Weight	3.3 mmHg^b 1.1 mmHg^b $.5 \text{ kg}^b$

[a]Effect significant $p < 0.05$
[b]High-intervention vs control group

Mhurchu et al. *(52)* randomly assigned 121 patients with hyperlipidemia to receive either three MI sessions or a standard dietary intervention, both of which were delivered by a dietitian. At 3 mo post-baseline, there were no group differences in dietary habits or BMI. Analysis of audiotaped counseling sessions indicated greater use of MI techniques such as reflective listening in the experimental condition, whereas more advice giving occurred in the standard intervention. As the authors suggested, the efficacy of MI may have been compromised because 80% of the sample was already making some dietary changes at baseline.

Woollard et al. *(57)* randomly assigned 166 hypertensive patients in general medical practices to one of three groups: a high-intensity MI intervention consisting of six 45-min sessions every fourth week; a low-intensity MI comprising a single face-to-face session plus five brief telephone contacts; or a control group receiving no MI counseling. All MI interventions were delivered by nurse counselors. Both intervention groups also received usual care plus an educational manual. After 18 wk, there were no significant differences between the two MI groups. However, the high-intensity MI group had significantly reduced their weight and blood pressure relative to the control group, whereas the low-intensity MI group significantly decreased its alcohol and salt intake relative to the control group. Physical activity and smoking were not significantly altered in any of the groups. A follow-up study by Woollard et al. *(50,51)* among 212 adults with high cardiovascular risk using a similar intervention protocol, again delivered by nurses, found no significant effects on blood pressure, weight, or serum lipids at 18 wk (not shown in table).

Harland et al. *(53)* recruited 523 adult patients from a general medical practice. Participants were sedentary but otherwise healthy. The study had four intervention groups. Two groups received a single 40-min MI session, and two groups received six 40-min MI sessions delivered over 12 wk. Approximately half the participants in the MI groups also received vouchers for free aerobics classes. There was also a control group that received neither MI nor vouchers. At the 12-wk follow-up, self-reported physical activity improved in the four aggregate intervention groups relative to the controls (38% improved vs 16%), but there were no significant differences between the "high" and "low" MI groups. Twelve months later, there were no significant differences in physical activity between the intervention groups, either combined or separately, relative to the control group. One limitation of this study is that participants in the "high" group, on average, attended only three MI sessions.

Resnicow et al. *(37)* conducted the Eat for Life (EFL) trial, a multicomponent intervention designed to increase fruit and vegetable consumption among African American adults recruited through black churches. Fourteen churches were randomly assigned to one of three treatment conditions: comparison; culturally tailored self-help (SH) intervention with one telephone cue; and SH intervention, one cue call, and three MI counseling calls. The cue calls were intended to increase the use of the SH intervention materials and were not structured as MI contacts. The MI counselors were either registered dietitians or dietetic interns. All counselors participated in three 2-h MI training sessions and received ongoing supervision. Fruit and vegetable intake was assessed at baseline and at 12 mo using three food frequency questionnaires (FFQs). Self-reported fruit and vegetable intake at 12 mo was significantly greater in the MI group than the comparison and SH-only groups. The net differences between the MI and the comparison group were 1.38, 1.03, and 1.21 servings of fruit and vegetables per day for the 2-item, 7-item, and 36-item FFQs, respectively. The net difference between the MI and SH group was 1.14, 1.10, and 0.97 servings for the 2-item, 7-item, and 36-item FFQs.

The Body & Soul project was a collaborative effort between two research universities, the national office of the American Cancer Society (ACS), and the National Cancer Institute (NCI). The Body & Soul intervention was constructed from two prior church-based behavior change programs, Black Churches United for Better Health *(62,63)* and Eat for Life. The Body & Soul intervention comprised several elements, including church-wide activities, distribution of self-help materials, and peer counseling. The peer counseling component was directly adapted from the MI protocol employed in the Eat for Life study. Whereas in Eat for Life the MI was delivered by trained dietitians, in Body & Soul MI was delivered by lay church members trained by project staff. These trained church members are subsequently referred to volunteer advisors. Churches were asked to identify individuals, preferably with a college degree or higher and a background in a "helping profession" (e.g., teacher, psychologist, nurse, counselor, social worker), who were willing to attend a 1.5-d training, make two intervention calls to at least five different church members, and undergo a tape-recorded evaluation to determine whether they met performance criteria. The training provided general skills in asking open-ended questions and reflective listening, as well as specific strategies to elicit discussion about fruit and vegetable consumption. At the end of the training, participants were audiotaped conducting a simulated encounter with another trainee using the semistructured protocol provided by the research team. Tapes were coded by two staff members experienced in MI. The coding system, based on the method developed by Miller and Mount (64), included 17 discrete skills, each scored on a scale of 1 to 7. Participants scoring a mean of 4.5 or higher across the 17 items were considered to possess adequate competence. Of the 88 individuals trained, 64 (73%) met competency criteria and were certified as volunteer advisors. Of those church members receiving at least one call, 72% reported being very satisfied with their volunteer advisors.

A total of 16 churches were randomized into an intervention or a comparison group of eight churches each. One comparison church dropped out, leaving 15 completing the baseline and follow-up surveys. One intervention "church" in California was an aggregate church that included five small, affiliated churches that were treated as a single unit for analytic purposes. All churches had a predominantly African American membership. The primary outcome for the study was fruit and vegetable intake, which was assessed by two self-report FFQs at baseline and 6 mo post-enrollment. One FFQ was the National Cancer Institute's 19-item fruit and vegetable assessing intake in the past month (65) and the second scale consisted of two items to assess usual fruit and vegetable intake on a daily basis (66). At baseline, a total of 1022 individuals were recruited across the 15 churches. Of the initial sample, 854 (84%) were assessed at 6 mo. At the time of the post-test, participants in the intervention group reported significantly greater consumption of fruit and vegetables than those in the comparison group. The adjusted post-test differences were 0.6 servings per day for the two-item measure and 1.2 servings per day for the 17-item measure. These differences equate to standardized effect sizes of 0.24 and 0.19 standard deviation units for the two-item and 17-item measures, respectively.

In a study by Bowen et al. (49), 175 participants from the Women's Health Initiative (WHI) dietary intervention study from three clinical centers were assigned randomly to either intervention or control status. Participants assigned to the intervention group received three individual MI counseling sessions with a dietitian, plus the usual WHI dietary modification intervention. Participants randomly assigned to the control group received only the usual WHI dietary modification intervention. The percent of energy from fat was estimated at baseline and again at 12 mo using an FFQ. The change in percent energy from fat between baseline and 12 mo was −1.2% for intervention subjects and +1.4% for control participants, which yielded a significant net difference of 2.6% ($p < 0.001$).

The final adult intervention reviewed is the recently reported Healthy Body/Healthy Spirit study (54). Healthy Body/Healthy Spirit was a multicomponent intervention to increase fruit and vegetable consumption and physical activity among a socioeconomically diverse sample of African Americans through black churches. The fruit and vegetable intervention was adapted from the Eat for Life trial. Sixteen churches were randomly assigned to three intervention conditions. Group 1 received standard educational materials; Group 2 received culturally targeted self-help nutrition and physical activity materials; and Group 3 received the same intervention as Group 2, plus four MI telephone counseling calls delivered over the course of 1 yr. The MI intervention was delivered by telephone by master's- or doctoral-level psychologists who received approx 16 h of initial training and 12 h of ongoing individual/group supervision. The four MI calls were delivered at approx 4, 12, 26, and 40 wk. Two of the four MI calls addressed fruit and vegetable intake, and two calls addressed physical activity. During the first and third calls, participants chose which topics they would like to address. If participants elected to address fruit and vegetable consumption during their first call, physical activity was discussed in the second call. This choice was repeated at the third call. Additional details regarding the MI intervention can be found elsewhere (54,67).

At baseline, a total of 1056 individuals were recruited across 16 churches, of which 906 (86%) were reassessed at 1 yr. The cohort had an average age of 46 (range 18–86) and was 76% female. The primary outcomes for Healthy Body/Healthy Spirit were self-reported fruit and vegetable intake and minutes of physical activity. At 12 mo, Groups 2 and 3 showed significant positive changes in both fruit and vegetable intake and physical activity. Changes were somewhat larger for fruit and vegetable intake. There was a clear additive effect for the MI calls on fruit and vegetable intake, but this effect was not replicated with physical activity. Because Groups 1 and 2 received no counseling, the effects of MI on fruit and vegetable consumption could be attributed to generic effects of attention or other elements of counseling not unique to MI.

Summary of Outcomes for Adult Diet and Activity Trials

With the exception of the studies by Mhurchu et al. (52) and Woollard et al. (50,51), each study reviewed showed a significant effect favoring the MI group on at least one main outcome. In all three studies in which MI was used to modify fruit and vegetable intake, significant effects were observed. In the four studies in which weight was at least a secondary target outcome, only one, by Woollard et al. (57), found a significant effect. Although Harland and colleagues (53) found a short-term effect of MI on physical activity, significant long-term outcomes in this study and Healthy Body/Healthy Spirit (54) were not observed. Effect sizes in positive studies generally were in the small to moderate range, 0.20 to 0.50, as defined by Cohen (68) (see Table 4).

RESEARCH PRIORITIES

The studies reviewed here indicate that MI has potential as a component of obesity prevention and treatment in medical practice. Data from youth and adult studies suggest that MI can be effective in modifying diet and, at least short-term, physical activity behaviors. However, data from randomized clinical trials are needed to establish the efficacy of MI for weight control.

To establish the efficacy of MI for weight control, several methodologic issues will have to be addressed. First, it is important to address intervention fidelity. Failure to assess and statistically control for treatment fidelity can result in type III error. This occurs when negative or weak results are due to poor intervention delivery but are erroneously attributed to the failure of the intervention itself. Few studies have provided evidence of counselor competence or fidelity to MI. This is complicated by the fact that there is considerable variability in how MI is conceptualized, executed, and assessed across studies. There are no widely accepted criteria for what comprises an MI intervention or for measuring how rigorously these components are administered.

An important question that should be examined is the extent to which the effects of MI-informed interventions can be attributed to MI *per se* as opposed to more generic elements of counseling such as attention effects and empathy. A related problem is that in several positive studies, internal validity is threatened by the fact that the MI interventions were often additive to other interventions. Client contact was often not comparable across conditions, as the comparison groups did not receive any "sham" or alternative counseling. Determining the efficacy of MI with high internal validity can be achieved by comparing MI head-to-head with other counseling methods while holding dose and delivery modality constant. An example of this is Project MATCH *(26)*. An important issue for pediatric obesity is determining the appropriate age at which to begin intervention directly with youth, as opposed to their parents, and when, if at all, parents should be included in the counseling *(46)*.

Challenge of Technology Transfer

Many of the strategies and programs recommended for the medical management of obesity were developed and tested under efficacy conditions *(70,71)*. Under these circumstances, interventions are generally delivered by highly skilled practitioners, who typically receive extensive training and supervision. The extent to which research-based interventions can be replicated under real-world conditions remains unclear. Whereas the primary "gatekeepers" for detection and treatment of obesity appear to be primary care physicians, many (if not most) of the successful interventions were conducted by psychologists or behavioral specialists. This is also true for MI interventions, where counselors were again highly trained behavioral specialists. More research is needed to develop and test MI-based interventions that *a priori* are designed for delivery by physicians that account for limitations of medical training, its implicit "disease" orientation, practice structure, and reimbursement guidelines.

Recast Obesity as a Cluster of Heterogeneous Conditions: Consider the Obesities

Perhaps, like cancer, obesity should be considered not as one disease but a rubric of many diseases, each with a unique etiology, course, and treatment. As noted by Epstein et al. *(71)*: "Treating obesity as a homogenous condition, with all participants receiving a common intervention, might contribute to the mixed treatment outcomes that are reported" (p. 566). Factors operative in obesity include age, gender, dietary patterns, physical activity, socioeconomics, psychosocial issues, metabolism, comorbidities, familial/genetic determinants, and race/ethnicity/cultural characteristics. With each of these factors having a greater or lesser influence on obesity on an individual case, classification and subclassification schemes should be developed to adequately describe the heterogeneity of the obesities.

The reasons for energy imbalance can be highly variable across individuals, and treatment programs can be better tailored to these individual differences. For example, excess caloric intake could be caused by consuming high-fat foods or foods high in simple carbohydrates. And for some "high-fat" food consumers, excess caloric intake could be attributed to one or two foods, whereas for others excess intake could be attributed to a variety of foods. In addition to focusing on specific foods, tailoring could also account for eating patterns such as consuming large serving sizes, rapid eating, eating second helpings, or eating at "all you can eat" establishments. The same applies to activity patterns. Despite the numerous potential differences in behavioral patterns, our current detection and treatment algorithms often fail to account for such micro-level individual differences. An advantage of MI is that with its emphasis on "pulling" rather than "pushing," clinicians are in a better position to tailor interventions to the behavioral and psychological needs of their clients.

Recast Obesity as a Behavioral Rather than Medical Condition: Flip Nexus of Care to Behavioral Professionals

"To treat malaria, go to a physician. To prevent it, consult a mosquito controller." Documenting the severe medical consequences of obesity can help motivate patients, practitioners, and policy makers to attend to the epidemic. However, despite its numerous and severe physiologic medical sequelae, the origins of obesity (and the recent increase in its prevalence) are largely social and behavioral. This raises questions about our current treatment paradigm. The medical profession has been (perhaps *de facto*, rather than by design) designated as the primary gatekeeper charged with stemming the epidemic. In the current model, behavioral and nutritional professions have largely been cast as secondary resources—as treatment adjuncts. This has considerable implications for how we conceptualize obesity and how we reimburse those who care for it. Given the behavioral origins of the condition, perhaps we should reconsider the nexus of professional responsibility. A model that casts behavioral professionals as the first line in clinical care would be more consistent with the underlying etiology. This paradigm shift, however, would require dramatic alterations in how managed care reimburses behavioral counseling, including a de-emphasis on the comorbidities of obesity and a greater focus on the underlying behavioral and psychological causes as well as alteration for how the public perceives the role of behavioral and psychological professions. As part of this reconceptualization, individuals, rather than being viewed as suffering from obesity, might be seen as having a particular eating or activity problem. Obesity becomes the symptom rather than the disease. Creation of an obesity treatment subspecialty within psychology and/or health education, not unlike what has been done with HIV and substance use specialists, should be considered.

CONCLUSION

Ultimately, the essential question may not be whether MI is effective for control of obesity, but rather how "effective," in what populations, at what dose, and at what cost. Which health care providers are best able to deliver MI with sufficient fidelity, how much training is needed to raise their competence to adequate levels, and how best to impart clinical skills at various career stages should also be explored. How different health care delivery systems may be willing and able to incorporate MI into training and clinical guidelines and how health care providers are reimbursed for training and delivery of MI also merits examination.

REFERENCES

1. Finkelstein E, Fiebelkorn I, Wang G. National medical spending attributable to overweight and obesity: How much, and who's paying? Health Affairs 2003;W3:219–226.
2. Wolf A, Colditz GA. Current estimates of the economic cost of obesity in the United States. Obes Res 1998;6(2):97–106.
3. Must A, Spadano J, Coakley EH, et al. The disease burden associated with overweight and obesity. JAMA 1999;282(16):1523–1529.
4. Dietz W. Health consequences of obesity in youth: childhood predictors of adult disease. Pediatrics 1998;101(Suppl):518–525.
5. Grizzard T. Undertreatment of obesity. JAMA 2002;288(17):2177.
6. Kushner RF. Barriers to providing nutrition counseling by physicians: a survey of primary care practitioners. Prev Med 1995;24(6):546–552.
7. Manson JE, Skerrett PJ, Greenland P, et al. The escalating pandemics of obesity and sedentary lifestyle. A call to action for clinicians. Arch Intern Med 2004;164(3):249–258.
8. Nawaz H, Adams ML, Katz DL. Physician-patient interactions regarding diet, exercise, and smoking. Prev Med 2000;31(6):652–657.
9. Galuska DA, Will JC, Serdula MK, et al. Are health care professionals advising obese patients to lose weight? JAMA 1999;282(16):1576–1578.
10. Simkin-Silverman LR, Gleason KA, et al. Predictors of weight control advice in primary care practices: patient health and psychosocial characteristics. Prev Med 2005;40(1):71–82.
11. Sciamanna C, Tate D, Lang W, et al. Who reports receiving advice to lose weight? Results from a multi-state survey. Arch Intern Med 2000;160::2334–2339.
12. Ma J, Urizar GG Jr, Alehegn T, et al. Diet and physical activity counseling during ambulatory care visits in the United States. Prev Med 2004;39(4):815–822.
13. Scott JG, Cohen D, DiCicco-Bloom B, et al. Speaking of weight: how patients and primary care clinicians initiate weight loss counseling. Prev Med 2004;38(6):819–827.
14. Kolasa KM. Strategies to enhance effectiveness of individual based nutrition communications. Eur J Clin Nutr 2005;59 Suppl 1:S24–S29; discussion S30.
15. Kolagotla L, Adams W. Ambulatory management of childhood obesity. Obes Res 2004;12(2):275–283.
16. Story MT, Neumark-Stzainer DR, Sherwood NE, et al. Management of child and adolescent obesity: attitudes, barriers, skills, and training needs among health care professionals. Pediatrics 2002;110(1):210–214.
17. Perrin EM, Flower KB, Garrett J, et al. Preventing and treating obesity: pediatricians' self-efficacy, barriers, resources, and advocacy. Amb Pediatr 2005;5(3):150–156.
18. Rogers L, Bailey J, Gutin B, et al. Teaching resident physicians to provide exercise counseling: a needs assessment. Acad Med 2002;77(8):841–844.
19. Huang J, Yu H, Marin E, et al. Physicians' weight loss counseling in two public hospital primary care clinics. Acad Med 2004;79:156–161.
20. Jelalian E, Boergers J, Alday CS, et al. Survey of physician attitudes and practices related to pediatric obesity. Clin Pediatr 2003;42(3):235–245.
21. Mihalynuk TV, Knopp RH, Scott CS, et al. Physician informational needs in providing nutritional guidance to patients. Fam Med 2004;36(10):722–726.
22. Miller WR. Motivational interviewing with problem drinkers. Behav Psychother 1983;11(2):147–172.
23. Miller W, Rollnick S. Motivational Interviewing: Preparing People to Change Addictive Behavior. Guilford Press, New York: 1991.
24. Rollnick S, Heather N, Gold R, et al. Development of a short "readiness to change" questionnaire for use in brief, opportunistic interventions among excessive drinkers. Br J Addiction 1992;87(5):743–754.
25. Heather N, Rollnick S, Bell A, et al. Effects of brief counselling among male heavy drinkers identified on general hospital wards. Drug Alcohol Rev 1996;15(1):29–38.
26. Kadden RM. Project MATCH: treatment main effects and matching results. Alcoholism Clin Exper Res 1996;20(8 Suppl):196A–197A.
27. Burke BL, Arkowitz H, Menchola M. The efficacy of motivational interviewing: a meta-analysis of controlled clinical trials. J Consult Clin Psychol 2003;71(5):843–861.
28. Dunn C, Deroo L, Rivara F. The use of brief interventions adapted from motivational interviewing across behavioral domains: a systematic review. Addiction 2001;96(12):1725–1742.

29. Colby SM, Monti PM, Barnett NP, et al. Brief motivational interviewing in a hospital setting for adolescent smoking: a preliminary study. J Consult Clin Psychol 1998;66(3):574–578.

30. Ershoff DH, Quinn VP, Boyd NR, et al. The Kaiser Permanente prenatal smoking cessation trial: When more isn't better, what is enough? Am J Prev Med 1999;17(3):161–168.

31. Stott NCH, Rollnick S, Pill RM. Innovation in clinical method: diabetes care and negotiating skills. Fam Pract 1995;12(4):413–418.

32. Miller WR. Motivational interviewing: research, practice, and puzzles. Addict Behav 1996;21(6):835–842.

33. Velasquez M, Hecht J, Quinn V, et al. Application of motivational interviewing to prenatal smoking cessation: training and implementation issues. Tobacco Cont 2000;9(Supp III):36–40.

34. Berg-Smith S, Stevens V, Brown K, et al. A brief motivational intervention to improve dietary adherence in adolescents. Health Educ Res 1999;14(3):399–410.

35. Smith D, Heckemeyer C, Kratt P, et al. Motivational interviewing to improve adherence to a behavioral weight-control program for older obese women with NIDDM. Diabetes Care 1997;20(1):52–54.

36. Emmons K, Rollnick S. Motivational interviewing in health care settings: opportunities and limitations. Am J Prev Med 2001;20(1):68–74.

37. Resnicow K, Jackson A, Wang T, et al. A motivational interviewing intervention to increase fruit and vegetable intake through black churches: results of the Eat for Life trial. Am J Pub Health 2001;91: 1686–1693.

38. Resnicow K, DiIorio C, Soet JE, et al. Motivational interviewing in health promotion: it sounds like something is changing. Health Psychol 2002;21(5):444–451.

39. Butler C, Rollnick S, Cohen D, et al. Motivational consulting versus brief advice for smokers in general practice: a randomized trial. Br J Gen Pract 1999;49:611–616.

40. Rollnick S, Miller WR. What is motivational interviewing? Behav Cogn Psychother 1995;23(4):325–334.

41. Rollnick S, Butler C, Cambridge J, et al. Consultations about behaviour change. BMJ 2005;331(7522): 961–963.

42. Carkhuff R. The Art of Helping. 7th ed. Human Resource Development Press, Amherst, MA: 1993.

43. Rollnick S, Mason P, Butler C. Health Behavior Change: A Guide for Practitioners. Churchill Livingstone (Harcourt Brace), London: 1999.

44. Bem D. Self-perception theory. In: Berkowitz L, ed. Advances in Experimetnal Social Psychology. Academic Press, New York: 1972; pp. 1–62.

45. Rollnick S, Butler CC, Stott N. Helping smokers make decisions: The enhancement of brief intervention for general medical practice. Patient Educ Counsel 1997;31(3):191–203.

46. Resnicow K. Obesity prevention and treatment in youth: what is known? In: Trowbridge FL, Kibbe D, eds. Childhood Obesity: Partnerships for Research and Prevention. ILSI Press, Washington, DC: 2002; pp. 11–30.

47. Knight KM, Bundy C, Morris R, et al. The effects of group motivational interviewing and externalizing conversations for adolescents with Type-1 diabetes. Psychol Health Med 2003;8(2):149–158.

48. Channon S, Smith VJ, Gregory JW. A pilot study of motivational interviewing in adolescents with diabetes. Arch Dis Child 2003;88(8):680–683.

49. Bowen D, Ehret C, Pedersen M, et al. Results of an adjunct dietary intervention program in the Women's Health Initiative. J Am Diet Assn 2002;102(11):1631–1637.

50. Woollard J, Burke V, Beilin LJ. Effects of general practice-based nurse-counselling on ambulatory blood pressure and antihypertensive drug prescription in patients at increased risk of cardiovascular disease. J Hum Hypertens 2003;17(10):689–695.

51. Woollard J, Burke V, Beilin LJ, et al. Effects of a general practice-based intervention on diet, body mass index and blood lipids in patients at cardiovascular risk. J Cardiovasc Risk 2003;10(1):31–40.

52. Mhurchu CN, Margetts BM, Speller V. Randomized clinical trial comparing the effectiveness of two dietary interventions for patients with hyperlipidaemia. Clin Sci 1998;95(4):479–487.

53. Harland J, White M, Drinkwater C, et al. The Newcastle exercise project: a randomised controlled trial of methods to promote physical activity in primary care. BMJ 1999;319(7213):828–832.

54. Resnicow K, Jackson A, Blissett D, et al. Results of the Healthy Body Healthy Spirit Trial. Health Psychol 2005;24(4):339–348.

55. Wasserman R, Slora E, Bocian A, et al. Pediatric research in office settings (PROS): a national practice-based research network to improve children's health care. Pediatrics 1998;102(6):1350–1357.

56. Resnicow K, Taylor R, Baskin M. Results of Go Girls: a nutrition and physical activity intervention for overweight African American adolescent females conducted through black churches. Obes Res 2005;13(10):1739–1748.

57. Woollard J, Beilin L, Lord T, et al. A controlled trial of nurse counselling on lifestyle change for hypertensives treated in general practice: preliminary results. Clin Exper Pharmacol Physiol 1995;22(6–7):466–468.

58. Resnicow K, Coleman-Wallace D, Jackson A, et al. Dietary change through black churches: baseline results and program description of the Eat for Life trial. J Cancer Educ 2000;15:156–163.

59. Resnicow K, Campbell MK, Carr C, et al. Body and soul. A dietary intervention conducted through African-American churches. Am J Prev Med 2004;27(2):97–105.

60. Hedges L, Olkin NI. Statistical Methods for Meta-Analysis. Academic Press, New York: 1985.

61. Dunn C, Deroo L, Rivara FP. The use of brief interventions adapted from motivational interviewing across behavioral domains: a systematic review.[see comment]. Addiction 2001;96(12):1725–1742.

62. Campbell MK, Motsinger BM, Ingram A, et al. The North Carolina Black Churches United for Better Health Project: intervention and process evaluation. Health Educ Behav 2000;27(2):241–253.

63. Campbell MK, Demark-Wahnefried W, Symons M, et al. Fruit and vegetable consumption and prevention of cancer: the Black Churches United for Better Health project. Am J Pub Health 1999; 89(9):1390–1396.

64. Miller W, Mount K. A small study of training in motivational interviewing: does one workshop change clinician and client behavior? Behav Cogn Psychother 2001;29:457–471.

65. Thompson FE, Kipnis V, Subar AF, et al. Evaluation of 2 brief instruments and a food-frequency questionnaire to estimate daily number of servings of fruit and vegetables. Am J Clin Nutr 2000;71(6):1503–1510.

66. Resnicow K, Odom E, Wang T, et al. Validation of three food frequency questionnaires and twenty four hour recalls with serum carotenoids in a sample of African American adults. Am J Epidemiol 2000;152:1072–1080.

67. Resnicow K, Jackson A, Braithwaite R, et al. Healthy Body/Healthy Spirit: Design and evaluation of a church-based nutrition and physical activity intervention using motivational interviewing. Health Educ Res 2002;17(2):562–573.

68. Cohen J. A power primer. Psychol Bull 1992;112(1):155–159.

69. Barlow SE, Dietz WH. Obesity evaluation and treatment: expert committee recommendations. Pediatrics 1998;102(3):E29.

70. NIH-NHLBI and the North American Association for the Study of Obesity. The Practical Guide: Identification, Evaluation, and Treatment of Overweight and Obesity in Adults: NIH, Pub Number 00-4084; 2000.

71. Epstein L, Myers M, Raynor H, et al. Treatment of pediatric obesity. Pediatrics 1998;101(3):554–570.

18

Weight-Loss Drugs

Current and on the Horizon

George A. Bray, MD, and Frank L. Greenway, MD

CONTENTS

INTRODUCTION
ALGORITHM FOR USING CURRENTLY AVAILABLE DRUGS
MEDICATIONS FOR OBESITY TREATMENT
CONCLUSIONS
REFERENCES

Summary

Obesity is increasing in prevalence and its medical liabilities are largely related to central adiposity and the associated insulin resistance. The present drugs available for the treatment of obesity and metabolic syndrome are few in number and limited in efficacy. This chapter reviews the drugs approved by the US Food and Drug Administration (FDA) to treat obesity, drugs approved by the FDA for other indications than weight loss, drugs in the late development process that have not been approved by the FDA, drugs in earlier stages of drug development for which clinical information is limited, drugs that have been dropped from development, and new potential drug targets for which essentially no clinical data yet exist. We also review the nonprescription products sold for the treatment of obesity and metabolic syndrome. The developmental pipeline of drugs for the treatment of obesity and the metabolic syndrome is rich. Because drugs to treat obesity are being developed in an era characterized by more sophisticated tools for drug development than existed when hypertension drugs were being developed, much faster progress in developing safe and effective drugs for obesity and metabolic syndrome is anticipated. With safe and effective drugs available, we anticipate that the chronic treatment of obesity with weight loss medication will become as well-accepted and prevalent as is the chronic drug treatment of hypertension and diabetes in the medical practice of today.

Key Words: Obesity; metabolic syndrome; development; drugs; prescription; over-the-counter.

INTRODUCTION

Although the drug treatment of obesity has at least a century-long history, progress in drug discovery related to obesity was given a new impetus by the discovery of leptin in 1994. This peptide demonstrated that obesity can be caused by a hormone deficiency and be reversed by replacement of that hormone *(1,2)*. Even before the discovery of leptin, obesity had been declared a chronic disease by a National Institutes of Health (NIH) consensus conference in 1985 *(3)*. In the 20th century, bad eating habits were

From: *Contemporary Endocrinology: Treatment of the Obese Patient*
Edited by: R. F. Kushner and D. H. Bessesen © Humana Press Inc., Totowa, NJ

considered a primary cause of obesity. As bad habits can be behaviorally extinguished over a 12-wk period of time, obesity medications approved before 1985 were approved for periods up to 12 wk as an adjunct to a lifestyle change program. Equating obesity with bad habits and the stigmatization of obesity slowed the chronic use of obesity medications as is done with other chronic diseases *(4)*. With the recognition that longer-term therapy was needed, clinical trials have been extended in length, and since 1990 three medications have been approved for the chronic treatment of obesity. One of them, dexfenfluramine, was withdrawn 2 yr later *(5,6)*.

ALGORITHM FOR USING CURRENTLY AVAILABLE DRUGS

Guidance on the use of medications to treat obesity can be found in a variety of sources *(7–9)*. One algorithm recently proposed is by the American College of Physicians *(9)*. It provides an organized approach and a framework to comment on drugs for the treatment of obesity. As a document prepared by physicians, it emphasizes the medical model in which drugs are used to treat symptoms. However, the algorithm shown in Fig. 1, from a National Heart, Lung, and Blood Institute (NHLBI) report, is a more versatile algorithm.

The first step is to measure height and weight to establish the body mass index (BMI) for the patient. If the BMI, the weight in kilograms divided by the square of the height in meters (kg/m^2) (weight in pounds divided by square of the height in inches times 703), is higher than 30, the patient is by definition in the obese category and medications can be considered. Not mentioned in this guideline is the essential next step of measuring waist circumference (for individuals with a BMI < 35 — if the BMI is above 35, the waist circumference will almost certainly be increased). The currently recommended upper limit for waist circumference is 102 cm (40 in.) for a man and 88 cm (35 in.) for a woman. Values above these numbers have the same meaning as a BMI > 30 kg/m^2.

Another important initial step is to assess the associated (comorbid) conditions by measuring blood pressure, glucose, and lipids, and, when indicated, performing other tests. With this laboratory panel and the waist circumference, the presence of metabolic syndrome can be diagnosed. This is best done using the criteria from the National Cholesterol Education Panel Adult Treatment III Guidelines that are shown in Table 1, although other classification schemes are available.

Once it is established that the patient is an appropriate candidate to lose weight and that he or she is motivated to do so, the next step is to set a weight loss goal. Most patients have an unrealistic view of how much weight they can lose. For them a weight loss of less than 15% would often be viewed as a failure. In contrast, the goal with monotherapy with the drugs described here that are currently available is not more than 10% for most patients. It is thus important for physician and patient alike to set a weight-loss goal for initial therapy that is not more than 10% and to set a lower limit for weight loss of not less than 5%, which will suggest that an alternative strategy is needed.

The next step is to be certain that the patient is "ready" to lose weight. Using ideas from psychology, we need to have the patient ready to work on weight loss, as opposed to not yet thinking about the problem. Once the weight goal is established and the patient is prepared to take charge of the weight-loss program, the next steps are to help develop lifestyle changes that will benefit the program. The most important of these are monitoring what is eaten, where it is eaten, and under what circumstances. A second element is to provide dietary advice. Replacing voluntary choices with "portion-controlled"

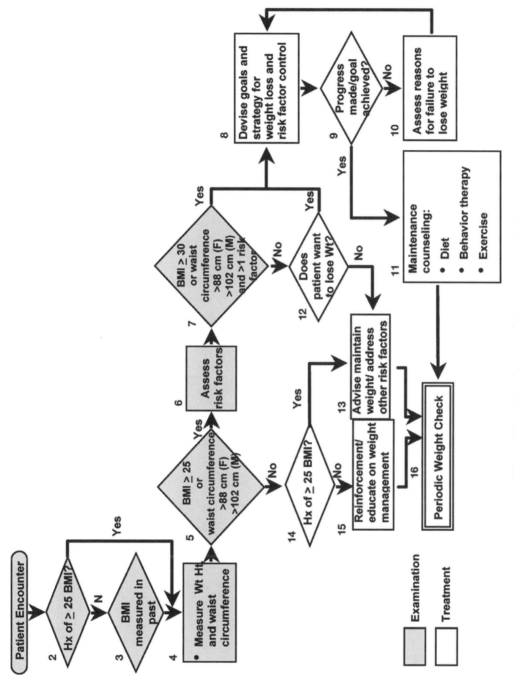

Fig. 1. Algorithm for use of drugs to treat obesity.

343

Table 1
Clinical Features of Metabolic Syndrome[a]

Risk factor	Defining level
Abdominal obesity (waist circumference)	
Men	>102 cm (>40 in.)
Women	>88 cm (>35 in.)
High-density lipoprotein cholesterol	
Men	<40 mg/dL
Women	<50 mg/dL
Triglycerides	≥150 mg/dL
Fasting glucose	≥110 mg/dL
Blood pressure	
Systolic	≥130 mm Hg
Diastolic	≥85 mm Hg

[a] Metabolic syndrome is present if 3 of the 5 risk factors are abnormal.
Modified from ref. *134*.

foods at one or more meals can be useful. There are frozen foods, ready-to-make food items, and meal replacements that can be used for this purpose. The patient also needs more exercise; one strategy is to have the patient get a pedometer, or "step-counter," and to records the number of steps taken, with the goal of gradually increasing it to 10,000 steps per day. When the patient returns, you establish whether the patient has met the goals. If so, the patient may continue as is, but if after 3 mo the patient fails to meet the goals, then medications may be considered.

The American College of Physicians (ACP) guidelines appropriately suggest discussing the pros and cons of medication with the patient and having a consent form signed for the use of medications to treat obesity. The algorithm then goes on to recommend six medications: orlistat, sibutramine, phentermine, diethylpropion, fluoxetine, and bupropion. Two other drugs, topiramate and zonisamide, are also mentioned in the ACP paper, but not included as "recommended" drugs in the algorithm. In our view, two of the drugs that are included in the algorithm, fluoxetine and bupropion, should be used only in special conditions. Fluoxetine is appropriate for the overweight patient who is depressed. Bupropion can be helpful in reducing or preventing weight gain when people try to stop smoking and when they are depressed. We will review each of these drugs below.

MEDICATIONS FOR OBESITY TREATMENT

Approved Medications

SIBUTRAMINE

Sibutramine is approved by the Food and Drug Administration for long-term use in the treatment of obesity. Sibutramine has been evaluated extensively in several multicenter trials lasting 6 to 24 mo; a meta-analysis of some of these trials is shown in Table 2 *(10–13)*. In a 6-mo dose-ranging study of 1047 patients, 67% treated with sibutramine achieved a 5% weight loss from baseline, and 35% lost 10% or more *(14)*.

Table 2
Meta-Analysis of Net Weight Loss With Sibutramine (Placebo Drug)

Author (Ref. no.)	Mean (95% CI)
Apfelbaum (10)	−5.70(95% CI −7.77 to −3.63)
Davis (13)	−3.00 (95% CI −4.55 to −1.45)
Hauner (11)	−5.30 (95% CI −6.83 to −3.77)
McNulty (12)	−4.80 (95% CI −6.02 to −3.58)
Wirth (16)	−4.00 (95% CI −5.01 to −2.99)

Adapted from ref. 5.

There was a clear dose-response effect in this 24-wk trial, and patients regained weight when the drug was stopped, indicating that the drug remained effective when used. Data from this multicenter trial are shown in Fig. 2 (14).

In a 1-yr trial of 456 patients who received sibutramine (10 mg or 15 mg/d) or placebo, 56% of those who stayed in the trial for 12 mo lost at least 5% of their initial body weight, and 30% of the patients lost 10% of their initial body weight while taking the 10-mg dose (8). In a third trial in patients who initially lost weight eating a very-low-calorie diet before being randomized to sibutramine (10 mg/d) or placebo, sibutramine produced additional weight loss, whereas the placebo-treated patients regained weight (8). The Sibutramine Trial of Obesity Reduction and Maintenance lasted 2 yr and provided evidence for weight maintenance (15). Seven centers participated in this trial, in which patients were initially enrolled in an open-label phase and treated with 10 mg/d of sibutramine for 6 mo. Of the patients who lost more than 8 kg, two-thirds were then randomized to sibutramine and one-third to placebo. During the 18-mo double-blind phase of this trial, the placebo-treated patients steadily regained weight, maintaining only 20% of their initial weight loss at the end of the trial. In contrast, the subjects treated with sibutramine maintained their weight for 12 mo and then regained an average of only 2 kg, thus maintaining 80% of their initial weight loss after 2 yr (16). Despite the higher weight loss with sibutramine at the end of the 18 mo of controlled observation, the blood pressure levels of the sibutramine-treated patients were still higher than in the patients treated with placebo.

The possibility of using sibutramine as intermittent therapy has been tested in a randomized, placebo-controlled trial lasting 52 wk (15). The patients randomized to sibutramine received one of two regimens. One group received continuous treatment with 15 mg/d for 1 yr, and the other had two 6-wk periods when sibutramine was withdrawn. During the periods when the drug was replaced by placebo, there was a small regain in weight that was lost when the drug was resumed. At the end of the trial, the continuous-therapy and intermittent-therapy groups had lost the same amount of weight.

Some trials have reported the use of sibutramine to treat patients with hypertension. In a 3-mo trial, all patients were receiving β-blockers with or without thiazides for their hypertension (17). The sibutramine-treated patients lost 4.2 kg (4.5%), compared with a loss of 0.3 kg (0.3%) in the placebo-treated group. Mean supine and standing diastolic and systolic blood pressure levels were not significantly different between drug-treated and placebo-treated patients. Heart rate, however, increased by 5.6 ± 8.25

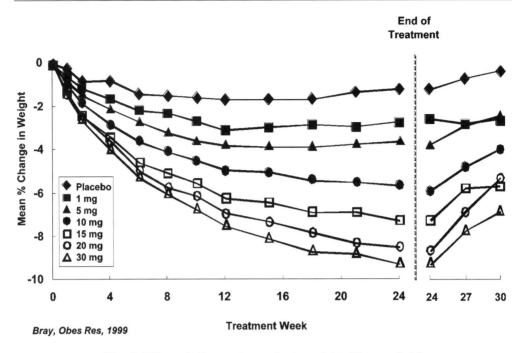

Fig. 2. Effect of sibutramine on body weight. (From ref. *14*)

(mean ± standard deviation) beats per minute in the sibutramine-treated patients, as compared with an increase of 2.2 ± 6.43 beats per minute in the placebo group. One 52-wk trial involved patients with hypertension whose blood pressure levels were controlled with calcium channel blockers with or without β-blockers or thiazides *(18)*. Sibutramine doses were increased from 5 to 20 mg/d during the first 6 wk. Weight loss was significantly greater in the sibutramine-treated patients, averaging 4.4 kg (4.7%), as compared with 0.5 kg (0.7%) in the placebo-treated group. Diastolic blood pressure levels decreased by 1.3 mmHg in the placebo-treated group and increased by 2 mmHg in the sibutramine-treated group. The systolic blood pressure levels increased by 1.5 mmHg in the placebo-treated group and by 2.7 mmHg in the sibutramine-treated group. Heart rate was unchanged in the placebo-treated patients, but increased by 4.9 beats/min in the sibutramine-treated patients.

Six studies with diabetic patients treated with sibutramine have been published *(19)*. In one study, patients were treated for 12 wk or 24 wk with sibutramine. In the 12-wk trial, patients with diabetes treated with sibutramine at 15 mg/d lost 2.4 kg (2.8%), compared with 0.1 kg (0.12%) in the placebo group *(20)*. In this study, hemoglobin A1C levels decreased 0.3% in the drug-treated group and remained stable in the placebo group. Fasting glucose values decreased by 0.3 mg/dL in the drug-treated patients and increased by 1.4 mg/dL in the placebo-treated group. In the 24-wk trial, the dose of sibutramine was increased from 5 to 20 mg/d over 6 wk *(21)*. Among those who completed the treatment, weight loss was 4.3 kg (4.3%) in the sibutramine-treated patients, compared with 0.3 kg (0.3%) in placebo-treated patients. Hemoglobin A1C levels decreased 1.67% in the drug-treated group, compared with 0.53% in the placebo-treated group. These changes in glucose and hemoglobin A1C levels were expected from the amount of weight loss associated with drug treatment.

Sibutramine has been studied as part of a behavioral weight-loss program. With minimal behavioral intervention, the weight loss was approx 5 kg (5%) over 12 mo. When behavior modification was added, the weight loss increased to 10 kg, and when a structured meal plan was added to the medication and behavioral modification, the weight loss increased further to 15 kg *(22)*.

Sibutramine has also been used in children and adolescents *(23–25)*. The trial by Berkowitz et al. *(23)* included 85 adolescents 13 to 17 yr of age with a BMI of 32 to 44 kg/m² who were treated for 6 mo. Weight loss in the drug-treated group was 7.8 kg, for an 8.5% reduction in BMI, compared with 3.2 kg for a 4.0% reduction in BMI. When the placebo group was switched to sibutramine after 6 mo, there was an additional significant weight loss in this group. In a multicenter trial, 498 adolescents aged 12 to 16 were randomized to receive either placebo or sibutramine for 12 mo. BMI was reduced by a mean of –7.9 kg/m² (–8.2%) in those treated with sibutramine, compared with –0.3 kg/m² (–0.8%) in those treated with placebo. Lipids and insulin sensitivity were improved, but there was no significant difference in blood pressure changes between the groups *(25)*.

Sibutramine is available in 5-, 10-, and 15-mg doses; 10 mg/d as a single dose is the recommended starting level, with titration up or down depending on response. Doses higher than 15 mg/d are not recommended. Of the patients who lost 2 kg (4 lb) in the first 4 wk of treatment, 60% achieved a weight loss of more than 5%, compared with less than 10% of those who did not lose 2 kg (4 lb) in 4 wk. Combining data from the 11 studies on sibutramine showed a reduction in triglyceride, total cholesterol, and LDL cholesterol levels and an increase in HDL cholesterol levels that were related to the magnitude of the weight loss.

ORLISTAT

Orlistat is a lipase inhibitor. In pharmacological studies, orlistat was shown to be a potent selective inhibitor of pancreatic lipase that reduces the intestinal digestion of fat. The drug has a dose-dependent effect on fecal fat loss, increasing it to approx 30% on a diet that has 30% of its energy as fat. Orlistat has little effect in subjects eating a low-fat diet, as might be anticipated from its mechanism of action *(8)*.

A number of 1- to 2-yr long-term clinical trials with orlistat have been published, and the results of a meta-analysis of these data are shown in Table 3 *(5)*. The results of a 2-yr trial are shown in Fig. 3 *(26)*. The trial consisted of two parts. In the first year, patients received a hypocaloric diet calculated to be 500 kcal/d less than the patient's requirements. During the second year, the diet was calculated to maintain weight. By the end of year 1, the placebo-treated patients lost 6.1% of their initial body weight and the drug-treated patients lost 10.2%. The patients were randomized again at the end of year 1. Those switched from orlistat to placebo gained weight from 10 to 6% below baseline. Those switched from placebo to orlistat lost weight from 6 to 8.1% below baseline, which was essentially identical to the 7.9% loss in the patients treated with orlistat for the full 2 yr.

In a second 2-yr study, 892 patients were randomized *(27)*. One group (97 patients) remained on placebo throughout the 2 yr, and a second group (109 patients) remained

Table 3
Meta-Analysis of Net Weight Loss With Orlistat (Placebo Minus Drug)

Author (year)	Mean (95% CI)
Davidson (1999)	–2.95 (95% CI –4.45 to –1.45)
Hauptman (2000)	–3.80 (95% CI –5.37 to –2.23)
Rossner (2000)	–3.00 (95% CI –4.17 to –1.83)
Sjostrom (1998)	–4.20 (95% CI –5.26 to –3.14)
Torgerson (2004)	–4.17 (95% CI –4.60 to –3.74)

Adapted from ref. 5.

on orlistat (120 mg three times per day) for 2 yr. At the end of 1 yr, two-thirds of the group treated with orlistat for 1 yr were changed to orlistat (60 mg three times per day) (102 patients), and the others were switched to placebo (95 patients) (27). After 1 yr, the weight loss was 8.67 kg in the orlistat-treated group and 5.81 kg in the placebo group (p < 0.001). During the second year, those switched to placebo after 1 yr reached the same weight as those treated with placebo for 2 yr (–4.5% in those with placebo for 2 yr and –4.2% in those switched to placebo during year 2).

In a third 2-yr study, 783 patients remained in the placebo or orlistat-treated groups at 60 mg or 120 mg three times per day for the entire 2 yr (28). After 1 yr with a weight-loss diet, the placebo group lost 7 kg, which was significantly less than the 9.6 kg lost by the group treated with 60 mg orlistat three times daily, or the 9.8 kg lost by the group treated with 120 mg orlistat three times daily. During the second year, when the diet was liberalized to a "weight maintenance" diet, all three groups regained some weight. At the end of 2 yr, the patients in the placebo group were 4.3 kg below baseline, the patients treated with 60 mg orlistat three times per day were 6.8 kg below baseline, and the patients who took 120 mg orlistat three times per day were 7.6 kg below baseline.

The final 2-yr trial that has been published evaluated 796 subjects in a general-practice setting (29). After 1 yr of treatment with 120 mg orlistat three times per day, the orlistat-treated patients (n = 117) had lost 8.8 kg, compared with 4.3 kg in the placebo group (n = 91). During the second year, when the diet was liberalized to "maintain body weight," both groups regained some weight. At the end of 2 yr, the orlistat group was 5.2 kg below their baseline weight, compared with 1.5 kg below baseline for the group treated with placebo.

The results of a 4-yr double-blind, randomized, placebo-controlled trial with orlistat have also been reported (30). A total of 3304 overweight patients, 21% of whom had impaired glucose tolerance, were included in this Swedish trial. The lowest body weight was achieved during the first year: more than 11% below baseline in the orlistat-treated group and 6% below baseline in the placebo-treated group. Over the remaining 3 yr of the trial, there was a small regain in weight, such that by the end of 4 yr, the orlistat-treated patients were 6.9% below baseline, compared with 4.1% for those receiving placebo. The trial also showed a 37% reduction in the conversion of patients from impaired glucose tolerance to diabetes; essentially all of this benefit occurred in the patients with impaired glucose tolerance at enrollment into the trial.

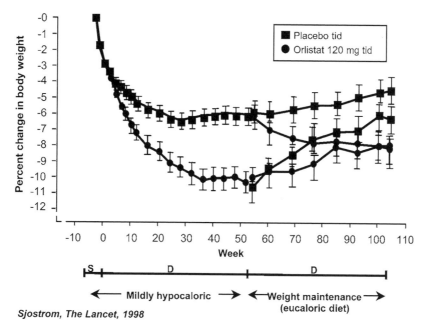

Fig. 3. Orlistat and body weight. (From ref. *26.*)

Weight maintenance with orlistat was evaluated in a 1-yr study *(8)*. Patients were enrolled if they had lost more than 8% of their body weight over 6 mo while eating a 1000 kcal/d (4,180 kJ/d) diet. The 729 patients were randomized to receive placebo or orlistat at 30, 60, or 120 mg three times per day for 12 mo. At the end of this time, the placebo-treated patients had regained 56% of their body weight, compared with 32.4% in the group treated with 120 mg orlistat three times per day. The other two doses of orlistat were not different from placebo in preventing the regain of weight.

Patients with diabetes treated with 120 mg orlistat three times daily for 1 yr lost more weight than the placebo-treated group *(31–33)*. The subjects with diabetes also showed a significantly greater decrease in hemoglobin A1C levels. In another study of orlistat and weight loss, investigators pooled data on 675 subjects from three of the 2-yr studies described previously in which glucose tolerance tests were available *(34)*. During treatment, 6.6% of the patients taking orlistat converted from a normal to an impaired glucose tolerance test, compared with 10.8% in the placebo-treated group. None of the orlistat-treated patients who originally had normal glucose tolerance developed diabetes, compared with 1.2% in the placebo-treated group. Of those who initially had normal glucose tolerance, 7.6% in the placebo group but only 3% in the orlistat-treated group developed diabetes.

In a further analysis, patients who had participated in previously reported studies were divided into the highest and lowest quintiles for triglyceride and HDL cholesterol levels *(35)*. Those with high triglyceride and low HDL cholesterol levels were labeled "syndrome X," and those with the lowest triglyceride levels and highest HDL cholesterol levels were the "non-syndrome X" controls. In this classification, there were almost no men in the non-syndrome X group, compared with an equal sex breakdown in the syndrome X group. In addition, the syndrome X group had slightly higher systolic and diastolic blood pressure levels and a nearly twofold higher level of fasting insulin. Besides weight loss, the only difference between the placebo and orlistat-treated patients was the decrease in LDL cholesterol levels in the patients treated with orlistat. However, the syndrome X subgroup showed a significantly greater decrease in triglyceride and insulin levels than those without syndrome X. Levels of HDL cholesterol increased more in the syndrome X group, but LDL cholesterol levels showed a smaller decrease than in the non-syndrome X group. All the clinical studies with orlistat have shown significant decreases in serum cholesterol and LDL cholesterol levels that usually are higher than can be accounted for by weight loss alone (8). One study showed that orlistat reduces the absorption of cholesterol from the GI tract, thus providing a mechanism for the clinical observations (36).

A multicenter trial tested the effect of orlistat in 539 obese adolescents (37). Subjects were randomized to placebo or 120 mg orlistat three times a day and a mildly hypocaloric diet containing 30% fat. By the end of the study, BMI had decreased 0.55 kg/m^2 in the drug-treated group but had increased 0.31 kg/m^2 in the placebo group. By the end of the study, weight had increased by only 0.51 kg in the orlistat-treated group, compared with 3.14 kg in the placebo-treated group. This difference was caused by differences in body fat. The side effects were gastrointestinal in origin as expected from the mode of action of orlistat.

Safety of Orlistat. Orlistat is not absorbed from the GI tract to any significant degree, and its side effects are thus related to the blockade of triglyceride digestion in the intestine (38). Fecal fat loss and related GI symptoms are common initially, but they subside as patients learn to use the drug (8). The quality of life in patients treated with orlistat may improve despite concerns about GI symptoms. Orlistat can cause small but significant decreases in fat-soluble vitamins. Levels usually remain within the normal range, but a few patients may need vitamin supplementation. Because it is impossible to tell which patients need vitamins, it is clinically appropriate to provide a multivitamin routinely with instructions to take it before bedtime. Orlistat does not seem to affect the absorption of other drugs except cyclosporin.

Combining Orlistat and Sibutramine. Because orlistat works peripherally to reduce triglyceride digestion in the GI tract and sibutramine works on noradrenergic and serotonergic reuptake mechanisms in the brain, their mechanisms of action do not overlap, and combining them might provide additive weight loss. To test this possibility, researchers randomly assigned patients to orlistat or placebo after 1 yr of treatment with sibutramine (Fig. 3) (39). During the additional 4 mo of treatment, there was no further weight loss. This result was a disappointment, but additional studies are needed.

PHENTERMINE AND DIETHYLPROPION: SYMPATHOMIMETIC DRUGS APPROVED FOR SHORT-TERM USE

Most of the data on phentermine, diethylpropion, benzphetamine, and phendimetrazine come from short-term trials (8). One of the longest of these clinical trials lasted 36 wk and compared placebo treatment with continuous phentermine or intermittent phentermine (40). Both continuous and intermittent phentermine therapy produced more weight loss than placebo. In the drug-free periods, the patients treated intermittently slowed their weight loss, only to lose more rapidly when the drug was reinstituted. Phentermine and diethylpropion are classified by the US Drug Enforcement Agency as schedule IV drugs;

benzphetamine and phendimetrazine are schedule III drugs. This regulatory classification indicates the government's belief that they have the potential for abuse, although this potential appears to be very low. Phentermine and diethylpropion are approved for only a "few weeks," which usually is interpreted as up to 12 wk. Weight loss with phentermine and diethylpropion persists for the duration of treatment, suggesting that tolerance does not develop to these drugs. If tolerance were to develop, the drugs would be expected to lose their effectiveness, and patients would require increased amounts of the drug to maintain weight loss. This does not occur.

Drugs Approved by FDA for Other Uses Than Weight Loss

Although sibutramine and orlistat are the only two medications approved for the long-term treatment of obesity, there is a great deal of activity in the pharmaceutical industry to develop new drugs or rediscover old ones to treat this disease. The prevalence of obesity is continuing to grow and new obesity drugs are clearly needed. One group of potential antiobesity drugs has approved indications for other purposes, but has been demonstrated to give weight loss. Bupropion, somatostatin, zonisamide, and topiramate are in this category. Although topiramate was being developed as an obesity drug, the manufacturers of others are not seeking an obesity indication, and the topiramate obesity development program was terminated in December 2004.

FLUOXETINE

Fluoxetine and sertraline are both selective serotonin reuptake inhibitors (SSRIs) approved for the treatment of depression. Sertraline gave an average weight loss of 0.45 to 0.91 kg in clinical trials for depression lasting 8 to 16 wk. Fluoxetine at a dose of 60 mg/d (three times the usual dose for treatment of depression) was evaluated in clinical trials by the Eli Lilly Company for the treatment of obesity. A meta-analysis of six studies showed a wide range of results, with a mean weight loss of 14.5 kg in one study and a weight gain of 0.40 kg in another (5). Goldstein et al. reviewed these trials, which included one 36-wk trial in type 2 diabetic subjects, a 52-wk trial in subjects with uncomplicated obesity, and two 60-wk trials in subjects with dyslipidemia, diabetes, or both (41). A total of 1441 subjects were randomized to fluoxetine (719) or placebo (722). Five hundred twenty-two subjects on fluoxetine and 504 subjects on placebo completed 6 mo of treatment. Weight loss in the placebo and fluoxetine groups at 6 mo and 1 yr were 2.2, 4.8, and 1.8, 2.4 kg, respectively. The regain of 50% of the weight during the second 6 mo of treatment on fluoxetine makes this drug inappropriate for the long-term treatment of obesity, which requires chronic treatment. Fluoxetine and sertraline, although not good antiobesity drugs, may be preferred for the depressed obese patient over some of the tricyclic antidepressants that are associated with significant weight gain.

BUPROPION

Bupropion is a norepinephrine and dopamine reuptake inhibitor that is approved for the treatment of depression and for smoking cessation. Gadde et al. reported a clinical trial in which 50 obese subjects were randomized to bupropion or placebo for 8 wk with a blinded extension for responders to 24 wk. The dose of bupropion was increased to maximum of 200 mg twice daily in conjunction with a calorie-restricted diet. At 8 weeks, 18 subjects in the bupropion group lost 6.2 ± 3.1 % of body weight compared with 1.6 $\pm 2.9\%$ for the 13 subjects in the placebo group ($p < 0.0001$). After 24 wk, the 14 responders to bupropion lost 12.9 ± 5.6% of initial body weight, of which 75% was fat as determined by dual-energy X-ray absorptiometry (DEXA) *(42)*.

Two multicenter clinical trials, one in obese subjects with depressive symptoms and one in uncomplicated obesity, followed this study *(43, 44)*. The study in obese patients with depressive symptom ratings of 10 to 30 on a Beck Depression Inventory randomized 213 subjects to 400 mg of bupropion per day and 209 subjects to placebo for 24 wk. The 121 subjects in the bupropion group who completed the trial lost 6.0 ± 0.5 % of initial body weight compared with 2.8 ± 0.5 % in the 108 subjects in the placebo group ($p < 0.0001$) *(43)*. The study in uncomplicated obese subjects randomized 327 subjects to bupropion 300 mg/d, bupropion 400 mg/d, or placebo in equal proportions. At 24 wk, 69% of those randomized remained in the study and the percent losses of initial body weight were 5 ± 1%, 7.2 ± 1%, and 10.1 ± 1% for the placebo, bupropion 300 mg, and bupropion 400 mg groups, respectively ($p < 0.0001$). The placebo group was randomized to the 300-mg or 400-mg group at 24 wk and the trial was extended to week 48. By the end of the trial the dropout rate was 41%, and the weight loss in the 300-mg and 400-mg bupropion groups was 6.2 ± 1.25% and 7.2 ± 1.5% of initial body weight, respectively *(44)*. Thus, it appears that nondepressed subjects may respond to bupropion with weight loss to a greater extent than those with depressive symptoms.

TOPIRAMATE

Topiramate is an antiepileptic drug that was discovered to give weight loss in the clinical trials for epilepsy. Weight losses of 3.9% of initial weight were seen at 3 mo and losses of 7.3% of initial weight were seen at 1 yr *(45)*. Bray et al. reported a 6-mo, placebo-controlled, dose-ranging study *(46)*. Three hundred eighty-five obese subjects were randomized to placebo or topiramate at 64, 96, 192, or 384 mg/d. These doses were gradually increased over 12 wk and were tapered in a similar manner at the end of the trial. Weight loss from baseline to 24 wk was 2.6, 5, 4.8, 6.3, and 6.3% in the placebo, 64-mg, 96-mg, 192-mg, and 384-mg groups, respectively. The most frequent adverse events were paresthesias, somnolence, and difficulty with concentration, memory, and attention *(46)*. This trial was followed by two multicenter trials *(47,48)*. The first trial randomized 1289 obese subjects to topiramate 89 mg/d, 192 mg/d, or 256 mg/d. This trial was terminated early owing to the sponsor's decision to pursue a time-release form of the drug. The 854 subjects who completed 1 yr of the trial before it was terminated by the sponsor lost 1.7, 7, 9.1, and 9.7% of their initial body weight in the placebo, 89-mg, 192-mg, and 256-mg groups, respectively. Subjects in the topiramate groups had significant improvement in blood pressure and glucose tolerance *(47)*. The second trial enrolled 701 subjects who were treated with a very-low-calorie diet to induce an 8% loss of initial body weight. The 560 subjects who achieved an 8% weight loss were randomized to topiramate 96 mg/d, 192 mg/d, or placebo. The sponsor terminated this study early too. At the time of early termination, 293 subjects had completed 44 wk. The topiramate groups lost 15.4 and 16.5% of their baseline weight, whereas the placebo group lost 8.9% *(48)*. Although topiramate is still available as an antiepileptic drug, the development program to obtain an indication for obesity was terminated by the sponsor owing to the associated adverse events.

Topiramate has also been evaluated in the treatment of binge-eating disorder. Thirteen women with binge-eating disorder were treated with a mean dose of 492 mg/d of topiramate. The binge-eating disorder symptoms improved and a weight loss was observed *(49)*. This open-label study was followed by a randomized controlled trial of 14 wk in subjects with binge-eating disorder. Sixty-one subjects were randomized to 25 to 600 mg/d of topiramate or placebo in a 1:1 ratio. The topiramate group had improvement in binge-eating symptoms and lost 5.9 kg at an average topiramate dose of 212 mg/d *(50)*. The 35 completers of this trial were given the opportunity to participate in an open-label extension. The topiramate-treated subjects continued to maintain improvement in binge-eating symptoms and weight *(51)*.

Topiramate has also been used to treat patients with Prader-Willi syndrome. Three subjects with Prader-Willi syndrome were treated with topiramate and had a reduction in the self-injurious behavior that is associated with this uncommon genetic disease *(52)*. A second study in seven additional subjects confirmed these findings *(53)*. A third study evaluated appetite, food intake, and weight. Although the self-injurious behavior improved, there was no effect on the other parameters *(54)*. Topiramate was also used to treat two subjects with nocturnal eating syndrome and two subjects with sleep-related eating disorder. There was an improvement in all subjects and there was an 11-kg weight loss over 8.5 mo with an average topiramate dose of 218 mg/d *(55)*.

ZONISAMIDE

Zonisamide is an antiepileptic drug that has serotonergic and dopaminergic activity in addition to inhibiting sodium and calcium channels. Weight loss was noted in the trials for the treatment of epilepsy. Gadde et al. performed a 16-wk randomized control trial in 60 obese subjects *(56)*. Subjects were placed on a calorie-restricted diet and randomized to zonisamide or placebo. The zonisamide was started at 100 mg/d and increased to 400 mg/d. At 12 wk, subjects who had not lost 5% of initial body weight were increased to 600 mg/d. The zonisamide group lost 6.6% of initial body weight at 16 wk compared with 1% in the placebo group. Thirty-seven subjects completing the 16-wk trial elected to continue to week 32 — 20 in the zonisamide group and 17 in the placebo group. At the end of 32 wk, the 19 subjects in the zonisamide group lost 9.6% of their initial body weight compared with 1.6% for the 17 subjects in the placebo group *(56)*. McElroy et al. evaluated zonisamide in an open-label prospective trial in subjects with binge-eating disorder. Fifteen subjects were treated with doses of 100 to 600 mg/d for 12 wk. The eight subjects who completed the trial had an average dose of 513 mg/d, experienced an improvement in their binge-eating symptoms, and lost significant weight *(57)*.

SOMATOSTATIN

Hypothalamic obesity has been associated with insulin hypersecretion *(58)*. Lustig treated eight children with obesity owing to hypothalamic damage with octreotide injections to decrease insulin hypersecretion. These children gained 6 kg in the 6 mo prior to octreotide treatment and lost 4.8 kg in the 6 mo on octreotide, an analog of somatostatin *(59)*. The weight loss was correlated with the reduction of insulin secretion on a glucose tolerance test. This open-label trial was followed by a randomized controlled trial of octreotide treatment in children with hypothalamic obesity. The subjects received 5 to 15 µg/kg/d octreotide or placebo for 6 mo. The children on octreotide gained 1.6 kg, compared with 9.1 kg for those in the placebo group *(60)*. This same group of investigators postulated that there might be a subset of obese subjects who were insulin hypersecretors and that these subjects would respond with weight loss to treatment with octreotide. Following an oral glucose tolerance test in which glucose and insulin were measured, 44 subjects were treated with long-acting octreotide-LAR 40 mg/mo for 6 mo. These subjects lost weight, reduced food intake, and had a reduced carbohydrate intake. Weight loss was greatest in those who hypersecreted insulin, and the amount of weight loss was correlated with the reduction in insulin hypersecretion *(61)*. In a controlled trial of octreotide LAR, 172 obese subjects who were shown to hypersecrete insulin during screening were randomized to doses of 20, 40, 60 mg/mo or placebo for 6 mo. The greatest weight loss was 3.8% of initial body weight in the high-dose group, an amount that does not meet the criteria for approval by the FDA *(62)*.

Octreotide has been shown to decrease gastric emptying *(63)*. Treatment with octreotide of Prader-Willi syndrome patients who have elevated ghrelin levels does not cause weight loss, but ghrelin levels are normalized. The reason for the lack of weight loss was postulated to be the reduction of PYY, a satiating gastrointestinal hormone that also decreased *(64)*.

METFORMIN

Metformin is a biguanide that is approved for the treatment of diabetes mellitus, a disease that is exacerbated by obesity and weight gain. This drug reduces hepatic glucose production, decreases intestinal absorption from the gastrointestinal tract, and enhances insulin sensitivity. In clinical trials where metformin was compared with sulfonylureas, it produced weight loss *(8)*. In one French trial, BIGPRO, metformin was compared to placebo in a 1-yr multicenter study in 324 middle-aged subjects with upper-body obesity and insulin resistance syndrome (metabolic syndrome). The subjects on metformin lost significantly more weight (1–2 kg) than the placebo group, and the study concluded that metformin may have a role in the primary prevention of type 2 diabetes *(65)*.

The best trial of metformin, however, is the Diabetes Prevention Program (DPP) *(66)* study of individuals with impaired glucose tolerance. The main part of this study included three treatment arms to which participants were randomly assigned, if they were over 25 yr of age, had a BMI above 24 (except Asian-Americans, who needed only a BMI ≥22) and had impaired glucose tolerance. The three primary arms included lifestyle ($N = 1079$ participants), metformin ($N = 1073$), and placebo ($N = 1082$). At the end of 2.8 yr, on average, the Data Safety Monitoring Board terminated the trial because the advantages of lifestyle and metformin were clearly superior to those of placebo. During this time the metformin-treated group lost 2.5% of their body weight ($p < 0.001$ compared with placebo), and the conversion from impaired glucose tolerance to diabetes was reduced by 31% compared with placebo. In the DPP trial, metformin was more effective in reducing the development of diabetes in the subgroup who were most overweight, and in the younger members of the cohort *(66)*. Although metformin does not produce enough weight loss (5%) to qualify as a "weight-loss drug" using the FDA criteria, it would appear to be a very useful choice for overweight individuals with diabetes or at high risk for diabetes. One area where metformin has found use is in treating women with polycystic ovary syndrome, where the modest weight loss may contribute to increased fertility and reduced insulin resistance *(67)*.

PRAMLINTIDE

Amylin is secreted from the β-cell along with insulin, and amylin is deficient in type 1 diabetes where β-cells are immunologically destroyed. Pramlintide, a synthetic amylin analog, was recently approved by the FDA for the treatment of diabetes. Unlike insulin and many other diabetes medications, pramlintide is associated with weight loss. In a study in which 651 subjects with type 1 diabetes were randomized to placebo or 60 µg subcutaneous pramlintide three or four times a day along with an insulin injection, the hemoglobin A1c decreased 0.29 to 0.34% and weight decreased 1.2 kg relative to placebo (68). Maggs et al. analyzed the data from two 1-yr studies in insulin-treated type 2 diabetic subjects randomized to pramlintide 120 µg twice a day or 150 µg three times a day (69). Weight decreased by 2.6 kg and hemoglobin A1c decreased 0.5% in the combined pramlintide-dose groups. When weight loss was then analyzed by ethnic group, African Americans lost 4 kg, Caucasians lost 2.4 kg, and Hispanics lost 2.3 kg; the improvement in diabetes correlated with the weight loss, suggesting that pramlintide is effective in ethnic groups with the greatest obesity burden. The most common adverse event was nausea, which was usually mild and confined to the first 4 wk of therapy.

EXENATIDE

Glucagon-like peptide-1 (GLP-1) is a protein derived from proglucagon and secreted by L-cells in the terminal ileum in response to a meal. GLP-1 decreases food intake and has been postulated to be responsible for the superior weight loss and superior improvement in diabetes seen with obesity bypass surgery (70,71). Increased GLP-1 inhibits glucagon secretion, stimulates insulin secretion, stimulates glycogenogenesis, and delays gastric emptying (72). GLP-1 is rapidly degraded by dipeptidyl peptidase (DPP)-4, an enzyme that is elevated in the obese. Obesity bypass operations increase GLP-1, but do not change the levels of DPP-4 (73).

Exendin-4 (exenatide) is a 39-amino-acid peptide that is produced in the salivary gland of the Gila monster lizard. It has 53% homology with GLP-1, but has a much longer half-life. Exenatide decreases food intake and body weight gain in Zucker rats while lowering HbA1c (74). Exenatide increases β-cell mass to a greater extent than would be expected for the degree of insulin resistance (75). Exenatide induces satiety and weight loss in Zucker rats with peripheral administration and crosses the blood–brain barrier to act in the central nervous system (76,77). In humans, exenatide reduces fasting and postprandial glucose levels, slows gastric emptying, and decreases food intake by 19% (78). The side effects of exenatide in humans are headache, nausea, and vomiting, which are lessened by gradual dose escalation (79). Exenatide at 10 µg/d subcutaneously or a placebo was given for 30 wk to 377 type 2 diabetic subjects who were failing maximal sulfonylurea therapy. The HbA1c fell 0.74% more than placebo, fasting glucose decreased, and there was a progressive weight loss of 1.6 kg (80). In ongoing open-label clinical trials, the weight loss at 18 mo is 4.5 kg without using behavior therapy or diet. Exenatide has been approved by the FDA for use in type 2 diabetics.

Drugs on the Near and Distant Horizons

Rimonabant is an orally active antagonist at the cannabinoid-1 receptor that is in the late stages of development, with approval by the FDA and a launch anticipated in 2006. The development of axokine has been terminated. Pramlintide and exenatide have been recently approved for the treatment of diabetes. Both these drugs give weight loss. There are other drugs in phase II, phase I, and earlier in development. There is less information about these compounds, but they generally fall into one of three categories: drugs acting on the central nervous system, drugs with a focus on the gastrointestinal tract, and metabolic regulators.

RIMONABANT

There are two cannabinoid receptors, CB-1 (470 amino acids in length) and CB-2 (360 amino acids in length). The CB-1 receptor has almost all the amino acids that comprise the CB-2 receptor, and additional amino acids at both ends. CB-1 receptors are distributed throughout the brain in the areas related to feeding, on fat cells, in the gastrointestinal tract, and on immune cells. Marijuana and tetrahydrocannabinol stimulate the CB-1 receptor and increase high-fat and high-sweet-food intake; fasting increases the levels of endocannabinoids, such as anandamide and 2-arachidonyl-glycerol. The rewarding properties of cannabinoid agonists are mediated through the mesolimbic dopaminergic system. Rimonabant is a specific antagonist of the CB-1 receptor, and inhibits sweet food intake in marmosets as well as high-fat food intake in rats, but not in rats fed standard chow. In addition to being specific in inhibiting highly palatable food intake, pair-feeding experiments in diet-induced obese rats show that the rimonabant-treated animals lost 21% of their body weight compared with 14% in the pair-fed controls. This suggests that, at least in rodents, rimonabant increases energy expenditure in addition to reducing food intake. CB-1 knockout mice are lean and resistant to diet-induced obesity. CB-1 receptors are upregulated on adipocytes in diet-induced obese mice, and rimonabant increases adiponectin, a fat cell hormone associated with insulin sensitivity (81).

The results of four phase III trials of rimonabant for the treatment of obesity have been presented. These reports are posted on the Sanofi website (82); only one exists in the form of a peer-reviewed publication at the time of this writing (82,83). The summary of these trials, therefore, comes primarily from these Sanofi press releases. The first trial to be announced was called the Rio-Lipids trial. This was a 1-yr trial that randomized 1018 obese subjects equally to placebo, 5 mg/d rimonabant, or 20 mg/d rimonabant. The subjects in this trial had untreated dyslipidemia, a BMI between 27 and 40, and a mean weight of 96 kg. Weight loss was 2% in the placebo group and 8.5% in the 20-mg rimonabant group. In the 20 mg/d rimonabant group, waist circumference was reduced 9 cm, triglycerides were reduced by 15%, and HDL cholesterol was increased by 23%, compared with 3.5 cm, 3%, and 12% respectively in the placebo group. In the 20 mg/d group the LDL particle size increased, adiponectin increased, glucose decreased, insulin decreased, C-reactive protein decreased, and metabolic syndrome prevalence was cut in half. There was no increase in depression or anxiety, and neither pulse nor blood pressure increased in contradistinction to sibutramine. Fifteen percent of subjects in the rimonabant 20 mg/d group dropped from the trial for adverse events. The most common adverse events were nausea and diarrhea, as one might expect from the location of the CB-1 receptors. Forty percent of the study cohort dropped out by 1 yr and 15% dropped in the high dose group for an adverse event.

In the second study, called Rio-Europe, 305 subjects were randomized to placebo, 603 subjects to 5 mg/d rimonabant and 599 subjects to 20 mg/d rimonabant for a 2-yr study. Weight loss at 2 yr in the placebo group was 2.5 kg compared with 7.2 kg in the 20 mg rimonabant group (83). The third study, Rio-North America, was also a 2-yr study that randomized 3040 obese subjects without diabetes to placebo, 5 mg rimonabant, or 20 mg rimonabant. At 1 yr, half the rimonabant groups were rerandomized to placebo. At 1 yr, weight loss was 2.8 kg in the placebo group and 8.6 kg in the 20 mg rimonabant group. The 2-yr results have not yet been published. It is anticipated that these three rimonabant studies will become available as peer-reviewed publications within the next year.

Leptin

The lack of leptin, a hormone derived from the fat cell, causes massive obesity in animals and man *(1,2)*. Its placement reverses the obesity associated with the deficiency state. The discovery of leptin generated hope that leptin would be an effective treatment for obesity. Leptin at subcutaneous doses of 0, 0.01, 0.05, 0.1, and 0.3 mg/kg daily were tested in 54 lean and 73 obese humans of both sexes *(84)*. Lean subjects were treated for 4 wk and lost 0.4 to 1.9 kg. Obese subjects were treated for 24 wk; a dose–response relationship for weight loss was seen, with the 0.3 mg/kg group losing 7.1 kg *(84)*. Pegylated leptin allows for weekly, rather than daily, injections. Although pegylated leptin at 20 and 60 mg/wk in obese subjects over 8 to 12 wk did not give any weight loss above placebo, pegylated leptin at 80 mg weekly combined with a very-low-calorie diet for 46 d gave 2.8 kg more weight loss in 12 subjects randomized to leptin compared to the 10 randomized to placebo ($p < 0.03$) *(85)*.

Leptin has been found to ameliorate many of the symptoms of lipodystrophy *(86)*. Nine female patients with lipodystrophy and a serum leptin level of less than 4 mg/mL were treated with recombinant methionyl human leptin for 4 mo. Eight of the women had diabetes. During treatment with leptin, the glycosylated hemoglobin decreased an average of 1.9%. During the 4 mo of therapy, triglyceride levels decreased by 60%. Liver volume was also reduced by an average of 28%, and resting metabolic rate also decreased significantly with therapy *(87)*. A reduced body weight is associated with decreased 24-h energy expenditure and decreased leptin and thyroid hormone levels. When body weight was reduced by 10%, circulating T3, T4, and leptin concentrations were decreased. All these endocrine changes were reversed by administration of "replacement" doses of recombinant human methionyl leptin. Total energy expenditure increased in all subjects during treatment with leptin, indicating that decreased leptin may account for some aspects of the endocrine adaptations to weight loss.

Axokine

Axokine is an analog of ciliary neurotrophic factor that, like leptin, acts through the STAT signaling pathway in the brain *(88)*. Axokine has been tested in two phase II studies, one in obesity and one in diabetes, in addition to one phase III study in obesity. The first multicenter 12-wk phase II study randomized 170 obese subjects with a BMI between 35 and 50. The optimal dose was 1 μg/kg, and this group lost 4.6 kg compared with a weight gain of 0.6 kg in the placebo group *(89)*. The second 12-wk phase II study randomized 107 overweight and obese type 2 diabetic subjects with a BMI between 35 and 50 *(90)*. Those subjects treated with the 1.0 μg/kg dose of axokine lost 3.2 kg compared with 1.2 kg in the placebo group ($p < 0.01$).

The 1-yr phase III trial with a 1-yr open-label extension randomized 501 subjects to placebo and 1467 subjects to axokine at a dose of 1 μg/kg/d *(90)*. Subjects had a BMI between 30 and 55, if their obesity was uncomplicated, or between 27 and 55, if their obesity was complicated by hypertension or dyslipidemia. At the end of 1 yr, the axokine group lost 3.6 kg, compared with 2.0 kg in the placebo group ($p < 0.001$), a difference that does not meet the FDA efficacy criteria for approval. The most common adverse events were mild and included injection site reactions, nausea, and cough. The most concerning finding, however, was that two-thirds of those receiving axokine developed antibodies after 3 mo that limited further weight loss, and there was no way to prospectively predict those who would develop the antibodies. Development of axokine has been terminated.

Drugs in Early Phases of Development

GROWTH HORMONE FRAGMENT

AOD9604 is a modified fragment of the amino acids in growth hormone from 177 to 191, and is orally active. This growth hormone fragment is said to bind to the fat cell, stimulating lipolysis and inhibiting reesterification without stimulating growth. A 12-wk multicenter trial randomized 300 obese subjects to one of five daily doses (1, 5, 10, 20, and 30 mg) of AOD9604 or placebo. The 1-mg dose was the most effective for weight loss. Subjects on the 1-mg dose lost 2.6 kg, compared with 0.8 kg in the placebo group, and the rate of weight loss was constant throughout the trial *(91)*. Phase III trials are evidently in the planning stages.

PYY 3-36

PYY 3-36 is a hormone produced by the L-cells in the gastrointestinal tract and is secreted in proportion to the caloric content of a meal. PYY 3-36 levels are lower when fasting and after a meal in the obese compared with the lean subjects. Caloric intake at a lunch buffet was reduced by 30% in 12 obese subjects and by 29% in 12 lean subjects after 2 h of PYY 3-36 infused intravenously *(92)*. Thrice-daily nasal administration over 6 d was well-tolerated and reduced caloric intake by about 30% while giving 0.6 kg weight loss *(93)*.

OXYNTOMODULIN

Oxyntomodulin, like PYY and cholecystokinin, is released from the GI tract and can inhibit food intake. In a study of healthy overweight and obese volunteers, participants self-administered saline or oxyntomodulin subcutaneously in a 4-wk randomized, double-blind, parallel-group protocol. Injections were given three times daily, 30 min before each meal, over a period of 4 wk. Body weight was reduced by 2.3 ± 0.4 kg in the treatment group, compared with 0.5 ± 0.5 kg in the control group ($p = 0.0106$). On average, the treatment group experienced an additional 0.45 kg weight loss per week. Oxyntomodulin reduced energy intake by 170 ± 37 kcal ($25 \pm 5\%$) at the initial study meal ($p = 0.0007$) and by 250 ± 63 kcal ($35 \pm 9\%$) at the final study meal ($p = 0.0023$). In this small, short-term trial, oxyntomodulin treatment produced a small weight loss and decreased food intake over a 4-wk period *(94)*.

CHOLECYSTOKININ

Cholecystokinin decreases food intake by causing subjects to stop eating sooner *(95)*. Although the relationship between cholecystokinin and satiety has been known for many years, development as a weight-loss agent has been slow owing to concerns regarding pancreatitis. As the human pancreas has no cholecystokinin-A receptors, an orally active compound that is a selective agonist of the cholecystokinin-A receptor is being evaluated in clinical trials, but no reports of those trials have yet appeared.

OLEOYLESTRONE

Oleoylestrone is a weakly estrogenic compound that is produced in fat cells, carried in the blood on HDL particles, and feeds back to the central nervous system to reduce food intake while maintaining energy expenditure. Oleoylestrone is orally active and has been used to treat one morbidly obese male without an accompanying weight loss program. Oleoylestrone was given in doses of 150 to 300 µmol/d in 10 consecutive 10-d courses of treatment separated by at least 2 mo. Weight dropped 38.5 kg and BMI dropped from 51.9 to 40.5 over 27 mo, and weight was still declining at the time of the report *(96)*. Oleoylestrone was well tolerated and there were no estrogenic side effects observed. Pharmaceutical company-sponsored phase I trials are presently in progress.

Serotonin 2C Receptor Agonist

Mice lacking the 5HT-2c receptor have increased food intake, because they take longer to be satiated. These mice also are resistant to fenfluramine, a serotonin agonist that causes weight loss. A human mutation of the 5HT-2c receptor has been identified that is associated with early-onset human obesity *(97,98)*. The FDA website lists, under ongoing clinical trials, a phase II trial of APD356, a serotonin 2C agonist. This is a multicenter, randomized, 4-wk trial in 400 obese subjects. No further information is available *(99)*.

Neuropeptide-Y Receptor Antagonists

Neuropeptide Y (NPY) is a widely distributed neuropeptide that has six receptors, Y-1 through Y-6. Neuropeptide Y stimulates food intake, inhibits energy expenditure, and increases body weight by activating Y-1 and Y-5 receptors in the hypothalamus *(100)*. Levels of NPY in the hypothalamus are temporally related to food intake and are elevated with energy depletion. Surprisingly, NPY knockout mice have no phenotype. NPY-5 receptor antagonists fall into two categories, those that reduce food intake and those that do not, but of those that do seem to do so through a mechanism separate from Y-5. Thus, Y-5 receptor antagonists do not appear promising as antiobesity agents *(101)*.

Y-1 receptor antagonists appear to have greater potential as antiobesity agents. A dihydropyridine neuropeptide Y-1 antagonist inhibited NPY-induced feeding in satiated rats *(102)*. Another Y-1 receptor antagonist, J-104870, suppressed food intake when given orally to Zucker rats *(103)*. A study measuring NPY in obese humans casts doubt on the importance of the NPY antagonists in the treatment of obesity in humans. Obese women had lower NPY levels than lean women and weight loss with a 400 kcal/d diet and adrenergic agonists (caffeine and ephedrine or caffeine, ephedrine, and yohimbine) did not change NPY levels at rest or after exercise *(104)*.

Melanin-Concentrating Hormone Receptor-1 Antagonist

Melanin-concentrating hormone (MSH) and α-MSH have opposite effects on skin coloration in fish, and excess melanin concentrating hormone blocks the effects of α-MSH when both are injected into the cerebral ventricles of rats *(105)*. MCH has two receptors, MCH-1 and MCH-2. Mice without the MCH-1 receptor have increased activity, increased temperature, and increased sympathetic tone *(106)*. Overexpression of the MCH-1 receptor and chronic infusion of an MCH-1 agonist cause enhanced feeding, caloric efficiency, and weight gain, whereas an MCH-1 antagonist reduces food intake and body weight gain without an effect on lean tissue *(107)*. MCH-1 antagonists reduce food intake by decreasing meal size, and also act as antidepressants and anxiolytics *(108,109)*. An orally active MCH-1 receptor antagonist that has good plasma levels and CNS exposure induced weight loss in obese mice with chronic treatment *(110)*. A number of other MCH-1 antagonists reduce food intake and body weight in experimental animals *(111)*. No human studies have been reported.

PANCREATIC LIPASE INHIBITOR

Although orlistat, a lipase inhibitor, is already approved for the treatment of obesity, ATL-962, another gastrointestinal lipase inhibitor, is also in development. A 5-d trial of ATL-962 in 90 normal volunteers was conducted on an inpatient unit. There was a three- to sevenfold increase in fecal fat that was dose-dependent, but only 11% of subjects had more than one oily stool. It was suggested that this lipase inhibitor may have fewer gastrointestinal adverse events compared with orlistat *(112)*.

Drugs No Longer Under Investigation or Withdrawn

PHENYLPROPANOLAMINE

Short-term studies with phenylpropanolamine were reviewed in 1992; weight loss was similar to the short-term weight loss seen with prescription obesity drugs *(113)*. The longest study of phenylpropanolamine lasted 20 wk. There was a 5.1-kg weight loss in the drug group and 0.4-kg weight loss in the placebo group, meeting the FDA criteria for a prescription weight loss drug of a greater than 5% weight loss compared with placebo *(114)*. Although phenylpropanolamine had a long history of safety in clinical trials dating to the 1930s, it was taken off the market because of an association with hemorrhagic stroke in women *(115)*.

EPHEDRINE

Ephedrine, combined with methylxantines, was used in the treatment of asthma for decades. A physician in Denmark noted weight loss in his patients taking this combination drug for asthma. The combination of 200 mg caffeine and 20 mg ephedrine given three times a day was subsequently approved as a prescription obesity medication in Denmark, where it enjoyed commercial success for more than a decade *(116)*. In 1994, legislation in the United States declared ephedra and caffeine to be foods, eligible to be sold as dietary herbal supplements. The use of this combination as an unregulated dietary supplement for the treatment of obesity was accompanied by reports of cardiovascular and neuropsychiatric adverse events, leading to the FDA declaring ephedra, the herbal form of ephedrine, as an adulterant *(117)*. Recently, courts in the United States have overturned the FDA decision to withdraw ephedra from the herbal market, at least in regard to ephedra doses of 10 mg or less, and the implications this legal decision may have on the availability of ephedra in the herbal dietary supplement market remain to be determined.

β-3 ADRENERGIC AGONISTS

In the early 1980s the β-3 adrenergic receptor was identified and shown, when stimulated, to increase lipolysis, fat oxidation, energy expenditure, and insulin action. Selective β-adrenergic agonists based on the rodent β-3 adrenergic receptor were not selective in humans, and the human β-3 adrenergic receptor was subsequently cloned and found to be only 60% homologous with rodents *(118)*. A β-3 adrenergic agonist selective for the human β-3 receptor, L-796568, increased lipolysis and energy expenditure when given as a single 1000-mg dose to obese men without significant stimulation of the β-2 adrenergic receptor *(119)*. A 28-d study with the same compound at 375 mg/d vs placebo in obese men gave no significant increase in energy expenditure, reduction in respiratory quotient, or changes in glucose tolerance. There was a significant reduction of triglycerides, however. This lack of a chronic effect was interpreted as either a lack of recruit-ment of β-3 responsive tissues, a downregulation of β-3 receptors, or both *(120)*. Thus, despite encouraging results from rodent trials, human trials of selective β-3 agonists have been disappointing.

BROMOCRIPTINE

Hibernating and migratory animals change their ability to store and burn fat based on circadian rhythms; these circadian rhythms are controlled by prolactin secretion. It has been postulated that obese and diabetic individuals have abnormal circadian rhythms. These abnormal rhythms favor fat storage and insulin resistance. Rapid-release bromocriptine (Ergocet®), given at 8:00 am, has been postulated to reverse this abnormal circadian rhythm and effectively treat diabetes and obesity. An uncontrolled trial of quick-release bromocriptine given orally for 8 wk significantly decreased 24-h plasma glucose, free fatty acid, and triglyceride levels from baseline *(121)*. This was followed by a controlled trial in which 22 diabetic subjects were randomized to quick-release bromocriptine or placebo. The hemoglobin A1c fell from 8.7 to 8.1% in the bromocriptine group and rose from 8.5 to 9.1% in the placebo group, a statistically significant differ-ence *(122)*. In an uncontrolled trial, 33 obese postmenopausal women reduced their body fat by 11.7% measured by skinfold thickness over 6 wk of treatment with quick-release bromocriptine *(123)*. This was followed by a controlled trial in which 17 obese subjects were randomized to rapid-release bromocriptine (1.6–2.4 mg/d) or a placebo for 18 wk. The bromocriptine group lost significantly more weight (6.3 kg vs 0.9 kg) and more fat as measured by skinfolds (5.4 kg vs 1.5 kg) *(124)*. The company developing Ergocet received an approvable determination by the FDA for quick-release bromocriptine to treat diabetes, but was asked to do additional safety studies. These studies were never performed, and the obesity development program proceeded no further.

ECOPIPAM

Ecopipam is an antagonist to dopamine 1 and 5 receptors. It was originally studied for the treatment of cocaine addiction *(125)*. Ecopipam was in development as an obesity drug but its development was recently terminated *(126)*.

New Areas for Drug Development

HISTAMINE-3 RECEPTOR ANTAGONISTS

Histamine and its receptors can affect food intake. Among the antipsychotic drugs that produce weight gain, binding to the H-1 receptor is higher than with any other monoam-ine receptor; histamine reduces food intake by acting on this receptor *(127)*. The search for drugs that can modulate food intake through the histamine system has focused on the histamine H3 receptor, which is an autoreceptor—that is, activation of this receptor inhibits histamine release, whereas blockade of the receptor increases histamine release. Both imidazole and nonimidazole antagonists of the H3 receptor have been published and shown to reduce food intake and body weight gain in experimental animals *(98,128)*.

MELANOCORTIN-4 RECEPTOR AGONISTS

Of the potential targets for drugs to treat obesity, the biological data favoring this receptor are among the strongest *(129)*. There are five melanocortin (MC) receptors that belong to the G protein-coupled 7-transmembrane family of receptors. The MC1 receptor is located primarily in skin and modulates pigmentation changes in response to α-MSH. The MC2 receptor is in the adrenal gland, where it responds to ACTH-modulating steroid production. The MC3 and MC4 receptors are primarily in the brain, where they are both involved in energy homeostasis. The final receptor, MC5, is located in exocrine tissues. The MC4 receptors in the brain are located in sites that affect feeding. In the hypothalamus, leptin-responsive neurons modulate MC4 expression, modifying energy balance. The MC4 receptor responds to α-MSH with a decrease in food intake. When animals are genetically engineered to remove expression of MC4 receptors, they become massively obese. The effect of α-MSH on the MC4 receptor can be blocked by agouti-related peptide (AgRP). Mice that overexpress AgRP or its equivalent agouti peptide (yellow mice) are obese. Numerous genetic variants of the MC4 receptor have been identified in humans that are associated in variable degrees of overweight and taller stature.

These biological observations have led to the search for agonists and antagonists to this receptor *(129)*. The first two, an agonist called melanotan-II (MT-II) and an antagonist called SHU-9119, are modifications of the core sequence of α-MSH. They demonstrate the viability of this strategy, as MT-II reduces food intake and body weight, whereas SHU-9119 as well as AgRP block this effect. Both peptide and nonpeptide agonists for the MC4 receptor have been developed, but no reports of clinical studies have emerged yet *(129)*.

MODULATORS OF ENERGY SENSING IN THE BRAIN

Recent developments suggest that the ratio of AMP to ATP in selected regions of the brain may play a role in modulating food intake and energy balance. The discovery that blockade of the fatty acid synthase with cerulenin, a naturally occurring product or a synthetic molecule (C-75) opened the door to these insights *(130)*. Fatty acid synthesis and oxidation are coordinately regulated. Adenosine 5-monophosphate activated kinase (AMPK) phosphorylates acetyl-Co-carboxylase to inhibit the enzyme that converts acetyl-CoA to malonyl CoA in the first step toward long-chain fatty acid synthesis. AMPK dephosphorylates malonyl Co-A decarboxylase, which activates this enzyme that lowers malonyl-CoA concentration. The net effect of these phosphorylations by AMPK is to convert substrate to oxidation rather than fatty acid synthesis. Cerulenin or C-75 blocks fatty acid synthase, which also blocks fat synthesis and activates fatty acid oxidation by activating carnitine palitoyl Co-A transferase-I. Injection of these fatty acid synthase inhibitors into animals produces a reduction in food intake and weight loss, suggesting the potential for future clinical drugs *(130)*.

GHRELIN ANTAGONISTS

The search for small orally absorbed peptides that could release growth hormone led to the identification in 1996 of the growth hormone secretogog (GHS) receptor, and the isolation in 1998 of ghrelin, the natural ligand for this GHS receptor. Ghrelin stimulates food intake in human subjects. Moreover, clinical trials with the small GH-stimulating peptides produced weight gain in human beings, suggesting that antagonists to this receptor might be useful in the treatment of obesity *(131)*. No clinical data are yet available.

11-β-HYDROXYSTEROID DEHYDROGENASE TYPE 1 INHIBITOR

Cortisol, the glucocorticoid secreted by the adrenal gland, can be inactivated through conversion to cortisone in peripheral tissues. Cortisone can be reactivated by the enzyme 11-β-hydroxysteroid dehydrogenase type 1. Mice in which this enzyme is overexpressed have increased amounts of fat in the abdomen, suggesting that modulation of this enzyme could be a target to selectively modulate visceral or central adiposity *(132)*.

ADIPONECTIN

Adiponectin, also called adipocyte complement-related protein (ACRP), is produced exclusively in fat cells, and is their most abundant protein. It has a long half-life in the blood and is of interest because its production and secretion by the fat cell is decreased as the fat cell increases in size. Higher levels of adiponectin are associated with insulin sensitivity and lower levels of adiponectin, as seen in obesity, are associated with insulin resistance. In experimental studies, adiponectin has been shown to reduce food intake when administered into the brain *(133)*. Although it is a large molecule, drugs that modulate its production, release, or action may be potential candidates for treating obesity.

CONCLUSIONS

Although the drugs currently available for the treatment of obesity are few in number and limited in efficacy, the pipeline for obesity drug development is very rich. Because drug development is more sophisticated today than in the past, we anticipate that the development of safe and effective drugs for the treatment of obesity will proceed at a more rapid pace than was the case for other chronic diseases, such as hypertension and diabetes, that now have safe and effective medications.

REFERENCES

1. Zhang Y, Proenca R, Maffei M, et al. Positional cloning of the mouse obese gene and its human homologue. Nature 1994;372(6505):425–432.
2. Halaas JL, Gajiwala KS, Maffei M, et al. Weight-reducing effects of the plasma protein encoded by the obese gene. Science 1995;269(5223):543–546.
3. NIH Consensus Development Conference Statement. Health Implications of Obesity. 1985.
4. Puhl RM, Brownell KD. Psychosocial origins of obesity stigma: toward changing a powerful and pervasive bias. Obes Rev 2003;4(4):213–227.
5. Li Z, Maglione M, Tu W, et al. Meta-analysis: pharmacologic treatment of obesity. Ann Intern Med 2005;142(7):532–546.
6. Anonymous. Dexfenfluramine for obesity. Med Lett Drugs Ther 1996;38(979):64–65.
7. Yanovski SZ, Yanovski JA. Obesity. N Engl J Med 2002;346(8):591–602.
8. Bray GA, Greenway FL. Current and potential drugs for treatment of obesity. Endocr Rev 1999;20(6):805–875.
9. Snow V, Barry P, Fitterman N, et al. Pharmacologic and surgical management of obesity in primary care: a clinical practice guideline from the American College of Physicians. Ann Intern Med 2005;142(7):525–531.
10. Apfelbaum M, Vague P, Ziegler O, et al. Long-term maintenance of weight loss after a very-low-calorie diet: a randomized blinded trial of the efficacy and tolerability of sibutramine. Am J Med 1999;106(2):179–184.
11. Hauner H, Meier M, Wendland G, et al. Weight reduction by sibutramine in obese subjects in primary care medicine: the SAT Study. Exp Clin Endocrinol Diabetes 2004;112(4):201–207.

12. McNulty SJ, Ur E, Williams G. A randomized trial of sibutramine in the management of obese type 2 diabetic patients treated with metformin. Diabetes Care 2003;26(1):125–131.

13. Davis JL. Use of sibutramine hydrochloride monohydrate in the treatment of the painful peripheral neuropathy of diabetes. Diabetes Care 2000;23(10):1594–1595.

14. Bray GA, Blackburn GL, Ferguson JM, et al. Sibutramine produces dose-related weight loss. Obes Res 1999;7(2):189–198.

15. James WP, Astrup A, Finer N, et al. Effect of sibutramine on weight maintenance after weight loss: a randomised trial. STORM Study Group. Sibutramine Trial of Obesity Reduction and Maintenance. Lancet 2000;356(9248):2119–2125.

16. Wirth A, Krause J. Long-term weight loss with sibutramine: a randomized controlled trial. JAMA 2001;286(11):1331–1339.

17. Sramek JJ, Leibowitz MT, Weinstein SP, et al. Efficacy and safety of sibutramine for weight loss in obese patients with hypertension well controlled by beta-adrenergic blocking agents: a placebo-controlled, double-blind, randomised trial. J Hum Hypertens 2002;16(1):13–19.

18. McMahon FG, Fujioka K, Singh BN, et al. Efficacy and safety of sibutramine in obese white and African American patients with hypertension: a 1-year, double-blind, placebo-controlled, multicenter trial. Arch Intern Med 2000;160(14):2185–2191.

19. Vettor R, Serra R, Fabris R, et al. Effect of sibutramine on weight management and metabolic control in type 2 diabetes: a meta-analysis of clinical studies. Diabetes Care 2005;28(4):942–949.

20. Finer N, Bloom SR, Frost GS, et al. Sibutramine is effective for weight loss and diabetic control in obesity with type 2 diabetes: a randomised, double-blind, placebo-controlled study. Diabetes Obes Metab 2000;2(2):105–112.

21. Fujioka K, Seaton TB, Rowe E, et al. Weight loss with sibutramine improves glycaemic control and other metabolic parameters in obese patients with type 2 diabetes mellitus. Diabetes Obes Metab 2000;2(3):175–187.

22. Wadden TA, Berkowitz RI, Sarwer DB, et al. Benefits of lifestyle modification in the pharmacologic treatment of obesity: a randomized trial. Arch Intern Med 2001;161(2):218–227.

23. Berkowitz RI, Wadden TA, Tershakovec AM, et al. Behavior therapy and sibutramine for the treatment of adolescent obesity: a randomized controlled trial. JAMA 2003;289(14):1805–1812.

24. Godoy-Matos A, Carraro L, Vieira A, et al. Treatment of obese adolescents with sibutramine: a randomized, double-blind, controlled study. J Clin Endocrinol Metab 2005;90(3):1460–1465.

25. Berkowitz RI, Fujioka K, Daniels SR, et al. Effects of sibutramine treatment in obese adolescents: aaaa randommmized trial. Ann Inst Med 2006;145:81–90.

26. Sjostrom L, Rissanen A, Andersen T, et al. Randomised placebo-controlled trial of orlistat for weight loss and prevention of weight regain in obese patients. European Multicentre Orlistat Study Group. Lancet 1998;352(9123):167–172.

27. Davidson MH, Hauptman J, DiGirolamo M, et al. Weight control and risk factor reduction in obese subjects treated for 2 years with orlistat: a randomized controlled trial. JAMA 1999;281(3):235–242.

28. Rossner S, Sjostrom L, Noack R, et al. Weight loss, weight maintenance, and improved cardiovascular risk factors after 2 years treatment with orlistat for obesity. European Orlistat Obesity Study Group. Obes Res 2000;8(1):49–61.

29. Hauptman J, Lucas C, Boldrin MN, et al. Orlistat in the long-term treatment of obesity in primary care settings. Arch Fam Med 2000;9(2):160–167.

30. Torgerson JS, Hauptman J, Boldrin MN, et al. XENical in the prevention of diabetes in obese subjects (XENDOS) study: a randomized study of orlistat as an adjunct to lifestyle changes for the prevention of type 2 diabetes in obese patients. Diabetes Care 2004;27(1):155–161.

31. Hollander PA, Elbein SC, Hirsch IB, et al. Role of orlistat in the treatment of obese patients with type 2 diabetes. A 1-year randomized double-blind study. Diabetes Care 1998;21(8):1288–1294.

32. Kelley DE, Bray GA, Pi-Sunyer FX, et al. Clinical efficacy of orlistat therapy in overweight and obese patients with insulin-treated type 2 diabetes: a 1-year randomized controlled trial. Diabetes Care 2002;25(6):1033–1041.

33. Miles JM, Leiter L, Hollander P, et al. Effect of orlistat in overweight and obese patients with type 2 diabetes treated with metformin. Diabetes Care 2002;25(7):1123–1128.

34. Heymsfield SB, Segal KR, Hauptman J, et al. Effects of weight loss with orlistat on glucose tolerance and progression to type 2 diabetes in obese adults. Arch Intern Med 2000;160(9):1321–1326.

35. Reaven G, Segal K, Hauptman J, et al. Effect of orlistat-assisted weight loss in decreasing coronary heart disease risk in patients with syndrome X. Am J Cardiol 2001;87(7):827–831.

36. Mittendorfer B, Ostlund RE Jr, Patterson BW, et al. Orlistat inhibits dietary cholesterol absorption. Obes Res 2001;9(10):599–604.

37. Chanoine JP, Hampl S, Jensen C, et al. Effect of orlistat on weight and body composition in obese adolescents: a randomized controlled trial. JAMA 2005;293(23):2873–2883.

38. Zhi J, Mulligan TE, Hauptman JB. Long-term systemic exposure of orlistat, a lipase inhibitor, and its metabolites in obese patients. J Clin Pharmacol 1999;39(1):41–46.

39. Wadden TA, Berkowitz RI, Womble LG, et al. Effects of sibutramine plus orlistat in obese women following 1 year of treatment by sibutramine alone: a placebo-controlled trial. Obes Res 2000;8(6): 431–437.

40. Munro J, MacCuish A, Wilson E, et al. Comparison of continuous and intermittent anorectic therapy in obesity. Br Med J 1968;1:352–354.

41. Goldstein DJ, Rampey AH Jr, Roback PJ, et al. Efficacy and safety of long-term fluoxetine treatment of obesity—maximizing success. Obes Res 1995;3 Suppl 4:481S–490S.

42. Gadde KM, Parker CB, Maner LG, et al. Bupropion for weight loss: an investigation of efficacy and tolerability in overweight and obese women. Obes Res 2001;9(9):544–551.

43. Jain AK, Kaplan RA, Gadde KM, et al. Bupropion SR vs. placebo for weight loss in obese patients with depressive symptoms. Obes Res 2002;10(10):1049–1056.

44. Anderson JW, Greenway FL, Fujioka K, et al. Bupropion SR enhances weight loss: a 48-week double-blind, placebo-controlled trial. Obes Res 2002;10(7):633–641.

45. Ben-Menachem E, Axelsen M, Johanson EH, et al. Predictors of weight loss in adults with topiramate-treated epilepsy. Obes Res 2003;11(4):556–562.

46. Bray GA, Hollander P, Klein S, et al. A 6-month randomized, placebo-controlled, dose-ranging trial of topiramate for weight loss in obesity. Obes Res 2003;11(6):722–733.

47. Wilding J, Van Gaal L, Rissanen A, et al. A randomized double-blind placebo-controlled study of the long-term efficacy and safety of topiramate in the treatment of obese subjects. Int J Obes Relat Metab Disord 2004;28(11):1399–1410.

48. Astrup A, Caterson I, Zelissen P, et al. Topiramate: long-term maintenance of weight loss induced by a low-calorie diet in obese subjects. Obes Res 2004;12(10):1658–1669.

49. Shapira NA, Goldsmith TD, McElroy SL. Treatment of binge-eating disorder with topiramate: a clinical case series. J Clin Psychiatry 2000;61(5):368–372.

50. McElroy SL, Arnold LM, Shapira NA, et al. Topiramate in the treatment of binge eating disorder associated with obesity: a randomized, placebo-controlled trial. Am J Psychiatry 2003;160(2):255–261.

51. McElroy SL, Shapira NA, Arnold LM, et al. Topiramate in the long-term treatment of binge-eating disorder associated with obesity. J Clin Psychiatry 2004;65(11):1463–1469.

52. Shapira NA, Lessig MC, Murphy TK, et al. Topiramate attenuates self-injurious behaviour in Prader-Willi syndrome. Int J Neuropsychopharmacol 2002;5(2):141–145.

53. Smathers SA, Wilson JG, Nigro MA. Topiramate effectiveness in Prader-Willi syndrome. Pediatr Neurol 2003;28(2):130–133.

54. Shapira NA, Lessig MC, Lewis MH, et al. Effects of topiramate in adults with Prader-Willi syndrome. Am J Ment Retard 2004;109(4):301–309.

55. Winkelman JW. Treatment of nocturnal eating syndrome and sleep-related eating disorder with topiramate. Sleep Med 2003;4(3):243–246.

56. Gadde KM, Franciscy DM, Wagner HR 2nd, et al. Zonisamide for weight loss in obese adults: a randomized controlled trial. JAMA 2003;289(14):1820–1825.

57. McElroy SL, Kotwal R, Hudson JI, et al. Zonisamide in the treatment of binge-eating disorder: an open-label, prospective trial. J Clin Psychiatry 2004;65(1):50–56.

58. Bray GA, Gallagher TF Jr. Manifestations of hypothalamic obesity in man: a comprehensive investigation of eight patients and a reveiw of the literature. Medicine (Baltimore) 1975;54(4):301–330.

59. Lustig RH, Rose SR, Burghen GA, et al. Hypothalamic obesity caused by cranial insult in children: altered glucose and insulin dynamics and reversal by a somatostatin agonist. J Pediatr 1999;135(2 Pt 1):162–168.

60. Lustig RH, Hinds PS, Ringwald-Smith K, et al. Octreotide therapy of pediatric hypothalamic obesity: a double-blind, placebo-controlled trial. J Clin Endocrinol Metab 2003;88(6):2586–2892.

61. Velasquez-Mieyer PA, Cowan PA, Arheart KL, et al. Suppression of insulin secretion is associated with weight loss and altered macronutrient intake and preference in a subset of obese adults. Int J Obes Relat Metab Disord 2003;27(2):219–226.

62. Lustig R, Greenway F, Velasquez D, et al. Weight loss in obese adults with insulin hypersecretion treated with Sandostatin LAR Depot. Obes Res 2003;11 (Suppl):A25.

63. Foxx-Orenstein A, Camilleri M, Stephens D, et al. Effect of a somatostatin analogue on gastric motor and sensory functions in healthy humans. Gut 2003;52(11):1555–1561.

64. Tan TM, Vanderpump M, Khoo B, et al. Somatostatin infusion lowers plasma ghrelin without reducing appetite in adults with Prader-Willi syndrome. J Clin Endocrinol Metab 2004;89(8):4162–4165.

65. Fontbonne A, Charles MA, Juhan-Vague I, et al. The effect of metformin on the metabolic abnormalities associated with upper-body fat distribution. BIGPRO Study Group. Diabetes Care 1996;19(9):920–926.

66. Knowler WC, Barrett-Connor E, Fowler SE, et al. Reduction in the incidence of type 2 diabetes with lifestyle intervention or metformin. N Engl J Med 2002;346(6):393–403.

67. Ortega-Gonzalez C, Luna S, Hernandez L, et al. Responses of serum androgen and insulin resistance to metformin and pioglitazone in obese, insulin-resistant women with polycystic ovary syndrome. J Clin Endocrinol Metab 2005;90(3):1360–1365.

68. Ratner RE, Dickey R, Fineman M, et al. Amylin replacement with pramlintide as an adjunct to insulin therapy improves long-term glycaemic and weight control in Type 1 diabetes mellitus: a 1-year, randomized controlled trial. Diabet Med 2004;21(11):1204–1212.

69. Maggs D, Shen L, Strobel S, et al. Effect of pramlintide on A1C and body weight in insulin-treated African Americans and Hispanics with type 2 diabetes: a pooled post hoc analysis. Metabolism 2003;52(12):1638–1642.

70. Small CJ, Bloom SR. Gut hormones as peripheral anti obesity targets. Curr Drug Targets CNS Neurol Disord 2004;3(5):379–388.

71. Greenway SE, Greenway FL 3rd, Klein S. Effects of obesity surgery on non-insulin-dependent diabetes mellitus. Arch Surg 2002;137(10):1109–1117.

72. Patriti A, Facchiano E, Sanna A, et al. The enteroinsular axis and the recovery from type 2 diabetes after bariatric surgery. Obes Surg 2004;14(6):840–848.

73. Lugari R, Dei Cas A, Ugolotti D, et al. Glucagon-like peptide 1 (GLP-1) secretion and plasma dipeptidyl peptidase IV (DPP-IV) activity in morbidly obese patients undergoing biliopancreatic diversion. Horm Metab Res 2004;36(2):111–115.

74. Szayna M, Doyle ME, Betkey JA, et al. Exendin-4 decelerates food intake, weight gain, and fat deposition in Zucker rats. Endocrinology 2000;141(6):1936–1941.

75. Gedulin BR, Nikoulina SE, Smith PA, et al. Exenatide (exendin-4) improves insulin sensitivity and β-cell mass in insulin-resistant obese fa/fa Zucker rats independent of glycemia and body weight. Endocrinology 2005;146(4):2069–2076.

76. Rodriquez de Fonseca F, Navarro M, Alvarez E, et al. Peripheral versus central effects of glucagon-like peptide-1 receptor agonists on satiety and body weight loss in Zucker obese rats. Metabolism 2000;49(6):709–717.

77. Kastin AJ, Akerstrom V. Entry of exendin-4 into brain is rapid but may be limited at high doses. Int J Obes Relat Metab Disord 2003;27(3):313–318.

78. Edwards CM, Stanley SA, Davis R, et al. Exendin-4 reduces fasting and postprandial glucose and decreases energy intake in healthy volunteers. Am J Physiol Endocrinol Metab 2001;281(1):E155–E161.

79. Fineman MS, Shen LZ, Taylor K, et al. Effectiveness of progressive dose-escalation of exenatide (exendin-4) in reducing dose-limiting side effects in subjects with type 2 diabetes. Diabetes Metab Res Rev 2004;20(5):411–417.

80. Buse JB, Henry RR, Han J, et al. Effects of exenatide (exendin-4) on glycemic control over 30 weeks in sulfonylurea-treated patients with type 2 diabetes. Diabetes Care 2004;27(11):2628–2635.

81. Bensaid M, Gary-Bobo M, Esclangon A, et al. The cannabinoid CB1 receptor antagonist SR141716 increases Acrp30 mRNA expression in adipose tissue of obese fa/fa rats and in cultured adipocyte cells. Mol Pharmacol 2003;63(4):908–914.

82. Website. http://en.sanofi-aventis.com/investors/p_investors.asp.

83. Van Gaal LF, Rissanen AM, Scheen AJ, et al. Effects of the cannabinoid-1 receptor blocker rimonabant on weight reduction and cardiovascular risk factors in overweight patients: 1-year experience from the RIO-Europe study. Lancet 2005;365(9468):1389–1397.

84. Heymsfield SB, Greenberg AS, Fujioka K, et al. Recombinant leptin for weight loss in obese and lean adults: a randomized, controlled, dose-escalation trial. JAMA 1999;282(16):1568–1575.

85. Hukshorn CJ, Westerterp-Plantenga MS, Saris WH. Pegylated human recombinant leptin (PEG-OB) causes additional weight loss in severely energy-restricted, overweight men. Am J Clin Nutr 2003;77(4):771–776.

86. Oral EA, Simha V, Ruiz E, et al. Leptin-replacement therapy for lipodystrophy. N Engl J Med 2002;346(8):570–578.

87. Rosenbaum M, Murphy EM, Heymsfield SB, et al. Low dose leptin administration reverses effects of sustained weight-reduction on energy expenditure and circulating concentrations of thyroid hormones. J Clin Endocrinol Metab 2002;87(5):2391–2394.

88. Anderson KD, Lambert PD, Corcoran TL, et al. Activation of the hypothalamic arcuate nucleus predicts the anorectic actions of ciliary neurotrophic factor and leptin in intact and gold thioglucose-lesioned mice. J Neuroendocrinol 2003;15(7):649–660.

89. Ettinger MP, Littlejohn TW, Schwartz SL, et al. Recombinant variant of ciliary neurotrophic factor for weight loss in obese adults: a randomized, dose-ranging study. JAMA 2003;289(14):1826–1832.

90. Website. www.regeneron.com/.

91. Website. www.metabolic.com.au/files/T5SH4035T6/ASX_%20AOD9604_result%20announcement.pdf.

92. Batterham RL, Cohen MA, Ellis SM, et al. Inhibition of food intake in obese subjects by peptide YY3-36. N Engl J Med 2003;349(10):941–948.

93. Brandt G, Sileno A, Quay S. Intranasal peptide YY 3-36: phase 1 dose ranging and dose sequencing studies. Obes Res 2004;12 (Suppl):A28.

94. Wynne K, Park AJ, Small CJ, et al. Subcutaneous oxyntomodulin reduces body weight in overweight and obese subjects: a double-blind, randomized, controlled trial. Diabetes 2005;54(8):2390–2395.

95. Pi-Sunyer X, Kissileff HR, Thornton J, et al. C-terminal octapeptide of cholecystokinin decreases food intake in obese men. Physiol Behav 1982;29(4):627–630.

96. Alemany M, Fernandez-Lopez JA, Petrobelli A, et al. [Weight loss in a patient with morbid obesity under treatment with oleoyl-estrone]. Med Clin (Barc) 2003;121(13):496–499.

97. Gibson WT, Ebersole BJ, Bhattacharyya S, et al. Mutational analysis of the serotonin receptor 5HT2c in severe early-onset human obesity. Can J Physiol Pharmacol 2004;82(6):426–429.

98. Nilsson BM. 5-Hydroxytryptamine 2C (HT2C) receptor agonists as potential antiobesity agents. J Med Chem 2006;49(14):4023–4034.

99. Website. www.clinicaltrials.gov/t/show/NCT00104507?order=1.

100. Parker E, Van Heek M, Stamford A. Neuropeptide Y receptors as targets for anti-obesity drug development: perspective and current status. Eur J Pharmacol 2002;440(2–3):173–187.

101. Levens NR, Della-Zuana O. Neuropeptide Y Y5 receptor antagonists as anti-obesity drugs. Curr Opin Investig Drugs 2003;4(10):1198–1204.

102. Poindexter GS, Bruce MA, LeBoulluec KL, et al. Dihydropyridine neuropeptide Y Y(1) receptor antagonists. Bioorg Med Chem Lett 2002;12(3):379–382.

103. Kanatani A, Hata M, Mashiko S, et al. A typical Y1 receptor regulates feeding behaviors: effects of a potent and selective Y1 antagonist, J-115814. Mol Pharmacol 2001;59(3):501–505.

104. Zahorska-Markiewicz B, Obuchowicz E, Waluga M, et al. Neuropeptide Y in obese women during treatment with adrenergic modulation drugs. Med Sci Monit 2001;7(3):403–408.

105. Ludwig DS, Mountjoy KG, Tatro JB, et al. Melanin-concentrating hormone: a functional melanocortin antagonist in the hypothalamus. Am J Physiol 1998;274(4 Pt 1):E627–E633.

106. Astrand A, Bohlooly YM, Larsdotter S, et al. Mice lacking melanin-concentrating hormone receptor 1 demonstrate increased heart rate associated with altered autonomic activity. Am J Physiol Regul Integr Comp Physiol 2004;287(4):R749–R758.

107. Shearman LP, Camacho RE, Sloan Stribling D, et al. Chronic MCH-1 receptor modulation alters appetite, body weight and adiposity in rats. Eur J Pharmacol 2003;475(1–3):37–47.

108. Kowalski TJ, Farley C, Cohen-Williams ME, et al. Melanin-concentrating hormone-1 receptor antagonism decreases feeding by reducing meal size. Eur J Pharmacol 2004;497(1):41–47.

109. Borowsky B, Durkin MM, Ogozalek K, et al. Antidepressant, anxiolytic and anorectic effects of a melanin-concentrating hormone-1 receptor antagonist. Nat Med 2002;8(8):825–830.

110. Souers AJ, Gao J, Brune M, et al. Identification of 2-(4-benzyloxyphenyl)-N-[1-(2-pyrrolidin-1-yl-ethyl)-1H-indazol-6-yl]acetamide, an orally efficacious melanin-concentrating hormone receptor 1 antagonist for the treatment of obesity. J Med Chem 2005;48(5):1318–1321.

111. Handlon A, Zhou H. Melanin-concentrating hormone-1 receptor antagonists. J Med Chem 2006;49:4017–4022.

112. Dunk C, Enunwa M, De La Monte S, et al. Increased fecal fat excretion in normal volunteers treated with lipase inhibitor ATL-962. Int J Obes Relat Metab Disord 2002;26 (suppl):S135.

113. Greenway FL. Clinical studies with phenylpropanolamine: a metaanalysis. Am J Clin Nutr 1992;55(1 Suppl):203S–205S.

114. Schteingart DE. Effectiveness of phenylpropanolamine in the management of moderate obesity. Int J Obes Relat Metab Disord 1992;16(7):487–493.
115. Kernan WN, Viscoli CM, Brass LM, et al. Phenylpropanolamine and the risk of hemorrhagic stroke. N Engl J Med 2000;343(25):1826–1832.
116. Greenway FL. The safety and efficacy of pharmaceutical and herbal caffeine and ephedrine use as a weight loss agent. Obes Rev 2001;2(3):199–211.
117. Shekelle PG, Hardy ML, Morton SC, et al. Efficacy and safety of ephedra and ephedrine for weight loss and athletic performance: a meta-analysis. JAMA 2003;289(12):1537–1545.
118. de Souza CJ, Burkey BF. Beta 3-adrenoceptor agonists as anti-diabetic and anti-obesity drugs in humans. Curr Pharm Des 2001;7(14):1433–1449.
119. van Baak MA, Hul GB, Toubro S, et al. Acute effect of L-796568, a novel beta 3-adrenergic receptor agonist, on energy expenditure in obese men. Clin Pharmacol Ther 2002;71(4):272–279.
120. Larsen TM, Toubro S, van Baak MA, et al. Effect of a 28-d treatment with L-796568, a novel beta(3)-adrenergic receptor agonist, on energy expenditure and body composition in obese men. Am J Clin Nutr 2002;76(4):780–788.
121. Kamath V, Jones CN, Yip JC, et al. Effects of a quick-release form of bromocriptine (Ergoset) on fasting and postprandial plasma glucose, insulin, lipid, and lipoprotein concentrations in obese non-diabetic hyperinsulinemic women. Diabetes Care 1997;20(11):1697–1701.
122. Pijl H, Ohashi S, Matsuda M, et al. Bromocriptine: a novel approach to the treatment of type 2 diabetes. Diabetes Care 2000;23(8):1154–1161.
123. Meier AH, Cincotta AH, Lovell WC. Timed bromocriptine administration reduces body fat stores in obese subjects and hyperglycemia in type II diabetics. Experientia 1992;48(3):248–253.
124. Cincotta AH, Meier AH. Bromocriptine (Ergoset) reduces body weight and improves glucose tolerance in obese subjects. Diabetes Care 1996;19(6):667–670.
125. Nann-Vernotica E, Donny EC, Bigelow GE, et al. Repeated administration of the D1/5 antagonist ecopipam fails to attenuate the subjective effects of cocaine. Psychopharmacology (Berl) 2001;155(4):338–347.
126. Bays H, Dujovne C. Anti-obesity drug development. Expert Opin Investig Drugs 2002;11(9):1189–1204.
127. Kroeze WK, Hufeisen SJ, Popadak BA, et al. H1-histamine receptor affinity predicts short-term weight gain for typical and atypical antipsychotic drugs. Neuropsychopharmacology 2003;28(3):519–526.
128. Leurs R, Bakker RA, Timmerman H, et al. The histamine H3 receptor: from gene cloning to H3 receptor drugs. Nat Rev Drug Discov 2005;4(2):107–120.
129. Nargund R, Strack A, Fong T. Melanocortin-4 receptor (MC4R) agonists for the treatment of obesity. J Med Chem 2006;49:4035–4043.
130. Shu IW, Lindenberg DL, Mizuno TM, et al. The fatty acid synthase inhibitor cerulenin and feeding, like leptin, activate hypothalamic pro-opiomelanocortin (POMC) neurons. Brain Res 2003;985(1):1–12.
131. Svensson J, Lonn L, Jansson JO, et al. Two-month treatment of obese subjects with the oral growth hormone (GH) secretagogue MK-677 increases GH secretion, fat-free mass, and energy expenditure. J Clin Endocrinol Metab 1998;83(2):362–369.
132. Morton NM, Paterson JM, Masuzaki H, et al. Novel adipose tissue-mediated resistance to diet-induced visceral obesity in 11 beta-hydroxysteroid dehydrogenase type 1-deficient mice. Diabetes 2004;53(4):931–938.
133. Masaki T, Chiba S, Yasuda T, et al. Peripheral, but not central, administration of adiponectin reduces visceral adiposity and upregulates the expression of uncoupling protein in agouti yellow (Ay/a) obese mice. Diabetes 2003;52(9):2266–2273.
134. National Cholesterol Education Program, National Heart, Lung, and Blood Institute, National Institutes of Health. Third report of the National Cholesterol Education Program (NCEP) Expert Panel on detection, evaluation, and treatment of high blood cholesterol in adults (adult treatment panel III): final report. Bethesda (MD): NHLBI; 2002. NIH Publication No. 02-5215.

19 Surgical Approaches and Outcomes

Treatment of the Obese Patient

George L. Blackburn, MD, PhD,
and Vivian M. Sanchez, MD

CONTENTS

INTRODUCTION
COMORBIDITIES
MECHANISMS OF ACTION IN WEIGHT-LOSS SURGERY
CURRENTLY PERFORMED SURGERIES
OUTCOMES
SAFETY AND EFFECTIVENESS
CONCLUSION
ACKNOWLEDGMENTS
REFERENCES

Summary

Weight-loss surgery is the only effective treatment for severe, medically complicated, and refractory obesity. It reverses, eliminates, or significantly ameliorates numerous life-threatening medical comorbidities that occur as part of the pathophysiology of obesity. Rapid changes in surgical technology and in demand for weight-loss surgery have made the field one of medicine's most dynamic. This chapter reviews available surgical procedures, their possible mechanisms of action through the enterohypothalamic endocrine axis, and their risks and outcomes.

Key Words: Bariatric surgery; weight loss surgery; morbid obesity; endocrinology; gastric bypass; laparoscopic adjustable band; gut hormones; type 2 diabetes.

INTRODUCTION

Candidates for bariatric surgery include those who are morbidly obese, with a BMI ≥ 40 kg/m^2, or those with a BMI ≥ 35 kg/m^2 and significant comorbidities [1]. In the United States, an estimated 8 to 10 million people suffer from morbid obesity [2]. Their numbers are increasing exponentially without any evidence of reaching a plateau or approaching a downward trend [1].

The growing prevalence of severe obesity has spurred concomitant growth in obesity surgery. Nguyen et al. [2] report a 450% increase in the number of bariatric operations performed in the United States between 1988 and 2002. Similar findings have been

From: *Contemporary Endocrinology: Treatment of the Obese Patient*
Edited by: R. F. Kushner and D. H. Bessesen © Humana Press Inc., Totowa, NJ

reported by Liu et al. *(3)* and Courcoulas et al. *(4)*. Most of the growth in bariatric surgery rates has occurred in relatively large, high-volume hospitals *(5)* that meet best-practice guidelines of more than 100 procedures per year. Other factors related to the safety and effectiveness of weight loss surgery focus on the clinical data infrastructure needed to assess and improve quality *(6,7)*.

COMORBIDITIES

Obesity is associated with substantially increased risk of morbidity and all-cause mortality from numerous comorbidities. These include type 2 diabetes, hypertension, dyslipidemia, cardiovascular disease, stroke, sleep apnea and other respiratory problems, gallbladder disease, fatty liver disease, osteoarthritis, and several forms of cancer. In addition to adverse health effects, people with obesity also suffer substantial social stigmatization and workplace discrimination *(6)*.

To facilitate assessment of obesity-related comorbidities in bariatric surgery patients, Ali et al. *(8)* have developed a clinically based, standardized system for scaled assessment of major comorbidities. By scoring each condition from 0 to 5, according to severity, this scheme allows for standardized preoperative characterization of a bariatric patient population and uniform postoperative longitudinal assessment of changes in comorbidities after weight-reduction surgery.

Weight loss improves or resolves many comorbid conditions. However, lifestyle and pharmaceutical treatments fail most people. Bariatric surgery is known to provide marked and lasting weight loss of 47.5 to 70.1% of excess body weight *(9)*. This is approx 25 to 30% of baseline body weight. Such results have been obtained in relative safety, with operative mortality equal to or less than that for other major operative procedures (about 0.5%) *(2,9)*.

MECHANISMS OF ACTION IN WEIGHT-LOSS SURGERY

Physiological Changes

There are two major categories of weight-loss surgery: gastric restriction and intestinal malabsorption. Restrictive operations create a small neogastric pouch and gastric outlet to decrease food intake. Malabsorptive procedures rearrange the small intestine in order to decrease the functional length or efficiency of the intestinal mucosa for nutrient absorption. Although the malabsorptive approach produces more rapid and profound weight loss than restrictive procedures, it also puts patients at risk of metabolic complications, such as vitamin deficiencies and protein–energy malnutrition *(10)*. Restrictive procedures are considered simpler and safer than their malabsorptive counterparts, but may result in a smaller amount of long-term weight loss.

Neuroendocrine Changes

One way bariatric surgery is thought to produce weight loss is through its effect on the enterohypothalamic endocrine axis *(12)*. Dramatic improvements in glycemic control have been observed in subjects with type 2 diabetes following bariatric surgery, specifically the Roux-en-Y gastric bypass (RYGB) procedure *(13–17)*. In many cases, normal fasting plasma glucose concentrations are achieved prior to substantial weight loss *(11,15,16)*. Data suggest that changes in circulating gut hormones may promote improvements in glycemic control, reductions in appetite, and subsequent weight loss following bypass surgery *(15,18,19)*.

A number of peptides released from the gastrointestinal tract have recently been shown to regulate appetite and food intake, effecting both orexigenic and anorexic outcomes through actions on the hypothalamic arcuate nucleus *(20,21)*. Peptides of interest include ghrelin, which increases expression of the orexigenic hypothalamic neuropeptide Y (NPY) and stimulates food intake in rodents and humans *(12,22)*; peptide YY (PYY), which acts within the arcuate nucleus to inhibit the release of NPY *(12)*; PYY_{3-36}, which has been known to induce satiety and reduce food intake *(23)*; and glucagon-like peptide 1 (GLP-1), which acts mainly as an incretin, promoting postprandial insulin release, improving pancreatic B-cell function, and inhibiting food intake in humans *(12)*. Pancreatic polypeptide (PP) has also been shown to inhibit food intake and promote energy expenditure *(24)*.

Le Roux et al. *(12)* have demonstrated a pleiotropic endocrine response to bariatric surgery, which might account for the appetite reduction that leads to long-term changes in body weight. Compared with lean and obese controls, postsurgical RYGB patients had increased postprandial plasma (PYY) and glucagon-like-peptide (GLP)-1, which favor enhanced satiety. Furthermore, those patients had early and exaggerated insulin responses, potentially mediating improved glycemic control. None of these effects was observed in patients losing equivalent weight through gastric banding. Leptin, ghrelin, and PP were similar in both surgical groups *(12)*.

CURRENTLY PERFORMED SURGERIES

Roux-en-Y Gastric Bypass

RYGB involves the creation of a small gastric pouch that is then connected to a distal segment of small intestine (alimentary limb). The remainder of the stomach is left *in situ* but is disconnected from the food stream. It reconnects with the alimentary limb at the jejunojejunostomy (Fig. 1). The restrictive component is based on the small pouch as well as the narrow aperture connecting the gastric pouch to the jejunum. The malabsorptive component is marginal at best, as only 20 to 50 cm of small bowel is bypassed. The altered anatomic configuration leads to changes in gut hormones that may be associated with satiety, gastric emptying, and weight loss. Gastric bypass can be performed laparoscopically (LRYGB) or via the open approach with similar success rates *(25,26)*. Mortality rates associated with gastric bypass surgery are reported to be between 0.3 and 2% *(27–29)*. Early complications associated with gastric bypass include leakage, bleeding, pulmonary embolus, gastrojejunal strictures, and death. Late complications include internal hernias, bleeding, ulcers, vitamin deficiencies, and anemia. To prevent nutritional deficiencies, gastric bypass patients must take a daily multivitamin (with iron), vitamin B_{12}, folate, and calcium.

Gastric Banding

The laparoscopic adjustable gastric band (LAGB) and the Swedish band are placed around the top portion of the stomach to reduce stomach size and thereby restrict the volume of ingested solid food. Both bands have been used widely throughout Europe, Australia, and South America for more than a decade, but only the LAGB has been

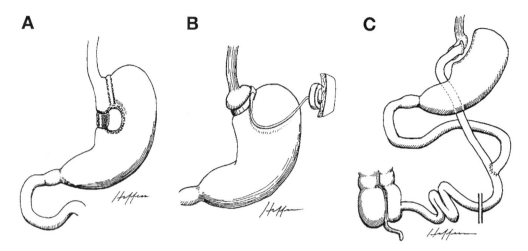

Fig. 1. Restrictive weight-loss surgeries. (**A**) Vertical banded gastroplasty. Both a band and staples are used to create a small stomach pouch. (**B**) Adjustable gastric banding. A band made of a special material is placed around the stomach near its upper end, creating a small pouch of the upper stomach and a narrow passage into the larger remainder of the stomach. (**C**) Roux-en-Y gastric bypass: a restrictive procedure in which a small proximal gastric pouch is created, followed by the creation of a jejunojejunostomy in a "Y" configuration to allow an end of the jejunum to be brought up and anastomosed to this proximal pouch. Drawings were rendered by A. Heffess and generously provided by E. C. Mun. Reprinted from ref. *12a*, with permission from the American Gastroenterological Association.

approved by the Food and Drug Administration for use in the United States since 2001. The band itself is made of silicone and is connected via plastic tubing to a port implanted in the patient's abdominal wall. The quantity of fluid placed into the port gradually increases the restriction on the stomach. Patients must have frequent follow-ups with their physicians to titrate the volume injected into the port. No alteration of the anatomy is required, and thus the procedure is completely reversible.

The mortality rate associated with the band is lower than it is with gastric bypass surgery, only 0.05%. The difference might be due to the absence of leaks and shorter operating times *(30)*. Complications associated with the band include erosions, slips, esophageal dilation, infections, and port problems. An average of 22% of patients with gastric banding require some kind of reoperation after 4 yr *(31)*.

Intragastric Balloon

The intragastric balloon (BioEnterics Intragastric Balloon, BIB), a temporary restrictive device implanted into the stomach endoscopically, promotes a feeling of satiety. In a study of more than 2500 patients, Genco et al. found a 34% loss of excess weight at 6 mo, with a complication rate of 2.8%. Many comorbidities were improved or resolved in more than 80% of patients *(32)*. After removal of the BIB, and with proper diet and exercise, the percentage of excess weight lost decreased from 39 to 26% at 1 yr, suggesting durable weight loss *(33)*. However, the device is not yet approved for use in the United States.

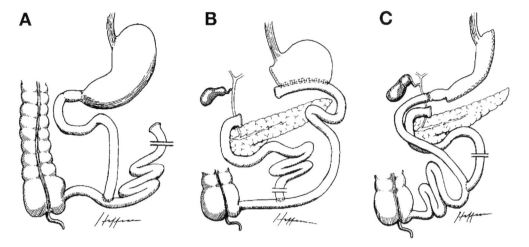

Fig. 2. Malabsorptive bariatric procedures. **(A)** Jejunoileal bypass. The first part of the jejunum is connected to the last portion of the ileum to bypass the area of the intestine where nutrients are absorbed;this procedure is no longer used. **(B)** Biliopancreatic diversion. Portions of the stomach are surgically removed. The small pouch that remains is connected directly to the last segment of the small intestine, bypassing both the duodenum and jejunum. **(C)** Duodenal switch. Biliopancreatic diversion that keeps the pyloric valve intact, maintaining a portion of duodenum in the food stream. Drawings rendered by A. Heffess and generously provided by E. C. Mun. Reprinted from ref. *12a*, with permission from the American GastroenterologicalAssociation.

Sleeve Gastrectomy

Still in its infancy, sleeve gastrectomy is a procedure currently being used as a bridge for surgery in patients with supermorbid obesity (BMI > 50) *(34)*. Laparoscopic sleeve gastrectomy (LSG) is a new procedure for weight loss with lower surgical risk than more complex surgeries, such as biliopancreatic diversion (BPD) with duodenal switch or RYGB *(34)*. The procedure, which is exclusively restrictive, involves removing 80% of the stomach, leaving behind only a sleeve of the stomach. LSG may be particularly well-suited for the most surgically challenging high-risk patients, defined as those who are super-super-obese (BMI > 60) and those with severe comorbidities. Such patients have higher perioperative morbidity and mortality with weight-loss surgery. Postoperative complications are not increased; however, they are more often fatal *(35)*. Milone et al. have shown mean weight loss of 45 kg and percentage excess weight loss (EWL) of 35% at 6 mo with sleeve gastrectomy *(36)*. Once weight is lost, surgery becomes less technically challenging and patients can then go on to have gastric bypass or another procedure.

Biliopancreatic Diversion

BPD is a malabsorptive procedure in which a distal gastrectomy and Roux-en-Y configuration are created with a short common limb. The duodenal switch (DS) procedure is similar to BPD, but a duodenojejunostomy is performed to limit marginal ulceration (Fig. 2). BPD is effective in inducing weight loss, particularly in super-obese patients (BMI > 50) *(37)*, but can cause significant complications *(38)*. It involves gastric resection and diversion of the biliopancreatic juices to the terminal ileum through an entero–entero anastomosis performed between the proximal limb of the transected jejunum and ileum, 50 cm proximal to the ileocecal valve. The distal end of the transected jejunum is anastomosed to the gastric pouch *(34)*.

Laparoscopic Mini-Gastric Bypass

Laparoscopic mini-gastric bypass (LMGB) has been proposed as a simple and effective treatment for morbid obesity *(39)*. It differs from RYGB in that it has a smaller dissection area and fewer anastomoses. The lower antecolic gastrointestinal anastomosis is thought to be much easier to perform than the high retrocolic or antecolic gastrointestinal anastomosis used in LRYGB. In LMGB, the use of one less anastomosis and the provision of a better blood supply to the gastric tube may decrease the incidence of leakage. Data suggest that LMGB is a simpler and safer procedure than LRYGB, with shorter operating time, reduced hospital stay, and significantly less postoperative pain *(40)*. However, there are controversies about the relative safety of the procedure— mainly the incidence of marginal ulcer and reflux esophagitis *(40)*.

OUTCOMES

Weight loss, possibly in association with changes in the gastrointestinal hormonal milieu, results in dramatic effects on the comorbid conditions of severe obesity *(1)*. Reversal or improvement have been seen for the following comorbidities: type 2 diabetes *(11)*, hyperlipidemia, hypertension, obstructive sleep apnea, weight-bearing osteoarthritis, gastroesophageal reflux disease, and depression. Reversal or improvement are reasonable and presumed for other comorbidities, including cardiac and peripheral vascular disease, and carcinomas of the breast, uterus, ovary, prostate, colon, pancreas, and liver *(10)*. There are also improvements in quality-of-life factors related to body image, personal hygiene, sexual activity, employment opportunities, and socioeconomic status *(1)*. Finally, growing epidemiological evidence suggests that weight-loss surgery may increase longevity *(41)*.

SAFETY AND EFFECTIVENESS

Rapid advances in bariatric surgical technology, coupled with rapidly expanding numbers of operations performed, have made the development and implementation of performance standards and patient safeguards a national priority. Although a focus on surgical volume and the setting in which surgery is performed is a necessary step, it falls short of what is required to protect the well-being of patients and the best interests of physicians and facilities.

Standardization of presurgical education, patient selection, perioperative care, and postsurgical support is essential to minimize risk to patients and avoid confounding in studies of surgical effectiveness *(6)*. Compatibility of database technology and consistency in data collection are likewise essential in the analysis of morbidity and mortality rates. Current variability in coding, information systems infrastructure, and database analyses *(29,42,43)* highlights the need for a nationwide perspective in addressing broad-based standards and outcome reporting. It also underscores the need for prospective, clinically derived outcome databases that will serve as a vehicle for quality improvement *(44)*, much like current systems for coronary artery bypass graft surgery established by the Society for Thoracic Surgeons *(45)*.

Efforts to address these shortfalls are part of a nationwide drive for quality control. Massachusetts was the first state to develop comprehensive evidence-based recommendations for best practices in weight loss surgery *(6)*. Many professional societies and other stakeholders have also moved forward with various patient protection and quality performance initiatives These include, among others, the American College of Surgeons (ACS), with its Bariatric Surgery Center Network Accreditation Program *(46)*; the Society of American Gastrointestinal Endoscopic Surgeons (SAGES) *(47)*; the American Society of Bariatric Surgeons (ASBS) *(48)*; Blue Cross Blue Shield of Massachusetts; and Aetna, Kaiser Permanente, Cigna, the California Association of Health Plans, HealthAmerica, and Blue Cross/Blue Shields in South Dakota, Wisconsin, North Carolina, and Idaho.

The ACS program, for example, is in-depth and comprehensive. Based on the Massachusetts Lehman Center report *(6)*, it specifies the necessary physical and human resources, clinical and surgeon credentialing standards, data reporting standards, and verification/approvals processes required to receive designation as an ACS Bariatric Surgery Center. Similarly, Blue Cross/Blue Shield of Massachusetts has based its reimbursement policy on the recommendations contained in the Lehman Center report. Such steps will serve as an impetus and a role model to others engaged in the practice of weight loss surgery and the delivery of required support services.

The Centers for Medicare and Medicaid Services (CMS) will also base reimbursement on evidence showing that open and laparoscopic RYGB, LAGB, and open and laparoscopic BPD/DS are reasonable and necessary for Medicare beneficiaries with a BMI ≥ 35, at least one comorbidity associated with obesity, and a history of unsuccessful medical treatment. Surgeries will be covered only if performed in ACS- or ASBS-certified facilities *(7)*.

CONCLUSION

Weight-loss surgery is fundamentally different from dieting. Changes in physiology resulting from the surgery reset energy equilibrium *(49)*, affect the complex weight-regulatory system at multiple levels, inhibit environmental influences on weight regulation, and defeat powerful mechanisms that are inappropriately active in obesity. Gastric bypass procedures, in particular, induce physiological and neuroendocrine changes that appear to affect the weight regulatory centers in the brain, suggesting alteration of the reward pathways in the central nervous system.

Researchers have begun to explore the molecular pathways responsible for these changes. As they identify those pathways and ascertain the differences between surgical and nonsurgical treatments, new therapeutic options will become available. In the interim, bariatric surgery has taken its place as a first-line treatment option for the rapidly increasing population of patients who suffer from life-threatening severe obesity.

ACKNOWLEDGMENTS

The authors thank Rita Buckley for editorial services in the preparation of this manuscript.

REFERENCES

1. Buchwald H. The future of bariatric surgery. Obes Surg 2005;15:598–605.
2. Nguyen NT, Root J, Zainabadi K, et al. Accelerated growth of bariatric surgery with the introduction of minimally invasive surgery. Arch Surg 2005;140:1198–1202.
3. Liu JH, Etzioni DA, O'Connell JB, et al. Inpatient surgery in California: 1990–2000. Arch Surg 2003;138:1106–1111.
4. Courcoulas A, Schuchert M, Gatti G, et al. The relationship of surgeon and hospital volume to outcome after gastric bypass surgery in Pennsylvania: a 3-year summary. Surgery 2003;134:613–621.
5. Birkmeyer NJ, Wei Y, Goldfaden A, et al. Characteristics of hospitals performing bariatric surgery. JAMA 2006;295:282–284.
6. Betsy Lehman Center for Patient Safety and Medical Error Reduction. Expert panel on weight loss surgery. Boston, Massachusetts Department of Public Health. Obes Res 2005;13:203–305.
7. Centers for Medicare and Medicaid Services. Medicare Coverage Database. Decision Memo for Bariatric Surgery for the Treatment of Morbid Obesity (CAG-00250R). Vol. 2006: US Department of Health and Human Services. Available at: http://www.cms.hhs.gov/mcd/viewdecisionmemo.asp?id=160. Accessed March 1, 2006.
8. Ali MR, Maguire MB, Wolfe BM. Assessment of obesity-related comorbidities: a novel scheme for evaluating bariatric surgical patients. J Am Coll Surg 2006;202:70–77. Epub 2005 Nov 18.
9. Buchwald H, Braunwald E, Avidor Y, et al. Bariatric surgery: a systematic review and meta-analysis. JAMA 2004;292:1724–1737.
10. Blackburn GL, Mun EC. Weight loss surgery and major cardiovascular risk factors. Nat Clin Pract Cardiovasc Med 2005;2:585–591.
11. Blackburn GL, Jones DB. Effective surgical treatment of diabetes for the obese patient. Current Diabetes Reports 2006;6(2):85–87.
12. le Roux CW, Aylwin SJ, Batterham RL, et al. Gut hormone profiles following bariatric surgery favor an anorectic state, facilitate weight loss, and improve metabolic parameters. Ann Surg 2006;243:108–114.
12a. Mun EC, Blackburn GL, Matthews JB. Current status of medical and surgical therapy for obesity. Gastroenterology 2001;120:669–681.
13. Pories WJ, Swanson MS, MacDonald KG, et al. Who would have thought it? An operation proves to be the most effective therapy for adult-onset diabetes mellitus. Ann Surg 1995;222:339–350.
14. Pories WJ, MacDonald KG, Jr., Morgan EJ, et al. Surgical treatment of obesity and its effect on diabetes: 10-y follow-up. Am J Clin Nutr 1992;55(2 Suppl):582S–585S.
15. Schauer PR, Burguera B, Ikramuddin S, et al. Effect of laparoscopic Roux-en Y gastric bypass on type 2 diabetes mellitus. Ann Surg 2003;238:467–484.
16. Clements RH, Gonzalez QH, Long CI, Wittert G, Laws HL. Hormonal changes after Roux-en Y gastric bypass for morbid obesity and the control of type-II diabetes mellitus. Am Surg 2003;70:1–4.
17. Blackburn GL. Solutions in weight control: lessons from gastric surgery. Am J Clin Nutr 2005;82(1Suppl):248S–252S.
18. Cummings DE, Weigle DS, Frayo RS, et al. Plasma ghrelin levels after diet-induced weight loss or gastric bypass surgery. N Engl J Med 2002;346:1623–1630.
19. Rubino F, Marescaux J. Effect of duodenal-jejunal exclusion in a non-obese animal model of type 2 diabetes: a new perspective for an old disease. Ann Surg 2004;239:1–11.
20. Schwartz MW, Morton GJ. Obesity: keeping hunger at bay. Nature 2002;418:595–597.
21. Schwartz MW, Woods SC, Porte D Jr, et al. Central nervous system control of food intake. Nature 2000;404:661–671.
22. Tschop M, Smiley DL, Heiman ML. Ghrelin induces adiposity in rodents. Nature 2000;407:908–913.
23. Batterham RL, Cohen MA, Ellis SM, et al. Inhibition of food intake in obese subjects by peptide YY3-36. N Engl J Med 2003;349:941–948.
24. Asakawa A, Inui A, Yuzuriha H, et al. Characterization of the effects of pancreatic polypeptide in the regulation of energy balance. Gastroenterology 2003;124:1325–1336.
25. Smith SC, Edwards CB, Goodman GN, et al. Open vs laparoscopic Roux-en-Y gastric bypass: comparison of operative morbidity and mortality. Obes Surg 2004;14:73–76.

26. Nguyen NT, Ho HS, Palmer LS, et al. A comparison study of laparoscopic versus open gastric bypass for morbid obesity. J Am Coll Surg 2000;191:149–155;discussion 155–157.

27. Shikora SA, Kim JJ, Tarnoff ME, et al. Laparoscopic Roux-en-Y gastric bypass: results and learning curve of a high-volume academic program. Arch Surg 2005;140:362–367.

28. Flum DR, Dellinger E. Impact of gastric bypass on survival: A population-based analysis. J Am Coll Surg 2004;199:543–551.

29. Flum DR, Salem L, Elrod JA, et al. Early mortality among Medicare beneficiaries undergoing bariatric surgical procedures. JAMA 2005;294:1903–1908.

30. Chapman AE, Kiroff G, Game P, et al. Laparoscopic adjustable gastric banding in the treatment of obesity: a systematic literature review. Surgery 2004;135:326–351.

31. Branson R, Potoczna N, Brunotte R, et al. Impact of age, sex and body mass index on outcomes at four years after gastric banding. Obes Surg 2005;15:834–842.

32. Genco A, Bruni T, Doldi SB, et al. BioEnterics Intragastric Balloon: the Italian experience with 2,515 patients. Obes Surg 2005;15:1161–1164.

33. Herve J, Wahlen CH, Schaeken A, et al. What becomes of patients one year after the intragastric balloon has been removed? Obes Surg 2005;15:864–870.

34. Regan JP, Inabnet WB, Gagner M, et al. Early experience with two-stage laparoscopic Roux-en-Y gastric bypass as an alternative in the super-super obese patient. Obes Surg 2003;13:861–864.

35. Fernandez AZ Jr, DeMaria EJ, Tichansky DS, et al. Experience with over 3,000 open and laparoscopic bariatric procedures: multivariate analysis of factors related to leak and resultant mortality. Surg Endosc 2004;18:193–197.

36. Milone L, Strong V, Gagner M. Laparoscopic sleeve gastrectomy is superior to endoscopic intragastric balloon as a first stage procedure for super-obese patients (BMI > or = 50). Obes Surg 2005;15:612–617.

37. Gagner M, Matteotti R. Laparoscopic biliopancreatic diversion with duodenal switch. Surg Clin North Am 2005;85:141–149, x–xi.

38. Kelly J, Tarnoff M, Shikora S, et al. Expert Panel on Weight Loss Surgery. Best practice recommendations for surgical care in weight loss surgery. Boston, MA: Betsy Lehman Center for Patient Safety and Medical Error Reduction, Massachusetts Department of Public Health; 2004. Obes Res 2005;13:227–233.

39. Rutledge R. The mini-gastric bypass: experience with the first 1,274 cases. Obes Surg 2001;11:276–280.

40. Lee WJ, Yu PJ, Wang W, et al. Laparoscopic Roux-en-Y versus mini-gastric bypass for the treatment of morbid obesity: a prospective randomized controlled clinical trial. Ann Surg 2005;242:20–28.

41. Christou NV, Sampalis JS, Liberman M, et al. Surgery decreases long-term mortality, morbidity, and health care use in morbidly obese patients. Ann Surg 2004;240:416–423.

42. Zingmond DS, McGory ML, Ko CY. Hospitalization before and after gastric bypass surgery. JAMA 2005;294:1918–1924.

43. Santry HP, Gillen DL, Lauderdale DS. Trends in bariatric surgical procedures. JAMA 2005;294:1909–1917.

44. Wolfe BM, Morton JM. Weighing in on bariatric surgery: procedure use, readmission rates, and mortality. JAMA 2005;294:1960–1963.

45. Ferguson TB Jr, Coombs LP, Peterson ED. Society of Thoracic Surgeons National Adult Cardiac Surgery Database. Preoperative beta-blocker use and mortality and morbidity following CABG surgery in North America. JAMA 2002;287:221–227.

46. Bariatric Surgery Center Network Accreditation Program. Vol. 2006: American College of Surgeons. Available at: http://www.facs.org/cqi/bscn. Accessed February 17, 2006.

47. SAGES Outcomes Initiative. Vol. 2006: Society of American Gastrointestinal Endoscopic Surgeons. Avaliable at: http://www.sages.org/outcomes.html. Accessed February 17, 2006.

48. Bariatric Surgery Centers of Excellence Program. Vol. 2006: Surgical Review Corporation. Available at: http://www.surgicalreview.org. Accessed February 17, 2006.

49. Blackburn GL, Waltman BA. Obesity and insulin resistance. In: McTiernan A, ed. Cancer Prevention and Management through Exercise and Weight Control. Marcel Dekker, New York: 2005;20:301–316.

20 Managing Micronutrient Deficiencies in the Bariatric Surgical Patient

Robert F. Kushner, MD

Contents

Introduction
Bariatric Surgical Procedures
Bariatric Surgery-Related Micronutrient Deficiencies
Prophylactic Management and Monitoring for Nutritional
    Deficiencies
Conclusion
References

Summary

Bariatric surgery is associated with development of several micronutrient deficiencies that are predictable based on the surgically altered anatomy and the imposed dietary changes. The three restrictive malabsorptive procedures—Roux-en-Y gastric bypass (RYGB), biliopancreatic diversion (BPD), and biliopancreatic diversion with duodenal switch (BPD/DS)—pose a greater risk for micronutrient malabsorption and deficiency than the purely restrictive laparoscopic adjustable silicone gastric banding (LASGB). Metabolic and clinical deficiencies of two minerals (iron and calcium) and four vitamins (thiamine, folate, vitamin B12, vitamin D) have been well described in the literature. This chapter reviews the pathophysiology, clinical presentation, screening tests, and treatment for each micronutrient deficiency. With careful monitoring and adequate supplementation, these deficiencies are largely avoidable and treatable.

Key Words: Bariatric surgery; micronutrient deficiency; Wernicke's encephalopathy; iron deficiency anemia; hypovitaminosis D; metabolic bone disease.

INTRODUCTION

Bariatric surgery has been endorsed as an acceptable weight loss option for patients with severe (also called extreme, morbid, or class III) obesity or those with moderate obesity who have comorbid conditions by several authoritative guidelines and conferences *(1–5)*. Between 1998 and 2002, the number of bariatric surgical procedures performed in the United States increased by more than five times, from approx 13,000 to 71,000, according to the Nationwide Inpatient Sample of the Healthcare Cost and Utilization Project *(6)*, and was expected to surpass 140,000 per year by 2004 *(7)*. The

From: *Contemporary Endocrinology: Treatment of the Obese Patient*
Edited by: R. F. Kushner and D. H. Bessesen © Humana Press Inc., Totowa, NJ

exponential growth in procedures is caused by several factors, including improved surgical techniques, reduction in the postoperative mortality rate, significant improvement in obesity-related comorbid conditions (8), increased media attention, and profitability. The upsurge in surgical procedures also reflects the increasing prevalence of severe obesity in the United States. Between 1986 and 2000, the prevalence of severe obesity (body mass index [BMI] $\geq$ 40 kg/m^2) quadrupled from about 1 in 200 adult Americans to 1 in 50; the prevalence of a BMI $\geq$ 50 increased by a factor of 5, from about 1 in 2000 to 1 in 400 (9). Approximately 5% of adult Americans are considered severely obese, with prevalence figures reaching 13.5% for African American women (10). It is therefore likely that health care professionals from all disciplines will encounter patients who have undergone a bariatric surgical procedure. Similarly, primary care physicians and endocrinologists will be expected to monitor and manage their patients on a long-term basis. Although physicians are trained to manage chronic diseases commonly associated with severe obesity, such as type 2 diabetes, obstructive sleep apnea, hypertension, mixed hyperlipidemia, and arthritis, among others, nutritional management following bariatric surgery is not routinely taught. The combined restrictive-malabsorptive surgical procedures—Roux-en-Y gastric bypass (RYGB), biliopancreatic diversion (BPD), and biliopancreatic diversion with duodenal switch (BPD/DS)—place patients at high risk for development of both macro- and micronutrient deficiencies unless they are properly counseled and supplemented. As most of the deficiencies can be identified early at a preclinical stage, early treatment will prevent or reduce symptoms and deficiency syndromes. This chapter will review the identification and management of the most common micronutrient deficiencies that may occur following restrictive-malabsorptive bariatric surgeries.

BARIATRIC SURGICAL PROCEDURES

Weight loss surgeries fall into one of two categories—restrictive and restrictive-malabsorptive (see Chapter 19 for illustrations of surgeries). Restrictive surgeries limit the amount of food the stomach can hold and slow the rate of gastric emptying. The vertical banded gastroplasty (VBG) is the prototype of this category but is currently performed on a very limited basis owing to a lack of effectiveness in long-term trials. Laparoscopic adjustable silicone gastric banding (LASGB) has replaced the VBG as the most commonly performed restrictive operation. The first banding device, the Lap-Band, was approved for use in the United States in 2001. In contrast to previous devices, the diameter of this band is adjustable by way of its connection to a reservoir that is implanted under the skin. Injection or removal of saline into the reservoir tightens or loosens the band's internal diameter, respectively, thus changing the size of the gastric opening. As there is no rerouting of the intestine with LASGB, the risk for developing miconutrient deficiencies is entirely dependent on the patient's diet and eating habits.

The three restrictive malabsorptive bypass procedures combine the elements of gastric restriction and selective malabsorption. The Roux-en-Y gastric bypass (RYGB) is the most commonly performed and accepted bypass procedure. It involves formation of a 10- to 30-mL proximal gastric pouch by either surgically separating or stapling the stomach across the fundus. Outflow from the pouch is created by performing a narrow (10 mm) gastrojejunostomy. The distal end of the jejunum is then anastomosed 50 to 150 cm below the gastrojejunostomy. "Roux-en-Y" refers to the Y-shaped section of small intestine

Table 1
Micronutrient Consequences of Bariatric Surgery

Deficiency of vitamins
  Thiamine
  Vitamin B_{12}
  Folic acid
  Vitamin D
Deficiency of minerals
  Iron
  Calcium

created by the surgery; the Y is created at the point where the pancreobiliary conduit (afferent limb) and the Roux (efferent) limb are connected. "Bypass" refers to the exclusion or bypassing of the distal stomach, duodenum, and proximal jejunum. RYGB may be performed with an open incision or laparoscopically.

The biliopancreatic diversion (BPD) is more complicated and less commonly performed than the RYGB. This operation involves a subtotal gastrectomy, leaving a much larger gastric pouch compared with the RYGB. The small bowel is divided 250 cm proximal to the ileocecal valve and connected directly to the gastric pouch, producing a gastroileostomy. The remaining proximal limb (biliopancreatic conduit) is then anastomosed to the side of the distal ileum 50 cm proximal to the ileocecal valve. In this procedure, the distal stomach, duodenum, and entire jejunum are bypassed, leaving only a 50-cm distal ileum common channel for nutrients to mix with pancreatic and biliary secretions.

BPD/DS is a variation of the biliopancreatic diversion that preserves the first portion of the duodenum. In this procedure, a vertical subtotal gastrectomy is performed and the duodenum is divided just beyond the pylorus. The distal small bowel is connected to the short stump of the duodenum, producing a 75- to 100-cm ileal–duodenal "common channel" for absorption of nutrients. The other end of the duodenum is closed, and the remaining small bowel connected onto the enteral limb at about 75 to 100 cm from the ileocecal valve.

BARIATRIC SURGERY-RELATED MICRONUTRIENT DEFICIENCIES

By definition, micronutrients are essential nutrients that are required in only small quantities (milligrams or micrograms) such as minerals, trace elements, and vitamins. The micronutrient deficiencies of the RYGB, BPD, and BPD/DS procedures are predictable based on the surgically altered anatomy. By bypassing the stomach, duodenum, and varying portions of the jejunum and ileum, malabsorption of thiamine, iron, folate, vitamin $B_{12,}$ calcium, and vitamin D may occur (Table 1). In general, the greater the malabsorption, the higher the risk of nutritional deficiencies. The prevalence of these deficiencies varies widely in the literature owing to differences in surgical technique, patient population, definition of deficiency, supplementation protocols, and length and completion of patient follow-up. For example, iron deficiency is reported to range from 20 to 49% and vitamin B_{12} deficiency from 26 to 70% (11–19). An accurate incidence of micronutrient deficiency following bariatric surgery will be obtained from the prospective National Institutes of Health (NIH)-sponsored Longitudinal Assessment of Bariatric Surgery (LABS) study that is currently under way *(20)*. In the following section, "at-risk" micronutrients will be reviewed considering pathophysiology, clinical presentation, screening tests, and treatment. Other recent review articles address the general topic of nutritional and metabolic problems following bariatric surgery *(21–26)*.

Micronutrient Deficiency

THIAMINE

Thiamine (vitamin B_1) is absorbed mainly in the jejunum, by both active and passive diffusion. Because the biological half-life of the vitamin is rather short (in the range of 9 to 18 d) and only a small percentage of a high dose is absorbed *(27)*, patients are at risk of developing deficiency syndromes after bariatric surgery. Over the past two decades, numerous case reports of thiamine deficiency have been reported following both restrictive and restrictive-malabsorptive surgeries *(28–45)*. An acute deficiency of thiamine associated with rapidly progressing clinical symptoms appears to result from a combination of restricted food intake and persistent intractable vomiting. Symptoms commonly occur 1 to 3 mo postoperatively, although they may occur later. The clinical presentation varies, but three conditions have been reported. Classical Wernicke's encephalopathy is the most common presentation and consists of double vision, nystagmus, ataxia, and a global confusion manifested by apathy, impaired awareness of the immediate situation, disorientation, inattention, and an inability to concentrate. Dry beriberi presents as bilateral, symmetric, lower extremity paresthesia, whereas wet beriberi manifests as high-output congestive heart failure, edema, and metabolic acidosis.

Several case series of neurologic complications following bariatric surgery have been published *(46–48)*. These authors describe a constellation of symptoms including mono- and polyneuropathy with weakness and/or paresthesias, burning feet syndrome, and hyporeflexia. Chang et al. *(48)* coined the acronym APGARS (acute postgastric reduction surgery neuropathy) to describe conditions with features of weakness, hyporeflexia, and vomiting. As all symptoms did not improve with thiamine treatment, the authors suggest that additional nutritional deficiencies may be involved in the etiology.

Thiamine status is best assessed by determining erythrocyte transketolase activity. Magnetic resonance imaging (MRI) is useful in confirming the diagnosis of acute Wernicke's encephalopathy. with a specificity of 93% *(49)*. With this test, increased T2 signal of paraventricular regions of the thalamus and increased T2 signal of periaqueductal regions of the midbrain are seen. However, treatment should not be delayed if a thiamine deficiency syndrome is suspected. Treatment with thiamine 100 mg iv or im for 7 to 14 d followed by 10 mg po daily is recommended for these syndromes until the patient fully recovers. To avoid deficiency, patients should be routinely discharged from the hospital receiving a chewable multiple vitamin–mineral supplement that contains between 1.5 and 1.8 mg thiamine.

IRON

Patients who have undergone restrictive malabsorptive procedures are at particular risk for developing iron deficiency and iron-deficiency anemia (IDA) owing to reduced iron absorption, decreased iron intake, and for menstruating women, increased iron losses. Surgical bypass of the duodenum and proximal jejunum decreases total iron uptake because the majority of iron absorption occurs in these regions *(50)*. Furthermore, acid secretion is nearly absent in the small gastric pouch *(51,52)*, which exacerbates the deficiency because both heme (found only in animal products) and nonheme (found in plants and dairy foods) iron depend on the acidic environment of the stomach for efficient absorption *(53)*. Specifically, nonheme iron requires an acidic pH to reduce it from the ferric (Fe^{2+}) to the ferrous (Fe^{3+}) state, thus increasing its solubility. Although heme iron is more soluble and readily absorbed than nonheme iron, it must be released from its protein structure by the acid and proteases present in gastric juice before absorption can occur *(54)*. In addition to decreased iron absorption, bariatric surgical patients typically consume less heme iron, owing to an intolerance of meat products *(11,55)*. Women with menorrhagia are particularly prone to develop iron deficiency and IDA from excessive menstrual blood loss. Menstrual iron losses range from 1.5 to 2.1 mg/d, bringing the recommended dietary allowances (RDA) for females between 19 and 50 years old to 18 mg/d compared with 8 mg/d for males *(56)*. Because of the combination of these factors, iron-deficiency anemia occurs postoperatively in 33 to 50% of patients, with a higher incidence in menstruating women *(13,14,57)*.

Iron deficiency may also be exacerbated in these patients as a result of a nutrient–nutrient inhibitory absorptive interaction between iron and calcium, another mineral that is routinely supplemented during the postoperative period. Most *(58–63)* but not all *(64,65)* studies show that nonheme- and heme-iron absorption is inhibited up to 50 to 60% when consumed in the presence of calcium supplements or with dairy products. Calcium at doses of 300 to 600 mg has a direct dose-related inhibiting effect on iron absorption. This has been seen with calcium carbonate, calcium citrate, and calcium phosphate. Studies by Hallberg et al. *(59,61)* suggest that the inhibitory effect is situated within the intestinal mucosal cells. These observations are particularly important for bariatric surgical patients who are routinely prescribed calcium supplements and advised to consume dairy foods high in calcium, such as milk, cheese, and yogurt. In these patients, it appears prudent to recommend that iron and calcium supplementation be separated by several hours to avoid inhibitory interaction.

Early functional symptoms of iron deficiency include fatigue, poor exercise tolerance, and decreased work performance *(66)*. Signs on physical examination include pale conjunctiva and spoon nails. Serum ferritin is the most sensitive indicator of iron status (normal values usually fall in the range of 20–300 µg/L) and is recommended for diagnosing early iron deficiency *(67)*. The concentration of serum ferritin reflects the size of the storage iron compartment, with each µg/L representing 8 to10 mg of storage iron *(53)*. However, caution is needed in interpreting ferritin concentration levels in the presence of acute and chronic inflammation, as ferritin is also an acute phase reactant. Thus, serum ferritin concentrations may fall within the normal range in individuals who have no iron stores. After the iron storage pool is depleted, there is an increase in total iron-binding capacity (TIBC), decreased serum transferrin saturation (serum iron concentration divided by TIBC × 100), followed by microcytosis (reduced mean corpuscular volume [MCV]), hypochromia (reduced mean corpuscular hemoglobin concentration [MCHC]), and anemia.

An unusual and fascinating symptom that is particularly associated with IDA is ice eating, or pagophagia, one of the most commonly reported forms of pica. Pica has been previously reported to occur with IDA of pregnancy *(68,69)*, gastrointestinal blood loss *(70)*, and sickle cell disease *(71)*. Our group recently reported the first five cases of pagophagia associated with RYGB surgery *(72,73)*. All patients were women between

34 and 45 yr old with menorrhagia. Onset of pica symptoms ranged from 1 mo to 23 mo postsurgery. Three of the patients described symptoms suggestive of pica when they were children and one during a previous pregnancy.

In order to prevent iron deficiency, all patients undergoing restrictive-malabsorptive surgeries should be prescribed a daily multivitamin–mineral supplement containing elemental iron. Often, supplementation with one prenatal vitamin and mineral tablet, which typically contains 28 to 40 mg elemental iron, is sufficient. High-risk individuals—for example, those who have preoperative iron deficiency or excessive blood loss or those who develop iron deficiency or any degree of anemia—require additional supplementation with an iron salt preparation containing ferrous sulfate, gluconate, or fumarate *(74)*. Typical dosing of iron therapy is 150 to 300 mg/d po given in two to three divided doses for 4 to 6 mo or until the serum ferritin reaches 50 µg/L. Coadministration with ascorbic acid (vitamin C), the best known reducing agent, is recommended to increase iron absorption *(75)*. In the presence of ascorbic acid, ferrous iron forms a soluble iron–ascorbic acid complex. In patients with profound iron deficits and severe anemia unresponsive to oral iron supplementation, intravenous administration of iron dextran (InFed®), ferric gluconate (Ferrlecit®) or ferric sucrose (Venofer®) will be required. Dosing calculations are available from one manufacturer (www.infed.com).

VITAMIN B$_{12}$

Vitamin B$_{12}$ (cobalamin) absorption requires a complex sequence of orchestrated metabolic steps within the gastrointestinal tract. In the stomach, food-bound vitamin B$_{12}$ is first dissociated from animal proteins by acid and peptic hydrolysis to liberate free vitamin B$_{12}$. Once released, the vitamin is avidly bound to R proteins, which are glycoproteins secreted by the salivary glands and the gastric mucosa. In the intestine, pancreatic proteases then degrade R proteins and permit vitamin B$_{12}$ to associate with intrinsic factor (IF), a glycoprotein that the parietal cells of the stomach secrete after being stimulated by food. The resulting IF–vitamin B$_{12}$ complex is then bound to specific receptors in the distal ileum, where absorption occurs *(27)*.

The restrictive-malabsorptive procedures disrupt several of these key steps. Vitamin B$_{12}$ deficiency may occur due to decreased acid and pepsin digestion of protein-bound cobalamins from food, incomplete release of vitamin B$_{12}$ from R proteins, and decreased availability of IF to form IF–vitamin B$_{12}$ complexes. Because the parietal cells that secrete acid and IF, and chief cells that secrete pepsinogen, are located primarily in the fundus and body of the stomach, the RYGB procedure essentially excludes food from the normal gastric digestive process. Acid secretion has been demonstrated to be virtually absent in the small pouch constructed from the gastric cardia *(51,52)*. Consequently, cobalamins are not liberated from protein and are not available for intestinal absorption. In all three restrictive-malabsorptive procedures, pancreatic secretions are diverted distally to mix with nutrients in a shortened common channel, thus affecting the vitamin's binding to IF and subsequent attachment to ileal IF–vitamin B$_{12}$ receptors.

Although B$_{12}$ deficiency is predictable, onset of signs and symptoms are typically delayed for months to years owing to prolonged hepatic storage of the vitamin. When they do occur, clinical effects of deficiency are similar to those of pernicious anemia—hematological and neurological. Hypersegmented polymorphonuclear leukocytes and macrocytic erythrocytes can be seen on peripheral blood smear, along with a macrocytic anemia. Neurological manifestations include sensory disturbances in the lower extremities (tingling and numbness); motor disturbances, including abnormalities in gait; and cognitive changes ranging from loss of concentration to memory loss and disorientation *(27)*.

Vitamin B_{12} status is most commonly and easily assessed by serum or plasma vitamin levels. The concentration of B_{12} in the serum or plasma reflects both the B_{12} intake and stores. The lower limit is considered to be approximately 120 to 180 pmol/L (170 to 250 pg/mL). However, a more sensitive biochemical indicator of deficiency is elevation of serum homocysteine and methylmalonic acid (MMA), levels that rise when the supply of B_{12} is low and virtually confirms the diagnosis.

All patients who undergo restrictive-malabsorptive procedures should receive pro-phylactic vitamin B_{12} supplementation to prevent deficiency. In contrast to the disrup-tion of food-bound B_{12} absorption, crystalline vitamin B_{12} (the form found in vitamin supplements) can be absorbed in the surgical patient, as approx 1% of orally adminis-tered crystalline cobalamin is absorbed by passive diffusion *(76,77)*. An oral dose of at least 200 times the RDA was shown to normalize mild vitamin B_{12} deficiency in older people assessed by reduction in plasma MMA concentration *(78)*. Oral treatment has also been effective in patients with pernicious anemia *(79)*. As a practical matter, patients should receive at least 500 µg B_{12} daily as a dietary supplement delivered orally as a tablet or liquid or sublingually; as a once-weekly nasal spray 500-µg cyanocobalamin gel (Nascobal®), or by im injection 100 µg monthly. The route of delivery is based on patient preference and monitoring of vitamin B_{12} status.

FOLATE

Folate deficiency occurs with lower frequency than vitamin B_{12} or iron deficiency; however, it should be considered when evaluating a patient who develops anemia. Folate is absorbed primarily from the proximal third of the small intestine after food folate polyglutamates are hydrolyzed to monoglutamates by intestinal brush border conjugases. Folate deficiency presents with many features similar to vitamin B_{12} deficiency, includ-ing hypersegmentation of the neutrophils, increased mean corpuscular volume (MCV), and macrocytic anemia. Inadequate folate intake first leads to a decrease in serum folate concentration, then a decrease in erythrocyte folate concentration, a rise in homocysteine concentration, then clinical hematological changes as mentioned above *(27)*. A serum folate concentration of less than 7 nmol/L (3 ng/mL) indicates negative folate balance. All patients undergoing a restrictive-malabsorptive bariatric operation should receive supplemental doses of folate to prevent deficiency. Supplements of folic acid are nearly 100% bioavailable. Typically, the amount of folate present in a general (400 µg) or prenatal multivitamin supplement (800 to 1000 µg) is adequate to prevent deficiency.

CALCIUM AND VITAMIN D

Calcium and vitamin D are considered together, as deficiency of both nutrients may result in metabolic bone disease and their metabolism is inter-related. A negative cal-cium balance may result from limited intake of calcium- and vitamin D-containing dairy products, and reduced fractional intestinal absorption owing to surgical bypass of the absorptive sites and vitamin D deficiency *(80)*. The latter factor is important because calcium is absorbed by an active transport process dependent on the action of 1,25-dihydroxyvitamin D (1,25(OH)$_2$D), which enhances calcium absorption primarily in the duodenum and jejunum *(81)* although most of the absorption occurs in the lower segment of the small intestine, the ileum *(82)*. Calcium is also absorbed by passive diffusion across the intestinal mucosa, which becomes important at high calcium intakes such as supplemental calcium (83).

Vitamin D deficiency may occur for the same reasons listed above for calcium deficiency—that is, reduced intake of vitamin D-fortified dairy products and malabsorption of vitamin D owing to mismixing of pancreatic and biliary juices in the distal small intestine. As vitamin D is fat-soluble, it must be incorporated into the intestinal micelle along with bile salts for absorption. However, the major source of vitamin D for most people comes from casual exposure to sunlight. Unlike any other vitamin, vitamin D_3 or cholecalciferol is photosynthesized by the skin by UVB radiation, converting 7-dehydrocholesterol to previtamin D_3 and eventually vitamin D_3 (81). In the liver, vitamin D undergoes hydroxylation at the 25-carbon position to form 25-hydroxy vitamin D (25(OH)D) and subsequently transported to the kidney for additional hydroxylation at the 1-carbon position to form $1,25(OH)_2D$, the biological active form of the vitamin. Several factors will impede the initial photosynthetic process, including living at northern latitudes, wearing sunscreen lotion, limited sun exposure, dark skin pigmentation (84), aging, and obesity itself (85–88). Several studies have demonstrated an inverse correlation between vitamin D concentrations and BMI or body fat percentage, suggesting decreased bioavailability of skin-derived vitamin D in obese individuals. Thus, severely obese individuals are predisposed to vitamin D insufficiency or deficiency prior to undergoing bariatric surgery.

Clinical deficiency of calcium or vitamin D owing to bariatric surgery cannot be detected on a routine chemistry panel, although an elevated alkaline phosphatase level and a low calcium or phosphorus level may be seen. Unless specifically monitored, the first indication of deficiency is likely to be a vertebral or wrist fracture secondary to development of osteoporosis or osteomalacia. Physiologically, chronic calcium deficiency causes the circulating ionized calcium concentration to decline, which triggers an increase in parathyroid hormone (PTH) synthesis and release. In turn, PTH acts on three organs to restore the circulating calcium concentration to normal. At the kidney, PTH promotes the reabsorption of calcium in the distal tubule. PTH affects the intestine indirectly by stimulating the production of $1,25(OH)_2D$. PTH also induces bone resorption, thereby releasing calcium into the blood (81). Chronic vitamin D deficiency results in secondary hyperparathyroidism, diagnosed by an elevated PTH level in the setting of low or normal serum calcium (84). Therefore, detection of subclinical calcium and/or vitamin D deficiency requires measurement of several nutrients, hormone levels, and biochemical markers of bone turnover that are not routinely assessed.

Serum 25(OH) vitamin D is the best indicator for determining adequacy of vitamin D intake, as it represents the combination of cutaneous production of vitamin D and the oral ingestion of both vitamin D_2 (ergocalcerferol or plant-based vitamin D) and vitamin D_3. 25(OH)D is not only the transport form of the vitamin D, but is also a direct measure of stores (90). In the current literature, severe vitamin D deficiency is identified as a 25(OH)D level of less than 5 to 8 ng/mL (12.5–20 nmol/mL) and mild deficiency or insufficiency as a serum level less than 20 ng/mL (50 nmol/mL) (91). However, there is debate about the exact cutoff values defining "deficiency" and "insufficiency," as these are static rather than functional definitions. When elevated PTH levels (secondary hyperparathyroidism) are used as a functional indicator of vitamin D deficiency, circulating levels of 25(OH)D of at least 30 ng/mL appear optimal (92,93). Biochemical monitoring of bone turnover includes measurement of bone formation markers—serum osteocalcin and bone-specific alkaline phosphatase, and the bone resorption marker— serum and urine peptide-bound N-telopeptide crosslinks of type 1 collagen (NTX) *(94)*. Assessment of bone mineral density and bone mineral content by dual energy X-ray absorptiometry (DEXA) remains the gold standard for the diagnosis of osteoporosis *(95)*.

Abnormalities in vitamin D and bone metabolism among patients undergoing restrictive-malabsorptive bariatric operations have been reported in numerous case series and case reports *(96–104)*. Although the studies are primarily observational, contain few patients, and are uncontrolled for diet and vitamin mineral supplementation, most studies document the occurrence of hypovitaminosis D and elevated PTH over the first 1 to 3 postoperative years, with a prevalence ranging from 30% *(98)* to 80% *(105)*. Many of the studies also show a corresponding elevation in alkaline phosphatase levels and biochemical markers of bone turnover. Several cases of severe secondary hyperparathyroidism with osteomalacia have been reported to occur from 9 to 17 yr postsurgery *(102,106)*. However, as weight reduction itself is associated with reduced bone mineral density (BMD) and bone mineral content (BMC) *(107)*, it is important to distinguish between the weight loss and malabsorptive effects of bariatric surgery. Pugnale et al. *(108)* showed that BMD of the cortical bone decreased significantly among 31 women who underwent a restrictive banding procedure without evidence of secondary hyperparathyroidism. Similarly, Guney et al. demonstrated that weight reduction causes bone loss among both diet-treated patients and those who underwent a restrictive vertical banded gastroplasty without a significant change in PTH levels *(109)*. In another study, six obese control patients were compared with four patients who underwent a RYGB and nine patients who received gastric banding *(101)*. The RYGB operation resulted in significant net loss of bone mass in comparison with the banding and obese control group. Unfortunately, a major limitation in most of the reviewed studies is the lack of baseline data, as obesity itself is associated with abnormalities in the PTH-vitamin D axis as discussed above. In the study by El-Kadre et al. *(99)*, 10% of patients had elevated PTH levels preoperatively, whereas the prevalence was 22% and 25% in the series by Johnson et al. *(104)* and Hamoui et al. *(100)*, respectively.

Inclusion of calcium- and vitamin D-containing dairy products in the postoperative diet is important. One serving of milk contains approx 300 mg calcium. However, many patients will avoid or limit dairy foods owing to lactose intolerance or lack of an acquired taste. Choosing Lactaid milk or adding lactase to dairy products will address the former problem. To avoid deficiency and supplement the diet, all patients should receive calcium supplements of at least 1200 to 1500 mg/d in divided doses, depending on the adequacy of dietary calcium. Postmenopausal, lactating, or pregnant women may require higher ranges owing to increased needs. Calcium citrate + vitamin D is the preferred preparation because it is more soluble than calcium carbonate in the absence of gastric acid production. Vitamin D is typically supplemented through a multivitamin–mineral tablet (400 IU) and the one to two servings of calcium + vitamin D tablets (400 to 800 IU) for a total daily supplemental dose of about 800 to 1200 IU vitamin D.

If vitamin D deficiency is detected, measurement of PTH should be obtained to provide a functional assessment. Treatment may involve recommending higher supplemental doses of calcium and vitamin D and reassessing in about 3 mo. In patients with severe vitamin D deficiency, initial repletion of stores with the vitamin D analog, ergo-

Table 2
Vitamin and Mineral Supplementation

Nutrient	DRI[a]	Childrens' chewable	Prescription Prenatal	Over-the-counter Prenatal
Folate (μg)	400	400	1000	800
Thiamine (mg)	1.2	1.5	1.8	1.84
Calcium (mg)	1200	100	200	200
Iron (mg)	18	18	28	27
Vitamin B_{12} (μg)	2.4	6	12	4
Vitamin D (IU)	400	400	400	400

[a]Dietary Reference Intake, highest value per individual group

calciferol, should be prescribed with 50,000 IU daily for 1 to 3 wk, followed by weekly or monthly administration until 25(OH)D and PTH levels are normalized (110). Monitoring of the alkaline phosphatase level and serum and urinary calcium should also be done.

OTHER DEFICIENCIES

Deficiencies of other micronutrients are likely to occur in patients who have undergone a restrictive malabsorptive operation, particularly the BPD and BPD/DS, although they are not well described. Slater et al. (111) observed an incidence of vitamin A deficiency of 52% at 1 yr, which increased to 69% by year four. Similarly elevated incidence rates of vitamin A deficiency were seen by Dolan et al. (112) at 1 to 1.5 yr after BPD or BPD/DS. At least two cases of symptomatic vitamin A deficiency have been reported following these procedures, occurring 18 mo and 24 mo postoperatively (113,114). Both patients presented with night blindness (nyctalopia), and one developed diffuse conjunctival xerosis with a Bitot's spot and diffuse punctuate keratitis of both corneas. As a fat-soluble compound, vitamin A, as well as the provitamin A carotenoids, is more likely to be malabsorbed with the BPD and BPD/DS procedures, which limit the exposure of food with biliopancreatic digestive secretions within a shortened common channel. A prenatal multiple vitamin–mineral supplement containing at least 5000 IU vitamin A should be provided on a daily basis. An incidence of serum vitamin E deficiency of 3 to 14% has been also reported by Slater and Dolan (111,112), although no clinical abnormalities have been reported.

PROPHYLACTIC MANAGEMENT AND MONITORING FOR NUTRITIONAL DEFICIENCIES

Nutritional management of the bariatric surgical patient must include prophylactic administration of vitamins and minerals to avoid deficiencies. As a practical manner, all patients should be discharged from the hospital receiving a chewable multiple vitamin–mineral supplement. After the first postoperative month, patients can be switched to a prescribed or over-the-counter prenatal supplement. Examples of products with nutrient

Table 3
Nutritional Monitoring of the Bariatric Surgical Patient

Routine tests
Complete blood count (CBC)
Chemistry profile
Liver function tests
Lipid panel
HbA1c (for diabetic patients)
Micronutrient tests
Ferritin (for iron status)
Folate
Vitamin B_{12}
25(OH)D
PTH (for calcium and vitamin D status)
DEXA (for calcium and vitamin D status)

content are shown in Table 2. Because the calcium, vitamin D, and vitamin B_{12} contents of the supplements are inadequate to meet postsurgical needs, all patients should receive additional calcium citrate + vitamin D 1200 to 1500 mg daily depending on dairy calcium, along with at least 500 µg vitamin B_{12}.

Monitoring of nutritional status should begin preoperatively. Table 3 displays a list of routine laboratory and micronutrient tests and procedures. Although no formal guidelines are available, it is reasonable to obtain all the micronutrient tests listed (except DEXA scan) preoperatively and at 6-mo intervals for the first 2 yr, followed by yearly assessments thereafter. Assessment of bone mineral density and screening for osteoporosis by DEXA should be considered for all patients because of the higher risk for development of metabolic bone disease. The timing and frequency of the DEXA test should be based on several factors, including gender, age and presence of other risk factors. Table 4 provides a summary of the assessment and treatment of micronutrient deficiencies. Once detected, deficiencies should be treated and monitored carefully. Patients at particularly high risk, such as women with menorrhagia or patients receiving corticosteroids, will likely require additional supplementation of selected nutrients.

CONCLUSION

Restrictive-malabsortive bariatric surgeries are associated with an increased risk of developing several micronutrient deficiencies. With judicious monitoring and adequate supplementation, these deficiencies are largely avoidable and treatable. However, the long-term sequelae of calcium and vitamin D malabsorption and development of metabolic bone disease remain a major concern. It is recommended that patients be screened preoperatively and at periodic intervals postoperatively. Identification of micronutrient deficiencies should be treated aggressively.

Table 4

Assessment and Treatment of Micronutrient Deficiencies

Nutrient	Deficiency conditions	Monitoring	Treatment
Thiamine (vitamin B_1)	Wernicke's encephalopathy Dry beriberi Wet beriberi	Low basal erythrocyte transketolase activity, enhanced response after TPP addition Increased T2 signal on MRI of brain in thalamus and midbrain	Acute deficiency Thiamine 100 mg iv or im × 7–14 d, then 10- mg po Prophylaxis 1.5–1.8 mg po qd
Iron	Iron-deficiency anemia (IDA)	Decreased serum ferritin (normal > 12 μg/L)	Deficiency 150–300 mg po qd, iv iron infusion Prophylaxis 28 mg po q d
Vitamin B_{12}	Macrocytic anemia Peripheral neuropathy	Low plasma or serum vitamin B_{12} (normal >300 pg/mL (>221 pmol/L) Elevated homocysteine level Elevated methylmalnotic acids (MMA)	Deficiency Vitamin B_{12} 1000 μg im q d x 1 wk, followed by 1000 μg every other wk × 4 Prophylaxis 500 μg po q d, intranasal 500 μg q wk, or 100 μg im q mo.
Calcium	Tetany Osteoporosis	Low serum calcium Elevated parathyroid hormone (PTH) level	Prophylaxis Calcium citrate 1200–1500 mg q d
Vitamin D	Osteomalacia	Low 25(OH)D level (normal >20–30 ng/mL) Elevated parathyroid hormone (PTH)	Prophylaxis Vitamin D 400–800 IU po q d Deficiency Ergocalciferol 50,000 IU po

REFERENCES

1. Gastrointestinal surgery for severe obesity. NIH Consens Dev Conf Consens Statement 1991 March 25–27. Am J Clin Nutr 1992;55:615S–619S.
2. National Heart, Lung, and Blood Institute (NHLBI) and National Institute for Diabetes and Digestive and Kidney Diseases (NIDDKD). Clinical guidelines on the identification, evaluation, and treatment of overweight and obesity in adults. The Evidence Report. Obes Res 1998;6(Suppl 2):51S–210S.
3. National Heart, Lung, and Blood Institute (NHLBI) and North American Association for the Study of Obesity (NAASO). Practical Guide on the Identification, Evaluation, and Treatment of Overweight and Obesity in Adults. NIH Publication number 00-4084. National Institutes of Health, Bethesda, MD: 2000.
4. Jones DB, Provost DA, De Maria EJ, et al. Optimal management of the morbidly obese patient. SAGES appropriateness conference statement. Surg Endosc 2004;18:1029–1037.
5. Buchwald H. Bariatric surgery for morbid obesity: health implications for patients, health professionals, and third-party payers. J Am Coll Surg 2005;200:593–604.
6. Encinosa WE, Bernard DM, Steiner CA, et al. Use and costs of bariatric surgery and prescription weight-loss medications. Health Affairs 2005;24:1039–1046.
7. Steinbrook R. Surgery for severe obesity. N Engl J Med 2004;350:1075–1079.
8. Buchwald H, Avidor Y, Braunwald E, et al. Bariatric surgery. A systematic review and meta-analysis. JAMA 2004;292:1724–1737.
9. Sturm R. Increase in clinically severe obesity in the United States, 1998–2000. JAMA 2003;163:2146–2148.
10. Hedley AA, Ogden CL, Johnson CL, et al. Prevalence of overweight and obesity among US children, adolescents, and adults, 1999–2002. JAMA 2004;291:2847–2850.
11. Avinoah E, Ovnat A, Charuzi I. Nutritional status seven years after Roux-en-Y gastric bypass surgery. Surgery 1992;111:137–142.
12. Amaral JE, Thompson WR, Caldwell MD, et al. Prospective hematologic evaluation of gastric exclusion surgery for morbid obesity. Ann Surg 1985;201:186–193.
13. Crowley LV, Seay J, Mullen G. Late effects of gastric bypass for obesity. Am J Gastroenterol 1984;79:850–860.
14. Halverson JD. Micronutrient deficiencies after gastric bypass for morbid obesity. Am Surg 1985;52:594–598.
15. Brolin RE, Gorman JH, Gorman RC, et al. Are vitamin B12 and folate deficiency clinically important after roux-en-y gastric bypass? J Gastrointest Surg 1998;2:436–442.
16. Brolin RE, Leung M. Survey of vitamin and mineral supplementation after gastric bypass and biliopancreatic diversion for morbid obesity. Obes Surg 1999;9:150–154.
17. Skroubis G, Sakellaropoulos G, Pouggouras K, et al. Comparison of nutritional deficiencies after roux-en-y gastric bypass and after biliopancreatic diversion with Roux-en-Y gastric bypass. Obes Surg 2002;12:551–558.
18. Schilling RF, Gohdes PN, Hardie GH. Vitamin B12 deficiency after gastric bypass surgery for obesity. Ann Intern Med 1984;101:501–502.
19. Provenzale D, Reinhold RB, Golner B, et al. Evidence for diminished B12 absorption after gastric bypass: oral supplementation does not prevent low plasma B12 levels in bypass patients. J Am Coll Nutr 1992;11:29–35.
20. Belle S. The NIDDK bariatric surgery clinical research consortium (LABS). SOARDS 2005;1:145–147.
21. Kushner R. Managing the obese patient after bariatric surgery: A case report of severe malnutrition and review of the literature. J Parental Enteral Nutr 2000;24:126–132.
22. Alvarez-Leite JI. Nutrient deficiencies secondary to bariatric surgery. Curr Opin Clin Nutr Metab Care 2004;7:569–575.
23. Mason ME, Jalagani H, Vinik AI. Metabolic complications of bariatric surgery: diagnosis and management issues. Gastroenterol Clin N Am 2005;34:25–33.
24. Fujioka K. Follow-up of nutritional and metabolic problems after bariatric surgery. Diab Care 2005;28:481–484.
25. Bloomberg RD, Fleishman A, Nalle JE, et al. Nutritional deficiencies following bariatric surgery: what have we learned? Obes Surg 2005;15:145–154.
26. Shuster MH, Vazquez JA. Nutritional concerns related to Roux-en-Y gastric bypass. Crit Care Nurs Q 2005;28:227–260.

27. Dietary Reference Intakes for thiamin, riboflavin, niacin, vitamin B6, folate, vitamin B12, pantothenic acid, biotin, and choline. Institute of Medicine. National Academy Press, Washington, DC: 1998.
28. MacLean JB. Wernicke's encephalopathy after gastric placation. JAMA 1982;248:1311.
29. Feit H, Glasberg M, Ireton C, et al. Peripheral neuropathy and starvation after gastric partitioning for morbid obesity. Ann Intern Med 1982;96:453–455.
30. Fawcett C, Young B, Holliday RL. Wernicke's encephalopathy after gastric partitioning for morbid obesity. Can J Surg 1984;27:169–170.
31. Viller HV, Ranne RD. Neurologic deficit following gastric partitioning: possible role of thiamine. JPEN 1984;8:575–578.
32. Somer H, Bergstrom L, Mustajoki P, et al. Morbid obesity, gastric placation and a severe neurological deficit. Acta Med Scand 1985;217:575–576.
33. Paulson GW, Martin EW, Mojzisik C, et al. Neurologic complications of gastric partitioning. Arch Neurol 1985;42:675–677.
34. Oczkowski WJ, Kertesz A. Wernicke's encephalopathy after gastroplasty for morbid obesity. Neurology 1985;35:99–101.
35. Salas-Salvado J, Garcia-Lorda P, Cuatrecasas G, et al. Wernicke's syndrome after bariatric surgery. Clin Nutr 2000;19:1356–1359.
36. Seehra H, MacDermott N, Lascelles RG, et al. Wernicke's encephalopathy after vertical banded gastroplasty for morbid obesity. BMJ 1996;312:434.
37. Mason EE. Starvation injury after gastric reduction for obesity. World J Surg 1998;22:1002–1007.
38. Cirignotta F, Manconi M, Mondini S, et al. Wernicke's-Korsakoff encephalopathy and polyneuropathy after gastroplasty for morbid obesity. Arch Neurol 2000;57:1356–1359.
39. Bozbora A, Coskun H, Ozarmagan S, et al. A rare complication of adjustable gastric banding: Wernicke's encephalopathy. Obes Surg 2000;10:274–275.
40. Toth C, Volt C. Wernicke's encephalopathy following gastroplasty for morbid obesity. Can J Neurol Sci 2001;28:89–92.
41. Chaves LC, Faintuch J, Kahwage S, et al. A cluster of polyneuropathy and Wernecke-Korsakoff syndrome in a bariatric unit. Obes Surg 2002;12:328–334.
42. Sola E, Morllas C, Garzon S, et al. Rapid onset of Wernicke's encephalopathy following gastric restrictive surgery. Obes Res 2003;13:661–662.
43. Loh T, Watson WD, Verman A, et al. Acute Wernicke's encephalopathy following bariatric surgery; clinical course and MRI correlation. Obes Surg 2004;14:129–132.
44. Nautiyal A, Singh S, Alaimo DJ. Wernicke's encephalopathy—an emerging trend after bariatric surgery. Am J Med 2004;117:804–805.
45. Towbin A, Inge TH, Garcia VF, et al. Beriberi after gastric bypass surgery in adolescence. J Pediatr 2004;145:263–267.
46. Abarbanel JM, Berginer VM, Osimani A, et al. Neurologic complications after gastric restriction surgery for morbid obesity. Neurology 1987;37:196–200.
47. Thaisetthawatkul P, Collazo-Clavell ML, Sarr MG, et al. A controlled study of peripheral neuropathy after bariatric surgery. Neurology 2004;63:1462–1470.
48. Chang CG, Adams-Huet B, Provost DA. Acute post-gastric reduction surgery (APGARS) neuropathy. Obes Surg 2004;14:182–189.
49. Antunwz E, Estruch R, Cardenal C, et al. Usefulness of CT and MR imaging in the diagnosis of acute Wernicke's encephalopathy. Am J Roentegenol 1998;171:1131–1137.
50. Conrad ME, Umbreit JN. Iron absorption and transport—an update. Am J Hematol 2000;64:287–298.
51. Smith CD, Herkes SB, Behrns KE, et al. Gastric acid secretion and vitamin B12 absorption after vertical Roux-en-Y gastric bypass for morbid obesity. Ann Surg 1993;218:91–96.
52. Behrns KE, Smith CD, Sarr MG. Prospective evaluation of gastric acid secretion and cobalmin absorption following gastric bypass for clinically severe obesity. Dig Dis Sci 1994;39:315–320.
53. Beard JL, Dawson H, Pinero DJ. Iron metabolism: a comprehensive review. Nutr Rev 1996;54:295–317.
54. Lash A, Saleem A. Iron metabolism and its regulation. A review. Ann Clin Lab Sci 1995;25:20–30.
55. Brolin RE, Robertson LB, Kenler HA, et al. Weight loss and dietary intake after vertical banded gastroplasty and Roux-en-Y gastric bypass. Ann Surg 1994;220:782–790.
56. Dietary Reference Intakes for vitamin A, vitamin K, arsenic, boron, chromium, copper, iodine, iron, manganese, molybdenum, nickel, silicon, vanadium, and zinc. A report of the panel on micronutrients, Dietary Reference Intakes. Food and Nutrition Board, Institute of Medicine. National Academy Press, Washington, DC: 2001.

57. Amaral JE, Thompson WR, Caldwell MD, et al. Prospective hematologic evaluation of gastric exclusion surgery for morbid obesity. Ann Surg 1985;201:186–193.
58. Monsen ER, Cook JD. Food iron absorption in human subjects IV. The effects of calcium and phosphate salts on the absorption of nonheme iron. Am J Clin Nutr 1976;29:1142–1148.
59. Hallberg L, Brune M, Erlandsson M, et al. Calcium: effect of different amounts on nonheme-and heme-iron absorption in humans. Am J Clin Nutr 1991;53:112–119.
60. Cook JD, Dassenko SA, Whittaker P. Calcium supplementation: effect on iron absorption. Am J Clin Nutr 1991;53:106–111.
61. Hallberg L, Rossander-Hulthen L, Brune M, et al. Calcium and iron absorption: mechanism of action and nutritional importance. Euro J Clin Nutr 1992;46:317–327.
62. Gleerup A, Rossander-Hulthen L, Gramatkovski E, et al. Iron absorption from the whole diet: comparison of the effect of two different distributions of daily calcium intake. Am J Clin Nutr 1995;61:97–104.
63. Minihane AM, Fairweather-Tait SJ. Effect of calcium supplementation on daily nonheme-iron absorption and long-term iron status. Am J Clin Nutr 1998;68:96–102.
64. Reddy MB, Cook JD. Effect of calcium intake on nonheme-iron absorption from a complete diet. Am J Clin Nutr 1997;65:1820–1825.
65. Grinder-Pederson L, Bukhave K, Jensen M, et al. Calcium from milk or calcium-fortified foods does not inhibit nonheme-iron absorption from a whole diet consumed over a 4-day period. J Clin Nutr 2004;80:404–409.
66. Andrews NC. Disorders of iron metabolism. N Engl J Med 1999;341:1986–1995.
67. Ross EM. Evaluation and treatment of iron deficiency in adults. Nutr Clin Care 2002;5:220–224.
68. Rainville AJ. Pica practices of pregnant women are associated with lower maternal hemoglobin level at delivery. J Am Diet Assoc 1998;98:293–296.
69. Simpson E, Mull JD, Longley E, et al. Pica during pregnancy in low-income women born in Mexico. West J Med 2000;173:20–24.
70. Rector WG. Pica: its frequency and significance in patients with iron-deficiency anemia due to chronic gastrointestinal blood loss. J Gen Intern Med 1989;4:512–513.
71. Ivascu NS, Sarnaik S, McCrae J, et al. Characterization of pica prevalence among patients with sickle cell disease. Arch Peds Adolesc Med 2001;155:1243–1247.
72. Kushner RF, Gleason B, Shanta-Retelny V. Reemergence of pica following gastric bypass surgery for obesity: a new presentation of an old problem. J Am Diet Assoc 2004;104:1393–1397.
73. Kushner RF, Shanta-Retelny V. Obes Surg 2005;15:1491–1495.
74. Brolin RE, Gorman JH, Gorman RC, et al. Prophylatic iron supplementation after Roux-en-Y gastric bypass. A prospective, double-blind, randomized study. Arch Surg 1998;133:740–744.
75. Rhode BM, Shustik C, Christou NV, et al. Iron absorption and therapy after gastric bypass. Obes Surg 1999;9:17–21.
76. Balk HW, Russell RM. Vitamin B12 deficiency in the elderly. Annu Rev Nutr 1999;19:357–377.
77. Rhode BM, Arseneau P, Cooper BA, et al. Vitamin B12 deficiency after gastric surgery for obesity. Am J Clin Nutr 1996;63:103–109.
78. Eussen SJPM, De Groot LCPM, Clarke R, et al. Oral cyanocobalamin supplementation in older people with vitamin B12 deficiency. A dose-finding trial. Arch Intern Med 2005;165:1167–1172.
79. Kuzminski AM, Del Giacco EJ, Allen RH, et al. Effective treatment of cobalamin deficiency with oral cobalamin. Blood 1998;92:1191–1198.
80. Riedt C, Brolin R, Shapses S. True fractional calcium absorption is decreased after Roux-en-Y gastric bypass. Obes Res 2004;12(supp):A33.
81. Wasserman RH. Vitamin D and the dual processes of intestinal calcium absorption. J Nutr 2004;134:3137–3139.
82. Charles P. Calcium absorption and calcium bioavailability. J Intern Med 1992;231:161–168.
83. Dietary Reference Intakes for calcium, phosphorus, magnesium, vitamin D, and fluoride. Institute of Medicine, National Academy Press, Washington, DC: 1997.
84. Looker AC. Body fat and vitamin D status in black versus white women. J Clin Endocrinol Metab 2005;90:635–640.
85. Wortsman J, Matsuika LY, Chen TC, et al. Decreased bioavailability of vitamin D in obesity. Am J Clin Nutr 2000;72:690–693.
86. Parikh SJ, Edelman M, Uwaifo GI, et al. The relationship between obesity and serum 1.12-dihydroxy vitamin D concentrations in healthy adults. J Clin Endocrinol Metab 2004;89:1196–1199.

87. Kamycheva E, Sundsfjord J, Jorde R. Serum parathyroid hormone level is associated with body mass index. The 5th Tromso study. Eur J Endocrinol 2004;151:167–172.

88. Arunabh S, Pollack S, Yeh J, et al. Body fat content and 25-hydroxyvitamin D levels in healthy women. J Clin Endocrinol Metab 2003;88:157–161.

89. Ahmad R, Hammond JM. Primary, secondary, and tertiary hyperparathyroidism. Otolaryngol Clin N Am 2004;37:701–713.

90. Whiting SJ, Calvo MS. Dietary recommendations for vitamin D: a critical need for functional end points to establish an estimated average requirement. J Nutr 2005;135:304–309.

91. Hickey L, Gordon CM. Vitamin D deficiency: new perspectives on an old disease. Curr Opin Endocrinol Diabetes 2004;11:18–25.

92. Hollis BW. Circulating 25-hydroxyvitamin D levels indicative of vitamin D sufficiency: implications for establishing a new effective dietary intake recommendation for vitamin D. J Nutr 2005;135:317–322.

93. Chapuy MC, Preziosi P, Maamer M, et al. Prevalence of vitamin D insufficiency in an adult normal population. Osteoporos Int 1997;7:439–443.

94. Rosen HN. Biochemical markers of bone turnover: clinical utility. Curr Opin Endocrinol Diabetes 2003;10:387–393.

95. Burke MS. Current roles and realities of noninvasive assessment of osteoporosis. Curr Opin Endocrinol Diabetes 2004;11:330–337.

96. Ott MT, Fanti P, Malluche HH, et al. Biochemical evidence of metabolic bone disease in women following Roux-en-Y gastric bypass for morbid obesity. Obes Surg 1992;2:341–348.

97. Newbury L, Dolan K, Hatzifotis M, et al. Calcium and vitamin D depletion and elevated parathyroid hormone following biliopancreatic diversion. Obes Surg 2003;13:893–895.

98. Diniz FHS, Diniz MTC, Sanches SRA,et al. Elevates serum parahormone after Roux-en-Y gastric bypass. Obes Surg 2004;14:1222–1226.

99. El-Kadre LJ, Rocha PR, de Almeida Tinoco AC, et al. Calcium metabolism in pre- and postmeno-pausal morbidly obese women at baseline and after laparoscopic Roux-en-Y gastric bypass. Obes Surg 2004;14:1062–1066.

100. Hamoui N, Anthone G, Crookes PF. Calcium metabolism in the morbidly obese. Obes Surg 2004;14:9–12.

101. von Mach MA, Stoeckli R, Bilz S, et al. Changes in bone mineral content after surgical treatment of morbid obesity. Metabolism 2004;53:918–921.

102. Prisco CD, Levine SN. Metabolic bone disease after gastric bypass surgery for obesity. Am J Med Sci 2005;329:57–61.

103. Coates PS, Fernstrom JD, Fernstrom MH, et al. Gastric surgery for morbid obesity leasds to an increase in bone turnover and a decrease in bone mass. J Clin Endocrinol Metab 2004;89:1061–1065.

104. Johnson JM, Maher JW, Samuel I, et al. Effects of gastric bypass procedures on bone mineral density, calcium, parathyroid hormone, and vitamin D. J Gastrointest Surg 2005;9:1106–1111.

105. Ybarra J, Sanchez-Hernandez J, Gich I, et al Unchanged hypovitaminosis D and secondary hyper-parathyroidism in morbid obesity after bariatric surgery. Obes Surg 2005;15:330–335.

106. Goldner WS, O'Dorisio TM, Dillon JS, et al. Severe metabolic bone disease as a long-term compli-cation of obesity surgery. Obes Surg 2002;12:685–692.

107. van Loan MD, Johnson HL, Barbieri TF. Effect of weight loss on bone mineral content and bone mineral density in obese women. Am J Clin Nutr 1998;67:734–738.

108. Pugnale N, Giusti V, Suter M, et al. Bone metabolism and risk of secondary hyperparathyroidism 12 months after gastric banding in obese pre-menopausal women. Int J Obes Relat Metab Disord 2003;27:110–116.

109. Guney E, Kisakol G, Ozgen G, et al. Effect of weight loss on bone metabolism: comparison of vertical banded gastroplasty and medical intervention. Obes Surg 2003;13:383–388.

110. Thomas MK, Demay MB. Vitamin D deficiency and disorders of vitamin D metabolism. Endocrinol Metab Clin North Am 2000;29:611–627.

111. Slater GH, Ren CF, Siegel N, et al. Serum fat-soluble vitamin D deficiency and abnormal calcium metabolism after malbsorptive bariatric surgery. J Gastrointest Surg 2004;8:48–55.

112. Dolan K, Hatzfotis M, Newbury L, et al. A clinical and nutritional comparison of biliopancreatic diversion with and without duodenal switch. Ann Surg 2004;240:51–56.

113. Hatzifotis M, Dolan K, Newbury L, et al. Symptomatic vitamin A deficiency following biliopancreatic diversion. Obes Surg 2003;13:655–657.

114. Lee WB, Hamilton SM, Harris JP, et al. Ocular complications of hypovitaminosis A after bariatric surgery. Ophthalmology 2005;112:1031–1034.

21 Lessons Learned From the National Weight Control Registry

James O. Hill, PhD, Holly R. Wyatt, MD, Suzanne Phelan, PhD, and Rena R. Wing, PhD

CONTENTS

INTRODUCTION
CHARACTERISTICS OF SUBJECTS
PREDICTORS OF SUCCESS IN LOSING WEIGHT
PREDICTORS OF WEIGHT-LOSS MAINTENANCE
PREDICTORS OF WEIGHT REGAIN
ARE THERE LESSONS TO BE LEARNED FROM THE NWCR?
EXCEPTIONS TO EACH WEIGHT-LOSS MAINTENANCE STRATEGY
ARE NWCR PARTICIPANTS DIFFERENT FROM THE AVERAGE PERSON
   TRYING TO LOSE WEIGHT?
WHAT TO DO AND HOW TO DO IT
REFERENCES

Summary

The National Weight Control Registry (NWCR) is a registry of more than 6000 individuals who have succeeded in long-term weight loss. This is the largest group of successful weight loss maintainers that has ever been studied. Over the past decade, we have identified many similarities in how these individuals are managing their body weight. We think this information can be useful in helping more people succeed at long-term weight management. We have eight recommendations for weight management based on our research: (1) treat weight-loss maintenance differently from weight loss; (2) make sure you are physically active during weight loss; (3) low-fat diets are best for preventing weight regain; (4) eat breakfast every day; (5) weigh yourself regularly and periodically keep diet and physical activity diaries; (6) get at least 1 h each day of physical activity; (7) maintain a consistent eating pattern; and (8) limit television viewing.

Key Words: Weight loss maintenance; obesity treatment; physical activity, National Weight Control Registry; breakfast; self-monitoring.

INTRODUCTION

The rise and fall of the popularity of low-carbohydrate diets is another indication that the public takes a short-term rather than a long-term approach to weight management. Many people seem willing to try each new popular diet, which usually involves relatively

From: *Contemporary Endocrinology: Treatment of the Obese Patient*
Edited by: R. F. Kushner and D. H. Bessesen © Humana Press Inc., Totowa, NJ

extreme diet changes, and often these diets seem to work for many people—at least for a while *(1,2)*. The problem is not in losing the weight in the first place, but in avoiding regaining the lost weight. The most likely reason that so many people who lose weight gain it back is because they are not able to sustain the behavioral changes they made to lose the weight. Losing weight is about short-term food restriction, but keeping weight off over the long term is about permanent lifestyle change. Our greatest challenge in treating obesity is not in producing weight loss but in maintaining the reduced weight once it is achieved.

A great deal of scientific research is directed toward developing and evaluating strategies for weight loss, but much less research is directed at developing and identifying strategies for maintenance of weight loss. In an effort to provide some of this information, we have been studying a unique group of successful weight-loss maintainers for more than a decade. These individuals have been successful not just in losing weight, but also in keeping it off for long periods of time. The group we are following currently consists of more than 6000 individuals who make up the National Weight Control Registry (NWCR). The NWCR began in 1994 to identify individuals who have succeeded in long-term weight-loss maintenance and to determine if we could identify common strategies used for weight loss and maintenance of weight loss. We have published 18 scientific articles about the individuals in the NWCR *(3–20)*.

To join the NWCR an individual must have maintained a weight loss of at least 30 lb for at least 1 yr. At present the average weight loss of the more than 6000 participants is more than 67 lb and the average length of time the weight loss has been maintained is about 6 yr.

The major intent of the NWCR research is to identify characteristics of successful weight-loss maintainers. This is not a prevalence study and these individuals do not constitute a random sample of those who have attempted weight loss. We recognize that the weight losses achieved in NWCR participants may be much greater than weight losses achieved by most people who attempt weight loss. However, we believe that there is value in learning from those who have been the most successful, and the NWCR represents the largest group of successful weight-loss maintainers that has ever been studied.

There are certainly other limitations to the NWCR. Individuals self-identify themselves as eligible for the NWCR and we only have retrospective self-reported information about them before weight loss. We ask that they provide some documentation, such as physician provided weight, pre–post pictures, and so on, but we do not vigorously evaluate this documentation for all participants. However, with a subgroup of NWCR participants, we did contact their physician or weight-loss counselor and found extremely good correspondence between the participant's self-reported weight and the verified weight. Additionally, most of the information is obtained from self-reports obtained through questionnaires that are mailed to participants; such information has been shown to underestimate energy intake and overestimate physical activity.

CHARACTERISTICS OF SUBJECTS

Most (80%) NWCR participants are female, with an average age of 45 yr. We have a low percentage (3%) of minorities in the NWCR. The majority (67%) of participants are married. The average pre-weight loss body mass index (BMI) of participants was 35 kg/m^2 and the average at time of entry into the NWCR was 25 kg/m^2. Thus, these individuals achieved an average decrease in BMI of 10 units.

PREDICTORS OF SUCCESS IN LOSING WEIGHT

Most NWCR participants reported that they used diet and physical activity to lose their weight (3). Fewer than 10% of participants lost weight with diet alone and fewer than 2% lost weight with physical activity alone. Somewhat surprisingly, there was no similarity in the types of diets used by the individuals to lose weight. We could find no particular diet that seemed to be used more than others for losing weight in this population. The fact that most of them used physical activity along with diet is interesting, particularly as adding physical activity to food restriction has minimal effects on weight loss (21).

PREDICTORS OF WEIGHT-LOSS MAINTENANCE

Unlike the differences for weight loss, many similarities are seen in how these individuals are maintaining their weight loss. We have identified five strategies that NWCR participants have in common.

Choosing Moderately Low-Fat, High-Carbohydrate Diets

We reported that the first 784 NWCR participants reported eating a diet containing 24% fat, 19% protein and 55% carbohydrate (3). We recently reported that dietary fat levels were increasing in those who entered the NWCR over the past 8 yr, from 24% to 29% (22). Even during the greatest popularity of the low-carbohydrate diets, most of the people entering the NWCR reported eating a low-fat diet to keep their weight off.

Frequent Self-Monitoring

A common characteristic among NWCR participants is that they weigh themselves frequently. Almost all of them weigh at least once a week and many weigh themselves daily (3).

Eating Breakfast

NWCR participants are breakfast eaters. Seventy-eight percent report eating breakfast 7 days a week and 90% eat breakfast 4 or more days a week. Only 4% report never eating breakfast.

Lots of Physical Activity

NWCR participants report engaging in very high levels of physical activity to maintain their weight loss. From self-reports we have estimated the average energy expenditure from physical activity to be about 2800 kcal/wk (3). This would correspond to about 1 h each day of moderate-intensity physical activity. Walking was the most frequently reported form of physical activity. We asked a subsample of NWCR participants to wear pedometers. We found that the average number of steps per day was about 11,000 (23).

Limiting TV Viewing

We recently reported (24) that NWCR participants spend a relatively minimal amount of their time watching television. A relatively high proportion (63.5%) of participants reported watching ≤10 h/wk upon entry in the NWCR. More than a third (38.5%) reported watching <5 h, whereas only 12.5% watched ≥21 h/wk. These data contract markedly from the national average of 28 h of TV viewing per week reported by American adults (25).

PREDICTORS OF WEIGHT REGAIN

We follow NWCR participants over time, and some participants do experience some weight regain. This has allowed us to examine factors that predict weight regain in these individuals. In general, increases in dietary fat intake and decreases in physical activity are associated with the greatest likelihood of weight regain *(4,8)*. We have also found that increases in TV viewing *(24)* and maintaining an inconsistent eating pattern *(18)* are related to greater risk of weight regain. Further, the duration of weight loss maintenance is a strong predictor of weight regain. The longer weight loss has been maintained, the less likely weight regain will occur *(4,8)*. Interestingly, people who had medical reasons for weight loss also appear to have better initial weight loss and maintenance over time *(18)*.

ARE THERE LESSONS TO BE LEARNED FROM THE NWCR?

We believe that results from the NWCR provide some important information for people trying to manage their weight and for health care professionals who are trying to help them with weight management. It must be emphasized that the results of the NWCR are correlational and cannot be used to establish cause and effect. Therefore it is important to evaluate NWCR results along with other information in the literature. With this caveat, we offer the following as lessons that can be learned from the NWCR.

Treat Weight-Loss Maintenance Differently From Weight Loss

It may make sense to treat weight management as having two phases — weight loss and maintenance of weight loss. Many people succeed in losing weight, but far fewer succeed in keeping it off. What works for losing weight may not work for keeping weight off. We are impressed at how little similarity we see in NWCR participants during weight loss but how much similarity we see during weight-loss maintenance.

It is clear that people can lose weight on many different types of diets *(1,2,26)*. In recent years, some of the popular diets *(1,2,26)* and some of the commercial weight-loss programs *(27)* have been scientifically evaluated and shown to produce weight loss. However, the problem for the popular diets and the commercial programs is that keeping the weight off is difficult *(1,2,26,27)*. The similarity of behaviors used by NWCR participants to keep weight off suggests that although weight can be lost using many different strategies, there may be less variability in how weight loss can be maintained.

Make Sure to Be Physically Active During Weight Loss

Successful weight loss maintainers used both diet and physical activity to lose weight. It is interesting to ask them if and how physical activity contributed to their long-term success in weight loss maintenance. Although the extra weight loss is probably quite small, physical activity could be important during weight loss because of its impact on body composition. Several studies have found that adding physical activity to food restriction serves to preserve lean body mass *(28)*, which could leave the participants with a higher rate of metabolism after weight loss than if they had used diet alone. Alternatively, as the NWCR participants report such high levels of physical activity during weight maintenance, physical activity during weight loss could be important because it is necessary to get them to the high levels of physical activity required to maintain their weight loss.

Low-Fat Diets Are Best for Preventing Weight Regain

Most successful weight-loss maintainers eat a low-fat, high-carbohydrate diet that is low in total calories. Even though there is great controversy in the literature over the best diet composition for maintaining a healthy body weight, the overwhelming majority of the NWCR participants report eating a diet with less than 30% fat and that is high in carbohydrate to keep their weight off. It is important to note that we did not see all NWCR participants eating a low-fat, high-carbohydrate diet to lose weight, suggesting that there can be more variety in weight-loss diets than in weight-loss maintenance diets.

Our results are consistent with many reports in the literature that low-fat, low-calorie diets may be best for long-term weight management. Perhaps the major impact of dietary fat is in helping individuals reduce their overall energy intake. Several studies have shown that diets high in fat lead to greater energy intake than lower-fat diets *(29–31)*. The tendency to overeat on higher-fat diets may be because of the higher energy density of these diets which is known to increase energy intake *(32)*.

Eat Breakfast Every Day

Skipping breakfast is not a good strategy for long-term weight maintenance. We believe that skipping breakfast is a common strategy used by many who are trying to lose weight in order to lower total daily energy intake. Our results from the NWCR would cast doubt on this as an effective strategy, at least for long-term weight-loss maintenance. NWCR participants rarely skip breakfast. There is a growing body of literature associating breakfast eating with lower BMI and with lower daily energy intake *(33,34)*. Consuming calories in the morning may have a more satiating effect than consuming calories later in the day *(35)*.

Weigh Yourself Regularly and Periodically Keep Diet and Physical Activity Diaries

Those who succeed in long-term weight-loss maintenance weigh themselves frequently. In trying to maintain a constant weight, it helps to know what you weigh. Almost all NWCR participants weigh themselves at least weekly, and most even more often. Similarly, many NWCR participants periodically keep diet and physical activity diaries. Frequent weighing and keeping records of food intake and physical activity promote awareness. If an individual is trying to maintain a constant weight, it seems to help to monitor weight frequently. This could serve as an "early warning system" allowing the person to modify food intake and/or physical activity when weight starts to increase. Similarly, because being vigilant in eating and physical activity behaviors is important for long-term weight loss maintenance, it helps to maintain awareness of those behaviors. Other studies in the literature support the benefit of dietary self-monitoring in weight management *(36,37)*.

Get at Least an Hour Each Day of Physical Activity

It is very difficult to maintain a significant weight loss without a lot of physical activity. NWCR participants are physically active and report an average of about 1 h per day of physical activity, or about 11,000 steps/d. Further, we have found that the more weight lost, the more physical activity reported (unpublished). The literature is consistent in that high levels of physical activity are perhaps the best predictor of long-term success in weight-loss maintenance *(38)*. Jakicic et al. *(39)* have shown in a perspective study that high levels of physical activity are better than low or moderate levels in maintaining weight loss after obesity treatment.

However, it is not clear why this is the case. Physical activity could be important simply because of its effects on energy balance. The more physical activity a person does, the more calories that can be consumed without weight gain. As energy requirements decrease with weight loss, a person who loses weight and does not increase physical activity may have to eat far less than before weight loss. Because food restriction is difficult for most people, increased physical activity may serve to allow the person to consume an amount of food that is sustainable. Alternatively, physical activity may have other metabolic effects that go beyond simply expending more energy. Some have suggested that there is a threshold of energy expenditure below which it is harder to match energy intake to energy expenditure *(40)*. Perhaps the high levels of physical activity seen in NWCR participants help get them above this threshold and makes matching energy intake and expenditure easier. Finally, high levels of physical activity may simply be a marker for achieving other lifestyle changes. People who are adherent to physical activity may also be more adherent to diet. Regardless of the reason, high levels of physical activity seem to be necessary for success in long-term weight-loss management.

Maintain a Consistent Eating Pattern

Most NWCR participants report that their eating is the same on weekends, weekdays, and on holidays/vacations throughout the year. Moreover, NWCR individuals who maintain a consistent diet regimen across the week and year appear more likely to maintain their weight loss over time. Allowing for flexibility in the diet may increase exposure to high-risk situations, creating more opportunity for loss of control.

Limit TV Viewing

Individuals in the NWCR spend a relatively minimal amount of their time watching TV. A relatively high proportion (63.5%) of individuals in this sample reported watching 10 or fewer hours per week upon entry into the NWCR. This is in stark contrast to the typical TV viewing behavior of American adults, who spend an average of 28 h per week watching TV *(25)*. These findings are consistent with a growing body of cross-sectional and prospective research showing that TV viewing is an independent correlate of weight status *(41–43)*. Thus, reducing common sedentary behaviors, such as watching TV, may help to promote long-term weight-loss maintenance. Although the effects of change in TV on weight gain have to be mediated by changes in either physical activity and/or dietary factors, it remains unclear which part of the energy balance equation is being affected by TV viewing in adults.

EXCEPTIONS TO EACH WEIGHT-LOSS MAINTENANCE STRATEGY

Even though the majority of NWCR participants show common behaviors, there are exceptions to each. For example, 4% of NWCR participants never eat breakfast and 9% report that they are maintaining weight loss with little or no physical activity. Further, with the recent popularity of low-carbohydrate diets, we are seeing more people (<10% of the population) who are maintaining a weight loss with a low-carbohydrate diet.

ARE NWCR PARTICIPANTS DIFFERENT FROM THE AVERAGE PERSON TRYING TO LOSE WEIGHT?

One potential criticism of the NWCR is that we have just captured people for whom weight loss is easy and that NWCR participants are somehow different from most over-weight and obese people who try to lose weight. Although we cannot conclusively determine whether or not this is the case, we do find that the majority of NWCR partici-pants were overweight as children or adolescents and that most have at least one over-weight or obese parent. It is generally thought that those with a family history of obesity and those who developed obesity as children may find weight loss to be more difficult than those without a family history of obesity or those who become obese later in life.

WHAT TO DO AND HOW TO DO IT

We think that the similarities we have identified in NWCR participants are supported by many other studies in the literature. Eating a low-fat diet, eating breakfast, self-monitoring, and being highly physically active are behaviors others have found to be important in maintaining weight loss. We believe that results from the NWCR can be useful both for people trying to lose weight and for health care providers who are helping them.

Although it is useful to see the behaviors that contribute to success, it remains a challenge to help more people achieve and maintain these behaviors. How, for example, do you help your sedentary patients get to the point where they are physically active for an hour each day—for the rest of their lives? We believe that our results are useful in identifying what to do to achieve success in long-term weight-loss maintenance, and to provide hope that weight-loss maintenance is possible. However, we still have the chal-lenge of helping more people achieve and maintain the behaviors that are consistent with maintenance of weight loss.

REFERENCES

1. Dansinger ML, Gleason JA, Griffith JL, et al. Comparison of the Atkins, Ornish, Weight Watchers, and Zone diets for weight loss and heart disease risk reduction: a randomized trial. JAMA 2005;293:43–53.
2. Foster GD, Wyatt HR, Hill JO, et al. A multi-center, randomized, controlled clinical trial of the Atkins diet. N Engl J Med 2003;348:282–290.
3. Klem ML, Wing RR, McGuire MT, et al. A descriptive study of individuals successful at long-term maintenance of substantial weight loss. Am J Clin Nutr 1997;66:239–246.
4. Shick SM, Wing RR, Klem ML, et al. Persons successful at long-term weight loss and maintenance continue to consume a low calorie, low fat diet. J Am Dietetic Assn 1998;98:408–413.
5. McGuire MT, Wing RR, Klem ML, et al. Long-term maintenance of weight loss: Do people who lose weight through various weight loss methods use different behaviors to maintain their weight? Int J Obes 1998:22:572–577.
6. Klem ML, Wing RR, McGuire MT, et al. Psychological symptoms in individuals successful at long-term maintenance of weight loss. Health Psych 1998;17:336–345.
7. Wyatt HR, Grunwald GK, Seagle HM, et al. Resting energy expenditure in reduced-obese subjects in the National Weight Control Registry. Am J Clin Nutr 1999;69:1189–1193.
8. McGuire MT, Wing RR, Klem ML, et al. What predicts weight regain among a group of successful weight losers? J Consul Clin Psych 1999;67:177–185.
9. McGuire MT, Wing RR, Hill JO. The prevalence of weight loss maintenance among American adults. Int J Obes 1999;12:1314–1319.
10. McGuire MT, Wing RR, Klem ML, et al. The behavioral characteristics of individuals who lose weight unintentionally. Obes Res 1999;7:485–490.

11. McGuire MT, Wing RR, Klem ML, et al. Behavioral strategies of individuals who have maintained long-term weight losses. Obes Res 1999;7:334–341.

12. Klem ML, Wing RR, Chang CH,et al. A case-control study of successful maintenance of a substantial weight loss: Individuals who lost weight through surgery versus those who lost weight through non-surgical means. Int J Obes 2000;24:573–579.

13. Klem ML, Wing RR, Lang W, et al. Does weight loss maintenance become easier over time? Obes Res 2000;8:438–442.

14. Wing R, Hill JO. Successful weight maintenance. Annual Rev Nutr 2001;21(33):323–341.

15. Wyatt HR, Grunwald GK, Mosca CL, et al. Long-term weight loss and breakfast in subjects in the National Weight Control Registry. Obes Res 2002;10:78–82.

16. Phelan S, Hill JO, Lang W, et al. Recovery from relapse among successful weight maintainers. Am J Clin Nutr 2003;78:1079–1084.

17. Gorin AA, Phelan S, Hill JO, et al. Medical triggers are associated with better short- and long-term weight loss outcomes. Prev Med 2004;39:612–616.

18. Gorin AA, Phelan S, Wing RR, et al. Promoting long-term weight control: does dieting consistency matter? Int J Obes 2004;28:278–281.

19. DelParigi A, Chen K, Salbe AD, et al. Persistence of abnormal neural responses to a meal in postobese individuals. Int J Obes 2004;28:370–377.

20. Raynor HA, Jeffery RW, Phelan S, et al. Amount of food group variety consumed in the diet and long-term weight loss maintenance. Obes Res 2005;13:883–890.

21. Wing RR. Physical activity in the treatment of the adulthood overweight and obesity: current evidence and research issues. Med Sci Sports Exerc 1999;31 (Suppl.):S547–S552.

22. Phelan S, Wyatt HR, Hill JO, and Wing R. Are the eating and exercise habits of successful weight losers changing? Obesity 2006;14:710–716.

23. Wyatt HR, Donahoo WT, Grunwald GK, et al. Average steps per day for long-term weight loss in the National Weight Control Registry. Obes Res 2001;9:192s (Abstract)

24. Raynor DA, Phelan S, Hill DO, and Wing RR. Television viewing and long-term maintenance: results from the National Weight Control Registry. Obesity 2006; in press.

25. Nielson Media Research 2000. Nielson Report on Television. Nielson Media Research, New York: 2000.

26. Stern L, Iqbal N, Seshadri P, et al. The effects of a low-carbohydrate versus conventional weight loss in severely obese adults: one-year follow-up of a randomized trial. Ann Intern Med 2004;140:778–785.

27. Heska S, Anderson JW, Atkinson RL, et al. Self help weight loss vs a structured commercial program: a randomized, controlled two-year trial. JAMA 2003;289:1799–1805.

28. Ballor DL, Keesey RE. A meta-analysis of the factors affecting exercise-induced changes in body mass, fat mass, and fat-free mass in males and females. Int J Obes 1991;15:717–726.

29. Lissner L, Levitsky DA, Strupp BJ, et al. Dietary fat and the regulation of energy intake in human subjects. Am J Clin Nutr 1987;46(6):886–892.

30. Stubbs RJ, Harbron CG, Murgatroyd PR, et al. Covert manipulation of dietary fat and energy density:effect on substrate flux and food intake in men eating ad libitum. Am J Clin Nutr 1995; 62(2):316–329.

31. Thomas CD, Peters JC, Reed GW, et al. Nutrient balance and energy expenditure during ad libitum feeding of high-fat and high-carbohydrate diets in humans. Am J Clin Nutr 1992;55(5):934–942.

32. Rolls BJ, Bell EA. Intake of fat and carbohydrate: role of energy density. Eur J Clin Nutr 1999;53 (suppl. 1):S166–S173.

33. Cho S, Dietrich M, Brown CJP, et al. The effect of breakfast type on total daily energy intake and body mass index: results from the third National Health and Nutrition Examination Survey (NHANES III). J Am Coll Nutr 2003;22:296–302.

34. Affenito SG, Thompson DR, Barton BA, et al. Breakfast consumption by African-american and white adolescent girls correlates positively with calcium and fiber intake and negatively with body mass index. J Am Diet Assn 2005;105:938–945.

35. deCastro JM. The time of day of food intake influences overall intake in humans. J Nutr 2004;134:104–111.

36. Linde JA, Jeffery JW, French SA, et al. Self weighing in weight gain prevention and weight loss trials. Ann Behav Med 2005;30:210–216.

37. Baker RC, Kirschenbaum DS. Self-monitoring may be necessary for successful weight control. Behav Ther 1993;24:377–394.

38. Saris WHM, Blair SN, van Baak MA, et al. How much physical activity is enough to prevent unhealthy weight gain? Outcome of the IASO 1st Stock Conference and consensus statement. Obes Rev 2003;4:101–114.
39. Jakicic JM, Marcus BH, Gallagher KI, et al. Effect of exercise duration and intensity on weight loss in overweight, sedentary women. A randomized trial. JAMA 2003;290:1323–1330.
40. Mayer J, Purnima R, Mitra KP. Relation between caloric intake, body weight and physical work: studies in an industrial male population in West Bengal. Am J Clin Nutr 1956;4:169–175.
41. Cameron AJ, Welborn TA, Zimmet PZ, et al. Overweight and obesity in Australia: The 1999–2000 Australian diabetes, obesity, and lifestyle study. Med J Aus 2003;178:427–432.
42. Hu FB, Li TY, Colditz GA, et al. Television watching and other sedentary behaviors in relation to risk of obesity and type 2 diabetes mellitus in women. JAMA 2003;290:1785–1791.
43. Jakes RW, Day NE, Khaw KT, et al. Television viewing and low participation in vigorous recreation are independently associated with obesity and markers of cardiovascular disease risk: EPIC-Norfolk population-based study. Eur J Clin Nutr 2003;57:1089–1096.

22 Pediatric Obesity

Lawrence D. Hammer, MD

CONTENTS

INTRODUCTION
EPIDEMIOLOGY
ETIOLOGIES
COMORBIDITIES
EVALUATION
BEHAVIORAL TREATMENT
PHARMACOLOGICAL TREATMENT
SURGICAL TREATMENT
PREVENTION
CONCLUSION
REFERENCES

Summary

Child obesity has increased dramatically in prevalence and severity over the past 40 yr. The tendency for obesity in childhood and adolescence to persist into adult life ties it to other risk factors for cardiovascular disease. This chapter will cover the epidemiology, evaluation, and management of child and adolescent obesity, with an emphasis on the impact of obesity as a life-span condition. The relationship between childhood obesity and other medical conditions will be reviewed. The impact of obesity psychologically, socially, and economically on the individual, family, and society will also be discussed. The bulk of the chapter will include information to assist the clinician in the evaluation of children and adolescents who are overweight and a description of the variety of medical, behavioral, and surgical approaches currently used in the management of this condition.

Key Words: Child obesity; adolescent obesity; overweight; body mass index; BMI, Stoplight Diet; gastric bypass; very low calorie diet; low carbohydrate; low glycemic; television; physical activity.

INTRODUCTION

This chapter will cover the epidemiology, evaluation, and management of child and adolescent obesity, with an emphasis on the impact of obesity as a life span condition. The relationship between childhood obesity and other medical conditions will be reviewed. The impact of obesity psychologically, socially, and economically on the individual, family, and society will be discussed. The bulk of the chapter will include information to assist the clinician in the evaluation of children and adolescents who are overweight

From: *Contemporary Endocrinology: Treatment of the Obese Patient*
Edited by: R. F. Kushner and D. H. Bessesen © Humana Press Inc., Totowa, NJ

and a description of the variety of medical, behavioral, and surgical approaches currently available.

Simply put, child obesity results when an excess of energy intake over energy expenditure results in deposition of adipose tissue. The energy balance of caloric intake and caloric expenditure in the pediatric age group, includes, not only basal metabolic rate, the thermic effect of food, and physical activity, but also a small contribution to ongoing growth.

EPIDEMIOLOGY

Obesity is increasing in prevalence and severity throughout the United States and the rest of the world. It affects all racial, ethnic, and socioeconomic groups. Changes in dietary patterns and physical activity probably account for this new "epidemic." Based on data from the survey years 1999 through 2002, 31.0% of youth ages 6 through 18 were at or above the 85th percentile for body mass index and 16.0% were at or above the 95th percentile for body mass index (BMI) (1).

Since the 1960s, the federal government has conducted a number of periodic nutrition surveys, currently referred to as the National Health and Nutrition Examination Surveys (NHANES). In all age groups, there has been steady increase in the prevalence of overweight over the past 40 yr. The most rapid increases in prevalence began to appear following the second NHANES (1976–1980), as seen in the increases of prevalence among white male adolescents by nine percentage points from the second NHANES to the third NHANES (1988–1991) with less dramatic, though significant, increases in rates for all other age and ethnic groups during that period of time (2). In particular, rates among African American and Hispanic children have increased more rapidly than for whites. In the 1999–2002 NHANES survey, the prevalence of overweight (BMI $\geq$ 95th percentile) was highest among Mexican American youth, with 22.1% of 6- to 19-yr-olds and 13.1% of 2- to 5-yr-olds so categorized by BMI, whereas among non-Hispanic whites, the comparable rates were 13.6% and 8.6% and among non-Hispanic blacks, 20.5% and 8.8%, respectively (1). During this same time period there has been a considerable increase in the caloric intake derived from snacks, soft drinks, and out-of-home meals. Adolescent females followed from before menarche until 4 yr post-menarche showed significantly greater increases in BMI if they consumed two or more fast-food meals out of their homes each week than those who ate fewer out-of-home meals (3), consistent with other studies showing a relationship between out-of-home fried food or fast-food intake and BMI (4,5). Likewise, portion sizes have increased steadily over the past 25 yr (6). Many popular fast-foods provide more than 1000 calories per meal. Soft drinks provide a particularly insidious source of extra calories to many children and adolescents (7).

At the same time, daily participation in physical activity and physical education has been steadily decreasing. Children spend the bulk of their time in low-intensity activity, with a great deal of time spent watching television (8), often in association with increased food consumption (9). Television viewing is increased among those children with a television in their bedroom, as early as the preschool years (10).

Defining Pediatric Overweight and Obesity

What is pediatric obesity? The Expert Committee on the Evaluation and Treatment of Childhood Obesity has defined pediatric obesity as "excess body weight (adipose tissue) associated with adverse health or psychological outcomes" *(11)*. BMI is used to assess the presence or risk of overweight. Children among whom the BMI exceeds the 95th percentile for age and gender are considered overweight. Those whose BMI falls between the 85th and 94th percentile for age and gender are considered "at risk" for overweight. In this chapter, the term "obesity" will be used in reference to the clinical condition as defined above, whereas the term "overweight" will be used in reference to patients, individually or as a group. Although BMI is not an ideal measure of body fatness, it represents a clear advance over reliance on skinfold thickness or other indirect measures of fatness in the clinical environment. Difficulties with reliability make skinfold measurement prone to error, especially as body fatness increases, and the BMI can be assessed quickly with each well-child visit *(12)*. For more precise estimation of body fatness, investigators are turning to dual-energy X-ray absorptiometry (DEXA), which is gaining acceptance in the research literature *(13)*. Use of densitometry and bioelectric impedance have not become widely accepted in studies of children and adolescents owing to practical limitations and variations in hydration and fat-free mass in this age group *(14)*. Another method for estimation of body fatness, air-displacement plethysmography, shows promise as a method for monitoring change in body fatness over time and is now becoming commercially available outside the research environment *(15)*.

Persistence, Sequelae, and Costs of Pediatric Overweight

Increased body fatness can occur at any age and may or may not persist. The longer a child is overweight, the more likely it is that he or she will be overweight as an adult. At any point in time the positive predictive value of early obesity increases with the age of the child but never reaches 100%. One of the most significant risks of childhood obesity is that it is a strong predictor of adult obesity and the medical complications associated with obesity in adult life, such as diabetes, hypertension, and hyperlipidemia. Early obesity is also a risk factor for later cardiovascular and metabolic morbidities. Although parental obesity is predictive of child and adolescent obesity, the contribution of parental obesity to this risk ratio diminishes in importance over time in relation to the child's own BMI *(16)*. The tendency for excess weight in childhood and adolescence to persist into adult life has been demonstrated in a variety of studies *(27–29)*. Thus, obesity persisting from early in life into the adult years should also be considered a risk factor for reduced lifespan, currently estimated at 4 to 9 mo of life lost but expected to increase in the future to 2 to 5 yr of potential life lost *(17)*.

Economic and social costs of obesity are quite high. Type 2 diabetes alone may account for as much as $30 billion in direct costs and $30 billion in indirect costs per year *(18)*. The cost of inpatient treatment for comorbid conditions associated with obesity has more than tripled over the past 20 yr. Health care-related costs for overweight and obesity in the United States exceed $90 billion per year and account for 9.1% of total US health expenditures *(19)*. A study of direct costs for obesity and related conditions in France showed that these costs represented about 11% of the total French health care system budget, split evenly between inpatient and outpatient care *(20)*.

The social consequences of obesity are also quite profound, affecting likelihood of employment, marriage, and educational attainment. Health-related quality-of-life scores are comparable to those of children diagnosed with cancer and worse than those of normal-weight peers or children with other chronic diseases.

A number of public health and prevention efforts are currently under way. It is important to understand the impact of policy decisions in each sector of government on access to physical activity through production, distribution, and quality. Zoning and other regulatory means may be available to increase safe opportunities for indoor and outdoor physical activity. Incentives and policy must be developed to promote the production and distribution of healthier foods. Economic tools may be used to modify institutional and organizational behaviors that directly or indirectly discourage healthier eating and physical activity. For example, regulation of food advertising during children's TV programs may be one approach to minimizing the promotion of sugared cereals and "junk foods."

ETIOLOGIES

Critical Growth Periods

There may be several "critical periods" during which adipose tissue development may be more of a factor in the long-term development of obesity *(21)*. Three such periods are the prenatal period *(22)*, the period of "adiposity rebound" *(23)*, and puberty *(24)*. Both high and low birthweights have been shown to correlate positively with rates of obesity later in life. Infants of diabetic mothers and other very large infants, as well as infants whose mothers were energy-deprived during the first two trimesters, are at significantly increased risk for hypertension, diabetes, and obesity later in life.

Examination of the pattern of change in BMI over the first 7 yr of life reveals a typical increase in BMI following the initial postinfancy nadir that occurs in the second to third year of life. The "adiposity rebound" then occurs between about 5 and 7 yr of age, with children whose adiposity rebound occurs earliest showing the greatest risk of obesity in the late teen years. Pubertal timing may also play a role in adiposity development, as early menarche has been shown to increase the risk of obesity and the metabolic syndrome *(25)*.

Genetics

Though accounting for a relatively small portion of obesity in the pediatric age group, a number of endocrine disorders and genetic syndromes can be causally linked to childhood obesity. Of note is that these disorders are generally accompanied by poor linear growth and developmental delay. Recent studies of large family pedigrees have also identified a number of genetic loci that appear to be associated with severe obesity *(103)*. One such genetic locus found in some obese individuals is that which encodes for the melanocortin 4 receptor *(104)*. It is also possible that alterations in the genes that control production of leptin and ghrelin may play a role in some cases of human obesity *(105)*. Leptin is a hormone secreted from adipocytes that moderates food intake and energy expenditure. Circulating levels correlate with body fat and BMI. Leptin increases in boys and girls from 5 to 15 yr of age, before the appearance of other pubertal hormones. Ghrelin is a gastric hormone that influences appetite and weight regulation.

Many investigators have attempted to develop and test risk factor models that include parental BMI as well as the child's BMI at various ages. For example, in one prospective British study, children with early adiposity rebound had parents with higher BMI and were more likely to have at least one obese parent *(26)*. In a US cohort, followed in the Fels Longitudinal Study, the probability of adult obesity increased in relation to child

BMI with the child's age at time of measurement a significant factor, in that the older the child with an elevated BMI, the more likely was that child to become an obese adult *(27)*. As mentioned above, Whitaker and colleagues have shown that both parent BMI and child BMI play important roles in predicting child to adult outcomes, with the parent's BMI having a decreasing influence and the child's BMI having an increasing influence over time *(16)*. These findings were echoed in another longitudinal cohort from the Quebec Family Study *(28)*. Prediction of adult BMI improves considerably after a child reaches 13 yr of age *(29)*.

The statistical contribution of parental BMI could be a result of environmental, rather than genetic, effects. In a study of parental eating attitudes and child BMI, parents who were both overweight and displayed high levels of disinhibited eating, coupled with a high level of dietary restraint on the Three Factor Eating Questionnaire *(30)*, had children with higher BMIs than those whose parents did not display disinhibited eating *(31)*. These parents may exert excessive control over their children's food consumption while themselves modeling excessive food intake *(32)*.

Impact of Food and Diet

Though very difficult to measure accurately, dietary excess remains the most likely explanation for most overweight children. Fast food is one such source of excess energy. Children who eat fast food, compared with those who do not, consume more total energy, more energy per gram of food, more total fat, more total carbohydrate, more added sugars, more sugar-sweetened beverages, less fiber, less milk, and fewer nonstarchy vegetables and fruits *(5)*. An association has been demonstrated between the presence of soda machines in schools and intake of sugared sodas by students *(33)*. Studies of dietary intake and adiposity development have not provided a consistent picture of the relationship between early patterns of intake and excessive weight gain, although a recent study involving an adult cohort from Spain demonstrated significant relationships between consumption of soft drinks, hamburgers, pizza, and sausages and subsequent weight gain *(34)*. In one pediatric study, protein intake at age 2 was predictive of BMI at age 8 and of early adiposity rebound *(35)*, whereas in another study, diet was not associated with change in BMI from 3 to 6 yr of age *(36)*.

An interesting literature has developed concerning parental feeding practices and beliefs and their relationship to child weight gain. In general, these studies support the notion that restrictive or overcontrolling parent feeding practices may increase the risk for later overweight, perhaps via an influence on the child's own development of feeding control *(32,37,38)*, whereas others have found no such relationship *(39)*. In two observational studies, encouragements to eat were associated with variation in BMI *(40,41)*.

Decreased Physical Activity

Both decreased physical activity and an increase in screen time likely contribute to the increasing prevalence of child and adolescent obesity. The majority of school age children in the United States do not participate in sufficient leisure-time physical activity during their nonschool hours. The amount of television viewing among young children and teens shows a significant positive correlation with increasing BMI *(42)*. A randomized controlled trial (RCT) that manipulated television viewing in elementary school children showed that children who reduced their time spent watching television increased their BMI at a slower rate than did children who did not reduce their television viewing

(43). An additional effect of television may be via its influence on buying and eating habits, as result of its powerful influence on children and the marketing of products to children during programming designed to be watched primarily by children. A longitudinal study of diet, physical activity, and TV viewing showed that TV viewing and physical activity predicted change in BMI from 3 to 6 yr of age, with no significant contribution of dietary intake to the prediction model *(36)*.

Behavioral Risk Factors

A prospective study of 150 children from birth to 9.5 yr of age examined the interplay of multiple proposed risk factors for child overweight and found that parent overweight was the largest factor but that the effect was mediated by child temperament. A risk factor was the presence of a "difficult" temperament, accompanied by tendencies to tantrum and parental tendencies to use food as a reward or behavioral contingency *(44)*. In the same study, coded videotapes of children observed during a meal with the parent also showed that maternal food offers, food presentations, and total prompts were all significantly related to child intake. Children who ate the fastest had mothers who delivered eating prompts at a higher frequency, suggesting that maternal interactions could encourage rapid eating or poor self-regulation during eating *(41)*.

Psychological Factors

A number of psychological factors may also influence eating behavior and weight gain. The prevailing social desirability of thinness leads many teens to engage in unhealthy weight-control practices. Dietary restraint, caloric restriction, exercise for weight-control purposes, and appetite suppressant/laxative use are all associated with an increased risk of obesity among female adolescents. In fact, weight reduction practices are more likely to result in weight gain than in weight loss in adolescent girls.

Food insecurity may be considered another psychological risk factor. In a sample of Hispanic school-age children, food supplies, children's at-home food consumption, and household food security were analyzed in relation to child BMI *(45)*. Although weekly food intake varied over the course of each month in food-insecure households, children's food intakes were not associated with the degree of food insecurity reported for the household and food insecurity was associated with lower child BMIs, rather than higher BMIs as had been previously shown for adults *(46)*.

COMORBIDITIES

Table 1 shows a list of medical conditions that are known to be associated with obesity in adult life. As indicated in the table, a number of these conditions are also commonly seen with severe overweight during childhood and adolescence.

Cardiovascular risk factors—including hyperinsulinemia, hypertension, and hyperlipidemia—begin to appear long before the adult years in overweight children and adolescents. Children with one or more cardiovascular risk factors may begin to show atherosclerotic changes in their coronary arteries at a young age. Children and adolescents between 5 and 17 yr of age whose BMI exceeds the 95th percentile are two to three times more likely to have one or more cardiovascular risk factors than children whose BMI is below the 95th percentile *(47)*. The clustering of metabolic disorders, often referred to as syndrome X or metabolic syndrome, can be seen in childhood and adoles-

Table 1
Medical Conditions Resulting From or Associated With Obesity*

Insulin resistance*
Type 2 diabetes*
Hypertension*
Dyslipidemia*
Coronary artery disease
Gallbladder disease
Cancer
Arthritis
Stroke
Asthma*
Sleep apnea*
Breathing difficulties*
Menstrual and pregnancy difficulties*
Hirsutism*
Surgical complications
Psychological disorders

* Indicates conditions also seen with some regularity in pediatric obesity.

cence. Its primary components include dyslipidemia, hypertension, hyperinsulinemia, and obesity. An analysis of data from the third NHANES found evidence of metabolic syndrome in 28.7% of youth with BMI in excess of the 95th percentile *(48,49)*. Non-insulin-dependent diabetes, as well as hyperinsulinemia, is growing in prevalence, in association with child overweight *(50)*. In one recent study, 84% of overweight patients entering a behavioral weight management program were hyperinsulinemic *(51)*. There has been considerable interest in the use of metformin as an approach to reducing the risk of these hyperinsulinemic patients going on to develop diabetes *(52)*.

The evaluation of the overweight child should include assessment for these various cardiovascular comorbidities as well as for liver disease, obstructive sleep apnea, and orthopedic disorders. For example, nonalcoholic fatty liver disease (NAFLD, sometimes also referred to as nonalcoholic steatohepatitis [NASH]) has been reported in up to two-thirds of overweight youth *(53,54)*. Likewise, obstructive sleep apnea is now known to be more common among overweight than nonoverweight youth *(55)*. Polycystic ovary syndrome (PCOS) commonly occurs in overweight adolescent females, although it can also occur in normal-weight individuals. PCOS is characterized by irregular menses, infertility, and hyperandrogenism, with other commonly occurring findings, including hirsutism, acne, acanthosis nigricans, and clitoromegaly *(56)*.

Slipped capital femoral epiphyses (SCFE) and other orthopedic syndromes appear to occur with increased frequency among overweight adolescents *(57)*. In one series, two-thirds of patients with Blount's disease were overweight *(58)* and up to half of patients with SCFE were overweight *(59,60)*.

Pseudotumor cerebri is a potentially vision-threatening condition that has been associated with obesity and recent weight gain *(61)*.

The psychological morbidity of obesity is difficult to measure and often unrecognized *(62)*. Psychological comorbidities include depression, anxiety, and binge eating. The stigma of obesity is manifested at all ages *(63,64)*, with significant psychosocial consequences in the adolescent years, associated with social isolation *(65)* and victimization *(66)*. Educational attainment and social outcomes are affected by excessive weight *(67)*. The stigma of obesity is linked to lower self-esteem and body esteem *(64)*. This stigma may also explain higher rates of depression. It may lead to self-blame and further feeling of guilt. Parents also blame themselves and feel stigmatized as a result of their overweight children. Studies of stigma associated with childhood obesity were performed in 1961 and replicated 40 yr later in 2001 *(68)*, at both times showing that children react to children who appear overweight more unfavorably than to children who appear to have a variety of physical disabilities.

As excessive body weight is often accompanied by body image disparagement, poor self-esteem, depression and anxiety, it is imperative that overweight children be screened for psychological comorbidities and referred if necessary to appropriately trained clinical psychologists or psychiatrists *(69)*. Overweight children and adolescents are also at risk of disordered eating, most commonly overeating and binge eating disorder *(70,71)*. Adolescents who overeat are more likely to be overweight or obese, to have dieted in the past year, to be trying to lose weight currently, and to express unhappiness and dissatisfaction with themselves. Health-related quality of life has been shown to be diminished in overweight youth *(72,73)*, particularly those with obstructive sleep apnea *(72)*.

EVALUATION

The evaluation of the overweight child should include a complete assessment of the child's medical condition and associated comorbidities. In addition, this evaluation should include the psychosocial impact of the child's weight, the child's eating behavior, physical activity, and sedentary behavior, as well as the child's and family's readiness to make changes in the home food environment and activities. The diet assessment should include a global assessment of a typical day, including meals, snack food, frequency, and types of restaurant and take-out food, opportunities for eating without adult supervision, either after school or weekends, and the adolescent's interest and access in social activities outside the home. Physical activity assessment should include both organized as well as unstructured vigorous activity, normal activities of daily living, sedentary behavior, and deterrents to activity. Although they are extremely uncommon, the evaluation of the child should include the assessment of rare causes, such as underlying genetic disorders. The presence of developmental delay, hypotonia, poor early weight gain and growth, and dysmorphic features, and should suggest further evaluation for Prader-Willi syndrome (PWS) or other genetic disorders (*see* Table 2). PWS is the most commonly recognized of the clinical obesity syndromes and results from the absence of normally expressed paternally derived genes in the chromosome region 15q11–q13. About 70% of affected individuals have a paternally derived interstitial deletion and about 25% have maternal disomy of chromosome 15, with the remaining 5% having an imprinting defect, with severity of the disorder varying with the genetic etiology *(74)*.

A number of medications, particularly some used in the treatment of neurologic and psychiatric disorders, have been associated with excessive weight gain. These include depakote and tegretol, two anticonvulsants, as well as a number of mood stabilizers and antidepressants, including lithium, risperdol, paroxetine, neurontin, and others.

Table 2
Clinical Syndromes That Include Obesity

Bardet-Biedel: short stature, developmental delay, hypogonadism, polydactyly of feet or hands, retinitis pigmentos

Cohen Syndrome: microcephaly, developmental delay, distinctive facies, long slender toes and fingers, occasional syndactyly

Carpenter Syndrome: acrocephaly, profound retardation, brachyclinosyndactyly of the hands

Cohen Syndrome: microcephaly, developmental delay, distinctive facies, long slender toes and fingers, occasional syndactyly

Cushing: short stature, "buffalo hump"

Hypothyroidism: growth delay, developmental delay, obstipation

Prader-Willi Syndrome: short stature, developmental delay, early FTT and hypotonia, hypogonadism, polyphagia, problems with behavioral control

Pseudohypoparathyroidism: short stature, round face, brachydactyly, developmental delay, delayed dental eruption

---

Taking the History

The process of history taking can be used to develop a narrative of the child's weight history, eating habits, important influences on eating and physical activity, and the family's role in supporting the factors contributing to the child's overweight. This narrative can then be used in the treatment process as a context for discussion of the food environment at home and the impact of the child's weight on his or her own health as well as on the family. For example, discussion of the child's weight history encourages parents to recognize important factors that, over time, may have contributed to excessive weight gain. Asking whether the child resembles any particular family members not only establishes the familial nature of the weight problem, but also allows parents to recognize some of the long-term health consequences of obesity, such as the presence of type 2 diabetes mellitus. Obesity rarely occurs in isolation. There are commonly other family members who have struggled with weight and whose experience can be valuable in helping to develop a realistic set of goals for the child and family. Inquiring as to what exactly concerns the parent about the child's weight helps to establish the motivating factors in seeking medical evaluation and treatment.

A very powerful portion of the history has to do with understanding ways in which the child's weight influences him or her directly, as well as how the weight affects the family. For example, the child may experience difficulty keeping up with others in athletic activities, be excluded from group activities, or may experience uncomfortable situations when shopping for clothing. Likewise, the presence of an overweight child may lead to parental disagreements over meals, family activities, vacation planning, and even attendance at family events. Such disagreements may add further stress to the child and contribute to difficulty engaging in productive strategies to modify the family's lifestyle and food environment. Another useful line of questioning concerns the parent's expectations or fears if the child's weight problem becomes a long-term problem. This question encourages parents to express their fears about the impact of the child's obesity on his or her life and to discuss ways in which their own experiences with weight may have influenced their decision to seek help with this problem. Many parents seek to protect their children from the misery they themselves have experienced in relation to their weight.

A narrative approach can be very effective in learning about the child's eating habits and physical activity. Gathering information about daily routines, meal times, typical meals, and, similarly, habits of physical activity, provides the clinician with a thorough understanding of the child and his environment, which is critical in determining which elements of a structured treatment program might be most salient to the specific child. Of course, additional detailed nutrition and physical activity data can be collected using 3- to 5-d diaries (or longer) of food intake and activity, as well as using food and activity frequency methodologies.

Physical Examination

A careful general physical examination is useful in the evaluation of the obese child. Such an examination yields identification of physical findings that may suggest an underlying endocrine syndrome or genetic disorder. The physical examination should include an overall assessment of the child's body habitus and notation of the pattern of fat distribution. Careful measurement of the height and weight of the child is important to rule out underlying short stature, which may indicate an associated endocrine or genetic abnormality. The presence of a buffalo hump, moon facies, short stature, and hypertension may suggest Cushing's syndrome (although many normal obese children have extra fat deposition over the upper back). Hypogonadism is present in a number of syndromes (Prader-Willi, Bardet-Biedl, and others). Short stature, short metacarpals and metatarsals, subcutaneous calcifications, and mental retardation are present in pseudohypoparathyroidism. The presence of acanthosis nigricans should be noted, although in overweight children, acanthosis is not a reliable predictor of hyperinsulinemia, with a sensitivity of only about 0.65 *(75)*.

Laboratory and Diagnostic Studies

Laboratory and diagnostic studies should be conducted as part of the initial evaluation to assess the patient's risk or presence of comorbidities. Such laboratory studies should include a fasting lipid profile, fasting insulin and glucose, and liver function tests. Should the history and physical examination suggest the presence of pseudotumor, a head CT scan should be ordered and consultation with a pediatric ophthalmologist arranged. Orthopedic complaints should lead to the use of relevant X-ray studies such as hip films to assess for slipped capital femoral epiphyses, and knee films to assess for the presence of Blount's disease. A sleep study should be ordered for patients with a history of apnea or snoring. An echocardiogram is important in patients whose degree of obesity may be causing cor pulmonale. Pulmonary function testing is indicated particularly for patients who complain of respiratory symptoms or shortness of breath with exercise. Indirect calorimetry is helpful in establishing baseline caloric requirements and when, during the course of treatment, weight loss is not progressing as might be expected from the diet and exercise history.

The Expert Committee also considered the need for referral guidelines in the evaluation and care of overweight children. The committee concluded that conditions that indicate consultation with a pediatric obesity specialist include pseudotumor cerebri, obesity-related sleep disorders, orthopedic problems, massive obesity, and obesity in children younger than 2 yr of age *(11)*.

BEHAVIORAL TREATMENT

In 1998, Dietz and Barlow published a protocol for the evaluation and treatment of child overweight based on the findings of an expert committee. This protocol calls for the assessment of BMI and for the presence of comorbidities of obesity *(11)*. The committee recommended that children 7 yr of age and older, with a BMI greater than or equal to the 85th percentile with complications of obesity or with a BMI greater than or equal to the 95th percentile, with or without complications, undergo evaluation and possible treatment. The committee also recommended that children between 2 and 7 yr of age with BMI greater than or equal to the 95th percentile, with complications, also undergo evaluation and possible treatment, while for those above the 85th or 95th percentiles and no complications, the emphasis should be on maintenance and prevention of further excessive weight gain.

Health professionals are often discouraged by the prospect of weight management. A study published of health professionals *(76)* found that a perceived lack of patient motivation and parent involvement presented a significant barrier to effective treatment, with feelings of treatment futility and lack of time, reimbursement, and lack of adequate support services also being cited as barriers. A consistent finding in the literature, and one that exemplifies the difficulty encountered by the clinician caring for an overweight child, is that parents often do not perceive their overweight children as overweight *(77)*, nor do they worry about the child's weight unless the child is being teased or experiencing a limitation in activity due to weight *(78)*.

Obesity is a problem that develops over time and is not easily treated. Unless the patient is experiencing life-threatening complications from severe obesity, the problem should be approached in a nonemergent fashion. Intervention for child obesity begins during the evaluation process. Involving the family in the evaluation gives the message that they are part of the solution. In the course of evaluation, it is important to assess the family's readiness to make the changes necessary to support the child's behavioral treatment program. Obesity is not the child's problem alone. The child lives within the family environment, and the family must be drawn into the process of evaluation and change; if the family appears to be dysfunctional, it is appropriate to delay the implementation of behavioral strategies until the family has had more extensive evaluation and entered into family counseling. Referral to a family therapist, particularly one familiar with many of the issues associated with obesity, can be extremely helpful.

For families who are capable of supporting the child's efforts, the initial strategies are focused on gradual alterations of the child's eating and physical activity. There are a number of behavioral strategies that are useful in the office-based approach to child obesity (Table 3). Over the past 20 yr, a number of behavioral treatment programs have been the subject of reports in the medical literature, all of which provide evidence of limited efficacy and long-term benefit *(79–81)*. Recently Kaiser Permanente has launched a massive population-based weight-management program *(82)*.

Intervention does not require calorie counting or specific calorie intake. An alternative approach is to categorize foods as more or less desirable and to set goals for the

Table 3
Characteristics of Successful Behavioral Treatments

Parent and family participation
Longer duration of treatment
Greater frequency of sessions
Dietary guidelines that are simple and explicit
Physical activity
Self-Monitoring
Use of goal and rewards both proximal and distal
Parent skills
Individualized problem-solving

reduction of less desirable foods and encouragement of more desirable foods. One such system of categorization is described in *The Stoplight Diet for Children (81)*, which categorizes food as "red light," "yellow light," and "green light." By identifying foods in this way, parents can support the child's efforts to reduce intake of "red light" foods and increase intake of foods from the other categories. Gradual reduction in intake of "red light" foods can be rewarded and sustained in association with goals of weight loss or maintenance.

Medical and behavioral therapies are the cornerstone of weight management in childhood and adolescence. Successful models of behavioral treatment have been shown to produce modest weight reduction with somewhat limited long-term efficacy. Treatment is known to be more effective in groups than when provided to individuals or family units alone. One group should consist of children or adolescents within a narrow age range (e.g., 8 to 12 yr) and a separate group should be conducted simultaneously, with at least one parent from each family. These groups should meet independently on a weekly basis, with some mixing of the two groups occurring from time to time to facilitate further communication within the family.

Perhaps the best follow-up data from group behavioral treatment can be found in the follow-up studies using the Stoplight Diet. Four follow-up studies targeted children between the ages of 6 and 12 yr, who participated in the group behavioral program along with at least one parent *(83)*. Ten-year follow-up of children participating in these four different family-based group behavior change studies that used the Stoplight Diet showed a significantly larger decrease in the percentage of overweight patients if their parents had also been targeted, as compared to controls whose parents were not also targeting weight loss. Another important finding was that a larger decrease was seen in children of nonobese parents than in patients whose parents were obese. At the 10-yr follow up assessments, 30% of patients no longer met the study's definition of obesity (now more comparable to the BMI-based categorization as overweight). Further analyses within these groups showed that parental weight change was a significant predictor of the child's weight change *(84)*.

Physical Activity

Just as behavioral approaches can be applied to support dietary change, so too can they be applied to encourage and reinforce changes in physical activity, be they lifestyle changes or organized physical activity. Most weight-loss experts advocate a combination of aerobic and strength exercises, combined with behavioral modifications and calorie reduction, for optimal results in weight reduction. A focus on screen time—such as television viewing, video game playing, and computer use—among children and adolescents is also helpful in encouraging increasing physical activity in the adolescent population *(85)*. In a school-based study involving a 6-mo classroom curriculum to reduce television viewing by third- and fourth-graders, a statistically significant decrease was found over the course of the study in change in BMI, triceps skin fold thickness, waist circumference, and waist-to-hip ratio in the intervention group as compared with controls. These studies highlight the importance of reducing sedentary behaviors to achieve effective weight control in the pediatric population *(43)*.

Reduced-Fat/Calorie-Deficit Diets

Although there have been fewer carefully controlled studies of dietary manipulation in the pediatric age group, a number of points can be made in regard to the application of reduced calorie diets for children and adolescents. These diets usually suggest that approx 20 to 30% of the daily caloric intake should come from dietary fats and that saturated fats be minimized. A good source of protein, such as meat, poultry, or fish, should be included in the daily diet. Soft drinks and juices should be avoided where possible. Carbohydrates should be selected from among whole-grain products rather than highly refined products.

Low Carbohydrate and Low Glycemic Index

There has been a dramatic increase in interest in use of diets low in carbohydrate content or having a low glycemic index (GI) to promote weight loss. (*See* Chapters 14 and 15 for discussion of these diets.) One 12-wk study in overweight adolescents showed significantly greater weight loss with a low-carbohydrate diet compared with a low-fat diet, with no adverse effects on lipid profiles in either group *(86)*. In a small study of 14 adolescents, those on a low- to moderate-GI diet lost significantly more weight and showed less of an increase in insulin resistance over a 12-mo period than did the adolescents assigned to a low-fat diet (25–30% of energy from fat) *(87)*. A low-GI diet may offer a more easily taught approach to dietary modification in the primary care setting than more traditional low-calorie/low-fat diets *(88)*.

Protein-Sparing Modified Fast

Sometimes referred to as very-low-calorie diets (VLCD) or "liquid diets," the protein-sparing modified fast (PSMF) is used on an inpatient or outpatient basis only for adolescents and adults suffering from very severe obesity. Studies published in the 1980s suggested that inpatient modified fasting could be used safely in treating severely obese patients *(89)* as long as careful monitoring of electrolytes and cardiac status was included in the treatment protocol. Little has appeared in the pediatric literature on the outpatient use of a VLCD, but at least one center has published one year follow-up results after a VLCD, followed by a program using a balanced hypocaloric diet and moderate-intensity exercise regimen *(90)*. These diets are known to carry a number of medical risks, including cholelithiasis, hyperuricemia, orthostatic hypotension, halitosis, and diarrhea. The diet typically allows for only 600 to 900 calories daily, with 1.5 to 2.5 g of protein per kilogram per day, with intakes of carbohydrate (20–40 g/d) and fat very restricted. If used on an outpatient basis, the PSMF requires very close medical monitoring, daily supplements, adequate water intake, and the frequent measurement of electrolyte levels in order to be safe.

PHARMACOLOGICAL TREATMENT

A limited number of medications are currently available in the pediatric age group for use as adjuncts to behavioral management. Sibutramine (Meridia) is currently available for the treatment of adolescents 16 yr of age or older. Sibutramine is a norepinephrine and serotonin reuptake inhibiter and has side effects that include hypertension, tachycardia, dry mouth, headache, constipation, and insomnia. When used in conjunction with a group-based behavioral therapy, sibutramine plus behavioral therapy led to a more rapid decline in BMI than behavioral therapy alone *(91)*. Sibutramine should not be administered in conjunction with monoamine oxidase inhibitors or other serotonin reuptake inhibitors. Another pharmaceutical alternative is orlistat (Xenical). Orlistat binds gut lipase and prevents hydrolysis of dietary fats into free fatty acids and monoacylglycerols. Its side effects, which often lead to discontinuation of the medication, include flatulence, diarrhea, steatorrrhea, and leakage of stool and a risk of fat-soluble vitamin deficiency *(92)*. A number of other drugs are used off-label, including metformin (Glucophage), bupropion (Wellbutrin), and topiramate (Topamax). Metformin is currently approved for use in the treatment of type 2 diabetes mellitus. It inhibits hepatic glucose production and increases insulin sensitivity. Its effectiveness as an adjunct to behavioral weight-loss therapy for adolescents is currently under investigation. Bupropion is a weak norepinephrine and serotonin and dopamine reuptake inhibitor and is more widely used as an antidepressant and adjunct to smoking cessation treatment. Topiramate is an anticonvulsant with a side-effect profile of weight loss in some patients. Somatostatin (Octreotide) is a suppressor of pancreatic insulin secretion and has been used in the management of intractable weight gain caused by hypothalamic obesity, as occurs following intracranial radiation or surgical therapy *(93)*.

SURGICAL TREATMENT

Surgical approaches to the management of obesity have been used in the adult population for many years. Progressive improvement in surgical technique and refinement in selection criteria have led to improvements in outcome with reductions in morbidity and mortality. Nevertheless, these operations all carry with them considerable risks, and outcome is dependent on the availability of excellent ongoing postoperative medical and surgical care. In general these procedures are irreversible, with the exception of the laparoscopic band. At this time, the laparoscopic band is not currently available for licensed use in the pediatric or adolescent age group. Early studies of gastric banding in the adolescent age group appear promising *(94)*.

Surgical procedures largely fall into two categories, malabsorptive or restrictive. A combination of these approaches, the Roux-en-Y, provides a combination of reduction in the volume of the stomach as well as a small intestinal bypass. Several authors have published their experience with the use of gastric bypass in the adolescent age group and have demonstrated the benefit of bypass in terms of both weight loss and resolution of presurgical comorbid conditions. These previous reports have been reviewed recently *(95,96)*, with the authors calling for additional follow-up studies to determine the efficacy and safety of bariatric surgery in the adolescent population and to guide selection of the optimal procedure for each patient. Complications are known to occur in the adolescent age group as in the adult age group, with both the Roux-en-Y and gastric band, with a need to monitor postoperative nutritional status for an extended period of time *(97)*. The use of restrictive and malabsorptive procedures for the management of adolescent obesity was reviewed by the American Pediatric Surgical Association and recommendations were subsequently published in *Pediatrics*, the official publication of the American Academy of Pediatrics *(98)*. The APSA recommended that gastric bypass procedures in the adolescent age group be performed only in an appropriate setting with a focus on children, such as a children's hospital, and with the informed assent of the teenager. The recommended criteria for performance of a Roux-en-Y gastric bypass include the presence of a BMI of 50 or greater, if no significant comorbidities are present, or with a BMI of at least 40 in the presence of at least one major comorbidity (as defined by the APSA), such as type 2 diabetes, sleep apnea, or pseudotumor cerebri. Additional requirements include evidence of skeletal maturation, generally seen in girls 13 yr of age or greater or boys 15 yr of age or greater, and the assessment of the patient by a qualified child psychiatrist or psychologist. This assessment should include an assessment of the patient's readiness to engage in this significant procedure and to commit to lifelong postoperative changes in dietary intake. It is also recommended that potential candidates participate in at least 6 mo of organized weight management before embarking on a surgical solution and that a comprehensive follow-up program must be available with a coordinated team approach to support the patient's ongoing behavioral and lifestyle changes postoperatively.

PREVENTION

No discussion of childhood obesity would be complete without attention to prevention. As there are no treatment approaches that have been shown to provide long-term remission from overweight and its consequences (surgery seems most promising despite its being most invasive), the obesity epidemic in the United States is not likely to abate until significant changes are made in the food environment and loss of activity in daily life so common in the United States and other developed countries. School-based prevention approaches offer the greatest demonstrated benefit, yet are costly and complex to implement *(43,99,100)*. The American Academy of Pediatrics has called for intensive research into a variety of behavioral and environmental initiatives and to the use of policy and regulation, where necessary, to affect eating behavior and physical activity, including changes in the built environment *(101)*. Robinson and Sirard have called for a paradigm shift in obesity-prevention research *(102)*, focusing on testing factors believed to be modifiable and, thus, subject to widespread implementation as part of any prevention efforts.

CONCLUSION

The prevalence of child obesity has increased dramatically over the past 40 yr. With increasing severity of overweight, rates of comorbidities, particularly type 2 diabetes mellitus, have also increased. The tendency for obesity in childhood and adolescence to persist into adult life ties it further to the metabolic syndrome and other risk factors for cardiovascular disease. The ultimate social and economic impact of this obesity epidemic is difficult to predict; however, there is an increasing demand for both early intervention and widespread efforts toward prevention. The evaluation of the overweight child requires a thorough examination of the family environment and the child's eating behavior and physical activity. Although group treatment appears to be most effective, most patients are managed individually within the context of the family. Relatively few clinical trials using obesity medications have been conducted in the pediatric age group and none have yielded dramatic results. Although limited in application to only the most severely affected adolescents, bariatric surgery is now being offered in a number of centers around the country; however, the long-term outcomes of bariatric surgery in this patient population have yet to be measured.

REFERENCES

1. Hedley AA, Ogden CL, Johnson CL, et al. Prevalence of overweight and obesity among US children, adolescents, and adults, 1999–2002. JAMA 2004;291:2847–2850.
2. Troiano RP, Flegal KM, Kuczmarski RJ, et al. Overweight prevalence and trends for children and adolescents. Arch Pediatr Adolesc Med 1995;149:1085–1091.
3. Thompson OM, Ballew C, Resnicow K, et al.Food purchased away from home as a predictor of change in BMI z-score among girls. Int J Obes 2004;28:282–289.
4. Taveras EM, Berkey CS, Rifas-Shiman SL, et al. Association of consumption of fried food away from home with body mass index and diet quality in older children and adolescents. Pediatrics 2005;116:518–524.
5. Bowman SA, Gortmaker SL, Ebbeling CB, et al. Effects of fast-food consumptionm on energy intake and diet quality among children in a national household survey. Pediatrics 2003;113:112–118.
6. Neilson SJ, Popkin BM. Patterns and trends in food portion sizes, 1977–1998. JAMA 2003;289:450–453.
7. Ludwig DS, Peterson KE, Gortmaker SL. Relation between consumption of sugar-sweetened drinks and childhood obesity: a prospective observational analysis. Lancet 2001;357:505–508.
8. Andersen RE, Crespo CJ, Bartlett SJ, et al. Relationship of physical activity and television watching with body weight and level of fatness among children. Results from the third National Health and Nutrition Examination Survey. JAMA 1998;279:938–942.
9. Matheson DM, Killen JD, Wang Y, et al. Children's food consumption during television viewing. Am J Clin Nutr 2004;79:1088–1094.
10. Dennison BA, Erb TA, Jenkins PL. Television viewing and television in bedroom associated with overweight risk among low-income preschool children. Pediatrics 2002;109:1028–1035.
11. Dietz WH, Barlow SE. Obesity evaluation and treatment: Expert committee recommendations. Pediatrics 1998;102(3):e29.
12. Dietz WH and Robinson TN. Use of the body mass index as a measure of overweight in children and adolescents. J Pediatr 1998;132:191–193.
13. Sopher AB, Thornton JC, Wang J, et al. Measurement of percentage of body fat in 411 children and adolescents: a comparison of dual-energy X-ray absorptiometry with a four-compartment model. Pediatrics 2004;113:1285–1290.

14. Goran MI. Measurement issues related to studies of childhood obesity: assessment of body composition, body fat distribution, physical activity, and food intake. Pediatrics 1998;101:505–518.

15. Elberg J, McDuffie JR, Sebring NG, et al. Comparison of methods to assess change in children's body composition. Am J Clin Nutr 2004;80:64–69.

16. Whitaker, R, Wright JA, Pepe MS, et al Predicting obesity in young adulthood from childhood and parental obesity. N Engl J Med 1997;337:869–873.

17. Olshansky SJ, Passaro DJ, Hershow RC, et al. A potential decline in life expectancy in the United States in the 21st century. N Engl J Med 2005;352:1138–1145.

18. Wolf AM, Colditz GA. Current estimates of the economic cost of obesity in the United States. Obes Res 1998;6:97–106.

19. Finkelstein EA, Fiebelkorn IC, Wang G. National medical spending attributable to overweight and obesity: how much, and who's paying. Health Aff (Millwood) 2003;[suppl W3]:219–226.

20. Levy E, Levy P, Le Pen C, et al. The economic cost of obesity: the French situation. Int J Obes Relat Metab Disord 1995;19(11):788–792.

21. Dietz WH. Critical periods in childhood for the development of obesity. Am J Clin Nutr 1994;59:955–959.

22. Oken E, Gillman MW. Fetal origins of obesity. Obes Res 2003;11:496–506.

23. Whitaker RC, Pepe MS, Wright JA, et al. Early adiposity rebound and the risk of adult obesity. Pediatrics 1998;101(3):E5.

24. Dietz WH. Overweight in childhood and adolescence. N Engl J Med 2004;350:855–857.

25. Frontini M, Srinivasan SR, Berenson GS. Longitudinal changes in risk variables underlying metabolic syndrome X from childhood to young adulthood in female subjects with a history of early menarche: the Bogalusa Heart Study. Int J Obes 2003;27:1398–1404.

26. Dorosty AR, Emmett PM, Cowin IS, et al, and the ALSPAC Study Team. Factors associated with early adiposity rebound. Pediatrics 2000;105:1115–1118.

27. Guo SS, Chumlea WC, Roche AF. Predicting overweight and obesity in adulthood from body mass index values in childhood and adolescence. Am J Clin Nutr 2002;76:653–658.

28. Campbell PT, Katzmarzyk PT, Malina RM, et al. Stability of adiposity phenotypes from childhood and adolescence into young adulthood with contribution of parental measures. Obes Res 2001;9:394–400.

29. Guo SS, Chumlea WC. Tracking of body mass index in children in relation to overweight in adulthood. Am J Nutr 1999;70(supp):145s–148s.

30. Stunkard AJ, Messick S. The three-factor eating questionnaire to measure dietary restraint, disinhibition and hunger. J Psychosom Res 1985;29:71–83.

31. Hood MY, Moore LL, Sundarajan-Ramamurti A, et al. Parental eating attitudes and the development of obesity in children. The Framingham Children's Study. Int J Obes 2000;24:1319–1325.

32. Francis LA, Birch LL. Maternal weight status modulates the effects of restriction on daughters' eating and weight. Int J Obes 2005;29:942–949.

33. Wiehe S. Sugar high. Arch Pediatr Adolesc Med 2004;158:209–211.

34. Bes-Rastrollo M, Sanchez-Villegas A, Gomez-Gracia E, et al. Predictors of weight gain in a Mediterranean cohort: the Seguimiento Universidad de Navarra Study. Am J Clin Nutr 2006;83:362–370.

35. Rolland-Cachera MF, Deheeger M, Akrout M, et al. Influence of macronutrients on adiposity development: a follow up study of nutrition and growth from 10 months to 8 years of age. Int J Obes 1995;19:573–578.

36. Jago R, Baranowski T, Baranowski JC, et al. BMI from 3–6 y of age is predicted by TV viewing and physical activity, not diet. Int J Obes 2005;29:557–564.

37. Faith MS, Scanlon KS, Birch LL, et al. Parent-child feeding strategies and their relationships to child eating and weight status. Obes Res 2004;12:1711–1722.

38. Faith MS, Berkowitz RI, Stallings VA, et al. Parental feeding attitudes and styles and child body mass index: prospective analysis of a gene-environment interaction. Pediatrics 2004;114:e429–e436. URL: www.pediatrics.org/cgi/doi/10.1542/peds.2003-1075-L.

39. Robinson TN, Kiernan M, Matheson DM, et al. Is parental control over children's eating associated with childhood obesity? Results from a population-based sample of third graders. Obes Res 2001;9:306–312.

40. Klesges RC, Malott JM, Bosche PF, et al. The effects of parental influences on children's food intake, physical activity, and relative weight. Int J Eating Dis 1986;5:335–346.

41. Drucker RR, Hammer LD, Agras WS, et al. Can mothers influence their child's eating behavior? J Dev Behav Pediatr 1999;20:88–92.

42. Robinson TN, Hammer LD, Killen JD, et al. Does television viewing increase obesity and reduce physical activity? Cross-sectional and longitudinal analyses among adolescent girls. Pediatrics 1993;91:273–280.
43. Robinson TN. Reducing children's television viewing to prevent obesity: a randomized controlled trial. JAMA 1999;282:1561–1567.
44. Agras WS, Hammer LD, McNicholas F, et al. Risk factors for childhood overweight: a prospective study from birth to 9.5 years. J Pediatr 2004;145:20–25.
45. Matheson DM, Varady J, Varady A, et al. Household food security and nutritional status of Hispanic children in the fifth grade. Am J Clin Nutr 2002;76:210–217.
46. Olson C. Nutrition and health outcomes associated with food insecurity and hunger. J Nutr 1999;129(supp):521s–524s.
47. Freedman DS, Dietz WH, Srinivasan SR, et al. The relation of overweight to cardiovascular risk factors among children and adolescents: the Bogalusa Heart Study. Pediatrics 1999;103:1175–1182.
48. Cook S, Weitzman M, Auinger P, et al. Prevalence of a metabolic syndrome phenotype in adolescents: findings from the third National Health and Nutrition Examination Survey, 1988–1994. Arch Pediatr Adolesc Med 2003;157:821–827.
49. Weiss R, Dziura J, Burgert TS, et al. Obesity and the metabolic syndrome in children and adolescents. N Engl J Med 2004;350:2362–2374.
50. Pinhas-Hamiel O, Dolan LM, Daniels SR, et al. Increased incidence of non-insulin-dependent diabetes mellitus among adolescents. J Pediatr 1996;128:608–615.
51. Kirk S, Zeller M, Claytor R, et al. The relationship of health outcomes to improvement in BMI in children and adolescents. Obes Res 2005;13:876–882.
52. Freemark M, Bursey D. The effects of metformin on body mass index and glucose tolerance in obese adolescents with fasting hyperinsulinemia and a family history of type 2 diabetes. Pediatrics 2001;107(4):e55. URL: http://www.pediatrics.org/cgi/content/full/107/4/e55.
53. Fishbein H, Miner DM, Mogren DC, et al. The spectrum of fatty liver in obese children and the relationship of serum aminotransferases to severity of steatosis. J Pediatr Gastroenterol Nutr 2003;36:54–61.
54. Xanthakos SM, Miles L, Bucuvalas J, et al. Histologic spectrum of NASH in morbidly obese adolescents differs from adults. Obes Res 2004;12:A211.
55. Chay OM, Goh A, Abisheganaden J, et al. Obstructive sleep apnea syndrome in obese Singapore children. Pediatr Pulmonol 2000;29:284–290.
56. Hillard PJA, Deitch H. Menstrual disorders in a college age female. Pediatr Clin N Am 2005;52:179–197.
57. Wilcox PG, Weiner DS, Leighley B. Maturation factors in slipped capital femoral epiphysis. J Pediatr Orthoped 1988;2:196–200.
58. Dietz WH, Gross WL, Kirkpatrick JA. Blount disease (tibia vara): another skeletal disorder associated with childhood obesity. J Pediatr 1982;101:735–737.
59. Kelsey JL, Acheson RM, Keggi KJ. The body build of patients with slipped femoral capital epiphysis. Am J Dis Child 1972;124:276–281.
60. Sorenson KH. Slipped upper femoral epiphysis. Acta Orthop Scand 1968;39:499–517.
61. Giuseffi V, Wall M, Siegel PZ, Rojas PB. Symptoms and disease associations in idiopathic intracranial hypertension (pseudotumor cerebri): a case-control study. Neurology 1991;41:239–244.
62. Britz B, Seigfried W, Ziegler A, et al. Rates of psychiatric disorders in a clinical study group of adolescents with extreme obesity and in obese adolescents ascertained via a population based study. Int J Obes Relat Metab Disord 2000;12:1707–1714.
63. Neumark-Sztainer D, Story M, Faibisch L. Perceived stigmatization among overweight African-American and Caucasian adolescent girls. J Adolesc Health 1998;23:264–270.
64. Pierce JW, Wardle J. Cause and effect beliefs and self esteem of overweight children. J Child Psychol Psychiatr 1997;38:645–650.
65. Strauss RS, Pollack HA. Social marginalization of overweight children. Arch Pediatr Adolesc Med 2003;157:746–752.
66. Pearce MJ, Boergers J, Prinstein MJ. Adolescent obesity, overt and relational peer victimization, and romantic relationships. Obes Res 2002;10:386–393.
67. Falkner NH, Neumark-Sztainer D, Story M, et al. Social, educational, and psychological correlates of weight status in adolescents. Obes Res 2001;9:32–42.
68. Latner JD, Stunkard AJ. Getting worse: the stigmatization of obese children. Obes Res 2003;11:452–456.

69. Zeller MH, Saelens BE, Roehrig H, et al. Psychological adjustment of obese youth presenting for weight management treatment. Obes Res 2004;12:1576–1586.
70. Isnard P, Michel G, Frelut ML, et al. Binge eating and psychopathology in severely obese adolescents. Int J Eat Disord 2003;34:235–243.
71. Stice E. Risk and maintenance factors for eating pathology: a meta-analytic review. Psychol Bull 2002;128:825–848.
72. Schwimmer JB, Burwinkle TM, Varni JW. Health-related quality of life of severely obese children and adolescents. JAMA 2003;289:1813–1819.
73. Swallen KC, Reither EN, Haas SA, et al. Overweight, obesity, and health-related quality of life among adolescents: the National Longitudinal Study of Adolescent Health. Pediatrics 2005;115:340–347.
74. Butler MG, Bittel DC, Kibiryeva N, et al. Behavioral differences among subjects with Prader-Willi syndrome and type I or type II deletion and maternal disomy. Pediatrics 2004;113:565–573.
75. Nguyen TT, Keil MF, Russell DL, et al. Relation of acanthosis nigricans to hyperinsulinemia and insulin sensitivity in overweight African American and white children J Pediatr 2001;138:474–480.
76. Story MT, Neumark-Stzainer DR, Sherwood NE, et al. Management of child and adolescent obesity: attitudes, barriers, skills, and training needs among health care professionals. Pediatrics 2002;110:210–214.
77. Jain A, Sherman SN, Chamberlain LA, et al. Why don't low income mothers worry about their preschoolers being overweight. Pediatrics 2001;107:1138–1146.
78. Baughcum AE, Chamberlin LA, Deeks CM, et al. Maternal perceptions of overweight preschool children. Pediatrics 2000;106:1380–1386.
79. Glenny A-M, O'Meara S, Melville A, et al. The treatment and prevention of obesity: a systematic review of the literature. Int J Obes Relat Metab Disord 1997;21:715–737.
80. Nemet D, Barkan S, Epstein Y, et al. Short- and long-term beneficial effects of a combined dietary-behavioral-physical activity intervention for the treatment of childhood obesity. Pediatrics 2005;115:e443–e449.
81. Epstein LH, Squires S. The Stoplight Diet for Children: An Eight-Week Program for Parents and Children. Little, Brown, Boston: 1988.
82. Histon TM, Goeldner JL, Bachman KH, et al. Kaiser Permanente's disease management approach to addressing the obesity epidemic. JCOM 2005;12:464–469.
83. Epstein L, Valoski A, Wing RR, et al. Ten-year outcomes of behavioral family based treatment for childhood obesity. Health Psychol 1994;13:373–383.
84. Wrotniak BH, Epstein LH, Paluch RA, et al. Parent weight change as a predictor of child weight change in family-based behavioral obesity treatment. Arch Pediatr Adolesc Med 2004;158:342–347.
85. Epstein LH, Paluch RA, Gordy CC, et al. Decreasing sedentary behaviors in treating pediatric obesity. Arch Pediatr Adolesc Med 2000;154:220–226.
86. Sondike S, Copperman N, Jacobson MS. Effects of a low-carbohydrate diet on weight loss and cardiovascular risk factors in overweight adolescents. J Pediatr 2003;142:253–258.
87. Ebbeling CB, Leidig MM, Sinclair KB, et al. A reduced-glycemic load diet in the treatment of adolescent obesity. Arch Pediatr Adolesc Med 2003;157:773–779.
88. Young PC, West SA, Ortiz K, et al. A pilot study to determine the feasibility of the low glycemic index diet as a treatment for overweight children in primary care practice. Ambulatory Pediatrics 2004;4:28–33.
89. Stallings VA, Archibald EH, Pencharz PB, et al. One year follow-up of weight, total body potassium, and total body nitrogen in obese adolescents treated with the protein sparing modified fast. Am J Clin Nutr 1988;48:91–94.
90. Sothern MS, Udall JN, Suskind RM, et al. Weight loss and growth velocity in obese children after very low calorie diet, exercise, and behavior modification. Acta Paediatr 2000;89:1036–1043.
91. Berkowitz R, Wadden TA, Tershakovec AM, et al. Behavior therapy and sibutramine for the treatment of adolescent obesity: a randomized controlled trial. JAMA 2003;289:1805–1812.
92. Chanoine JP, Hampl S, Jensen C, et al. Effect of orlistat on weight and body composition in obese adolescents. JAMA 2005;293:2873–2883.
93. Lustig RH, Hinds PS, Ringwald-Smith K, et al. Octreatide therapy of pediatric hypothalamic obesity: a double blind, placebo-controlled trial. J Clin Endocrinol Metab 2003;88:2586–2592.
94. Widhalm K, Diedtrich S, Prager G. Adjustable gastric banding surgery in morbidly obese adolescents: experiences with eight patients. Int J Obes 2004;28:s42–s45.
95. Inge TH, Zeller M, Lawson ML, et al. A critical appraisal of evidence supporting a bariatric surgical approach to weight management for adolescents. J Pediatr 2005;147:10–19.

96. Apovian CM, Baker C, Ludwig DS, et al. Best practice guidelines in pediatric/adolescent weight loss surgery. Obes Res 2005;13:274–282.

97. Shuster MH, Vazquez JA. Nutritional concerns related to Roux-en-Y gastric bypass. Crit Care Nurs Q 2005;28:227–260.

98. Inge TH, Krebs NF, Garcia VF, et al. Bariatric surgery for severely overweight adolescents: concerns and recommendations. Pediatrics 2004;114:217–223.

99. Luepker RV, Perry CL, McKinlay SM, et al. Outcomes of a field trial to improve children's dietary patterns and physical activity. JAMA 1996;275:768–776.

100. Yin Z, Gutin B, Johnson MH, et al. An environmental approach to obesity prevention in children: Medical College of Georgia Fit Kid Project year 1 results. Obes Res 2005;13:2153–2163.

101. American Academy of Pediatrics, Committee on Nutrition. Prevention of pediatric overweight and obesity. Pediatrics 2003;112:424–430.

102. Robinson TN, Sirard JR. Preventing childhood obesity: a solution-oriented research paradigm. Am J Prev Med 2005;28(Supp 2):194–201.

103. Pérusse L, Rankinen T, Zuberi A, et al. The human obesity gene map: the 2004 update. Obes Res 2005;13:381–490.

104. Barsh GS, Farooqi IS, O'Rahilly S. Genetics of body-weight regulation. Nature 2000;404:644–651.

105. Lustig RH. Pediatric endocrine disorders of energy balance. Rev Endocr Metab Disord 2005;6:245–260.

Index

A

Abdominal muscle
  premenopausal women, 136f
Abdominal subcutaneous fat
  measurement, 137f, 138
  waist circumference, 126f
Acanthosis nigricans, 205
Accelerometers, 155
Acetyl CoA carboxylase 2
  energy expenditure, 164–165
Acne
  eflornithine, 233
  flutamide, 233
  OCP, 233
  ornithine decarboxylase inhibitor, 233
ACRP. See Adipocyte complement-related protein (ACRP)
Activity. See Physical activity
Activity energy expenditure (AEE)
  children, 161–162
Activity thermogenesis, 156–157
Adenosine monophosphate activated
  kinase (AMPK), 71, 73
Adipocyte complement-related protein
  (ACRP), 363
Adiponectin, 59, 72–74, 363
  sensitivity index, 74
Adipose tissue
  endocannabinoids, 59
  as endocrine organ, 61f
  IL-6, 77–78
  inflammatory alterations
    obesity, 74–75
  metabolism, 75–76
  monocyte chemoattractant protein-1, 78
  pathology-associated changes, 76–77
Adiposity
  regional patterns
    IR, 90–91
  visceral, 91
    measurement, 137, 137f
    waist circumference, 126f
Adiposity signal integration
  appetite neuroregulation, 9–10
Adjustable gastric banding, 372f
AEE. See Activity energy expenditure (AEE)

Age
  BMI, 124
  waist circumference, 126
Agouti-related peptide (AgRP), 11t, 28,
  56, 362
Air-displacement plethysmography, 407
Amenorrhea
  PCOS, 222–223
Amitriptyline, 204
AMPK. See Adenosine monophosphate
  activated kinase (AMPK)
Amylin
  satiety, 8
Anabolic effector systems
  appetite neuroregulation, 10–11
Anemia
  iron-deficiency, 382–383
Anovulation
  treatment, 229t
Anthropometry, 122–124
Antidepressant drugs, 204
Antidiabetic drugs, 204
Antiepileptic drugs, 204
Anti-obesity drugs
  PCOS, 231–232
Antipsychotic drugs, 204
Anxiety, 213
  pediatric obesity, 411
AOD9604, 358
Appetite neuroregulation, 3–18
  adiposity signal integration, 9–10
  anabolic effector systems, 10–11
  catabolic effector systems, 14–18
  CNS regulation by adiposity signals
    and effector pathways, 6–7
  CNS regulation of food intake, 4–5
  dual-centers hypothesis, 4–5
  energy homeostasis central signals,
    10–14
  energy intake control, 7–8
  satiety, 7–8
Arcuate nucleus (ARC), 28, 107
  endocannabinoids, 55–56
ATL-962, 360
Axokine, 357
  appetite neuroregulation, 16

B

Balloon
    intragastric, 372
Bardet-Biedl syndrome
    pediatric obesity, 413t, 414
Bariatric surgery, 214, 369–375
    calcium deficiency, 385–386
    currently performed, 371–374
    iron deficiency, 382–384
    malabsorptive, 373f
    mechanisms of action, 370–371
    micronutrient deficiencies, 379–390, 380t
        assessment and treatment, 390t
        prophylactic management and
            monitoring, 388–389, 389t
    neuroendocrine changes, 370–371
    obesity comorbidities, 370
    outcomes, 374
    physiological changes, 370
    procedures, 381–382
    safety, 374–375
Behavioral risk factors
    pediatric obesity, 410
Behavioral therapy
    DPP, 250–251
β-Adrenergic agonists, 360–361
β3-Adrenergic receptors
    energy expenditure, 163
11-β-hydroxysteroid dehydrogenase type
    1 inhibitor, 79–80, 363
BIA. *See* Bioelectric impedance analysis (BIA)
Biking, 187
Biliopancreatic diversion, 373–374, 373f, 380
Binge eating
    pediatric obesity, 411–412
Bioelectric impedance analysis (BIA), 132
Biomarkers
    inflammatory
        low-carbohydrate diets, 303–304
Blood pressure
    low-carbohydrate diets, 306
Blood tests
    PCOS, 222t
Blount's disease
    pediatric obesity, 411
BMC. *See* Bone mineral content (BMC)
BMD. *See* Bone mineral density (BMD)
BMI. *See* Body mass index (BMI)

Body composition
    BMI, 129
    measurement, 202
Body diameters, 130
Body image disparagement
    pediatric obesity, 412
Body mass index (BMI), 122–123, 123f,
        175, 200t, 201t
    age, 124
    body composition change, 129
    defined, 198–199
    diabetes, 177–178
    employment, 181t
    pediatric, 407–408
    pediatric obesity, 407, 410
    shifting, 176
    weight-loss drugs, 342
Body & Soul project, 332
Body weight
    DPP, 246f
    orlistat, 349f
Bone mineral content (BMC), 387
Bone mineral density (BMD), 387
Brain
    coronal section, 5f
    endocannabinoids, 57–58
    energy sensing modules, 362–363
Breakfast
    NWCR, 397, 399
Bromocriptine, 361
Buffalo hump
    pediatric obesity, 413t
Bupropion, 205, 351–352
    pediatric obesity, 418

C

Cafeteria diets
    lactation, 104
Calcium
    deficiency
        bariatric surgery, 385–386
        treatment, 390t
    supplementation, 388t
Caloric sweeteners, 189f
Calories
    vs carbohydrates
        low-carbohydrate diets, 301–303
    reduced-fat/calorie-deficit diets
        pediatric obesity, 417

Calorimetry
  direct, 152
  indirect, 152–153
CAM. *See* Cell-adhesion molecule (CAM)
Cancer, 205
Cannabinoid
  intrahypothalamic, food intake, 56
  ligands, endogenous, 52
  receptors, 49, 50–51
    distribution, 52
Carbamazepine, 204
Carbohydrate. *See also* Low-carbohydrate
    diets
  vs calories
    low-carbohydrate diets, 301–303
  containing foods
    chemical structure vs glycemic
        index, 282–283
    classification, 282–285
    debate, 285
    glycemic load vs glycemic index,
        283–285, 284t
  low
    pediatric obesity, 417
Carpenter syndrome
  pediatric obesity, 413t
CART. *See* Cocaine-amphetamine-related
    transcript (CART)
Catabolic effector systems
  appetite neuroregulation, 14–18
CB1, 49–52
CB2, 49–52
CB1 antagonists
  clinical use, 61–62
CC. *See* Clomiphene citrate (CC)
CCK. *See* Cholecystokinin (CCK)
Cell-adhesion molecule (CAM)
  intracellular, low-carbohydrate diets, 304
Central nervous system (CNS)
  adiposity signals and effector path-
      ways, 6–7
  food intake regulation, 4–5
Children. *See* Pediatric obesity
Cholecystokinin (CCK), 28, 29t, 358
  energy homeostasis, 10
  mechanism of action, 36–37
  satiety, 8
Cholesterol
  PCOS, 222t

Ciliary neurotrophic factor (CNTF), 11t
  appetite neuroregulation, 16
Clomiphene citrate (CC)
  infertility, 232
Clozapine, 204
CNS. *See* Central nervous system (CNS)
CNTF. *See* Ciliary neurotrophic factor
    (CNTF)
Cobalamin
  deficiency
    bariatric surgery, 384–385
    treatment, 390t
  supplementation, 388t
Cocaine-amphetamine-related transcript
    (CART), 11t, 28, 56
  appetite neuroregulation, 14
Cohen syndrome
  pediatric obesity, 413t
Communication styles
  motivational interviewing, 324–325
Comorbidities
  bariatric surgery, 370
Computed tomography (CT)
  tissue size quantification, 134–135
Contraceptive pill, oral
  acne, 233
Coronary artery disease, 205
Corticotropin-releasing hormone (CRH),
    11t, 56
  appetite neuroregulation, 15
C-reaction protein (CRP)
  low-carbohydrate diets, 304
CRH. *See* Corticotropin-releasing hor-
    mone (CRH)
Critical growth periods
  pediatric obesity, 408
CRP. *See* C-reaction protein (CRP)
CT. *See* Computed tomography (CT)
Cushing syndrome, 203, 204
  pediatric obesity, 413t
Cyproterone acetate
  acne, 233

D

Daily energy expenditure, 154f
Daytime hypersomnolence, 205
Degenerative joint disease, 205
Depakote
  pediatric obesity, 412

Depression, 213
  pediatric obesity, 411
Developmental delay
  pediatric obesity, 412
DEXA. *See* Dual-energy X-ray
    absorptiometry (DEXA)
DGAT. *See* Diacylglycerol transferase
    (DGAT)
Diabetes. *See also* Type 2 diabetes melli-
    tus
  BMI, 177–178
  education, 190t
  health care providers, 191–192
  obesity, 180t–182t
    insurance, 180t
    treatment, 189–192
  PCOS, 220–221
  sibutramine, 346
  socioeconomic disparities, 178–183
Diabetes Prevention Program (DPP),
    245–259
  behavioral therapy, 250–251
  body weight changes, 246f
  clinical practice intervention, 247–248
  costs, 258
  diabetes cumulative incidence, 246f
  diet, 252–255
  drugs, 257
  exercise, 255–256, 256f
  goals, 248–250, 250f
  leisure physical activity, 246f
  metabolic syndrome and lifestyle
      changes, 258–259
  weight maintenance, 258
Diacylglycerol transferase (DGAT)
  energy expenditure, 164
Diaries
  diet, 399
  physical activity, 399
Dietary Intervention Study in Children
    (DISC), 329
Diethylpropion, 350–351
Diet-induced thermogenesis, 156
Diets. *See also* Low-carbohydrate diets
  cafeteria, 104
  changes, 187–188
  diaries, NWCR, 399
  DPP, 252–255
  energy density, 268f, 268t
    clinical interventions, 272–273
    defined, 266–268

experimental studies, 269–271, 271f
foods, 273–274, 275t, 277t–278t
population-based studies, 268–269
reduction, 265–278
reduction strategies, 273–276
values, 267f, 267t
  Internet tools, 211t
  lactation, 104
  liquid, 417–418
  low fat, 399
  pediatric obesity, 409, 417–418
  preventing weight regain, 399
  reduced-fat/calorie-deficit, 417
  studies, 329–330
  very-low-calorie, 254, 417–418
Direct calorimetry, 152
Directing style
  MI interviews, 325
DISC. *See* Dietary Intervention Study in
    Children (DISC)
DLW. *See* Doubly labeled water (DLW)
DMN. *See* Dorsomedial nucleus (DMN)
Dopamines
  endocannabinoids, 57–58
Dorsomedial nucleus (DMN), 28
Doubly labeled water (DLW), 153–154
DPP. *See* Diabetes Prevention Program
    (DPP)
Driving, 187
Dual-centers hypothesis
  appetite neuroregulation, 4–5
Dual-energy X-ray absorptiometry
    (DEXA), 132–134, 407
Duodenal switch, 373f
Dynamic blood tests
  PCOS, 222t
Dyslipidemia, 326
  motivational interviewing, 329–334
Dysmorphic features
  pediatric obesity, 412

E

Eat for Life (EFL), 332
Eating patterns
  NWCR, 400
Ecopipam, 361
Ectopic fat, 88
  computed tomography, 139
  liver and muscle, 95–96
  MRI, 141
  MRS, 141–142

ED. *See* Erectile dysfunction (ED)
Education
    diabetes, 190t
        obesity, 180t–182t
EEPA. *See* Energy expended in physical
    activity (EEPA)
EFL. *See* Eat for Life (EFL)
Eflornithine
    acne, 233
11-β-hydroxysteroid dehydrogenase type
    1 inhibitor, 79–80, 363
Employment
    BMI, 181t
Endocannabinoids
    adipose tissue, 59
    anabolic actions, 55–56
    arcuate nucleus, 55–56
    biology, 52–53
    brain reward systems, 57–58
    CB1 knockout animals, 56–57
    characteristics, 60t
    constitutive release, 54–55
    distribution, 53
    dopamines and serotonin, 57–58
    energy expenditure, 59
    energy homeostasis, 49–62
    gastrointestinal tract, 59–60
    hypothalamus, 55–56
    intrahypothalamic cannabinoids
        increase food intake, 56
    liver, 60
    opioids, 58
    palatability, 57
    peripheral metabolism, 58–60
    retrograde neurotransmitters, 53–54
    sustained weight loss, 58–59
    synthesis and degradation, 52–53
Endocrine organ
    adipose tissue, 61f
Endogenous cannabinoid ligands, 52
Energy density
    diet, 268f, 268t, 269–274
Energy expended in physical activity
    (EEPA), 210
Energy expenditure
    acetyl CoA carboxylase 2, 164–165
    assessment, 210–211
        obesity, 210–211
    β3-adrenergic receptors, 163

components, 155–156
    daily, 154f
    DGAT, 164
    endocannabinoids, 59
    energy intake, 152f
    measurement, 151–152, 213
    molecular mechanisms, 162–165
    obesity etiology, 158–161
    pediatric obesity, 161–162
    resting, 210
    total
        leisure-time physical activity
            (LTPA), 313f
        physical activity, 312–313
    total daily, 155
        in pediatric obesity, 161–162
Energy homeostasis
    CCK, 10
    central signals
        appetite neuroregulation, 10–14
    endocannabinoids, 49–62
    insulin, 10
    signals controlling, 50f
Energy intake
    assessment, 209–210
    control, 7–8
    energy expenditure balance, 152f
Energy metabolism
    genes, 162t
Enterostatin
    satiety, 8
Ephedrine, 360
Erectile dysfunction (ED), 205
Ergocet, 361
Esophagitis
    reflux, 205
Ethnic groups
    obesity, 199–202
    waist circumference, 209t
Ethnicity
    BMI, 124
    diabetes and obesity, 180t
Exenatide, 355
Exendin-4, 355
Exercise
    DPP, 255–256, 256f
    Internet tools, 211t
    mode, 316–317
    PCOS, 234

prescription development for weight
   control, 316–317
progression to prevent weight regain,
   315f
weight regain, 315f
Expectations, 213

F

Fasting blood tests
   PCOS, 222t
Fat. *See also* Ectopic fat
   abdominal subcutaneous
      measurement, 137f, 138
      waist circumference, 126f
   absolute loss, 131f
   distribution, gender, 131f
   glucose-induced inhibition, 93
   kidney, 144
   obesity, 131f
   oxidation, 92
      low, 160–161
      timing, 93–94
   pancreas, 143
   pediatric obesity, 417
   pericardial, 142–143
   perivascular, 143
   reduced-fat/calorie-deficit diets, 417
Fatty liver, 140f
Fetus
   hormones, 103
   insulin, 103
FFA. *See* Free fatty acids (FFA)
FFQ. *See* Food frequency questionnaires
   (FFQ)
Finasteride
   acne, 233
Fitness
   waist circumference, 126
Fluoxetine, 344, 351
Flutamide
   acne, 233
Folate
   deficiency, bariatric surgery, 385
   supplementation, 388t
Following style
   MI interviews, 325
Food. *See also* Carbohydrate, containing
   foods
   CNS regulation, 4–5
   diet energy density, 273–274, 275t,
      277t–278t

insecurity, 410
intake, 4–5, 56
intrahypothalamic cannabinoids, 56
pediatric obesity, 409, 410
pyramid, low-glycemic, 291, 294t
supply, 187–188
   price indices, 188f
Food frequency questionnaires (FFQ), 332
Free fatty acids (FFA), 60, 87–96
   glucose substrate competition, 91
   metabolism, 93
Fruits
   price indices, 188

G

GABAergic neuron
   CB1 receptors, 53f
Gabapentin, 204
Gallstones, 205
Gastrectomy
   laparoscopic sleeve, 373
   sleeve, 373
Gastric banding, 371–372
   adjustable, 372f
   laparoscopic adjustable silicone, 381
Gastric bypass. *See also* Roux-en-Y gastric
      bypass (RYGB)
   laparoscopic mini, 374
Gastrin-releasing peptide (GRP)
   satiety, 8
Gastrointestinal tract
   endocannabinoids, 59–60
Gastroplasty
   vertical banded, 372f, 381
GBP. *See* Adiponectin
Gelatin-binding protein (GBP). *See*
      Adiponectin
Gender, 180t–183t
   fat distribution, 131f
   waist circumference, 126
Genetics
   energy metabolism, 162t
   pediatric obesity, 408–409
Gestation, 101–106
Ghrelin, 11t, 28, 29t
   antagonists, 362
   appetite neuroregulation, 13–14
   mechanism of action, 39–40
   in physiology and disease, 41

GIP. *See* Glucose-dependent insulinotropic polypeptide (GIP)
Glicentin-related pancreatic peptide (GRPP), 37f
GLP1. *See* Glucagon-like peptide-1 (GLP1)
Glucagon-like peptide-1 (GLP1), 11t, 28, 29t, 38–39, 285, 355, 371
   satiety, 8
Glucophage, 205, 229t, 354
   PCOS, 230
   pediatric obesity, 418
Glucose
   PCOS, 222t
Glucose-dependent insulinotropic polypeptide (GIP), 285
Glucose-FFA substrate competition, 89–91
Glucose-induced fat inhibition, 93
Glucose-to-insulin ratio
   PCOS, 222t
Glucose tolerance test, 225f
Glycemic index, 281–294
   body weight regulation, 286–288
   carbohydrate-containing foods, 282–285, 284t
   clinical utility experimental evidence, 289–290
   food, 293t–294t
   physiological changes, 287f
   practical application, 291–292
   proposed physiological mechanisms, 285–289
   short-term weight loss, 289–290
   weight-independent mechanisms for disease risk, 287–288
   weight loss long-term efficacy, 290–291
Go Girls, 328–329
Gonadotropins
   infertility, 232–233
Growth hormone fragment, 358
Growth periods, 408
GRP. *See* Gastrin-releasing peptide (GRP)
GRPP. *See* Glicentin-related pancreatic peptide (GRPP)
Guiding style
   MI interviews, 325
Gut hormones, 29t
   gut–adipose interaction, 42
   gut–brain interaction, 41
   gut–gut interaction, 41–42
   synergism and antagonism, 41–42

Gut peptides, 27–43
   anorexigenic, 31–39
   appetite regulation, 30f
   central pathways, 28–31
   hypothalamic circuitry, 28–31
   orexigenic, 39–41
   peripheral signals, 31

H

HDL. *See* High density lipoprotein (HDL)
Headaches
   morning, 205
Health care access
   socioeconomic disparities, 189–190
Health care providers
   diabetes, 191–192
Healthy Body/Healthy Spirit, 333–334
Healthy Lifestyles Study (HLS), 324–328
Hepatic steatosis
   IR, 95
High density lipoprotein (HDL)
   PCOS, 222t
Hirsutism
   PCOS, 223–224
   treatment, 229t, 233, 234–235
Histamine-3 receptor antagonists, 361
HLS. *See* Healthy Lifestyles Study (HLS)
Homeostasis model assessment (HOMA), 206
Hormones. *See also* Gut hormones
   corticotropin-releasing, 56
   fetus, 103
   growth, 358
   melanin-concentrating
      appetite neuroregulation, 13
      receptor-1 antagonist, 359
   parathyroid, 386
   thyroid-stimulating, 204
17-Hydroxyprogesterone
   PCOS, 222t
Hydroxysteroid dehydrogenase type 1 inhibitor, 79–80, 363
Hyperandrogenemia
   PCOS, 223–224
Hyperandrogenism
   PCOS, 223–224
Hyperglycemia, 286
   maternal, 103

Hyperinsulinemia, 205
    maternal, 103
    PCOS, 220–221
    pediatric obesity, 410
    treatment, 229t
Hyperlipidemia, 205
    pediatric obesity, 410
Hypersomnolence
    daytime, 205
Hypertension, 205
    pediatric obesity, 410
    sibutramine, 345
Hypocretin/orexin, 11t
    appetite neuroregulation, 13
Hypothalamus, 28
    endocannabinoids, 55–56
    obesity, 204
Hypothyroidism, 204
    pediatric obesity, 413t
Hypotonia
    pediatric obesity, 412

I

IDA. *See* Iron-deficiency anemia (IDA)
IDEEA. *See* Intelligent Device for Energy
        Expenditure and Activity (IDEEA)
IL. *See* Interleukin (IL)-6
ILS. *See* Intensive lifestyle intervention (ILS)
IMCL. *See* Intramyocellular content of
        lipids (IMCL)
Income
    diabetes and obesity, 180t
Indirect calorimetry, 152–153, 213
Infertility
    clomiphene citrate, 232
    gonadotropins, 232–233
    PCOS, 222–223
        treatment, 232–233
    treatment, 229t, 232–233
Inflammatory biomarkers
    low-carbohydrate diets, 303–304
Insulin, 6, 204
    energy homeostasis, 10
    fetus, 103
    PCOS, 222t
    physiological effects, 93
    postnatal influences, 106
    sensitivity and glycemic control
        low-carbohydrate diets, 306–307
Insulin hypothesis
    PCOS, 220–221

Insulin resistance (IR), 87, 205
    adiposity regional patterns, 90–91
    FFA infusion inducing, 89–90
    hepatic steatosis, 95
    history, 88–89
    IMCL, 95
Insulin-sensitizing agents
    PCOS, 229–230
Insurance
    diabetes and obesity, 180t
Intelligent Device for Energy Expendi-
        ture and Activity (IDEEA), 155
Intensive lifestyle intervention (ILS)
    DPP, 247–248, 255–256
Interleukin (IL)-6
    adipose tissue, 77–78
    low-carbohydrate diets, 304
Internet tools
    diet, 211t
    exercise, 211t
Intimidation factor, 324–325
Intracellular cell-adhesion molecule
    low-carbohydrate diets, 304
Intragastric balloon, 372
Intrahypothalamic cannabinoids
    food intake, 56
Intramyocellular content of lipids
        (IMCL), 95, 142
IR. *See* Insulin resistance (IR)
Iron deficiency
    bariatric surgery, 382–384
    treatment, 390t
Iron-deficiency anemia (IDA), 382–383
Iron supplementation, 388t

J

Jejunoileal bypass, 373f

K

Ketoconazole
    PCOS, 234
Kidney fat, 144

L

L-796568, 360–361
Lactation, 101–106
    cafeteria diets, 104
Laparoscopic adjustable silicone gastric
        banding (LASGB), 381
Laparoscopic mini-gastric bypass
        (LMGB), 374
Laparoscopic sleeve gastrectomy (LSG), 373

LASGB. *See* Laparoscopic adjustable
    silicone gastric banding (LASGB)
Lateral hypothalamic area (LHA), 4
LDL. *See* Low density lipid (LDL)
Leisure-time physical activity (LTPA),
    186–187, 313
    DPP, 246f
Leptin, 6, 60–61, 357
    energy expenditure, 163
    energy homeostasis, 10
    fetus, 103–104
    long-term weight loss, 72
    postnatal influences, 106
LHA. *See* Lateral hypothalamic area (LHA)
Lifestyle
    DPP, 258–259
        intensive intervention, 247–248,
            255–256
    PCOS, 234
Lipids, 222t
    low-carbohydrate diets, 303–304
Liquid diets
    pediatric obesity, 417–418
Listening
    reflective, 323
Lithium, 204
    pediatric obesity, 412
Liver
    endocannabinoids, 60
    fat, 140f
        ectopic, 95–96
        measurement, 138–142
Liver disease
    nonalcoholic fatty
        pediatric obesity, 411
LMGB. *See* Laparoscopic mini-gastric
    bypass (LMGB)
Look AHEAD, 247–248
Low-activity thermogenesis, 159–160
Low-carbohydrate diets, 299–308
    blood pressure, 306
    calories vs carbohydrates, 301–303
    CAM, 304
    CRP, 304
    fasting lipids, 303–304
    IL-6, 304
    inflammatory biomarkers, 303–304
    insulin sensitivity and glycemic
        control, 306–307
    lipoprotein subfractions, 304–305
    weight loss efficacy, 300–303

Low density lipid (LDL)
    PCOS, 222t
Low fat diets
    preventing weight regain
        NWCR, 399
Low-glycemic food pyramid, 291, 294t
Low metabolic rate
    obesity, 158–159
Low sympathetic nervous system
    activity, 160
LSG. *See* Laparoscopic sleeve gastrec-
    tomy (LSG)
LTPA. *See* Leisure-time physical activity
    (LTPA)

M

Macronutrients, 188, 189f
    balance, 92
Magnetic resonance imaging (MRI)
    tissue size quantification, 135
Magnetic resonance spectroscopy (MRS), 138
Maternal diet
    obesity, 101–102
Maternal environment, 101–106
Maternal hyperglycemia, 103
Maternal hyperinsulinemia, 103
MCR. *See* Melanocortin receptors (MCR)
Melanin-concentrating hormone (MSH), 11t
    appetite neuroregulation, 13
    receptor-1 antagonist, 359
Melanocortin-4 receptor agonists, 361–362
Melanocortin receptors (MCR), 28–29
Melanocortins
    appetite neuroregulation, 16–17
Meridia, 257, 344–347
    body weight, 346f
    diabetes, 346
    hypertension, 345
    net weight loss, 345t
    orlistat, 350
    pediatric obesity, 418
Metabolic imprinting, 100
Metabolic inflexibility
    biochemical determinants, 94–95
Metabolic syndrome, 206–209
    clinical diagnosis, 207t
    clinical features, 344t
    defined, 208t
    lifestyle changes
        DPP, 258–259
    pediatric obesity, 410–411

Metabolism
  adipose tissue, 75–76
  endocannabinoids, 58–60
  FFA, 93
  obesity, 158–159
Metformin, 205, 229t, 354
  PCOS, 230
  pediatric obesity, 418
MI. *See* Motivational interviewing (MI)
Micronutrient deficiencies
  bariatric surgery, 379–390, 380t
    assessment and treatment, 390t
    prophylactic management and
      monitoring, 388–389, 389t
Mineral supplementation, 388t
Minoxidil
  PCOS, 234
Mirtazapine, 204
Monocyte chemoattractant protein-1
  adipose tissue, 78
Mood stabilizers, 204
Morning headaches, 205
Motivational interviewing (MI)
  adult diet and activity trials, 330t–331t
  communication styles, 324–325
  dyslipidemia and diabetes studies,
    329–334
  medical settings, 321–336
  obesity
    conceptual and pragmatic issues, 325
    prior studies, 326–334
  research priorities, 334–336
  technology transfer, 335
  values list for counseling parents of
    overweight children, 325t
MRI. *See* Magnetic resonance imaging (MRI)
MRS. *See* Magnetic resonance spectroscopy (MRS)
MSH. *See* Melanin-concentrating hormone (MSH)
Muscle
  ectopic fat, 95–96

N

NAF. *See* Nonalcoholic fatty liver disease
  (NAF)
NASH. *See* Nonalcoholic steatohepatitis
  (NASH)
National Weight Control Registry
  (NWCR), 395–401
    lessons learned, 398–400
    subject characteristics, 396
    weight-loss maintenance strategy
      exceptions, 400
    weight loss maintenance success
      predictors, 397
    weight loss success predictors, 397
    weight regain predictors, 398
NEAT. *See* Nonexercise activity thermo-
  genesis (NEAT)
Neuromedin B
  satiety, 8
Neurontin
  pediatric obesity, 412
Neuropeptide Y (NPY), 11t, 28, 56, 371
  appetite neuroregulation, 10–12
  receptor antagonists, 359
Neuroregulation. See Appetite
  neuroregulation
Nonalcoholic fatty liver disease (NAF)
  pediatric obesity, 411
Nonalcoholic steatohepatitis (NASH)
  pediatric obesity, 411
Nonexercise activity thermogenesis
  (NEAT), 157
NPY. *See* Neuropeptide Y (NPY)
NWCR. *See* National Weight Control
  Registry (NWCR)

O

Obesity. *See also* Pediatric obesity
  absolute fat loss, 131f
  adipokines, 69–80
  adipose tissue, 74–75
  anthropometry and body composition
    change, 129
  assessment, 195–215
    allied health professionals, 214
  behavioral condition, 336
  body composition imaging, 134–138
  body composition measurement, 121–144
  clinical practice evaluation, 195–200
  clinicians, 198
  costs, 197
  defined, 198–200
  diabetes, treatment, 189–192
  endocrine causes, 204–205
  energy expenditure, 151–165
  epidemiology, 195–196

ethnic groups, 199–202
health complications assessment, 205–210
heterogeneous conditions, 335–336
hypothalamic, 204
importance, 197–198
inflammatory alterations, 74–75
laboratory evaluation, 206
medications causing, 204–205
morbidity and mortality, 196–197
perinatal period, 99–109
prevalence, 195–196
secondary causes, 204–210
severe trends, 176–177
socioeconomics, 175–192
surgery, 369–375
treatment, 229t
Obesity epidemic
health and cost consequences, 175–179
Obstructive sleep apnea, 205
OCP. See Oral contraceptive pills (OCP)
Octreotide, 353–354
pediatric obesity, 418
satiety, 8
Offspring
postnatal influences, 104–106, 105t
prenatal influences, 102–103, 103t
Olanzepine, 204
Oleolyestrone, 358–359
Oligomenorrhea
PCOS, 222–223
Open-circuit spirometry, 153
Opioids
endocannabinoids, 58
Oral contraceptive pills (OCP)
acne, 233
Oral glucose tolerance test
PCOS, 222t
Orexin, 11t
appetite neuroregulation, 13
Orlistat, 257, 347–350
body weight, 349f
net weight loss, 348t
pediatric obesity, 418
safety, 350
sibutramine, 350
Ornithine decarboxylase inhibitor
acne, 233
Ovarian hypothesis
PCOS, 220

Ovarian-suppressive therapies
PCOS, 228–229
Overweight
pediatric persistence, sequelae, costs,
408–409
Oxyntomodulin (OXM), 28, 29t, 37–38, 358

P

PAI-1. See Plasminogen activator inhibi-
tor-1 (PAI-1)
PAL. See Physical activity level (PAL)
Pancreas fat, 143, 143f
Pancreatic lipase inhibitor, 360
Pancreatic polypeptide (PP), 28, 29t, 35–
36, 371
fold family of peptides, 31–35
Parathyroid hormone (PTH), 386
Paraventricular nucleus (PVN), 28, 107
Parent counseling, 325t
Paroxetine
pediatric obesity, 412
PCOS. See Polycystic ovary syndrome
(PCOS)
Pediatric obesity, 405–420
AEE, 161–162
anxiety, 411
behavioral risk factors, 410
behavioral treatment, 415–418, 416t
binge eating, 411–412
BMI, 407–408, 410
body image disparagement, 412
buffalo hump, 413t
clinical syndromes including, 413t
comorbidities, 410–412, 411t
defined, 407–408
depression, 411
developmental delay, 412
diet, 409
dysmorphic features, 412
energy expenditure, 161–162
activity, 161–162
epidemiology, 406–408
etiology, 408–410
evaluation, 412–413
food insecurity, 410
genetics, 408–409
history taking, 413–414
hyperinsulinemia, 410
hyperlipidemia, 410

hypertension, 410
hypothyroidism, 413t
hypotonia, 412
laboratory and diagnostic studies,
    414–415
liquid diets, 417–418
lithium, 412
low carbohydrates, 417
metabolic syndrome, 410–411
MI studies, 326, 327t
NASH, 411
neurontin, 412
nonalcoholic fatty liver disease, 411
orlistat, 418
PCOS, 411
pharmacological treatment, 418
physical examination, 414
prevention, 419
    websites, 420t
sibutramine, 347
social consequences, 407
surgical treatment, 418–419
syndromes, 413t
Pediatric overweight
    persistence, sequelae, costs, 408–409
Pedometers, 155
Peptides. *See also* Glucagon-like peptide-
    1 (GLP1); Gut peptides
    agouti-related, 28, 56, 362
    gastrin-releasing
        satiety, 8
    glicentin-related pancreatic, 37f
    proglucagon-derived
        appetite neuroregulation, 15
Peptide YY (PYY), 31–32, 371
    mechanism of action, 33–34
    normal physiology and disease, 34–35
Peptide YY3-36 (PYY3-36), 28, 29t, 32, 358
Pericardial fat, 142–143
Perinatal environment
    brain development, 106–107
Peripheral (ovarian) hypothesis
    PCOS, 220
Peripheral metabolism
    endocannabinoids, 58–60
Perivascular fat, 143
Phentermine, 350–351
Phenylpropanolamine, 360
Physical activity, 212

during active weight loss, 398
diaries, 399
DPP, 246f
energy expended, 210
intensity vs volume, 317–318
leisure-time, 186–187, 246f, 313
long-term weight loss and weight-loss
    maintenance, 314–316
NWCR, 397, 398, 399–400
obesity, 311–318
pediatric obesity, 409–410, 412, 416–417
preventing weight gain, 313–314
self-reported assessments, 154–155
short-term weight loss, 314
spontaneous, 157
studies, 329–330
total energy expenditure, 312–313
weight loss and weight regain preven-
    tion, 314–316
Physical activity level (PAL), 159–160
Physician advice
    diet and physical activity, 191t
Pioglitazone, 229t
    PCOS, 231
Plasminogen activator inhibitor-1 (PAI-1)
    adipose tissue, 79
Plethysmography
    air-displacement, 407
Polycystic ovary syndrome (PCOS), 205,
    219–235
    acne treatment, 233
    anti-obesity drugs, 231–232
    cardiovascular risk factors, 226–227
    central hypothesis, 220
    cholesterol, 222t
    diabetes, 220–221
    diagnostic criteria, 221t
    dynamic blood tests, 222t
    etiology, 220–221
    exercise, 234
    fasting blood tests, 222t
    glucose-to-insulin ratio, 222t
    HDL, 222t
    hirsutism, 223–224
        treatment, 233, 234–235
    17-hydroxyprogesterone, 222t
    hyperandrogenemia/
        hyperandrogenism, 223–224
    hyperinsulinemia, 220–221

infertility, 222–223
    treatment, 232–233
insulin, 222t
insulin hypothesis, 220–221
insulin-sensitizing agents, 229–230
ketoconazole, 234
lifestyle, 234
long-term consequences, 224–228
malignancy, 227–228
metformin, 230
minoxidil, 234
nonfertility treatments, 233
obesity, 226
oligomenorrhea/amenorrhea, 222–223
oral glucose tolerance test, 222t
ovarian-suppressive therapies, 228–229
pediatric obesity, 411
peripheral (ovarian) hypothesis, 220
pregnancy complications, 228
surgery, 234
tests, 222t
treatment, 228–235, 229t
type 2 diabetes mellitus, 224–226
ultrasound, 224
Polypeptides
    glucose-dependent insulinotropic, 285
    pancreatic, 35–36, 371
POMC. See Pro-opiomelanocortin (POMC)
Portable devices
    energy assessment, 155
PP. See Pancreatic polypeptide (PP)
Prader-Willi syndrome (PSW)
    pediatric obesity, 412, 413t, 414
Pramlintide, 354–355
Pregnancy
    PCOS, 228
Premenopausal women
    abdominal muscle, 136f
Price indices
    food supply, 188f
Proglucagon-derived peptides, 11t
    appetite neuroregulation, 15
Proglucagon gene products, 37–38
Prolactin
    PCOS, 222t
Pro-opiomelanocortin (POMC), 11t, 28, 107
Protein-sparing modified fast
    pediatric obesity, 417–418
P-selectin
    low-carbohydrate diets, 304

Pseudohypoparathyroidism
    pediatric obesity, 413t
Pseudotumor cerebri
    pediatric obesity, 411
PSW. See Prader-Willi syndrome (PSW)
Psychological assessment, 214
Psychological factors
    pediatric obesity, 410
Psychotic drugs, 204
PTH. See Parathyroid hormone (PTH)
PVN. See Paraventricular nucleus (PVN)
PYY. See Peptide YY (PYY)

Q

Quantitative insulin sensitivity check
    (QUICK), 306
Quetiapine, 204

R

Race/ethnicity
    BMI, 124
    diabetes and obesity, 180t
Reduced-fat/calorie-deficit diets
    pediatric obesity, 417
REE. See Resting energy expenditure (REE)
Reflective listening, 323
Reflux esophagitis, 205
Resting energy expenditure (REE), 210, 312
Resting metabolic rate (RMR), 156, 210
Rimonabant, 355–356
RIO Trials, 61–62, 62f
Risk factors
    behavioral, pediatric obesity, 410
    glycemic index, 287–288
    PCOS, 226–227
Risperdol
    pediatric obesity, 412
Risperidone, 204
RMR. See Resting metabolic rate (RMR)
Rosiglitazone, 229t
    PCOS, 231
Roux-en-Y gastric bypass (RYGB), 370–371,
    371, 372f, 381–382
    pediatric obesity, 419
RYGB. See Roux-en-Y gastric bypass
    (RYGB)

S

Safety
    bariatric surgery, 374–375
    orlistat, 350

Satiety
  amylin, 8
  appetite neuroregulation, 7–8
  CCK, 8
  enterostatin, 8
  GLP1, 8
  GRP, 8
  neuromedin B, 8
SCFE. *See* Slipped capital femoral epiphyses (SCFE)
Self esteem
  pediatric obesity, 412
Serotonin, 11t
  appetite neuroregulation, 15–16
  endocannabinoids, 57–58
Serotonin 2C receptor agonist, 359
Serotonin reuptake inhibitors, 204
Severe obesity
  trends, 176–177
Short-term weight loss
  glycemic index, 289–290
Sibutramine, 257, 344–347
  body weight, 346f
  diabetes, 346
  hypertension, 345
  net weight loss, 345t
  orlistat, 350
  pediatric obesity, 418
Skeletal muscle
  measurement, 138–139
    mass, 136–137
Skinfolds, 132
Skin tags, 205
Sleep apnea, 205
Sleeve gastrectomy, 373
Slipped capital femoral epiphyses (SCFE)
  pediatric obesity, 411
SLIVGTT. *See* Stable-label IV glucose tolerance test (SLIVGTT)
Snoring, 205
SNS. *See* Sympathetic nervous system (SNS)
Soft drinks
  price indices, 188
Somatostatin, 353–354
  pediatric obesity, 418
  satiety, 8
SPA. *See* Spontaneous physical activity (SPA)
Spirometry
  open-circuit, 153

Spironolactone
  acne, 233
Spontaneous physical activity (SPA), 157
Sports, 185f
SR 141716, 61
Stable-label IV glucose tolerance test (SLIVGTT), 307
Steatohepatitis
  nonalcoholic
    pediatric obesity, 411
Stoplight Diet, 416t
Sugars
  price indices, 188
Sulfonylurea, 204
Supermarkets, 191
Sustained weight loss
  endocannabinoids, 58–59
Sweeteners
  caloric, 189f
Sweets
  price indices, 188
Sympathetic nervous system (SNS)
  low activity, 160
Sympathomimetic drugs, 350–351
Syndecan-3
  appetite neuroregulation, 17–18
Syndrome X. *See* Metabolic syndrome

T

Tape position
  waist, 203f
TDEE. *See* Total daily energy expenditure (TDEE)
TEE. *See* Total energy expenditure (TEE)
TEF. *See* Thermic effect of food (TEF)
Tegretol
  pediatric obesity, 412
Television, 185f
  viewing, 397, 400
Testosterone
  PCOS, 222t
TGZ. *See* Troglitazone (TGZ)
Thermic effect of food (TEF), 156, 303, 312
Thermogenesis
  activity, 156–157
  diet-induced, 156
  low-activity, 159–160
Thiamine
  deficiency
    bariatric surgery, 382
    treatment, 390t
  supplementation, 388t

Thiazolidinedione, 204, 229t
  PCOS, 230–231
Thyroid-stimulating hormone (TSH), 204
Time
  exercise, 183–188
Tissue area
  imaging, 135
Tissue volume and mass
  imaging, 135
TNF. *See* Tumor necrosis factor (TNF)-{a}
Topamax, 205, 352–353
  pediatric obesity, 418
Topiramate, 205, 352–353
  pediatric obesity, 418
Total daily energy expenditure (TDEE), 155
  in pediatric obesity, 161–162
Total energy expenditure (TEE)
  leisure-time physical activity (LTPA), 313f
  physical activity, 312–313
Total testosterone test
  PCOS, 222t
Transportation, 187
Triglycerides
  PCOS, 222t
Troglitazone (TGZ)
  PCOS, 231
TSH. *See* Thyroid-stimulating hormone (TSH)
Tumor necrosis factor (TNF)-α, 74
  adipose tissue, 76–77
  low-carbohydrate diets, 304
TV viewing
  NWCR, 397, 400
Type 2 diabetes mellitus, 205
  cost, 407
  glucose-induced fat inhibition, 93
  glucose metabolism, 244
  hepatic steatosis, 95
  IMCL, 95
  metabolic inflexibility, 94–95
  PCOS, 224–226
  prevention, 243–259
  weight loss in IGT, 244–245

U

Uncoupling protein
  energy expenditure, 164
Urinary stress incontinence, 205
Urocortin, 11t, 15

V

Valproate, 204
Valproic acid, 204
Vascular cell adhesion molecule (VCAM), 74
VAT. *See* Visceral adiposity (VAT)
VCAM. *See* Vascular cell adhesion molecule (VCAM)
Vegetables
  price indices, 188
Ventromedial hypothalamus (VMH), 4–6
Ventromedial nucleus (VMN), 28
Vertical banded gastroplasty, 372f, 381
Very-low-calorie diets, 254
  pediatric obesity, 417–418
Very-low-density lipoprotein VLDL), 304
Visceral adiposity (VAT), 91
  measurement, 137, 137f
  waist circumference, 126f
Visceral fat
  waist circumference, 130f
Vitamin
  supplementation, 388t
Vitamin A
  deficiency
  bariatric surgery, 388
Vitamin B1
  deficiency
    bariatric surgery, 382
    treatment, 390t
  supplementation, 388t
Vitamin B 12
  deficiency
    bariatric surgery, 384–385
    treatment, 390t
  supplementation, 388t
Vitamin D
  deficiency
    bariatric surgery, 385–388
    treatment, 390t
  supplementation, 388t
VMH. *See* Ventromedial hypothalamus (VMH)
VMN. *See* Ventromedial nucleus (VMN)

W

Waist circumference, 124–125, 125f, 128f
  abdominal subcutaneous fat, 126f
  age, 126
  body composition change, 129

defined, 199
ethnic groups, 209t
fitness, 126
gender, 126
increased disease risk, 202t
visceral fat, 130f
Waist-to-hip ratio (WHR), 127–128
  body composition change, 129
  visceral fat, 130f
Walking, 187
Web tools
  diet, 211t
  exercise, 211t
Weighing
  NWCR, 399
Weight control
  DPP, 246f, 258
  exercise, 316–317
  orlistat, 349f
Weight gain
  physical activity, 313–314
  prevention, 314–316
Weight history
  assessment, 202–203
Weight loss, 253–254
  drugs, 341–363
    algorithm, 342–343, 343t
    BMI, 342
    early development, 358–359
    new development areas, 361–362
    withdrawn from investigation, 360
  long-term efficacy
    glycemic index, 290–291
  low-carbohydrate diets, 300–303

maintenance
  strategy exceptions, 400
  success predictors, 397
  vs weight loss, 398
orlistat, 348t
physical activity, 314–316
short-term
  glycemic index, 289–290
success predictors, 397
sustained
  endocannabinoids, 58–59
Weight maintenance
  DPP, 258
Weight regain
  exercise, 315f
  predictors, 398
Wellbutrin, 205, 351–352
  pediatric obesity, 418
WHI. See Women's Health Initiative (WHI)
WHR. See Waist-to-hip ratio (WHR)
Women's Health Initiative (WHI), 333

X

Xenical, 257, 347–350
  body weight, 349f
  net weight loss, 348t
  pediatric obesity, 418
  safety, 350
  sibutramine, 350

Y

Y receptor superfamilies, 32t

Z

Zonisamide, 344, 351, 353